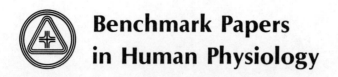

Benchmark Papers
in Human Physiology

Series Editor: L. L. Langley
School of Medicine
University of Missouri–Kansas City

PUBLISHED VOLUMES

HOMEOSTASIS: Origins of the Concept
   L. L. Langley
CONTRACEPTION
   L. L. Langley
MICROCIRCULATION
   Mary P. Wiedeman
CARDIOVASCULAR PHYSIOLOGY
   James V. Warren
PULMONARY AND RESPIRATORY PHYSIOLOGY, PART I
   Julius H. Comroe, Jr.
PULMONARY AND RESPIRATORY PHYSIOLOGY, PART II
   Julius H. Comroe, Jr.
INFANT NUTRITION
   Doris H. Merritt

RELATED TITLES IN OTHER BENCHMARK SERIES

HORMONES AND SEXUAL BEHAVIOR (Benchmark Papers in Animal
   Behavior)
   Carol Sue Carter

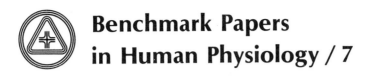

Benchmark Papers in Human Physiology / 7

A BENCHMARK ® Books Series

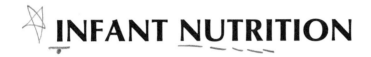

INFANT NUTRITION

Edited by

DORIS H. MERRITT

**Indiana University–Purdue University
at Indianapolis**

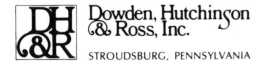

Dowden, Hutchinson & Ross, Inc.

STROUDSBURG, PENNSYLVANIA

Distributed by

HALSTED
PRESS

A Division of
John Wiley & Sons, Inc.

LIBRARY OF CONGRESS CATALOGING IN PUBLICATION DATA

Main entry under title:
Infant nutrition.
  (Benchmark papers in human physiology ; 7)
  Includes index.
  1. Infants—Nutrition—Addresses, essays, lectures.   I. Merritt, Doris H.
RJ216.15   612'.39   76-21831
ISBN 0-87933-125-9

Exclusive Distributor: **Halsted Press**
A Division of John Wiley & Sons, Inc.
ISBN: 0-470-98918-1

ACKNOWLEDGMENTS
AND PERMISSIONS

ACKNOWLEDGMENT

THE AMERICAN SOCIETY OF BIOLOGICAL CHEMISTS, INC.—*Journal of Biological Chemistry*
  Milk as a Source of Water-Soluble Vitamine

PERMISSIONS

The following papers have been reprinted with permission of the authors and copyright holders.

ALMQUIST AND WIKSELL—*Acta Paediatrica*
  The Prothrombin Content in Relation to Early and Late Feedings of the Newborn: A Preliminary Report

THE AMERICAN ACADEMY OF PEDIATRICS—*Pediatrics*
  Comparative Study of Adequacy of Protein from Human Milk and Cow's Milk in Promoting Nitrogen Retention by Normal Full-Term Infants
  Role of Linoleic Acid in Infant Nutrition: Clinical and Chemical Study of 428 Infants Fed on Milk Mixtures Varying in Kind and Amount of Fat

THE AMERICAN MEDICAL ASSOCIATION
  American Journal of Diseases of Children
    The Carbohydrate Metabolism of the Normal New-Born Infant: II. The Effect on the Concentration of the Blood Sugar of Feeding Various Sugars to New-Born Infants
    Choice of Formulas Made by Three Infants Throughout the Nursing Period
    Comparison and Interpretation on a Caloric Basis of the Milk Mixtures Used in Infant Feeding
    Hunger in the Infant
    Infantile Scurvy: The Blood, the Blood-Vessels and the Diet
    Milk or Formula Volume Ingested by Infants Fed ad Libitum
    Milk Sugar in Infant Feeding: A Study of the Effects of the Routine Use of Milk Sugar in Infant Feeding
    Physiology and Pathology of the Digestion of Fat in Infancy: Their Application to Infant-Feeding
    The Relation of Calcium and Phosphorus in the Diet to the Absorption of These Elements from the Intestine
    Respiratory Metabolism in Infancy and in Childhood: XXI. Daily Water Exchange of Normal Infants
    The Rôle of Mineral Salts in the Metabolism of Infants
    Some Studies on Sugar in Infant Feeding
    Studies in the Adaptation of an Artificial Food to Human Milk
    Twenty-Four-Hour Metabolism of Two Normal Infants with Special Reference to the Total Energy Requirements of Infants
    Use of Ferric and Ferrous Iron in the Prevention of Hypochromic Anemia in Infants

Acknowledgments and Permissions

Journal of the American Medical Association
 The Artificial Feeding of Athreptic Infants
 Boiled Versus Raw Milk: An Experimental Study of Milk Coagulation in the Stomach,
   Together with Clinical Observations on the Use of Raw and Boiled Milk
 Nutritional Disturbances in Infancy Due to Overfeeding
 Prevention of Anorexia in Children
 Protein Nutrition in Pediatrics
 The Relative Value of Different Varieties of Vitamin D Milk for Infants: A Critical Inter-
   pretative Review

FEDERATION OF AMERICAN SOCIETIES FOR EXPERIMENTAL BIOLOGY—*Proceedings*
 Pyridoxine Deficiency in the Human Being

THE JOHNS HOPKINS UNIVERSITY PRESS—*Bulletin of the Johns Hopkins Hospital*
 Studies on the Protein Metabolism of Infants: II. Tryptophane Requirement of the Infant

LITTLE, BROWN AND COMPANY—*Lancet*
 An Experimental Investigation on Rickets

THE C. V. MOSBY COMPANY—*Journal of Pediatrics*
 The Metabolic Basis for the Individualized Feeding of Infants, Premature and Full-Term
 Reaction of 150 Infants to Cold Formulas
 The Retentions of Nitrogen, Calcium, and Phosphorous of Infants Fed Sweetened
   Condensed Milk
 Whole Lactic Acid Evaporated Milk Does Not Require a Refrigerator

SOUTHERN MEDICAL ASSOCIATION—*Southern Medical Journal*
 Results of Three Years Experience with a New Concept of Baby Feeding

STATE MEDICAL SOCIETY OF WISCONSIN—*Wisconsin Medical Journal*
 A Simplified Infant Feeding Formula: A Report of the Use of Irradiated Evaporated
   Milk and Water in 2,004 Cases

SERIES EDITOR'S FOREWORD

As Dr. Merritt says in her Preface, infant nutrition is a remarkably broad subject; it was therefore a major task to reduce its scope to the demands of a Benchmark volume. An editor was required who was not only completely versed in the literature of infant nutrition but one blessed with terseness, discipline, and authority. This is why I asked Doris Merritt to undertake the task.

There is a saying that to get something done and to get it done well and on time, ask a busy person. This adage fits Doris Merritt perfectly: she has always been busy; she always does things well; and she finishes them on schedule. Physician, wife of a physician, mother of bright, vigorous children, in control of a crisply run household, investigator, administrator, and a member of many national committees, she agreed to tackle this subject. She has brought to it not only the benefit of her knowledge of the field but also her personal experience of infant nutrition, and, quite importantly, her great warmth as a compassionate human being.

The field of infant nutrition has always been fused and confused with myth, superstition, ignorance, fad, and religion. At one time, of course, there was no substitute for breast feeding. As knowledge developed, so did substitutes. On the one hand was the effort to perfect those substitutes; on the other was the growing and still not concluded discussion of the relative merits of breast and bottle feeding. Just this morning an article in the newspaper proclaimed that dental caries are related to infant nutrition. The gravamen of the article is that bottle feeding and other infant preparations contain a higher level of glucose than does maternal milk; consequently the infant develops a taste for glucose and this does him in, or at least his teeth, later in life. The interesting point is that the field remains controversial, and not terribly noted for a high level of investigation or proclamation. In this volume, Dr. Merritt traces that controversy, the myths, the fads, the superstitions, the confusion, and leads us through the maze, after which we emerge with an understanding of how we got to today's concepts and what those concepts are. It is a noteworthy presentation and a highly satisfying one.

L. L. LANGLEY

PREFACE

In retrospect, I marvel at the casual way in which I accepted Dr. Langley's invitation to prepare a Benchmark volume on infant nutrition. The briefest perusal of the tables of contents in the early medical literature revealed that the only other topic covering an equal magnitude of print was that of infectious disease! It was apparent that some curtailment of scope and self-discipline in selection was in order if I was to limit choices to anything like a manageable number. As a result, I elected to focus solely on material related to artificial feeding of the normal full-term infant under six months of age.

This proved to be a rewarding decision, for there is much to be learned from this literature. Ours, for example, is not the first generation of pediatricians to debate the use of saturated and/or unsaturated fatty acids (and which ones?) in the infant's formula. Nor are we alone in our concern for what proportion of calories in the diet should be contributed by carbohydrate or protein. Many of the concepts underlying successful total parenteral feeding for the premature or the infant unable to take fluids by mouth were recorded for the first time within the pages reprinted here.

Having reached my conclusions, I most naturally turned to the preceptor of my early training, Dr. Jerome S. Harris, Professor of Pediatrics, Duke University School of Medicine, and confessed to him what task I had had the temerity to undertake. After reassuring me that the task was indeed impossible without narrowing it down to a well-defined area, he then reviewed the manuscript, managing with his usual perspicacity to reinstate an important omission. In addition, Dr. Harris provided an introduction to Dr. Harry Gordon, Grover Powers Professor of Pediatrics, Albert Einstein College of Medicine, whose incomparable work in the field of infant nutrition illuminates all facets of our current knowledge. Dr. Gordon, with more kindness than I had any right to expect, gave generously of his time in critiquing the review and extending my selections while further contributing to my personal education with some early Talmudic references to breast feeding. To these men and to Dr. Norman Kretchmer, Director of the National Institute of Child Health and Human Development, who was also generous in his comments, I can never say a sufficient "thank you."

Preface

An undertaking of this comprehensive nature obviously owes a debt of gratitude to a number of people. Among others whose assistance was of high order are the able librarians at the Indiana University School of Medicine who, with a limited budget, have maintained a remarkable collection, both historical and current. To Ms. Mary Jane Laatz, Ms. Virginia Humnicky and Ms. Nina Campbell belong the credit for making much of the reference work a pleasure. Dr. Morris Green and Dr. Joseph Fitzgerald of the Indiana University School of Medicine Department of Pediatrics were most helpful in allowing me the use of their private reprint collections. Dr. Wolfgang Zeman, Director of the Indiana University School of Medicine division of neuropathology, donated much precious time translating the early German material for me. Dr. John Silverio, Director of Clinical Nutrition of Wyeth Laboratories, provided a most practical bibliography. My secretary, Ms. Gwen Allen, patiently tracked authors, living and dead; and Mr. William Spencer, Special Assistant to the Vice President of Indiana University, provided real editorial finesse.

Reference has been made to the terseness of my chapter introductions; I can assure you that it was intentional. The articles are reproduced not only for their inherent contributions to medical science, but for their illustration of a literate medical style that is fast disappearing, if not already vanished, from our scientific journals. The objectivity of the data collection and the conclusions are clear despite a total disregard for the sterile academic prose style imposed by today's editors. To savor the essence of this literature, it must be read. The index is designed for those who want only the facts.

This volume, then, is more than a historical chronical; from every point of view it is good reading. It was a great adventure to collect; I hope that it will prove equally thought-provoking to read.

DORIS H. MERRITT

CONTENTS

Contents

PART III: CARBOHYDRATES

PART IV: FATS

PART V: MINERALS AND WATER

Contents

CONTENTS BY AUTHOR

INTRODUCTION

The current preoccupation with food fads is as ancient as civilization. To improve his own longevity and productivity, man has continually sought to alter his physical and spiritual condition, and that of his offspring, through nutrition. All begins with infant feeding. Perhaps on no other subject in the early medical literature was so much written and so little said. Scant scientific evidence was available. Editorial observation and comment based on opinion, biased observation, and partially or ill controlled studies were dictums accepted as axioms until the mid-1800s.

The first records relate to the obvious substitute for the biologic mother, the wet nurse. "And Pharaoh's daughter said unto her, take this child away, and nurse it for me, and I will give thee thy wages. And the woman took the child and nursed it" (*Exodus: 2:9*). Wet nursing, ubiquitous through the centuries, endowed certain women lacking other means of support with a built-in career.

Wet nurses all too often came from the ranks of prostitutes. Not only might they be diseased, they frequently exercised a deleterious effect upon a household. For example, the wet nurse often received a better diet than other servants, a cause of discontent, and was likely to be taken more into confidence of the new mother because of the nurse's close relationship to the baby. It was further noted that men, however moral, may fall prey to the wiles of such women at this particular time in their married lives. Exhaustive discussions on the selection and perils of employing a wet nurse and the caveats related thereto were pervasive until the early part of the twentieth century.

1

On the other hand, if a wet nurse were needed and not available, precious little else was. "Behold, a virgin shall conceive, and bear a son...butter and honey shall he eat"(*Isaiah 7:15*). Reference is often made to pap, a bread soaked in milk or wine, and other short-term substitutes. Pemell (1653) provides some choices. Almond milk is one. A recipe for "borrage water" calls for 4 ounces of syrup of violets or 1½ ounces of syrup of citrons, mixed together with 5 or 6 drops of spirit of vitriol and given to the child 2 or 3 spoonfuls at a time. Barley water made with poppy seeds, not a very satisfactory solution, is first recommended in this work.

Some championed the method of direct feeding from domestic animals. That Romulus and Remus thrived suckling a wolf's teats was commonly known apocrypha. Orion presumably did as well with a bear. The more conventional human infant, however, faced other problems. Consider Routh (1879):

> Some precautions, however, are necessary at first, as a child may be injured by the violence of the movements of the untrained animal. For instance, it is difficult to admit the prudence of allowing a child to suck a mare, and even with some cows such a proceeding would be highly hazardous. The most natural way would be to select a cow known for her gentle disposition, and then if the child were not held by a person to the udder, it might be placed on a raised bed, which would stand in front of the cow's hind legs, so that she would be prevented from moving. The nipple might be taken hold of, and thus the child be fed directly from the breast. The udder, however, of the cow would be too large for a small child to suck, and therefore, speaking practically, a goat would be the animal selected. The goat could be easily overpowered and tied down, its feet enveloped in some cloth, and the child, till such time as the goat became accustomed to the plan and allowed it to be done without hinderance, could be allowed to suck the udder directly.

There was, in short, ample incentive for the development of an adequate, nutritious mother's milk substitute.

The possibility of satisfactory artificial feeding of the normal newborn became a realistic goal in the middle to late nineteenth century, when chemical techniques were developed for determining the constitutents of human and animal milk. Scientific formulations, providing the normal infant with a milk from other than the human breast on which it would thrive, have evolved over a fifty-year span, beginning in the late 1800s. The work of Biedert (1905) in Germany, followed by the studies of Finklestein and Meyer (1910; Finklestein, 1912) and Czerny and Keller (1909), are most often quoted as the basis of the science of artificial feeding. No reprints or translations of their writings are provided in this book because of their length and detail. Studies along similar lines were being conducted and reported almost simultaneously in the United States.

That it was desirable to build the ingredients and proportions of the infant's formula to mimic breast milk on a firm scientific basis was almost the sole undisputed and accepted principle underlying these studies. What constituted that scientific basis was the subject of intense written and oral debate. Partisans of the "percentage" school of Rotch warred untiringly with the "caloric" contenders, exemplified by Powers (1935) and by Brennemann (1923, 1949) in his extension of the Czerny and Keller (1909) studies. One intricate Solomon-like solution was offered by Cowie (1912), who combined the caloric and percentage approach in a graphic system of charting that undoubtedly doubled the exuberance with which some practitioners must have turned to the simpler formulas and proprietary preparations.

The success of proprietary preparations, due largely to private entrepreneurship and integrity, supported much of the research responsible for progress in nutrition. Acknowledgments are made to Ross Laboratories, Mead Johnson, the Borden Company, and Wyeth, to name only a few of the contributors to research that resulted in the wholesome milks for infants now commercially available. It is interesting and perhaps unfortunate that use of these preparations has become a status symbol in some developing countries, where the economy can ill afford substitutes for readily available, and far more economical, breast milk.

With the application of principles and experience in practice, the printed record captures the excitement of discovery, the vigor of championship, and the acrimony of dissent. Meigs, Rotch, Brennemann, Holt, Howland, Powers, Jacobi, Marriott—the founders of pediatrics—all made practical contributions, some of benchmark significance, to infant feeding and nutrition, most of them prior to 1930. Under the circumstances, Meyer's comment, in an excellent review of the standards of artificial feeding in 1955, evokes no surprise. "It may come as a relief to those who think they have not kept up with the current literature and practice of infant feeding to learn that *no fundamental* changes have been made in our knowledge in this field since 1935."

What has been added to the general body of knowledge since the middle 1930s are refinements of understanding and modification of precise formulas designed to be used in specialized circumstances. No attempt is made in this volume to cover the elegant studies of metabolism and feeding in the premature, postsurgical, or life-support parental feeding, the sophisticated artificial deletion or substitution diets for the baby with allergy or inborn errors of metabolism, or the studies of intestinal transport mechanisms that undoubtedly will provide the base for a better means of managing the infants who still fail to thrive.

This collection is chiefly concerned with normal full-term infant nutritional requirements and with those studies that provided the standards for our accepted proprietary and home-prepared formulas—the safety, efficacy, and availability of which are now so readily taken for granted.

Because the feeding of infants has generated a considerable amount of literature, the selection and organization of materials for this finite volume has required an editorial mixture of the judgmental and the arbitrary. Many worthy articles could not be included. As for organization, the outline of general topics, or sections, concerns modified whole milk, protein, carbohydrate, fat, minerals and water, vitamins, bases for feeding (hunger, energy, metabolism), safety and cleanliness, and hunder, appetite, and freedom of choice.

Part I

MODIFIED WHOLE MILK

Editor's Comments
on Papers 1 Through 4

As the techniques were developed to establish the chemical composition of human milk, by Biedert in Germany and Meigs in the United States, it was only a step to the analysis of all other animal milks, in the hope of finding one that would be similar to human milk, without the necessity for adaptation. From ass to elephant, from rabbit to reindeer, the chemical composition of animal milks was exhaustively detailed. The logistics of supply and the relative similarity of most animal milk contents clearly dictated the practicality of the cow as the animal of choice.

It was Meigs who popularized the scientific basis for modification of cow's milk to provide a digestible infant formula. In his early attempts (see Paper 1) he called attention to the fact that by diluting the "villain" casein with water, one also was diluting the fat and the sugar, consequently making it necessary to add sugar along with the water. Thus, the door was opened to allowing each physician to prescribe, publish, and justify his own formulation while vilifying, in professional phraseology, the formulas of his colleagues.

Building on Meigs' early efforts came the architect of the complex school of "percentage" feeding, Rotch, whose prescriptions, the fulfilling of which was not to be entrusted to the mother, were formulated in his own milk laboratory (Paper 2). Nothing escaped his scrutiny—the quality of the farmer's feed, the species of animal, the precise percentages of protein, fat, and carbohydrate contained in the individual milking, all to be modified in a precise manner as necessary. The formulas varied from baby to baby and week to week. His method flourished with the mathematically inclined, and that the babies also flourished on the formulas was undeniable. Whether this was due to the exactitude of the prescription or the cleanliness of the preparation is uncertain.

Much early discussion of the digestibility of artificial formulas in the United States centered on observation of the curds produced by the various milks: thin and fine from breast milk, large and hard from cow's milk. Theories for the origin of the hard curds produced by cow's milk multiplied in American literature, along with outright denial of their existence in the European literature. It was Brennemann, revered father of pediatrics, along with Meigs and Rotch, who solved the mystery surrounding the presence of curds in the stools of American infants and their absence from those of European infants (Paper 3). As he observed, there was only one possible explanation for the discrepancy between equally competent observers: the Americans used raw milk, while the Germans used boiled milk. Thus it was that the path was cleared to using a simple dilution of boiled milk as the basis for an infant formula while chemical protein modifiers, such as rennin, fell into disuse.

Shortly thereafter, Marriott underscored the value of the hydrogen ion in the modification of the curd and introduced the addition of lactic acid in formulas, first for the athreptic infant (Paper 4), and four years late, in 1923, with comments as to its bacterial growth inhibiting qualities, as a practical means of feeding any normal infant. This experience, coupled with the fine chemical study of Clark (1915), which proved the value of an acidified mixture, finally disproved the theories held by the proponents of an alkaline formula. The simple, inexpensive evaporated milk formula known to the Duke University pediatrics house staff during the 1950s as "idiot's delight" because it was almost impossible to prepare improperly reflects the principles laid down by Marriott in 1919.

By that time, however, it was known that the process of preparing evaporated milk in itself modified the curd, and that the lactic acid was used primarily to slow bacterial multiplication in homes without refrigeration, rather than to enhance digestibility.

Reprinted from *Phila. Med. Times*, 660–664 (July 1, 1882)

MILK ANALYSIS

Arthur V. Meigs, M.D.

The Pennsylvania Hospital

GENTLEMEN,—In addressing you this evening I desire to lay before you the results of some experiments made in the last year with milk, and to detail a method for its analysis which I have devised. If my results are correct,—and I am quite satisfied they are,—they will prove useful in putting upon a more settled basis the much-vexed question of the artificial feeding of infants; and my method of analysis offers a rapid means of determining with certainty and exactitude whether any given specimen of commercial milk has been adulterated. The question of the composition of milk may seem, to any one who has not investigated the subject, one upon which ample and exact information may be had by turning to any one of the many standard works on physiological chemistry. That this is not the case, in regard to human milk at least, an examination of a number of books has convinced me. The most widely different results are quoted without comment by different authors, and in some instances there are placed upon the same page, in parallel columns, figures so different that an examination of them makes it plain that both cannot be correct. Two of the most widely quoted analyses are those of Vernois and Becquerel, and of Simon, whose results, which are nearly identical, seem to me to be certainly incorrect. These analyses are taken as standard by Carpenter, Kirke, Marshall, Edward Smith, Kehrer, Gorup-Besanez, and others. The time is too short for me at present to make a detailed statement of their processes, or to attempt to show what I consider to be the fallacious portions. It will be sufficient to say that Vernois and Becquerel do not separate each of the constituents of milk by itself, but satisfy themselves in determining the amount of casein simply by difference; that is, when they come to the stage of analysis at which they desire to separate the casein and sugar, they attempt to precipitate the casein and filter off the sugar; then they estimate the amount of sugar in the filtrate, and assume that what is not sugar is casein. Any one who will repeat their process will find, I think, a large proportion of sugar left on the filter, and this they class as casein, thereby making the percentage of casein much larger, and that of sugar much less, than it actually is. Simon attempts to separate the casein and sugar by the addition of an excess of alcohol to a concentrated watery solution of the two. If a concentrated solution of milk-sugar in water is treated with an excess of alcohol, a part of the sugar is precipitated. This precipitation of sugar doubtless took place in Simon's experiments, and caused him to class a portion of the sugar as casein. Mr. Wanklyn, who has written the best book with which I am acquainted upon "Milk Analysis," says, "Milk exhibits great constancy of composition. . . . The milk of an animal has probably very much the same constancy of composition as the blood of the animal. . . . As will be readily comprehended, this constancy of composition is a cardinal fact in milk analysis. If milk were variable in strength, as urine is, chemical analysis would fail to detect the watering of milk." Mr. Wanklyn confines himself to the examination of cow's milk ; but if what he says of cow's milk is true, why should the case be different with human milk? Why should human milk vary so much as the analyses of different chemists would lead us to believe, when such great uniformity of composition is exhibited by the milk of the cow? I will quote three analyses of human milk to show how widely at variance are the results of different chemists : first, one by Henri and Chevallier, then that of Vernois and Becquerel (the mean of eighty-nine analyses), and, last, one from the *Practitioner* (vol. xxvi., 1881), by Messrs. Dolan and Wood, of Halifax.

	H. and C.	V. and B.	D. and W.
Water.....	87.95	88.908	89.045
Fat.........	3.55	2.666	1.764
Casein	1.52	3.924	7.005
Sugar......	6.50	4.364	1.921
Ash........	.45	.138	.265
	100.000	100.000	

(The analysis of Henri and Chevallier, it will be observed, does not add up quite correctly. It is quoted as found in the work of Gorup-Besanez.)

It is impossible that these three analyses can all be correct. I cannot believe that human milk ever contained, as Messrs. Dolan and Wood state, seven per cent. of casein and less than two per cent. of sugar. The method they pursued was to estimate the sugar by the use of Fehling's solution, and calculate the casein by difference. The copper test, I am convinced, is not to be depended upon as a means of quantitative analysis if there is no way of proving the results arrived at, and when an unknown quantity of sugar is to be determined. In support of this belief, I may state that I once sent two solutions of milk-sugar of known strength to a reputable sugar-chemist, and asked him to estimate the amounts contained by means of the copper test. In both instances he concluded that the solutions contained about one-third less than was actually the case.

I agree with Mr. Wanklyn that milk usually exhibits great uniformity of composition. This is particularly the case with that which we get from dealers, for then it is always the milk of many cows mixed together ; and of course the mixed milk of a whole herd is not liable to the same variations as would be the milk of any one individual cow. There is one point, however, upon which I must differ from him, and it is that I believe the fat to vary very much, although the other constituents do exhibit great uniformity in their amounts.

My own analyses prove quite to my satisfaction—and this is the point I particularly desire to bring to the attention of the Society—that human milk never contains more than from seven-tenths of one, to one and a half per cent. of casein, and about seven per cent. of sugar. Now, if this be true, how different is human milk in its composition from the idea commonly accepted by the profession ! In many books upon physiological chemistry the results of Vernois and Becquerel are quoted as being the mean of eighty-nine analyses, and therefore they are given the first place in authority. A comparison of their figures and those of Simon with any ordinary analysis of cow's milk shows almost an identity, the only difference of any considerable amount being in the quantities of ash given ; and yet who is prepared to say that human and cow's milk are identical? I quote for comparison an analysis of "average country milk," as given by Mr. Wanklyn ("Milk Analysis," etc., New York, D. Van Nostrand, 1874), and with it the mean result, as given by Vernois and Becquerel (incorrect, in my opinion), of eighty-nine analyses of human milk. (Mr. Wanklyn's figures have been reduced to percentage.)

	Wanklyn.	V. and B.
Water	87.551	88.908
Fat.................	3.071	2.666
Casein............	4.043	3.924
Sugar.............	4.626	4.364
Ash	.709	.138
	100.000	100.000

Some chemists have attempted to show that the difference lies in the casein, that of cow's milk being unlike that found in human milk. The fact seems to me to be plain, whatever may be the differences between the two caseins, that the milk of the woman contains only one-third as much as that of the cow. The question is often asked, Why does human milk coagulate so much less readily and so differently from cow's milk ? The answer is that it contains a much less proportion of casein, the coagulable matter. Human milk cannot form the large leathery coagula so often produced in cow's milk, because the casein is relatively dissolved in a so much greater quantity of water. Biedert (*Virchow's Archiv*, Bd. lx., 1874) has written an elaborate and much-quoted article to prove the difference between the caseins contained in human and cow's milk, and makes a very strong case, but fails to notice the great and cardinal difference, that the proportion of casein is much less in the one than in the other. Casein is in its nature akin to albumen, and every physician has noticed the different effects produced when albuminous urines containing different amounts of albumen are boiled or treated with acid. If the amount of albumen is small, the coagulation takes place in the form of a mere opalescence of the fluid, the coagula are individually so small that they cannot be seen ; whereas if the amount of albumen be large, the coagulation takes place in heavy white flakes. Why can we not accept so plain an explanation of the different coagulability of the two milks, that the one contains much less coagulable matter than the other, rather than seek for some far-away difference in the chemical composition of the casein ?

Casein is universally acknowledged to be the element in cow's milk which the infant stomach finds most difficult of digestion; and yet most physicians and nurses forget that in diluting milk to reduce the proportion of casein they reduce also the proportion of fat much below the amount contained in healthy human milk, and the sugar still lower, because, even in its normal condition, human milk contains much more sugar than does cow's milk. Therefore cow's milk, in order to make it a proper food for infants, should be reduced one-half or two-thirds with water, and cream and sugar added to make the fat and sugar amounts equal those contained in healthy human milk. The giving of pure cow's milk to new-born infants, as advised by M. Parrot, is altogether inadmissible, both because experience shows that infants so fed do not thrive, and on the theoretical ground that cow's milk is too unlike human milk to be a good food for the new-born infant. I wish, then, to be clearly understood to assert, as the result of my experiments, that human milk contains only from seven-tenths of one, to one and a half per cent. of casein and

about seven per cent. of sugar, and that it never contains, as is the commonly accepted belief, nearly four per cent. of casein, for which latter belief I think the erroneous and widely quoted results of Vernois and Becquerel and of Simon are largely responsible.

To carry out the method of analysis I propose, 15 c.c. of milk are required. The first step is to discharge from a pipette 5 c.c. of milk into a small platinum dish, and at once weigh it and note the weight. This dish is then placed in a water-bath, and the water kept at the boiling-point until the milk is completely dried and ceases to lose weight. This takes, as Mr. Wanklyn points out, about three hours, when 5 c.c. of milk are used. (I have found most convenient as a water-bath a common skillet, and into this I place a disk of copper, with holes in it, of such a size as to hold the platinum dishes to be used, the whole being floated upon copper air-chambers soldered to the under side of the disk. This apparatus may be left for hours in the bath without any watching, and yet the platinum dishes are constantly immersed in the boiling water.) As soon as the weight becomes constant, it must be noted, and the contents are then incinerated, best over a blast-flame, and the weight again noted. (In incinerating, the heat used must at first be moderate, and then gradually increased.) This ends the work upon the first 5 c.c., and gives the amounts of water, solids not ash, and the ash. At the same time that the first 5 c.c. are weighed, 10 c.c. must be weighed in another dish, care being taken, of course, that the weight is exactly twice that of the 5 c.c. This is poured into a high, narrow bottle (the ordinary 100 c.c. graduated bottle answers the purpose), and 20 c.c. of distilled water added, this being used to wash all the milk from the vessel in which it has been weighed into the bottle. To this are now added 20 c.c. of ether. The bottle must then be tightly stoppered and agitated violently for five minutes; 20 c.c. of alcohol are then added, and it is agitated for five minutes more. If it is then set down for a few minutes, the contents will be found to have separated into two layers: on top will be found ether, containing fat in solution, and below will be a mixture of part of the ether, the alcohol, and the water, containing coagulated casein in suspension and the sugar in solution. The ethereal solution, which is on top, is then drawn off with a pipette, as nearly as can be done without disturbing the lower layer; 5 c.c. of ether are poured on to mix with what fat is left, and this drawn off. Ether I have usually poured on and drawn off five times, 5 c.c. being used each time, so as to remove all the fat. The ethereal solution of fat is now dried over warm water, and finally, for a few minutes, over boiling water : the resulting weight—that of the dish being deducted— is, of course, the weight of the fat. We have now left in the bottle the sugar and casein, with the salts. The contents are carefully washed into a large platinum dish, and dried over the water-bath. The dried residue is treated with boiling water, and the dish and contents placed aside to settle. The undissolved casein soon settles to the bottom, and the clear solution of sugar is poured off. The solution of sugar is now again dried, and the same process repeated, the sediment being added to that which was obtained before. This must be done four or five times, until it is found that when boiling water is poured upon the dried sugar it dissolves completely, no flocculi of casein being seen in the solution. The casein residue is then, after being dried, treated once or twice with boiling water, to wash out any sugar that may have been left in it, care being taken that none of the solid casein is poured off with the matter dissolved. This sugar is added to that formerly obtained, and the two substances are then ready for the final drying, which must be done over the water-bath, and continued until they cease to lose weight sensibly. The two residues are then incinerated over the blast-flame, and the loss in the burning gives the weights of the casein and sugar.

The only error that strikes me as possible in this method is that a small portion of soluble albumen may be classed as sugar. I do not think, however, that this occurs, for I have tried in every way to separate such a substance from my sugar residue, and never succeeded in obtaining any appreciable quantity. The method possesses many advantages: it is more exact than any other I have tried, the loss being usually only a small fraction of one per cent. ; then it should be valuable as offering a scientifically exact but rapid method of determining the amount of fat. The exact amount of fat in any given sample of milk can be determined in at most half an hour to an hour. When a full proximate analysis is made, the process is very tedious, taking from three to five days to be completed. If, however, it is not necessary to separate the casein and sugar,—as is the case in examining commercial milk,—an analysis can be completed in about three or four hours. The pouring of milk into the street, as has lately been done in some of our cities, because it failed to show a certain specific gravity when tested with the lactometer, is a great outrage ; for an analysis which will show the amount of water, fat, and ash is the only true test of milk. The idea of separating the fat by means of ether and alcohol was suggested to my mind by the perusal of an article by Ed. J. Hallock (*American Journal of Pharmacy*, October 1, 1874). The use of the reagents in the proportions suggested by him, however, fails to effect the purpose, as any one can see who will try the process ; for the oil-globules are set free instead of being dissolved in ether, as happens when my proportions are used, and they only partially rise to the top, many becoming entangled in the meshes of the coagulated casein and remaining thus distributed through the fluid. The method I propose also extracts the fat more perfectly than that used by chemists generally, of extracting it with ether from the dried residue. This I have proved by actual experiment, taking two samples of the same milk. When the fat was extracted from the dried residue of 10 c.c. of milk, 270 milligrammes only were obtained, whereas my own method gave 305 milligrammes. This difference is large enough to be a matter of great importance where such small quantities are used as is often the case in milk analysis.

In calculating results it is easiest to bring the amount of each constituent up to what is contained in 100 c.c. This is done by multiplying the amounts of water and ash by twenty, as they are arrived at by the use of 5 c.c., and those of fat, casein, and sugar by ten, as they are arrived at by the use of 10 c.c. of milk. The sum of the amounts of the different constituents will be found to be from one hundred and one to one hundred and three, as the milk happens to be of high or low specific gravity. A use of the simple rule of three enables one easily from this to calculate the quantities in parts of one hundred (percentage). I append five analyses of human milk, which I have made with great care, and which I believe to be as nearly correct as may be:

Water	87 1c6	87 695	89.038	83.001	87 306
Fat	4.370	3.682	2.412	9.045	4.498
Casein	1.268	.938	.730	.787	1.083
Sugar	7.120	7.568	7.703	7.669	6.996
Ash	.136	.117	.117	.098	.117
	100.000	100.000	100.000	100.000	100 000

The error in these analyses was, in No. 1, seventy-eight thousandths of one per cent. in excess; in No. 2 there was no error; in No. 3 the loss was forty-eight thousandths of one per cent.; in No. 4 there was a loss of forty-nine thousandths of one per cent.; and in No. 5 there was twenty-nine thousandths of one per cent. in excess.

Condensed milk, in my opinion, enjoys its high reputation as an infant food because, when used as it commonly is, the proportions of casein and sugar approximate more nearly to those contained in human milk than in the usual dilutions of cow's milk; and it fails because it gives the infant too little fat, and because no preserved food can be so good as the same substance when fresh. Another grave objection to its use is that as children get older the quantity given them is increased, and they get much too large an amount of saccharine food, and become very fat, the fat being soft like that of persons who drink too much malt liquor.

In conclusion, I will reiterate that the result of my experiments has been to convince me that human milk contains only about one-third as much casein as cow's milk, and that in order to make the latter a proper food for infants we must dilute it with water and add cream and sugar. The main object of this paper has been to state my conviction that human milk never contains more than the quantity I have so often mentioned of casein; and this observation I consider as new, for, although Henri and Chevallier and some other writers have before arrived at nearly the same analytical results, yet I know of no one who has stated that human milk contains only this quantity, and never more, thereby denying the correctness of most previous analyses. If time proves my view to be correct, I think it must make a change in the views of the profession upon the proper mode of feeding infants. On some ·future occasion I hope to publish precise directions as to my view of the proper combination of cow's milk, cream, water, and sugar, to be used as food for new-born infants.

1322 WALNUT STREET.

2

Reprinted from *Boston Med. Surg. J.*, **127**, 56–58 (July 21, 1892)

IMPROVED METHODS OF MODIFYING MILK FOR INFANT FEEDING

T. M. Rotch, M.D.

Harvard University

It is not my purpose to enter upon the question of whether cow's milk represents the best medium for the artificial preparation of an infant's food, or whether if this be accepted, it is necessary to modify this medium. These questions I have already dealt with in an article written in 1887. The opinion expressed at that time, that an ideal artificial food should be a close copy of good average human breast milk, I at present see no reason for changing.

It seems to me now as it did then that the best and most satisfactory work which can be done in solving the intricate question how and what to substitute for human milk can be most wisely accomplished by perfecting the materials with which we are to work. Purity of material and an exact knowledge of the elements which compose the material are essential and primary qualifications for ultimate success. When these are once known and mastered, it becomes a mere question of mechanics and mathematics to make the especial combinations which we are seeking after. In the light of the precise and advanced investigations which have been carried on in almost every other branch of medicine, it is most remarkable that such simple and self-evident truths as have just been stated, should have been practically ignored, although acknowledged. I repeat that it is most remarkable that in this present time and place, and so far as I know at no other place in the world, it is possible for a prescription to be written for the elements which are contained in human milk, and various precise combinations to be made with these elements. For the first time in the history of infant feeding are we enabled to change the strength of the elements which we are using, as precisely as we have for years been accustomed to see accomplished in pharmacy.

It is with the idea that it may be of some interest to the medical profession to understand the various steps by which we have arrived at these important results, that I have ventured to prepare a brief paper on this subject.

Assuming that average human milk is the combination of elements which we had best endeavor to copy, it is self-evident that a knowledge of this secretion must be understood not only chemically but physiologically and clinically. The details of this knowledge I shall not now dwell upon, as it would be but a repetition of a careful study of the subject which I incorporated in a paper read before the New York Academy of Medicine in 1889.

We must, however, understand that the combination of elements represented in human milk is exceedingly varying, not only as a whole but in its different parts. We must acknowledge that infants thrive not on a staple and uniform fluid, but on one which in its changes adapts itself to the digestive functions of the individual. Thus only shall we be able to understand that proprietary foods, no matter how exact in their composition, should be relegated to oblivion as unworthy of the notice of the practical physician of the present day. Thus only shall we acknowledge that an artificial food should be written as precisely for by prescription as the combinations of drugs which we are continually sending to the pharmacist.

By way of illustration, then, I beg leave to draw your attention to Diagram I which represents some analyses of human milk, any one of which although possibly a good food for numbers of infants, would be liable to prove ill adapted to certain individuals.

DIAGRAM I.

HUMAN MILK ANALYSES (*Harrington*).

	1	2	3	4	5	6	7
Fat	4.0%	4.5%	3.0%	2.0%	4.0%	4.37%	2.96%
Milk sugar	6.5	7.0	6.0	6.0	6.0	6.30	5.78
Albuminoids	2.0	3.0	1.5	2.0	1.0	3.27	1.91
Mineral matter	..	..	..	..	..	0.16	0.12
Total solids,	..	..	..	..	..	14.10	10.77
Water	..	..	..	..	..	85.90	89.23
	100.0	100.0	100.0	100.0	100.0	100.00	100.00

Many infants would digest and thrive on Analyses I and II, but the average infant would be most likely to do well on Analysis III, while an individual with an especially highly developed function for digesting the albuminoids and a poorly developed function for disposing of fat would do well on Analyses IV and poorly on Analyses V. Analyses VI and VII represent the milk of a mother and a wet nurse. The infant that was fed by its mother on VI digested the high fats and albuminoids perfectly and has grown into a rugged and finely developed child having been nursed on this milk for a year. This infant would have digested Analysis VII, but probably would not have been so well nourished by it, judging from similar cases in my clinical experience. The infant that is now being fed on Analysis VII is digesting well and thriving on the low fats and albuminoids, while when it was attempted to feed it on a stronger milk such as VI, nervous symptoms and mal-assimilation resulted.

In this way clinical facts supply us with numerous illustrations which force us to the conclusion that we must in cases of difficult digestion, increase or diminish all or part of the percentages according to the infant's especial functional idiosyncrasy. In our endeavor to make a close copy, however, of this varying human milk, we must not only deal with the percentages of its elements but with its characteristics as a whole.

What are these characteristics?

A fluid consisting of about 88 parts water and 12 parts solids; slightly alkaline; sterile; free from extraneous matter, such as dirt of any kind; of a temperature on entering the infant's mouth of about 100° F; and with its total solids made up of fat (2 to 4½ per cent.), milk sugar (5 to 7 per cent.), albuminoids (1 to 3½ per cent.), and mineral matter (0.1 to 0.2 per cent.).

Assuming that cow's milk is the best medium to modify in copying the above-mentioned characteristics, the question arises which breed of cow is best adapted for our purposes? It has been found that the finer breeds of cows from the Channel Islands are not so rugged and are more liable to contract diseases, such as tuberculosis than the more common animals represented by Durham, Devon, Ayrshire and Holstein. The characteristic analysis of the finer breeds, such as Jersey and Guernsey is represented in Diagram II in comparison with the commoner breeds; the difference being seen to be mostly in the fat percentage and slightly in the albuminoids. (It may be well to state here that the albuminoid percentage in pure Holsteins is also a little raised.)

DIAGRAM II.

COW'S MILK ANALYSES.

	Jersey, Guernsey.	Durham, Ayrshire, Devon, Holstein.
Fat	5.50%	4.00%
Milk sugar	4.50	4.50
Albuminoids	4.25	4.00
Mineral matter	0.65	0.65
Total solids,	14.90	13.15
Water	85.10	86.85
	100.00	100.00

It is for future research to determine whether there is a qualitative as well as a quantitative difference between the secretion of the finer and more common breeds, but at present it would seem wiser in choosing our medium for modification, to select the milk of common cows. Practical experience has shown that the mixed milk of a carefully selected herd of a mixed breed of Durham, Devon, Ayrshire and Holstein. will produce the most satisfactory results as to stability and quantity of percentages. Such a herd, 60 in number, has been under my observation for the past six months and careful expert analyses have established the fact that we can rely on a very near approach to the percentages as they appear in

DIAGRAM III.

AVERAGE MILK FROM SELECTED COMMON HERD.

Fat	3.75%
Milk sugar	4.30
Albuminoids	4.00
Mineral matter	0.65
Total solids,	12.70
Water	87.30
	100.00

The food, drinking-water, stable accommodations and care of this herd is under expert supervision, and in order that the uniformity of the milk shall be preserved,

any change in the food is made by slight degrees and the salt is given in regular amounts and immediately after the milking. Only the morning milk is used and the time the cows are milked to the time the milk is delivered, at a laboratory here in Boston, is just three hours. The cows are carefully groomed, the hands of the milkers are well washed and the milk is received directly into glass pails and delivered at the laboratory in glass jars insulated against heat and cold. In this way we have at our command a fluid which is exceptionally clean, to an unusual degree free from contamination, and of a known chemical percentage.

The problem which now meets us is by what method we shall modify this pure fresh milk so as to resemble in its reaction cleanliness, sterility and chemical percentage, not any especial formula, but any reasonable prescription which the physician may write for. This has been accomplished by still further increasing our materials or rather subdividing the pure material (whole milk) which we have as a comparatively stable medium at our command.

Diagram IV represents the chemical percentages, determined by numerous expert analyses, of the various materials used; these materials thus in their turn being definite products, known as the pharmacist knows his drugs, and ready to be combined in various proportions according to the prescription, by means of exact mathematical rules.

DIAGRAM IV.

STABLE MATERIALS FOR PRESCRIPTION COMBINATIONS.

	Cream.	Separated Milk.
Fat	16.00%	0.26%
Milk sugar	4.00	4.40
Albuminoids	3.60	4.00

Distilled water. Milk-sugar solution, 20%. Freshly-prepared lime-water.

The means adopted in an especial laboratory for not only separating the fat from the whole milk but for obtaining a uniform fat percentage corresponding to the general mathematical formula employed for making the combinations, was a peculiarly finely-made and exact separator imported from Stockholm. With this machine running at a speed of 6,800 revolutions in the minute, it was found that if required, practically the entire quantity of fat in the whole milk could be extracted leaving in one of the trial analyses only thirteen one hundreths of one per cent. of fat in the resulting separated milk.

As a further proof of the accuracy of the separator and the above mentioned formula used for making the various prescription combinations required, the four analyses represented in Diagram V were made.

DIAGRAM V.

ANALYSES MADE FOR VERIFICATION OF THE MECHANICAL AND MATHEMATICAL WORK ON WHOLE MILK, CREAM AND SEPARATED MILK.

	Original Whole Milk.	Cream.	Separated Milk.	Recombined Whole Milk.
Fat	2.85%	18.21%	0.24%	2.75%
Milk sugar	4.05	3.76	4.35	4.05
Albuminoids	4.34	3.33	4.19	4.33
Mineral matter	0.66	0.62	0.72	0.68
Total solids,	11.90	25.92	9.50	11.81
Water	88.10	74.08	90.50	88.19
	100.00	100.00	100.00	100.00

The whole milk used in this experiment happened to be received from the farm at a time before the feeding of the cows had been sufficiently regulated to produce the higher fat percentage shown in Diagram III and now used for prescriptions. A portion of this whole milk was placed in a bottle and another portion in the separator. The resulting cream was placed in a second bottle and the separated milk in a third bottle. A combination, by the formula, was then made of the cream and the separated milk, with the idea of reproducing the whole milk contained in bottle one. This combination was placed in a fourth bottle. The four bottles were then given to Dr. Harrington to determine how nearly the percentages in bottle four would correspond to those in bottle one. The result as seen in Diagram V was so satisfactory that I then wrote the prescription represented in Diagram VI; had the milk modifier put it up and sent it to Dr. Harrington. The resulting analysis is also shown in

DIAGRAM VI.

	Prescription.	Analysis.
Fat	4.00%	3.92%
Milk sugar	7.00	6.95
Albuminoids	1.50	1.03

Since making the above analysis much greater accuracy as regards the albuminoids has been accomplished.

These experiments showed so conclusively that it is possible to put up a milk prescription accurately that I considered the chemical part of the process a success. The question of the reaction of the milk next had to be attended to. This is also something which will have to be worked out more fully in the future, but the probability is that the cows can be so bred and fed that they can be made to secrete a neutral or slightly alkaline milk. The reaction of this especial herd's milk was found to be so much less acid than the milk which I have ordinarily used, that where formerly I have had to use one-sixteenth part lime water, I now have to add only one-twentieth part, and even a smaller quantity will probably be sufficient for many milkings in the year. Another advantage to be found in the mechanism of the separator is that it removes effectually any dirt which may have fallen into the milk during the milking or the transportation. Cream also from the separator has, of course, the advantage of being just as fresh as the milk, in this case, being only between three and four hours old.

We now come to the subject of sterilization which has held such a prominent position in the history of artificial feeding during the past five or six years. As is usual in new discoveries in any branch of medicine much enthusiasm and an exaggerated idea that we had at last found a universal panacea for all evils of the past, was expressed by the exponents of sterilization. In my article on feeding in Keating's "Cyclopædia of the Diseases of Children," I stated that sterilization was but one factor in the problem which we had to deal with and that all the other factors which had been solved in the past must still be made use of if we expected to evolve a successful artificial food. The pendulum is now apparently swinging somewhat in the opposite direction and we are at present in danger of underrating a great and important adjunct to the feeding problem. The objections to sterilization are the boiled milk taste and the possible lowering of the nutritive properties of the milk sterilized, by coagulation of the coagulable portion of the albuminoids. In copying human milk we must remember that although the infant on the breast is being fed with a sterile food, it is a raw food and not one which has been heated to

212° F. That is, that sterility does not necessarily mean sterilization. With the view of meeting this question at once, for it is exceedingly important that infant modified milk sent out from a laboratory should be in a condition to keep without ice for 24 hours, I have had a series of bacteriological examinations made by Dr. Ernst, and I am also indebted to Dr. Henry Jackson for valuable work and information on the subject.

As the results of these bacteriological examinations are not yet conclusive, I shall reserve their detailed description for a later paper and shall now merely refer to a few general deductions which I have been able to make from them. On referring to the valuable work of Professor Leeds on this subject, published in the *American Journal of Medical Sciences*, June, 1891, we find that if the temperature of the milk is kept below 171° F., coagulation of the albuminoids to a degree which would be detrimental to digestion does not take place.

It was shown by Dr. Ernst's experiments that when the milk was heated to 167° F., it was as practically sterile for twenty-four hours as when it was heated to 212° F. This observation has been found to hold good when applied to the testing of the milk in the laboratory, where by means of a large sterilizer with a thermometer attachment a high or low temperature can be obtained at will. Heating the milk then to 167° F. avoids coagulation, to a great degree lessens the boiled milk taste, sterilizes sufficiently for a twenty-four hours' infant feeding, preserves the milk for transportation and allows the lime water, when needed, to be mixed with the milk at the laboratory before sterilizing. This latter modification could not be done when a temperature of 212° F. was used, on account of the reaction which took place with the milk sugar.

We have then, by perfecting this new method of modifying milk, an important instrument placed at our disposal, for aiding us to carry out exactly whatever line of thought we may choose to follow in our cases of artificial infant feeding.

3

Copyright ©1913 by the American Medical Association
Reprinted from *JAMA*, **60**(8), 575–582 (1913)

BOILED VERSUS RAW MILK:
An Experimental Study of Milk Coagulation in the Stomach, Together with Clinical Observations on the Use of Raw and Boiled Milk

Joseph Brennemann, M.D.
Chicago

Milk, alone of all foods, enters the stomach a liquid and becomes there a more solid food. This hidden and insidious solidness, if I may use the term, is peculiarly characteristic of raw cow's milk, as compared with boiled cow's milk, or human milk. The housewife and the dairyman are practically familiar with the fact that boiled milk forms a different curd from raw milk. We, on the other hand, have quite ignored the fact that raw and boiled milk are not identical foods. If we have thought of it at all it has been rather from a bacteriologic than from a physiologic point of view. And yet boiled cow's milk forms in the stomach, as does human milk, nearly a liquid food; while raw cow's milk, as I shall hope to demonstrate, is not even a soft food, but a solid food, so solid, in fact, that, unless modified in some way and given in careful moderation, it commonly forms hard masses that pass undigested throughout the whole alimentary tract and appear as hard curds in the stools.

It is exactly in these hard curds that one has the most tangible evidence that raw and boiled milk are not interchangeable clinical and experimental factors. It will be remembered that Talbot[1] demonstrated from various angles that these "hard tough curds" were casein derivatives, that is, "casein curds," in contradistinction to the small, soft, white curds that are "fat curds." Meyer and Leopold,[2] representing the Finkelstein school, denied the existence of a casein curd, basing their conclusions on the analysis they had made and on metabolism experiments. There was only one possible explanation for this discrepancy between equally compe-

tent observers about so simple a phenomenon; the hard curds that Talbot and other American clinicians described did not occur in Leopold and Meyer's experience. Talbot used raw milk, Meyer and Leopold used boiled milk exclusively, and the hard curd is essentially a raw-milk phenomenon, as pointed out independently by Ibrahim[3] and myself.[4] Meyer then fed a number of babies raw milk and promptly for the first time in his enormous experience saw these hard curds, and at once granted their casein origin. After being impressed again and again by the striking differences in the behavior of raw milk and boiled milk, first in the clinic and then in laboratory and stomach experiments, I cannot help feeling that other differences in clinical results will be cleared up, as in this case, if we have in mind that raw milk and boiled milk are not identical foods.

In the former paper[4] I offered as an explanation, as did also Ibrahim,[3] for the invariable occurrence of these hard curds when enough raw milk was fed, that, while

1. Talbot, F. B.: Composition of Large Curds in Infants' Stools, Boston Med. and Surg. Jour., June 11, 1908, p. 205; The Composition of Small Curds of Infants' Stools, Boston Med. and Surg. Jour., Jan. 7, 1909, p. 13; Casein Curds of Infant' Stools, Arch. Pediat., December, 1910, p. 919; Casein Curds in Infants' Stools, Biologic Proof of Their Casein Origin, Arch. Pediat., June, 1910, p. 440.
2. Meyer, L. F., and Leopold, J. S.: The So-Called Casein Masses in Infants' Stools, Arch. Ped'at., October, 1909, p. 773, and February, 1910, p. 126.
3. Ibrahim, J.: Kaseinklumpen im Kinderstuhl in Zusammenhang mit Rohmilchernährung, Monatsschr. f. Kinderh., 1911, x, No. 2.
4. Brennemann, Joseph: A Contribution to Our Knowledge of the Etiology and Nature of Hard Curds in Infants' Stools, Am. Jour. Dis. Child., May, 1911, p. 341.

boiled milk formed fine soft curds in the stomach, raw milk formed large hard curds that under given conditions would be passed through the whole digestive tract before they were completely digested. The evidence for this explanation was twofold:

1. Experiments *in vitro*. When rennin is added to raw milk in a beaker at a proper temperature the milk will quickly form a dense hard coagulum that separates rapidly and completely from the whey. Boiled milk under the same conditions coagulates less slowly, separates less completely and forms a soft, finely divisible curd that differs but little from a thick liquid.

2. The clinical observation that babies fed on raw cow's milk will at times vomit hard, leathery curds of enormous size.

A third observation, made since that time, makes this explanation even more probable. In a series of babies I have found that if raw milk is injected by rectum and retained for a time, the next bowel movement will contain typical hard curds, indistinguishable from those that occur when raw milk is fed by mouth. If the milk was returned in a short time the curds were soft and white; if after four or five hours, they were smaller and harder, more brownish or amber-colored, and more rounded or bean-shaped, an exact parallel to what occurs when these curds are present clinically. Thus in diarrhea, in which they are rushed through rapidly, they resemble more nearly a fresh-milk coagulum. As a condition of constipation is approached and they pass through more slowly they contract longer and are therefore harder, are more stained and are more rounded. If a portion of the feces of one of these babies is added to milk, the latter will coagulate as with rennin. The identical nature of the process of curd formation in the two cases can hardly be doubted. With boiled milk no such typical hard curds were formed in the rectum.

The interest now naturally drifted away from the hard curds to the processes going on in the stomach that produced them. The difference in coagulation of raw and boiled milk as shown in the beaker could not be applied forthwith to the stomach. One must assume, until the opposite is proved, that a living organ, lined with an active mucous membrane, with a complex specific secretion and a constant peristaltic motion, acts otherwise on ingested milk than would a motionless glass beaker. Czerny[5] has maintained, for example, that the constant motion of the stomach prevents the formation of large hard curds. That motion does not prevent the formation of large hard curds is evident from experiments *in vitro* when the milk and rennin are constantly stirred or shaken. In fact, the curds thus formed are always large, with raw milk, and peculiarly hard; often, indeed, the whole curd content of the beaker is collected in one hard mass. Whether there are other conditions present in the stomach that cause milk to act differently there than in a beaker can be determined only by a study of what goes on in the stomach itself.

Such a study presents difficulties that are greater than one would at first imagine. The stomach-tube, on account of the size of the curds, is worse than useless, because its use can lead only to erroneous conclusions. The use of an emetic introduces an element that is objectionable because unnatural, and is accompanied by discomforts that practically prohibit its use. Both are peculiarly contra-indicated in an infant, and the use of an emetic, especially in the presence of large hard curds, would not be wholly free from danger.

5. Czerny, A.: Des Kindes Ernährung, Ernährungs-Störungen und Ernährungs-Therapie, 1909, Franz Deuticke, Leipsic und Berlin.

While debating in my mind how these difficulties could be overcome, I discovered a healthy young adult, with normal digestion, and according to an analysis by Dr. Buhlig, with normal stomach contents, who could promptly, with little effort and a minimum of trauma to the curds, empty the stomach by the simple method of passing the finger into the throat. I intended at first to have this done only twice, once with raw milk and once with boiled milk, but the process was so free from serious discomfort, the disclosures so interesting, and the subject so willing, that about forty experiments were made with raw and boiled milk and with various "milk modifiers." While these observations were made on the adult, and only such application must be made to the infant as known identical physiologic conditions would warrant, nevertheless they can at least form a working basis for clinical observation in the infant.

In all of these experiments, unless otherwise stated, one quart of certified milk was taken in a period of about five minutes, at a temperature of about 95 F., on an empty stomach before breakfast, and was returned at the end of thirty minutes. One quart was a simple measure and represented about the amount, relatively, that a baby would take at one feeding. When "boiled" milk was used it was milk boiled actively for five minutes in a single boiler and then cooled to 95 F. as before.

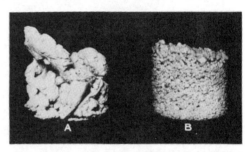

Fig. 1.—*A*, curds of one quart of raw fat-free milk returned from the stomach after thirty minutes; *B*, curds of one quart of boiled fat-free milk returned from the stomach after thirty minutes. (The glass jars in which the specimens in this and the following illustrations were placed do not show in the reproductions. All pictures of specimens are one-half their actual size.)

After examining the returned contents, 40 per cent. formaldehyd solution was added up to 10 per cent. After standing for from six to twelve or more hours the curds were hard, and were then washed, dried and placed in jars as here shown. The preserved specimens are all smaller than the fresh ones, very much so when returned in thirty minutes, because they contracted considerably after being returned, while those remaining in the stomach much longer contracted very little.

REPORT OF EXPERIMENTS

EXPERIMENT 1 (Fig. 1 *B*).—A quart of boiled fat-free milk, returned in thirty minutes, had curdled in fine, small, easily divisible, soft masses, that were of about the consistency of good custard, and were perfectly separated from the whey even after standing for some time.

EXPERIMENT 2 (Fig. 1 *A*).—Same as Experiment 1, except that one quart of raw fat-free milk was used. There was complete separation of curd and whey. In the clear straw-colored whey there were lying enormous, distinctly isolated curds that were firm and more or less rubbery, could be handled easily without breaking, and resembled exactly the curds I had become familiar with in beaker experiments when the milk and rennin were stirred constantly. So large and firm were these curds that they caused a sensation of alarm as they passed the throat. The average size was from that of a hazelnut to that of a walnut; many were 2 inches long, and one was 3 inches long and for the greater part of its length was 1 inch in diameter.

EXPERIMENT 3.— Same as Experiment 2, using raw whole milk. The result was the same except that the whey was a little milkier, and the curds somewhat yellower, softer and even larger than before. One curd was 4 inches long. Another came into the throat, stuck for a while, had to be reswallowed, and resisted all further attempts at delivery.

EXPERIMENT 4.—Same as Experiment 3, except that the raw whole milk was returned in one hour instead of thirty minutes. About a pint was returned. There was complete separation, as before, of curd and whey, but the latter was more turbid, was distinctly bitter and contained more mucus. The curds were somewhat smaller than before, were less angular, more rounded and firmer, and many had bizarre shapes, evidently arising from the coalescing of several curds. There were many more fine curds than before.

EXPERIMENT 5 (Fig. 2 A).—Same as Experiments 3 and 4, except that the raw whole milk was returned at the end of two hours. About a pint was returned. This was much more bitter than in the previous experiments, and had a decided taste and odor of vomitus for the first time. The whey was decidedly

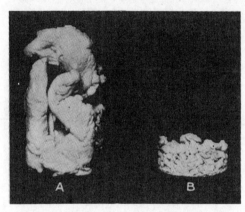

Fig. 2.—A, curds of one quart of raw whole milk returned from the stomach after two hours; B, curds of one quart of boiled whole milk returned from the stomach after two hours.

turbid. There were few small curds, but the remaining curds were larger and harder to return than in any other experiment in the whole series. One curd, from one-half to three-quarters of an inch thick, was 5 inches long and extended laterally 2½ inches at one end and 1½ inches at the other end. Another was banana-shaped, 1 inch in diameter and 3 inches long. Another was 2½ by 1½ by ¾ inches. They were all smooth and rounded, as if the sharp corners had been packed down.

EXPERIMENT 6 (Fig. 2 B).—Same as Experiment 5, except that boiled whole milk was used. Returned in two hours. There was so little whey that it was necessary to drink a glass of water to be able to return all of the curds. The curds were still abundant, averaged from a pea to a small hazelnut in size, and were larger and firmer than when returned in thirty minutes.

EXPERIMENT 7 (Fig. 3 B).—Same as Experiment 6, except that the boiled whole milk was returned in three hours. Contents could not be returned without drinking water. Were reported "bitter and sour." About a tablespoonful of rather soft, round curds were returned, that were about the size of sand grains, with a few as large as a pea. A large mass of mucus floated on top of the water with gray, feathery, stringy

masses of milk tangled up in it. The stomach was thus nearly empty after three hours, with boiled milk.

EXPERIMENT 8 (Fig. 3 A).—Same as Experiments 3, 4 and 5, except that the raw whole milk was returned in five hours. A glass and a half of water was required to return it. It was reported that the returned fluid was very "bitter" even in this dilution, but especially that "it left a horrid taste in the mouth as after taking vinegar." The liquid was very turbid and was filled with feathery whitish strings of mucus radiating out in parallel lines from the remaining curds to which they were intimately attached. There were still about ten curds an inch or more in length, and from half an inch to an inch in breadth. One was over 2 inches long. All were rounded or almond-shaped and firmer than in any preceding experiment. Some had, again, bizarre shapes, and looked as if eaten into, an appearance that is characteristic of the large, hard, yellowish curds of infants' stools. There were few small curds. Thus with raw milk there were still large curds after five hours.

EXPERIMENT 9 (Fig. 4 B).—One quart of whole milk was pasteurized by heating twenty minutes at 155 F. and was

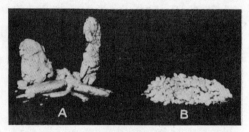

Fig. 3.—A, curds of one quart of raw whole milk returned from the stomach after five hours; B, curds of one quart of boiled whole milk returned from the stomach after three hours.

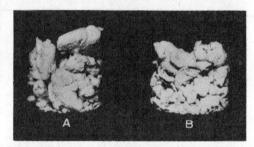

Fig. 4.—A, curds of one pint of raw whole milk returned from the stomach after thirty minutes; B, curds of one quart of pasteurized whole milk returned from the stomach after thirty minutes

returned in thirty minutes. The result lay between that of raw and boiled milk but much nearer the former. There was complete separation of curd and clear whey as with raw milk. The curds were not so massive but had all the characteristics of raw milk curds.

So far in each experiment the quart of milk was taken in about five minutes. To meet the objection that a baby does not take its milk in this way, but slowly over a period of from ten to twenty minutes, the following test was made:

EXPERIMENT 10.—A quart of raw whole milk was sipped slowly in a period of forty-five minutes, and returned thirty minutes later. One pint of clear whey, without bitter taste, was returned and contained only one small curd. Two glasses of water were returned clear with no curds. For some time a "heavy feeling" was felt under the lower end of the sternum. Five hours later, with two glasses of water, half a dozen curds were returned, that were each about the size of a large almond, and resembled closely those of Experiment 8.

To exclude the possibility of coincidence this experiment was repeated four times:

EXPERIMENT 11.—Duplicate of Experiment 10. Result exactly the same except that there were no curds after thirty minutes or after five hours.

EXPERIMENT 12.—Same as Experiments 10 and 11, but sipped only thirty minutes. Result the same. Only one curd after thirty minutes. No attempt was made to return the contents after five hours.

EXPERIMENT 13.—Same as Experiments 10, 11 and 12 except that one pint of raw whole milk was sipped in thirty minutes. Results exactly the same. Half a pint of clear whey was returned after thirty minutes. No curds then or five hours later.

EXPERIMENT 14.—Same as Experiment 13, but sipped in twenty minutes. Result the same except that the returned whey contained six or seven curds the size of unshelled almonds. This is at least suggestive that the shorter period of sipping is causing curds to return.

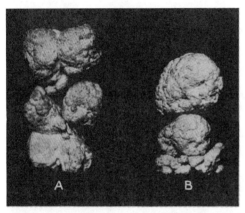

Fig. 5.—*A*, large curds formed in the beaker when raw whole milk and rennin solution were slowly mixed and stirred over a period of forty-five minutes and stirred for thirty minutes longer. Note coalescence of large curds. *B*, same as *A* except that raw fat-free milk was used. Only two very large curds and a few very small ones formed.

This astounding and most unexpected result to my mind admits of only one interpretation, that drinking raw milk very slowly favors the formation of a smaller number of curds so large that they cannot be returned. The large amount of unmistakable whey was positive evidence that the milk had coagulated completely as raw milk always does, and it is unthinkable that the curd could have passed on and left the whey. The absence of bitter taste, that is, peptonization, would alone exclude such a possibility. That they had not passed on was evident, too, from the fact that in the first case, at least, curds were returned after five hours.

Further evidence that this explanation is the correct one was obtained in two ways: (1) by repeating the sipping experiments with diluted raw milk, or with undiluted boiled milk, instead of undiluted raw milk; and (2) by duplicating the experiment in the laboratory. Diluted raw milk and undiluted boiled milk, even if they showed the same tendency to form larger curds if sipped, would still not be likely to form curds large enough not to be returnable.

EXPERIMENT 15.—Sipped in forty-five minutes a mixture of 1 pint of raw whole milk and 1 pint of water. The whey was returned clear with a large amount of curd practically indistinguishable in amount and size from those found when equal parts of raw whole milk and water were taken in five minutes. (See Experiment 19.)

EXPERIMENT 16.—One quart of boiled whole milk sipped in forty-five minutes and returned in thirty minutes. Large amount of curd returned, indistinguishable again from that of former experiment in which boiled whole milk was taken in five minutes.

The evidence from the laboratory was equally positive and demonstrated, once more, the striking parallelism between coagulation behavior in the stomach and in the test-tube. The laboratory experiment, furthermore, can be seen throughout the process, and offers an evident explanation for this phenomenon.

EXPERIMENT 17 (Fig. 5 *B*).—A vessel was set in water, over a heater, and kept at a temperature of from 100 to 105 F. To this was slowly added, over a period of forty-five minutes, from one vessel a quart of raw fat-free milk and from another a solution of 60 grains of chymogen (a proprietary preparation containing rennin) in 1 ounce of water. The mixture was stirred gently and constantly during this time and for thirty minutes after all the milk and ferment had been mixed. In five or ten minutes after the beginning of the experiment a fine flocculent coagulum began to form. The small curds formed during the process of stirring gradually united with one another into larger masses, which in turn attracted other smaller curds, until at the end of the experiment the clear whey contained two large round firm curds, one the size of a tennis-ball, the other that of a golf-ball. Neither, I feel sure, could have been returned from the stomach. Outside of these two large balls there were only a few small curds, such as those that were occasionally returned in the sipping experiments.

EXPERIMENT 18 (Fig. 5 *A*).—To exclude, again, the possibility of coincidence the experiment was repeated exactly with raw whole milk. In this case the coagulation was for some reason less rapid, the whey less clear as would be expected, but the result was otherwise identical. Practically all of the curd was collected into six round firm balls, each about the size of an English walnut.

The explanation for this phenomenon becomes evident as one watches coagulation experiments. Two curds brought into contact with one another almost immediately coalesce, so that practically no line of cleavage is left. This tendency seems proportional to the freshness of the curds. Thus in the last two experiments one could gradually see two or more curds predominating over the rest and uniting to them the small nascent curds as they came into contact with them. This accounts for the fact that not infrequently the curd of milk and rennin, stirred constantly in a beaker, will form in one large hard ball. This union of curds is well shown in the specimen of the six balls of the second experiment that were allowed to lie together in a graduate for a few seconds before formaldehyd solution was added. They were quite inseparable.

It is probable that such coalescence of curds takes place less readily in the stomach. Two stomach curds if brought in contact show relatively little tendency to unite. This seems to be due to the coating of mucus over the curds, and is probably proportional to the amount of the latter. Indeed, if curds united as readily in the stomach as they do in the beaker, it would be hard to see how their union into one large curd could possibly be avoided, when we consider how peculiarly favorable the peristaltic movements of the stomach as shown in recent *x*-ray work are for pressing the contents together. That curds do unite, however, in the stomach is shown in the sipping experiments and in the facts that the largest curds occurred after two hours and that many large curds are manifestly a union of several smaller curds.

When we come to consider the question of whether boiled milk differs clinically and therapeutically from raw milk, it will be of interest, first, as bearing directly on this question, to see what happens in the stomach when the various empirically time-honored "milk-modifiers" are used. It is certainly an interesting fact in this connection that nearly all "milk-modifiers" such as dilution with water, cereal water dilution, alkalinization, condensation, drying, souring, peptonization, the use of pegnin or other lab-ferments, all have one thing in common: they prevent in one way or another the formation of a large hard curd in the stomach. Have we not been told emphatically too by Finkelstein[6] that *Eiweissmilch,* which also has been modified in this way, does not work well, in fact can work disastrously when the curd is not fine? The following experiments were made along this line:

EXPERIMENT 19 (Fig. 6 *A*).—Dilution. A mixture of 1 pint each of raw whole milk and water was returned in thirty minutes. There was complete separation of curd and whey, but the

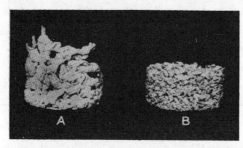

Fig. 6.—*A*, curds of raw whole milk diluted with an equal amount of water and returned from the stomach in thirty minutes; *B*, same as *A*, with barley-water substituted for water.

latter was somewhat turbid. The curds were much smaller, softer and more friable than with undiluted milk. Although many of them were from 1 to 1½ inches long, they were peculiarly thin, often membrane- or ribbon-like, and all seemed spongy or porous. There was also a large amount of crumbly detritus.

EXPERIMENT 20.—Same as Experiment 19, except that the milk was boiled and the mixture was returned in one hour. There was so little whey that it was necessary to drink water. About a level tablespoonful of soft fine curd, about like coarse sand, was returned.

EXPERIMENT 21.—A mixture of 8 ounces of raw whole milk and 24 ounces of water was returned in thirty minutes. This did not differ much from the dilution of 1 to 1, but the curds were a little smaller and still more porous or spongy looking. The latter condition seemed characteristic of diluted milk.

EXPERIMENT 22 (Fig. 6 *B*).—Barley-water. A mixture of 1 pint of barley-water (one-half ounce of barley flour to 1 pint of water boiled twenty minutes in a single boiler) and 1 pint of raw whole milk was returned in thirty minutes. The curds were small, like fine gravel, of peculiarly uniform size, with few as large as peas. About a third of them floated. They were greenish-gray in color. They were much finer even than with the 1:3 dilution with water, and were about the same size as those of undiluted boiled milk.

6. Finkelstein, H., and Meyer, L. F.: Ueber Eiweissmilch, Jahrb. f. Kinderh., May and June, 1910.

EXPERIMENT 23.—Sodium citrate, 2 grains to the ounce, was added to 1 quart of raw fat-free milk and returned in thirty minutes. There was no separation whatever of curds and whey even after standing for some time. The milk was simply thickened like a good cream soup, with no distinct curd formation, except an occasional small floccule.

EXPERIMENT 24.—Sodium citrate, 1 grain to the ounce, was taken in 1 quart of raw whole milk and returned in thirty minutes. The returned fluid looked like pale bluish milk, and the curds were soft, scraggly looking, about midway in size and consistency between those of raw and those of boiled milk.

EXPERIMENT 25.—Sodium citrate, 1 grain to the ounce of milk, that is, 16 grains in a mixture of 1 pint of raw whole milk and 1 pint of water, was returned in one hour. The separation of curd and whey was much more complete than in Experiments 23 and 24. The curds were about the size of coarse sand or fine gravel, and nearly all floated. The reaction was practically the same as in Experiment 20, with equal parts of boiled milk and water.

EXPERIMENT 26.—Sodium bicarbonate, 2 grains to the ounce, in 1 quart of raw whole milk, was returned in thirty minutes. The result was indistinguishable from that when an equal amount of sodium citrate was used, except that the returned fluid was yellow, probably because whole milk was used. The mixture was so nauseating and hard to take that only 28 ounces could be swallowed. Large amounts of gas were returned during the process, sometimes bringing milk with them. For some time there was annoying belching and a feeling of fulness. These objectionable features were of course wholly absent with the sodium citrate.

EXPERIMENT 27.—Lime-water, 5 per cent., that is, 30 ounces of raw whole milk with 1½ ounces of lime-water, was returned in thirty minutes. There was distinct separation of curds and whey, but the latter was rather milky, though not so much so as with the sodium salts. The curds were about the size of those of milk with 1 grain of sodium citrate to the ounce, that is, about midway between those of raw and boiled milk. They were, however, peculiarly soft, scraggly and friable, so that they could hardly be picked up without breaking.

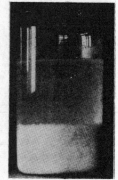

Fig. 7.— Stomach contents returned thirty minutes after drinking one quart of a 1:10 watery solution of condensed milk.

EXPERIMENT 28.—Lime-water 10 per cent., under the same conditions as in Experiment 27. The result was the same, except that the curds, while perhaps not smaller, were even thinner, more ribbon-like or flaky, more soft and friable than in the preceding experiment, and were described as subjectively "the softest yet." The returned contents were said to have a "very sweet taste."

EXPERIMENT 29 (Fig. 7).—Condensed milk, 1 quart of 1:10 dilution with water, was returned in thirty minutes. The curd formed a fine soft flocculent precipitate like fine white sand. This quickly settled to the bottom like a fine sediment leaving about an equal amount of nearly clear water above it.

EXPERIMENT 30.—Buttermilk. One pint of milk ripened with *Bacillus bulgaricus* was returned in one hour. About 10 ounces were returned. There was no perceptible change, but it was said to have been "sourer up than down."

No tests were made with powdered milk foods, or with *Eiweissmilch,* but there can be no doubt what the result would be.

It is, of course, necessary to confirm these results in other cases before one can assume that they are of unquestionable general application, and I attempted to duplicate some of the experiments on myself. Using the same method was wholly unsuccessful and the following was resorted to as the nearest imitation:

EXPERIMENT 30 (Fig. 8 A).—One quart of raw whole milk was swallowed in five minutes, and thirty minutes later one-tenth grain of apomorphin was taken hypodermically. The result was satisfactory in about ten minutes, and the curds and whey were exactly as in the other case except that they were somewhat smaller. This may be accounted for, to some extent, by the comparatively prolonged and violent time required to deliver the curds that at this stage are still quite breakable. The narcotic effect of the drug was, however, so violent for many hours that it seemed wiser to use only one twentieth of a grain in the remaining two attempts, with the result that, while the nausea was as intense, it was not so productive as with the larger dose.

EXPERIMENT 31 (Fig. 8 B).—A quart of boiled whole milk was returned after thirty minutes with about 2 ounces of curd that was exactly as in the other person, except that the curds were rather finer.

An attempt to return a quart of raw whole milk after four hours was not convincing. A small amount of turbid fluid was returned with some nearly disintegrated curds. Whether there were larger ones that were not returned is uncertain, as the effect of the drug was inadequate.

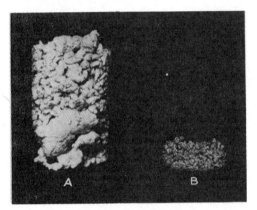

Fig. 8.—Same as Figure 1 in a second individual. *A*, raw whole milk; *B*, boiled whole milk.

The criticism that these findings may be largely individual in this case, and were only unsatisfactorily corroborated in a second case, must be admitted, and yet this applies rather to absolute than to the really more pertinent relative findings, such as the comparative coagulation of raw and boiled milk. To what extent these findings in the adult apply in the infant is difficult to estimate. Since we know, however, that all of the ferments of the adult are present and active in the stomach of the baby it is not unfair to assume that, in all probability, the same relative reactions take place there as in the adult. These limited observations must be taken only as a working hypothesis for further clinical and experimental observation.

The really important question, after all, is not how raw milk and boiled milk coagulate in the beaker or in the stomach, but how the person reacts clinically to raw and to boiled milk. On account of the enormous individual factor in infant-feeding it is peculiarly difficult to generalize, and yet it seems to me that certain clinical differences stand out conspicuously. For many years we used raw milk almost exclusively at North-

western University; for the last few years I myself have used raw or boiled milk according to what seemed to me indications, and somehow the indications for boiled milk seem to have increased at the expense of those for raw milk. In spite of a natural leaning toward raw milk, I find myself giving a large proportion of my babies, unless in florid health, boiled milk, and have frequently found myself in the position of many a mother who has told me, "I'm very anxious to get away from the boiling (or the soda), but I can't get farther than just so far and then I go back again." In this discussion I use "boiled" and "citrated" milk as practically synonymous because I have been unable to satisfy myself in what respects they differ from one another clinically, although I feel sure that there are differences.

DIFFERENT EFFECTS OF RAW AND BOILED MILK

While it has been a matter of surprise to me how frequently individual babies have no trouble with raw milk when one would expect it theoretically, nevertheless I am convinced that there are certain symptoms which are common with the use of raw milk and which disappear when the milk is boiled. This conviction, primarily the result of clinical observation, antedated the experiments I have here recorded.

1. The hard or tough curd of infants' stools is the most demonstrable clinical difference between raw and boiled milk. It can be produced in every infant by giving it enough raw milk, and it will promptly disappear when the milk is boiled. In feeding babies a considerable quantity of casein, as one must when using simple milk dilutions without cream, such curds are by no means infrequent. Ibrahim[3] found that on simply changing the milk from boiled to raw in the ordinary mixtures of ten of his babies the hard curds appeared in three. Their incidence among different clinicians with the same material is directly dependent on the amount of raw casein they give.

These curds are nearly always accompanied by other evidences of indigestion, especially diarrhea. Exceptionally they are found embedded, like seeds, in an apparently normal or nearly normal movement, but even then they usually represent a state of unstable equilibrium; either they tend to disappear or they increase and the stools become dyspeptic. Whether these curds are the result of some other factor in raw milk that produces dyspeptic symptoms, or whether they themselves mechanically produce these symptoms remains to be demonstrated. The fact remains that they occur on raw milk and are accompanied by indigestion, and that they disappear, always, and with them the indigestion when the milk is boiled.

These curds can occur, apparently (Ibrahim,[3] Courtney[7]) on boiled milk in a much attenuated form. This in no way lessens their significance, clinically, as a raw milk phenomenon, for in several years of search I have only once seen fine thread-like hard curds on boiled milk. That they may occur in small form in diarrheas with rapid peristalsis is quite consistent with the coagulation findings I have reported. Furthermore, one must not forget the possibility of error in the kitchen, or the fact that "boiling" is a term capable of varying interpretations, and that the difference in temperature between milk just beginning to simmer and milk welling up actively is from 20 to 30 F., and that the longer the "boiling" the more marked the influence on coagulation.

7. Courtney, Angelina M.: Studies on Infant Nutrition. 11. The Hard or Casein Curds in Infants' Stools, Am. Jour. Dis. Child., January, 1912, p. 1.

2. Diarrhea and dyspepsia. It is a time-honored empiricism that babies with diarrhea, or with any gastro-intestinal disturbance accompanied by diarrhea, and during convalescence from diarrhea, stand boiled milk much better than raw milk. That raw milk will cause diarrhea and dyspeptic stools, and that boiled milk will cure the condition are likewise matters of common observation. In making hard curds experimentally in babies, as recorded in my former paper, indigestion with diarrhea occurred regularly whenever I gave a baby enough raw milk to produce a good output of curds, and quite as regularly there was a prompt return to normal when the milk was boiled. The question rather forces itself on us whether the proverbial constipation from boiled milk is not due to the fact that boiled milk is more readily digested and completely assimilated than raw milk.

3. Vomiting. Here again the evidence is quite positive that many cases of vomiting when raw milk is fed are promptly relieved, as one might expect theoretically, when the milk is boiled or citrated. It is evident that raw milk is peculiarly contra-indicated in the vomiting of pyloric stenosis.

4. Colic and discomfort are among the most manifest and frequent symptoms arising from the use of raw milk. We are all familiar with the fact that a great many babies that are in constant distress, either having a great deal of colic, or crying almost constantly when awake and sleeping restlessly and brokenly, are promptly made comfortable when their food is changed from a raw milk to a boiled or citrated milk, or, what is still more striking, to a condensed milk, either liquid or powdered. If babies could talk they could unfold many a tale of their sufferings in trying to digest a strictly modern scientific, raw-milk formula and of their immediate relief on receiving a very unscientific food from a tin can.

A surgeon of my acquaintance is accustomed to drink about 20 ounces of milk at bedtime. When he takes it boiled he is perfectly comfortable; when he takes it raw he has an uncomfortable night and a diarrhea the next day. Few adults drink so much milk at a time and it is impossible to estimate how frequent such disturbances would occur if they did. The baby, on the other hand, with its far greater proneness to colic and diarrhea, takes six or seven such feedings a day instead of one.

If time permitted, an abundance of clinical evidence could be presented to show how frequent all of these symptoms are when raw milk is fed to an infant, and how often they disappear when the milk is boiled.

The disturbances that I have just enumerated are all of a purely digestive, and not of a metabolic or bacterial nature. In other words, raw milk often produces an indigestion that is relieved when the patient takes boiled milk. Whether this is due alone to the difference in coagulation or to some other difference between raw and boiled milk remains to be determined. The fact that boiled and citrated milk are peculiarly alike in their effect on digestion, though they have nothing else in common except the fact that in them the coagulation of casein is inhibited, would lead one to think that the determining factor in raw-milk dyspepsia is the nature of the coagulum.

CASEIN DIGESTION

This leads, much as one would like to avoid it, directly to the old question, that like Banquo's ghost "will not down," Is the casein of cow's milk difficult to digest by the baby? It is interesting, in the light of these newer observations on raw and boiled milk, to review how this question has been answered in various places and at various times.

Biedert[8] himself, the first great exponent of the difficulty of digestion of the casein of cow's milk, was also the great champion of the protein origin of the curds in infants' stools. That Biedert used raw milk to an extent sufficient to make himself familiar with the "hard tough curds" of our later literature can hardly be doubted when we read his description of weissbräunlich-gelbliche Brocken und Knollen that occur with "poor casein digestion." It is interesting to note that he recommended as curative three foods for which Czerny took him severely to task because of their apparent diversity; ramogen (a German proprietary condensed milk), breast-milk and buttermilk, three foods that have, however, one thing in common that now again seems rational enough—they all form a very fine curd in the stomach.

The later German pediatricians with few exceptions came to the conclusion, and correctly so, that the casein of cow's milk produced no recognizable clinical disturbance in their experience, an experience practically limited to boiled milk. If the German pediatricians had used raw milk, this whole question would not so long have seemed so puzzling; nor would it have been answered so positively in the negative.

In England the casein of cow's milk is considered a serious disturber in infant-feeding, but it really gives the Englishman no trouble because he uses sodium citrate to produce a fine curd.

The French pediatrician likewise has no trouble with the casein of cow's milk; in fact, he rather likes undiluted whole milk for his babies, but he lays more stress than any one else on lait stérilisé, even though he puts the emphasis on the sterilization rather than on the inhibition in coagulation. It is interesting that almost nowhere else than in France has the idea of using undiluted milk in feeding young infants found any favor, and in France the milk is always boiled, and to some extent in England where it is citrated.

In this country, where some of us use raw milk, some boiled milk, some both and some neither, our ideas have clashed. In using low protein, high fat, raw-milk mixtures the casein gives comparatively little trouble. With simple whole-milk mixtures the high casein is apt to make trouble unless the milk is boiled or otherwise modified. It is again an interesting fact that Jacobi, who has always used simple milk mixtures, notably 1 : 1 mixtures, has also always boiled his milk, and has used cereal waters as diluents; and in the stormy controversies that have centered about this subject, Jacobi for nearly half a century has stood out alone and unmoved as a rock.

Our own experience at Northwestern University is not without interest in this connection. Our departure from the percentage system, in which we rarely encountered "hard curds," to simple diluted whole-milk mixtures was accompanied in a great measure by a change to boiling the milk. This led us, too, to believe that there was "no clinical picture that we could recognize as casein indigestion." A few attempts to feed raw fat-free milk during the skim-milk epoch when "hard curds" that were evidently casein curds gained their greatest ascendency quickly showed us that our conclusion did not apply to raw milk. Of boiled milk it was as true as ever. It seems to me that we are justified in answer-

8. Biedert, P.: Die Kinderernährung im Säuglingsalter, Ferdinand Enke, Stuttgart, 1905, p. 225.

ing this whole question, in the light of our present knowledge, by saying that the difficulty that the baby encounters in digesting cow's milk casein gives rise to recognizable symptoms only when the milk is fed raw.

The digestive disturbances caused by the casein of raw milk, as here interpreted, are of course wholly distinct from those serious derangements of digestion and metabolism of the fat, the carbohydrates and the whey salts with which we have become so familiar through the works of Czerny and Finkelstein and their schools. Neither have they anything to do with bacterial activity. The questions further of transmission of disease through raw milk, and its influence on the intestinal flora and other similar considerations, lie beyond the scope of this discussion.

EFFECT OF BOILING MILK

I can hardly conclude without a brief consideration of whether boiling makes milk a less valuable or even a harmful food, especially to the infant. This consideration naturally includes four points:

1. Boiling changes practically every constituent of milk and many of its properties. Czerny[5] enumerates eleven changes and yet favors boiled milk, as does nearly every German and French pediatrician. An exhaustive analysis of the whole subject has recently appeared by an English student, Lane-Claypon,[9] who sums up the whole matter in the end by saying that "such small differences as have been found in the nutritive value of raw and boiled milk have been in favor of boiled milk." While this method of studying the subject is not of great value, nevertheless one must admit that there is not one particle of real evidence that babies in general do less well on boiled than on raw milk.

2. Hardly a single modern text-book in English, German or French even mentions boiled milk as a factor in producing rickets, and the whole question would long ago have died a natural death but for the alderman and the philanthropist.

3. Scurvy, that rare, easily recognizable and promptly curable condition, is probably and undeservedly more responsible than anything else for the present strong prejudice against heating milk. The fact that scurvy is commonly associated with the prolonged use of a dead food has led us to blame all dead foods, without careful discrimination as to the nature of the food in other respects. The German and French writers do not consider boiled milk an important factor, but rather conserved and canned foods, or milk boiled for a long time, and even treat scurvy with milk that has been boiled only a short time.[10] There is furthermore so much evidence that scurvy occurs only in children with a peculiar predisposition to the disease that this may indeed be the important factor. The fact that boiled milk is not so important a factor in the etiology of scurvy as are other things is shown strikingly in the fact that scurvy is, if anything, less prevalent in Germany, and much less in France, than with us. While this may be due in part, or wholly, to the alarming popularity in this country of condensed and evaporated milk infant foods, nevertheless the French writers, especially, are unanimous in saying that they do not see scurvy in infants fed on boiled milk. I will quote only one out of many that might be quoted. Anderodias[11] says:

> In the consultations for nurslings in which we feed sterilized milk, as in those of Budin, Variot and Maygrier, one has yet to see an infant with scurvy; while abroad, in England, and in America especially, where laboratory milk is commonly employed, the cases of scurvy are very frequent.

4. Perhaps the most wide-spread objection to boiled milk is constipation. While mothers are much concerned about constipation, the physician has rather a friendly feeling toward it, and in fact often considers it, as compared with diarrhea, rather a domestic than a medical problem.

I cannot refrain from quoting at this point the impressive words of one of the greatest French masters. Budin,[12] in 1905, after years of extensive experience with undiluted sterilized milk, says:

> So-called whole milk dyspepsia is absolutely unknown to us. . . . Neither do we encounter rickets. . . . Since all of our milk is sterilized we see practically no manifestations of tuberculosis. As to scurvy, concerning which so much has been said in recent times, we have up to the present seen not a single case.

CONCLUSIONS

I wish to emphasize the fact that I am not advocating the use of boiled milk, or of raw milk as a routine measure, but I believe that each has its indications. I have endeavored to show that raw milk and boiled milk are clinically very different foods; that the most striking difference between them as shown experimentally is in their reaction to rennin; that the casein of raw milk, unless modified so that it will not form hard, large, coagula offers serious difficulties in digestion that are not present in boiled milk; and lastly that these differences between raw and boiled milk should always be borne in mind in comparing clinical, therapeutic and experimental results in infant-feeding and elsewhere.

4529 Woodlawn Avenue.

9. Lane-Claypon, Janet E.: Report to the Local Government Board on the Available Data in Regard to the Value of Boiled Milk as a Food for Infants and Young Animals, New Series No. 63, Darling and Son, Ltd., Bacon St., E., London, 1912, pp. 60.
10. Since this article was put in type I have seen one case of scurvy in an infant of 9 months with the most marked involvement of the gums that I have ever seen. By feeding it undiluted whole milk boiled for five minutes, and without using fruit juices, etc., the child made just as prompt recovery as I would have expected with the employment of all the usual antiscorbutic measures.

4

Reprinted from JAMA, **73**(16), 1173–1177 (1919)

THE ARTIFICIAL FEEDING OF
ATHREPTIC INFANTS

W. McKim Marriott, M.D.
St. Louis

The term "athrepsia," as used in this paper, refers to that well known condition of extreme malnutrition of infants otherwise known as "marasmus," "infantile atrophy," or "dekomposition."

PATHOGENESIS OF ATHREPSIA

The essential factors in the pathogenesis of the condition, as determined by recent investigation, are discussed elsewhere,[1] and they need now only be referred to briefly. The condition of athrepsia may be considered as the end result of an insufficient intake or of a failure to utilize food in sufficient amount to supply the demands of the body; in other words, a condition of virtual starvation. In this condition the volume flow of the blood, that is to say, the amount of blood flowing through a given portion of the body per minute, is diminished. This diminished volume flow, it has been shown, is dependent, in part at least, on a decreased blood volume, seemingly the result of a decreased protein content of the plasma and consequent inability of the blood to maintain its water content. There is an atrophy of the blood as well as of the rest of the body.

PRINCIPLES OF TREATMENT

The obvious remedy for the condition is food, and very considerable amounts of food, for the energy requirement of such infants is high, and there is the need for replacing much lost tissue. Many of these infants will not begin to gain until they have received as much as 150 or 200 calories per kilogram of body weight, but unfortunately the tolerance for food is low. The intestinal tract and digestive glands supplied by an atrophied, poorly circulating blood are functionally weak. Digestion and absorption of food is necessarily poor. Unabsorbed food remaining in the intestinal tract of a weak infant is "gunpowder" which requires only the proper "match," bacterial or otherwise, to precipitate a catastrophe. We are confronted then, with the problem of feeding a large amount of food to an infant whose intestinal tract may be incapable of caring for even small amounts of ordinary food.

THE INJECTION OF GLUCOSE

Food may, of course, be introduced parenterally, but this method of administration has definite limitations. Carbohydrate, in the form of glucose, is the only food that it is practicable to administer parenterally. Pure amino acids or fat emulsions are theoretically suitable for intravenous administration, but are not practical in the present circumstances. Intravenous injection of glucose is a valuable and temporary expedient when the need for food is imperative. The few extra calories introduced in this way occasionally seem to be sufficient to turn the tide in favor of the infant.

Something may be done toward increasing the tolerance of the infant for food. This tolerance, of course, rises as the nutrition and circulation improve, but it is possible to shorten to a great extent the period of repair. This is accomplished by increasing the blood volume and as a result, the volume flow. This may be done by blood transfusions or by the intravenous injection of a gum acacia saline mixture.[2] It is necessary to repeat the transfusions or injections at fairly frequent intervals. Whether or not these procedures are carried out, we still have before us the necessity for providing a food which contains the elements essential to nutrition and which can be fed in large amounts without causing gastro-intestinal disturbances. Breast milk, of course, meets the indication; but breast milk is not always available.

USE OF LACTIC ACID MILK

It has been a matter of common experience that infants suffering from gastro-intestinal disturbances are able to take larger amounts of milk artificially soured by lactic acid organisms than they can of sweet milk. We have come to regard buttermilk and protein milk as our chief reliance in the feeding of infants with gastro-intestinal disturbances. Buttermilk, that is to say, fat-free lactic acid milk, is low in caloric value; and although a useful food during a period of lowered tolerance, is not a food on which an athreptic infant will gain weight consistently. The caloric value may be increased by the addition of sugar and starch, and favorable results from the feeding of such a mixture have been reported. Protein milk is also a food invaluable for certain purposes, but of relatively low caloric value; and even when enriched by sugar addition it is not especially well adapted to the feeding of markedly athreptic infants, particularly those under 3 months of age, for any length of time.

* From the Department of Pediatrics, Washington University, and the St. Louis Children's Hospital.
* Read before the Section on Diseases of Children at the Seventieth Annual Session of the American Medical Association, Atlantic City, N. J., June, 1919.

1. Marriott, W. McKim: Proc. Am. Ped. Soc., 1919.

2. The solution used is composed of gum acacia, 10 gm.; glucose, 5 gm., and physiologic sodium chlorid solution, enough to make 100 c.c. The solution should be centrifuged a short time before using, as a slight sediment tends to collect. From 10 to 20 c.c. of the solution per kilogram of body weight are injected very slowly into the sinus or into a surface vein.

In selecting a food for athreptic infants, we determined on a lactic acid milk as a basis. There would seem to be no very good reason *a priori* why the fat or, at any rate, all of the fat, should be removed from lactic acid milk. Surely the 2.5 per cent. of fat in protein milk is perfectly well tolerated. Buttermilk is ordinarily fed undiluted to even young infants with fairly good results, thus demonstrating that the concentration of sugar, protein and whey constituents contained in whole milk is not in itself harmful. A certain amount of fat can be tolerated by almost any infant, especially in a lactic acid milk mixture. On this assumption we have fed undiluted lactic acid milk containing amounts of fat up to the amount contained in whole milk, and have been convinced that the great majority of weak, athreptic infants tolerate extremely well undiluted whole lactic acid milk in fairly large amounts, one fifth of the body weight or more per day. For infants under 2 months of age we have usually fed the lactic acid milk somewhat diluted, but the evidence is not conclusive that such dilution is essential.

ADDITION OF CARBOHYDRATE

Having demonstrated to our satisfaction that whole lactic acid milk is well tolerated, we cautiously tried the addition of carbohydrate to the lactic acid milk in order further to increase the caloric value. The sugar selected for such a purpose must be one which does not readily undergo fermentation or which, if fermentable, will be so rapidly absorbed that but little fermentation can occur before absorption. The dextrins are not readily fermentable; they are easily split into maltose and glucose by intestinal enzymes but apparently not more rapidly than the end product can be absorbed; therefore little fermentable material is present in the intestinal tract at any one time. Glucose itself is absorbed with astonishing rapidity, as has been demonstrated by intestinal loop experiments on animals. On the other hand, glucose is very readily fermentable, and for this reason has not been extensively used in infant feeding. Weill and Dufourt[3] have fed considerable amounts of glucose to infants in the attempt to render the stools acid, but in no case was it possible to do so, presumably because the glucose was absorbed before a great deal of fermentation had occurred. The products of the action of lactic acid organisms on glucose are quite innocuous. On theoretical grounds, it would seem that if glucose were fed in combination with lactic acid milk there would be a fair chance of its being absorbed before being attacked by intestinal organisms capable of producing harmful fermentation products. Experiments *in vitro* have shown that in such a mixture the common bacterial inhabitants of the intestinal tract are unable to flourish. In view of the considerations just mentioned, it would seem that a mixture of glucose and dextrin would be an ideal form of carbohydrate for our purpose. Maltose is usually present in ordinary mixtures of glucose and dextrin. In moderate amounts it is well tolerated by infants.

THE ADVANTAGES OF CORN SYRUP

Commercial "glucose," otherwise known as "corn syrup," is a mixture of dextrin, glucose and maltose. Of the total carbohydrate present, dextrin makes up approximately 55 per cent., the remainder being maltose, 30 per cent., and glucose, 15 per cent.[4] From its

3. Weill and Dufourt: La Nourrisson 2: 65, 1914.
4. Wesener and Teller: J. Indust. and Engin. Chem. 7: 1009, 1916.

composition, such a mixture would seem to be well adapted for the purpose desired. An additional advantage of corn syrup is that it is cheap and is obtainable everywhere. We have added carbohydrate in the form of commercial corn syrup to the whole lactic acid milk fed to athreptic infants, and the results were as would have been anticipated. There was little or no tendency to diarrhea, even when as much as 10 per cent. of carbohydrate was added. The stools remained firm, formed and pasty, averaging from one to three a day. In the case of some infants there seemed to be almost no limit to the amount of carbohydrate that could be added to such a milk mixture. Thus we have added a sufficient amount of carbohydrate to cause a distinct glycosuria and have continued the feeding of such large amounts for long periods of time without there being the least tendency to diarrhea or vomiting, and this in the case of extremely weak and emaciated infants, previously suffering from prolonged diarrhea. Not only has it been possible to add this form of carbohydrate to whole lactic acid milk mixtures with impunity, but corn syrup in 5 per cent. solution may be given almost ad libitum between feedings as a means of supplying further calories.

METHOD OF PREPARATION OF LACTIC ACID MILK AND CORN SYRUP MIXTURES

Whole milk is sterilized by boiling, cooled to room temperature, inoculated with a culture of Bulgarian bacillus or other lactic acid producing organisms, and incubated over night. A properly prepared whole lactic acid milk is thick, creamy and homogeneous. Too long a period of incubation or too high a temperature results in the separation of curds and whey.

The corn syrup we have used has been an ordinary commercial variety. Such a syrup contains from 80 to 85 per cent. of carbohydrate by weight or, as its specific gravity is high (approximately 1.40), it contains from 110 to 120 per cent. of carbohydrate by volume. The thick syrup is somewhat difficult to handle and to mix with milk. It is more convenient to prepare a diluted syrup. Mixing 45 volumes of the thick syrup with 55 volumes of water gives a thin syrup containing approximately 50 per cent. of carbohydrate. One hundred c.c. of this by volume may be considered as containing 50 gm. of carbohydrate. Such a thin syrup is measured in a graduate and added to the whole lactic acid milk. The mixture should not be agitated sufficiently to separate the fat as butter. The mixture is not further sterilized, but is kept in a refrigerator until used. As such mixtures are very thick, a nipple with a large hole must be used in feeding.

THE FEEDING OF THE MIXTURES

In feeding formulas of the type described, it is advisable to begin with a mixture of equal parts of whole lactic acid milk and buttermilk (fat-free lactic acid milk) or, in the case of infants convalescing from diarrhea, on buttermilk alone. If such a mixture is well tolerated, the proportion of whole lactic acid milk in the mixture is increased until straight whole lactic acid milk is fed in most instances. The addition of the syrup is then begun, 3 per cent. of sugar being added at first; if no diarrhea occurs, the sugar percentage is gradually increased, depending on the infant's tolerance and on the amount of food necessary to cause a gain in weight. Fairly large amounts of the corn syrup can often be given to advantage.

The number of ounces of the milk mixture given at a feeding should be approximately the same as if breast milk were fed. We have used four-hour feeding intervals almost exclusively.

RESULTS OBTAINED

Up to the present time, we have fed the enriched whole lactic acid milk mixtures to forty infants varying in age from 1½ months to 18 months, the majority being between 2 and 5 months of age, at the time the feeding was begun. The period of time over which different infants received the formula varied from four days to eight weeks.

All of the infants were undernourished—the majority markedly so. About half of those observed had recently suffered from diarrhea. Four were syphilitic; fifteen suffered from other infections during the period they were on the formula. The infections included pyelitis, otitis media, pertussis and bronchopneumonia.

Little difficulty was experienced in making the infants take the food. Some older infants refused the food at first, but later took it eagerly. There were mechanical difficulties in feeding two infants with cleft palates. They did not at first seem able to swallow well the very thick mixture; later they took it without difficulty.

The amount of carbohydrate *added* to whole lactic acid milk varied up to 10 per cent. or over, the total sugar content up to as high as 15 per cent. The total added carbohydrate has been as high as 3 ounces a day. The amount of added carbohydrate has been greater in our more recent cases, as we have become convinced of its relative harmlessness. The result, as far as improvement of the nutritional conditions were concerned, have been distinctly better with the increased amount of added carbohydrate.

Vomiting, other than the spitting up of very small amounts immediately after a feeding, was unusual. In almost every instance it could be accounted for by the onset of an acute infection. Two infants with cleft palates vomited if the food was forced, and one infant with syphilis of the central nervous system vomited at intervals. This infant also had convulsions from time to time, and it seemed a reasonable assumption that the vomiting was of central origin.

THE CHARACTERISTIC STOOLS

The characteristic stools of the infants fed on the mixture described were light brown, formed, and pasty when mashed with the spatula. The number averaged from one to three a day. Several infants had stools looser than normal for a day or two at a time, but the stools again resumed their usual character without a change in food. Two infants with bronchopneumonia, one with pyelitis, and one very athreptic infant dying in collapse, developed a diarrhea during the last few hours of life. Aside from these four, only three infants developed a sufficient degree of diarrhea to warrant a change of formula, and all were returned to the same formula after a period and did well. Two of these had at a previous time suffered from diarrhea while on breast milk. None of the infants developed a condition at all suggestive of "intoxication."

THE GAIN IN WEIGHT

A gain in weight of the infants fed on whole lactic acid milk mixtures began when a sufficient caloric intake was reached, and generally continued steadily for days and weeks, interrupted only by acute infections. Some infants continued to gain even through febrile periods. The number of calories required before an infant would gain weight consistently was often high. Few infants whose weight was as low as 50 per cent. of the normal weight for the age gained on less than 160 calories per kilogram, and many required 200 calories or more. The gain in weight of these infants was not due to a process of "water logging." The gain continued over too long a period, and the flesh was firm and elastic. There was no tendency to edema, and none of the excessive flabbiness observed in condensed milk babies which one might expect in infants fed on a high carbohydrate intake. It might be well to draw attention to the fact that although the food here described contains a high percentage of carbohydrate, it is also high in protein and in fat, the relative proportions not being unlike those of ordinary milk mixtures. It is essentially a concentrated food, and therein lies its chief advantage. If an infant can take only a limited number of ounces at a feeding and only a limited number of feedings in the twenty-four hours and yet requires a large caloric intake, the only solution is to give him a food containing a large number of calories per ounce. The mixtures described have a fuel value of from 25 to 30 calories to the ounce, a larger amount than is contained in breast milk or in any of the usual milk formulas that could be fed with safety.

CONCLUSION

We wish to emphasize the fact that we do not consider the type of feeding here described as a panacea for infants. Whole lactic acid milk enriched with the carbohydrates of commercial corn syrup is simply a type of food that enables one to administer a considerable amount of nutriment in an easily assimilable form to infants needing a large amount of food but having an intolerant gastro-intestinal tract. Aside from this, there are no mysterious virtues in such a mixture.

ABSTRACT OF DISCUSSION

DR. FRITZ B. TALBOT, Boston: There is much in Dr. Marriott's paper which gives food for thought. One point he brought out, which I think bears repetition, is that children under weight require more calories per kilogram of body weight than the child of normal or average weight. That is borne out both in practice and in the basal metabolism. There is one point, however, which he neglected to state in his paper, and as he read it I thought of atrophic children I have seen, most of whom have subnormal temperatures. If such children are warmed up they frequently commence to gain weight, if they get enough calories. It must be remembered that if the amount of sugar is raised beyond a certain point it will not be absorbed and diarrhea will result. Of course, Dr. Marriott is dealing with another type of sugar than what is ordinarily used, and it is quite conceivable that the limit of absorption of this sugar is higher than that for those in ordinary use.

DR. ALFRED F. HESS, New York: About one year and one-half ago, I had an oportunity to feed some children on corn sugar. At that time, as you know, there was a great want of sugar in the community, and the Division of Chemistry in the Department of Agriculture, Washington, asked me whether I would see how corn sugar was digested by infants. I tried about twelve infants on the regular milk mixtures with the addition of 5 per cent. corn sugar instead of the ordinary cane sugar. These babies varied in age from about 2 months to 1 year. They were kept on this sugar for a period of about three months, and they all did exceedingly well. After the war was over and the shortage of sugar no

l·nger existed, we went back to cane sugar. I did not use
the syrup, but just used the ordinary cane sugar. It is
always cheaper than cane sugar and could be sold for a
great deal less, but is always less than the cane sugar. Dr.
Marriott has raised the question of whether this sugar· is
absorbed better. If it is absorbed to a greater extent it is
of course of greater value. This can be determined readily
by metabolism experiments.

Dr. J. P. Crozer Griffith, Philadelphia: I asked the chief
resident physician of the Children's Hospital of Philadelphia
several months ago what diet he would choose if he were
obliged to select one kind of diet for these marantic babies.
Without hesitation he answered, "buttermilk." By this I
mean the usual buttermilk mixture with flour and sugar,
which is now being used so much by physicians, and I hope
will be used more and more because it is such a valuable
preparation. I was very glad, indeed, to hear Dr. Marriott's
paper corroborate my own experience with the lactic acid
preparations of milk, and regarding the ability of the child
to take a high percentage of carbohydrate. With the ordinary preparation of buttermilk, wheat flour and saccharose,
referred to, the carbohydrate runs up to 10 or 11 per cent.,
or even more. I have had a decided fear of the high percentage of fat which Dr. Marriott has been using, believing
that one of the values of the buttermilk food was the small
amount of butter fat in it. However, experience must be the
teacher in that matter, and Dr. Marriott's observation seems
to show that the fat after all can be borne better than we
supposed. It will be interesting to test this further. Dr.
Marriott spoke about the food preparations containing lactic
acid being more digestible. This has been my own experience. The fact that it is often difficult to have the parents
prepare buttermilk properly at their homes makes me desir-
ous, in hospital practice. of placing the infants on some other
food as soon as possible. We have tried often to get away
from the buttermilk mixture by making one of similar composition by using skimmed milk instead of buttermilk; but
repeatedly we have found it was not tolerated as well. The
only difference was that of the lactic acid content present.

Dr. C. G. Kerley, New York: Dr. Marriott's method of
using lactic acid milk impressed me very favorably. I have
used a great deal of lactic acid milk and protein milk but
never after the fashion that the doctor has followed. I have
usually employed the fat free lactic acid milk or one with a
low percentage of fat in intestinal disorders, under which
conditions it is extremely valuable. When the diarrhea sub-
sides, other feeding is instituted. I have not been successful
in using lactic acid milk as a general diet in young infants.
I confess I would not have had the courage to use the milk
in quite the strength that Dr. Marriott used it. I will be
much interested in giving this scheme a trial. As regards
the carbohydrates, it is quite necessary in feeding very delicate malnutrition infants to give a high percentage of carbohydrates. I usually prescribe the carbohydrate equal to 10
or 12 per cent., this being made up of the sugar that is in
the milk, lactose or maltose and starch. Thin, emaciated
infants, very much under weight, require from sixty to sixty-
five calories to the pound. As regards the milk used in
these cases, I prefer the evaporated unsweetened product. I
find this much easier of assimilation than fresh cow's milk,
regardless of the way in which it may be handled.

Dr. James Hoyt Kerley, New York: Dr. Marriott
undoubtedly has had splendid results with his carbohydrate
feedings in marasmic infants. It seems to me, however, that
the trouble is often caused by the protein. The casein in
cow's milk forms a hard curd, while in mother's milk it forms
a flocculent curd. I have had great success with evaporated
milk, in which the milk has been heated to a high degree,
and the protein molecule was broken into many fine particles,
which do not form the hard curds in the infant's stomach as
is the case with cow's milk. An ounce of evaporated milk
is equal to two and one-half ounces of cow's milk, so there
is no difficulty in keeping up the caloric value. Dextrimaltose or lactose is added to the evaporated milk mixture
in suitable proportions to obtain the requisite percentage of
carbohydrates, just as is done with the lactic acid milk.

Dr. H. F. Helmholz, Chicago: I have been very much
interested in Dr. Marriott's results, especially as we, too,
have been interested in the sugar tolerance of atrophic
infants. During the summer of 1915 we used this product in
one of our stations in feeding about 125 babies with very

good success. We used it as we would use a sugar and flour
mixture. The difficulty of preparing the food with the syrup
in the homes was such that we found it practically impossible to use it. If Dr. Marriott can show us how it can be
used in the homes, it certainly would be a help in our infant
welfare work, because it seems to me, from what he has said
and from our experience, that it would be a cheap and very
excellent food to use in infant welfare work.

Dr. Lewis Webb Hill, Boston: One of the most important things in infant feeding is a proper understanding of
the use of the sugars. Often we feed altogether too little
carbohydrate to our babies, being afraid of producing sugar
fermentation. I was, therefore, greatly interested to hear
Dr. Kerley say that he often uses from 10 to 12 per cent. in
feeding his babies, as I do myself in many cases. Some
years ago Dr. Talbot and I investigated sugar metabolism in
a baby by gradually increasing the amount of sugar in the
food, from 5 to 14 per cent., and keeping the other food constituents constant. We found that the feeding of high sugar
increased the nitrogen and salt retention up to a certain
point (14 per cent. sugar), when the baby developed a diarrhea. The way that high carbohydrate works beneficially is
probably by sparing the protein, and by allowing the baby to
store and retain more nitrogen and probably more salts than
he would on a low carbohydrate diet. I am in the habit
sometimes of feeding my babies on a rather low protein diet,
just enough to cover the nitrogen needs, and supplying most
of the fuel in the form of carbohydrate, usually as a mixture
of dextrimaltose and lactose. Several years ago Dr. Dunn
and Dr. Porter worked along these lines at the Infant's Hospital in Boston, and they found their babies could take from
10 to 12 and even 14 per cent. sugar in many cases without
any harm, and with marked gain in weight. I believe that
in constipated babies, especially those with small alkaline,
rather foul stools, we need not be afraid of feeding high
sugars. The baby must be watched carefully, of course, during the high sugar feeding, and if spitting up or diarrhea
develops, the sugar must be reduced. The point is, however,
that many babies do a great deal better on a high sugar diet
(much higher than is ordinarily given) than on a low or a
moderate amount of sugar, and we should not follow slav-
ishly any set rule as to the maximum sugar that should be
fed to babies.

Dr. Thomas C. McCleave, Oakland, Calif.: I was very
much interested in Dr. Marriott's paper, because I have been
pondering how we can give more carbohydrate to certain
children. I would like to ask as to the intervals of feeding
he has used in these children, and to put in the form of a
suggestive question the possibility that perhaps the secret of
his being able to give these children the large amount of fat
that he is able to give them is dependent on the particular
type of mixture he is giving them. It seems to be the whole
success of his scheme. He has described his mixture of corn
syrup, dextrin, maltose and dextrose. The whole explanation of the success of his scheme is dependent on the composition of his mixture.

Dr. W. McKim Marriott, St. Louis: The point raised
is quite interesting in the light of some of the work we have
been doing. I mentioned the fact that in the pathogenesis of
this condition there is a greatly diminished volume of the
flow of the blood sometimes down to as low as one-eighth of
the normal. As the flow is increased by feeding, the subnormal temperatures rise and the infants begin to gain. In the
preparation of these milk mixtures in the home we find the
vacuum bottle convenient. The whole milk is boiled, cooled
down to incubator temperature, inoculated and poured into
the vacuum bottle and left over night. In the morning it is
ready for use. As to the feeding intervals, we have used
four hour intervals, six feedings in twenty-four hours; none
more frequently than that. With those four hour feeding
intervals we were able to give up to 280 calories per kilogram, so it was not necessary to feed any more frequently.
I draw attention to the fact also that these mixtures are
quite elastic. One does not have to use the undiluted milk
and add so much carbohydrate. The milk may be diluted,
or the fat diminished. Of course, I realize that children of
this type are likely to develop diarrhea and have to be
watched. We made it a practice in the hospital to have the
stools saved and to have the resident informed if there was
a loose stool, so although we were feeding very high carbohydrate we felt that if we could stop it at the time one loose
stool occurred no particular harm would be done.

Part II

PROTEIN

Editor's Comments
on Papers 5 Through 8

The practical pediatrician of the late nineteenth and early twentieth centuries concerned himself with the provision of a milk made to conform as closely as possible to that from the human breast. He evaluated the effect of his formulations on observations of growth and weight gain, combined with minute examination of the stool consistency. "Stool gazing" was an expected and accepted clinical practice and a cross for the house staff to bear. Concurrently, the biochemist, the nutritionist, and the more scientifically trained pediatrician turned their attention from the composition of the milk to the protein requirements of the growing organism.

Using rats as experimental subjects, Osborne and Mendel (1915) obtained their supporting data for the concept of a "protein minimum" for animals. They hypothesized that the percentage of calories provided by the protein and the balance of its amino acid constituents were pivotal.

With a constant energy intake the amount of protein available for constructive functions will be limited by the "law of minimum." For example, a diet containing 20 percent of the calories

> ingested in the form of some protein relatively deficient in an
> essential amino-acid may supply enough of that amino-acid to
> satisfy the requirements of the animal for maintenance and
> growth; whereas one containing only 10 percent of its calories
> in the form of the same protein, with an equivalent energy in-
> take, may not supply enough.

They further concluded that the nutritive value of certain proteins
was better than that of others. Lactalbumin, for example, appeared
superior to casein when measured in terms of rat growth.

Harrison's studies of nitrogen retention in human infants
(Paper 5) substantiated the hypotheses of Osborne and Mendel. He
clearly demonstrated for the first time that increasing the amount
of protein in the infant's diet without increasing the caloric intake
did not result in an increased storage of protein. Similarly, he did
not feel that his experiments allowed quantitation of the daily protein minimum. Indeed, the appropriate allowance for daily intake
is still a matter of debate among those with differing and well-
documented opinions. In a 1959 review of the protein allowances
for young infants, Gordon and Ganzon add little to Levine's conclusion (Paper 6), merely reiterating that infants thrive on protein
intakes that vary considerably in amount and source: i.e., breast
milk, contrasted with artificial feeding mixtures, which customarily
have a higher protein allowance than that of the breast.

Paper 7, on the tryptophane requirement of the infant, is an
example of the fine contributions made by investigators from the
New York University College of Medicine, Department of Pediatrics, in collaboration with others. Although an entire volume
could be devoted to this aspect of protein nutrition in children, one
sample must suffice.

Finally, Fomon's study (Paper 8) concludes that the adequacy
of protein from human milk and cow's milk is similar, insofar
as promoting nitrogen retention—the scientific Q.E.D. of the
empirical observation.

5

THE RETENTIONS OF NITROGEN, CALCIUM, AND PHOSPHORUS OF INFANTS FED SWEETENED CONDENSED MILK

HAROLD E. HARRISON, M.D.

NEW HAVEN, CONN.

THE minimal protein requirement of infants has never been actually determined. It has been generally assumed, however, that infants fed cow's milk require a considerably greater intake of protein than do breast-fed infants. A nursing infant receives about 8 per cent of his total calories in protein, whereas an artificially fed infant is said to require at least 12 per cent of his calories in protein.[1] This difference in protein requirement is explained by the higher lactalbumin content of human milk since Osborne and Mendel[2] demonstrated that less lactalbumin than casein was necessary to maintain normal growth in the rat. Edelstein and Langstein[3] attempted to prove that these findings were valid also for the human infant, but owing to the inherent difficulties of the method employed, their results were not entirely conclusive. No other similar experiments have been reported.

Although experimental evidence is lacking, most writers on infant nutrition attribute the nutritional disturbances occasionally seen in infants fed cow's milk mixtures providing less than 12 to 15 per cent of the calories in protein to deficiency of protein. Sweetened condensed milk which contains about 10 per cent of its calories in protein is frequently cited as an example of a feeding inadequate in protein. It is well known, however, that many modifications of cow's milk designed to resemble human milk, and consequently low in protein, are used for infant feeding without any evidences of impaired nutrition.

The nitrogen balances of infants fed a cow's milk mixture low in protein should afford an indication of the adequacy of the intake of protein. The present study was, therefore, undertaken to determine the retention of nitrogen of infants fed a cow's milk mixture providing about 10 per cent of the calories in protein. Sweetened condensed milk was used, but the results probably apply to other cow's milk modifications of similar protein content.

METHOD

The subjects of the experiments were five healthy infants ranging from four to seven months of age. Their nitrogen balances were determined first when given diluted sweetened condensed milk and then

From the Department of Pediatrics, Yale University School of Medicine and the Pediatric Service of the New Haven Hospital and Dispensary.

This work was aided by a grant from the Borden Company, New York, N. Y.

Presented in abstract before the Society for Pediatric Research, May 7, 1935.

when fed an equal number of calories in the form of a cow's milk mixture providing about 15 per cent of the calories in protein. This consisted of unsweetened evaporated milk diluted with an equal volume of water to which was added sucrose to make up 6 per cent by weight of the total mixture. In addition, one infant was studied during a third period on a feeding of diluted evaporated milk without added sugar which supplied 20 per cent of the calories in protein. The percentage of distribution of calories of the feeding mixtures used is shown in Table I. Both the sweetened condensed milk and the evaporated milk mixtures were supplemented with 8 c.c. of cod liver oil and 30 c.c. of orange juice daily. The total calories fed were sufficient to allow normal gain of weight and ranged from 100 to 120 calories per kilogram. Since sweetened condensed milk mixtures are relatively low in calcium and phosphorus, the retentions of these elements were also determined in addition to the retention of nitrogen.

Each infant was fed the milk mixture to be studied for at least ten days before the balance determinations. Following this foreperiod, the infants were placed on metabolism frames permitting the quantitative collection of urine and feces. The metabolism periods were of seven

TABLE I

PERCENTAGE DISTRIBUTION OF CALORIES

	PROTEIN	FAT	CARBOHYDRATE
Sweetened condensed milk	10	25	65
Evaporated milk and 6 per cent sucrose	15	40	45
Evaporated milk	20	55	25
Breast milk	8	47	45

days each. Carmine red was used to mark the feces. Aliquots of the milk mixture fed were taken for analysis. The food, feces, and urine were analyzed for nitrogen by the Kjeldahl method, calcium by a modification of the McCrudden method,[4] and phosphorus by the gravimetric magnesium pyrophosphate method.[4] The accuracy of the urine collections was checked by the determination of creatinine in each twenty-four-hour specimen. During each period the variations in the daily creatinine excretion were less than 10 per cent of the average for the period. The gain in weight of the infants was also noted.

RESULTS

The experimental results are summarized in Table II. The data are expressed in terms of twenty-four-hour periods.

The rate of gain in weight was satisfactory in all of the experiments, ranging from 19 to 41 gm. per day, and was essentially the same during the periods of feeding with sweetened condensed milk and with evaporated milk.

In four of the five experiments the retentions of nitrogen during the periods of low protein feeding were approximately equal to the retentions obtained with the higher levels of protein. The constancy of retention of nitrogen is quite strikingly shown by the subject E. M., who retained the same amount of nitrogen when 10 per cent, 15 per cent or 20 per cent of the calories were provided in protein. One subject, H. B., showed a considerably greater retention of nitrogen during the evaporated milk period.

The sweetened condensed milk feedings supplied only about two-thirds as much calcium and phosphorus as the mixtures of evaporated milk and sucrose. Less calcium was retained during the periods of lower calcium intake except in one experiment. The retentions of phosphorus corresponded approximately to those expected from the calcium and nitrogen balances, i.e.,

$$\text{P retention} = \frac{\text{Ca retention}}{2} + \frac{\text{N retention}^5}{17.4}$$

TABLE II

DAILY NITROGEN, CALCIUM, AND PHOSPHORUS BALANCES

SUB-JECT	AGE MO.	WEIGHT GM.	FEED-ING	WT. GAIN GM.	N INT. GM.	N RET. GM.	CA INT. GM.	CA RET. GM.	P INT. GM.	P RET. GM.
W. K.	5	7,655	C.M.*	+35	2.92	+1.19	0.67	+0.22	0.55	+0.18
		9,600	E.M.+S.†	+36	4.46	+1.22	1.04	+0.33	0.82	+0.24
H. B.	7	7,915	C.M.	+39	2.65	+0.64	0.64	+0.24	0.52	+0.16
		8,670	E.M.+S.	+36	4.47	+1.12	1.04	+0.16	0.83	+0.17
T. B.	6	7,915	C.M.	+41	2.55	+0.96	0.57	+0.23	0.47	+0.17
		8,660	E.M.+S.	+40	4.38	+0.87	1.05	+0.32	0.79	+0.16
T. T.	5	7,260	C.M.	+23	2.60	+0.82	0.58	+0.17	0.47	+0.14
		7,720	E.M.+S.	+39	4.38	+0.82	1.05	+0.21	0.79	+0.14
E. M.	4	6,025	C.M.	+35	2.40	+0.82	0.56	+0.17	0.42	+0.13
		6,765	E.M.+S.	+19	4.02	+0.83	1.06	+0.20	0.73	+0.14
		7,455	E.M.‡	+29	5.63	+0.80	1.37	+0.24	1.02	+0.15

*C.M., diluted sweetened condensed milk.
†E.M. + S., diluted evaporated milk with 6 per cent sucrose.
‡E.M., diluted evaporated milk without added sucrose.

DISCUSSION

The failure of four of the subjects to show increased retention of nitrogen when the protein calories were increased from 10 to 15 per cent of the total calories indicates that the lower level of protein was sufficient to permit the maximum possible protein storage. The one subject, H. B., who showed less retention of nitrogen during the sweetened condensed milk period may not have been adjusted to the low protein feeding at the time the collection of urine and feces was started, since he showed increasing daily retentions of nitrogen during the period of low protein feeding. However, if this lower retention of 0.64 gm.

nitrogen daily be accepted, it still compares favorably with the reported retention of nitrogen of breast-fed infants. According to the literature, the daily nitrogen balance of healthy infants fed human milk averaged 0.56 gm.[6] Swanson[7] determined the retention of nitrogen of an infant fed human milk for a period of almost six months and found the average daily retention to be 0.54 gm. When sufficient calories are given, cow's milk mixtures which provide 10 per cent of the calories in protein apparently satisfy the infant's protein requirements. Increasing the protein in the diet above this level without increasing the calories does not result in increased storage of protein. The greater retention of nitrogen of artificially fed infants as compared with breast-fed infants, and especially of infants fed concentrated milk mixtures, may be associated with a higher intake of calories rather than of protein. Nelson[8] and Jeans and Stearns[9] found that the retentions of nitrogen of infants fed undiluted milk or evaporated milk mixtures were greater than those of infants fed diluted milk mixtures. The infants receiving the concentrated mixtures were given more calories as well as more protein than the infants receiving the diluted milk feedings.

No conclusions as to the protein minimum, meaning by this term, the lowest level of dietary protein permitting the maximum retention of protein, can be drawn from the present experiments. The fact that one subject showed a relatively low retention of nitrogen when given the 10 per cent protein feeding may indicate that this level is close to the minimum for infants fed cow's milk.

The nitrogen balances of the infants given sweetened condensed milk feedings do not support the commonly expressed belief that sweetened condensed milk is an inadequate food for infants because of its low content of protein. It is possible that the poor results of sweetened condensed milk feedings may have been due to deficiency of vitamins rather than of protein. This is in accord with the findings of De Sanctis and Craig[10] and Wolf and Sherwin[11] who reported normal growth and development in infants fed sweetened condensed milk supplemented with additional sources of vitamins C and D.

The lower intake of calcium and phosphorus during the periods of feeding with sweetened condensed milk was apparently associated with smaller retentions of these elements. This should not necessarily be interpreted as signifying that sweetened condensed milk is inadequate with respect to calcium and phosphorus. It has been observed many times that infants fed cow's milk supplemented with vitamin D show much greater retentions of calcium and phosphorus than do breast-fed infants. This is true even when the balance studies are carried out for long periods of time.[7, 12, 13, 14] Swanson[7] over a period of three months found that the daily retention of calcium of an infant fed human milk supplemented with cod liver oil averaged 0.08 gm. daily, whereas that of an infant fed a cow's milk mixture plus cod liver oil averaged 0.29 gm.

35

daily. Neither of these infants showed any evidences of rickets. Greater retentions of calcium and phosphorus can be obtained in infancy by increasing the amount of these elements in the diet, as the studies of Nelson[15] and Jeans and Stearns[9] show, but there is no evidence that this increased retention of calcium and phosphorus is necessary. Although the retentions of calcium and phosphorus of infants fed sweetened condensed milk supplemented with cod liver oil are less than those obtained with higher intakes of calcium and phosphorus, they are, nevertheless, considerably greater than those reported in normally growing breast-fed infants and are probably adequate.

SUMMARY

The retentions of nitrogen, calcium, and phosphorus of five infants ranging from four to seven months of age were determined when fed cow's milk mixtures providing 10, 15, and in one case 20 per cent of the calories in protein. The 10 per cent protein feeding consisted of diluted sweetened condensed milk. The feedings were all supplemented with orange juice and cod liver oil.

With an adequate intake of calories, the protein requirements of the infants were apparently satisfied when 10 per cent of the calories were provided by protein.

The retentions of calcium and phosphorus of infants fed sweetened condensed milk supplemented with cod liver oil were less than the retentions observed when the amounts of calcium and phosphorus in the diet were increased but were, nevertheless, considered sufficient to permit normal growth.

REFERENCES

1. White House Conference on Child Health and Protection. Report of the Commission on Growth and Development, Part III, Nutrition, New York, 1932, The Century Co.
2. Osborne, T. B., and Mendel, L. B.: J. Biol. Chem. 20: 351, 1915.
3. Edelstein, F., and Langstein, L.: Ztschr. f. Kinderh. 20: 115, 1919.
4. Peters, J. P., and Van Slyke, D. D.: Quantitative Clinical Chemistry, Vol. II. Methods, Baltimore, 1931, Williams and Wilkins Co.
5. Albright, F., Bauer, W., Roper, M., and Aub, J. C.: J. Clin. Investigation 7: 139, 1929.
6. Czerny, A., and Keller, A.: Das Kindes Ernährung, Ernährungstörungen und Ernährungstherapie, Vol. I, Leipzig, 1925, Franz Deuticke.
7. Swanson, W. W.: Am. J. Dis. Child. 43: 10, 1932.
8. Nelson, M. V.: Am. J. Dis. Child. 39: 701, 1930.
9. Jeans, P. C., and Stearns, G.: Am. J. Dis. Child. 46: 69, 1933.
10. De Sanctis, A. G., and Craig, J. D.: Arch. Pediat. 48: 439, 1931.
11. Wolf, M., and Sherwin, C. P.: Arch. Pediat. 40: 397, 1923.
12. Daniels, A. L., Stearns, G., and Hutton, M. K.: Am. J. Dis. Child. 37: 296, 1929.
13. Boldt, F., Brahm, C., and Andresen, G.: Arch. f. Kinderh. 87: 277, 1929.
14. Rominger, E., and Meyer, H.: Monatschr. f. Kinderh. 34: 408, 1926.
15. Nelson, M. V.: Am. J. Dis. Child. 42: 1090, 1931.

6

Reprinted from *JAMA*, **128**(4), 283–287 (1945)

PROTEIN NUTRITION
IN PEDIATRICS

S. Z. Levine, M.D.
New York

In addition to the many functions subserved by protein in adults, this foodstuff serves the special function in the child of providing basic building materials for the manufacture of tissues during growth. Protein also acts by virtue of its chemical and physiologic properties as a therapeutic agent in certain ailments peculiar to infancy and childhood; less commonly it may be biologically harmful when administered to children in its native state.

PROTEIN NEEDS FOR GROWTH

Protein needs for human growth are both qualitative and quantitative. Knowledge of these needs stems from studies on animals (notably the young white rat) and human observations including dietary surveys, measurements of nitrogen balance and creatinine excretion in urine and estimations of the rate and composition of growth at varying levels of protein intake and at different ages. Dietary prescription to meet these needs depends on such dietary factors as the biologic value of the proteins (amino acid mixture) ingested, their coefficients of digestibilit the degree of preparatory heating, the caloric, vitamin and mineral intake, sulfonamide medication [1] and such physiologic factors as pregnancy, puberty, the menarche, lactation, the state of nutrition and health, and age. Besides these known

From the New York Hospital and the Department of Pediatrics, Cornell University Medical College.

1. Martin, G. J.: Mixtures of Pure Amino Acids as Substitutes for Dietary Protein, Proc. Soc. Exper. Biol. & Med. **55**: 182 (March) 1944.

conditioning factors, other issues of a more controversial nature preclude complete acceptance of currently established protein quotas for human growth: (a) the questionable validity of transposing to infants and children experimental data and conclusions derived from young animals and human adults;[2] (b) lack of acceptable clinical criteria for defining optimal as against average and maximal nutrition and protein requirements; (c) a paucity of quantitative information of the composition of essential amino acid mixtures conducive to optimal human growth.[3]

In the present state of knowledge an adequate protein intake for the infant and child may be defined as one which contains all the known essential (and perhaps nonessential) amino acids in sufficient amounts and in palatable and digestible form to cover maintenance needs and to provide in addition the surplus for protein deposition within the body compatible with normal growth.

Qualitative Considerations.—Proof is convincing that the young white rat grows in normal fashion when the sole source of dietary protein consists of a mixture of the following ten highly purified amino acids: arginine,[4] histidine, isoleucine, leucine, lysine, methionine, phenylalanine, threonine, tryptophan and valine.[5] Applicability of these results to other animals and to human beings is suggested by recent observations on the nitrogen balance of dogs,[6] infants[7] and adults[8] and on the manufacture of hemoglobin and serum proteins by animals and man[9] receiving natural proteins, amino acid mixtures as such or as casein hydrolysates. The nitrogen studies showed that positive nitrogen balances of similar magnitude resulted on equivalent intakes, irrespective of the source of dietary nitrogen. Pending long term observations of growth curves and physical fitness of infants and children receiving pure mixtures of essential amino acids, final proof is lacking that the rest of the protein molecule and its fourteen or more constituent amino acids are of no nutritional impor-

tance.[10] Furthermore, quantitative data on the relative importance of each of the essential amino acids are still sparse. The absolute amounts and percentage composition of amino acid mixtures conducive to optimal human growth are not yet known. Reliance for growth and maintenance of health remains with the natural protein foodstuffs; use of purified amino acid mixtures

TABLE 1.—*Percentage Amino Acid Composition of Proteins in Some Foods Commonly Used by Infants and Children* *

| | Milk † | | | | White Bread |
	Lactalbumin	Casein	Egg	Meat	
Nitrogen	16.0	16.0	16.0	16.0	16.0
Arginine	3.5	4.1	7.0	7.2	3.5
Histidine	2.0	2.5	2.4	2.1	2.3
Isoleucine	4.5	6.5	5.3	3.4	2.8
Leucine	12.2	12.1	19.0	12.1	11.2
Lysine	8.0	6.9	6.0	7.6	2.8
Methionine	2.8	3.5	3.5	3.3½	2.2
Phenylalanine	5.6	5.2	5.2	4.5	5.1
Threonine	5.3	3.9	4.9	5.3	2.8
Tryptophan	2.3	1.8	1.1	1.2	1.3
Valine	4.0	7.0	4.4	3.4	3.1

All values determined on a basis of 16 per cent nitrogen.
* Block, R. J., and Bolling, D.: The Amino Acid Composition of Proteins and Foods, Springfield, Ill., C. C Thomas, Publisher, 1945.
† The protein content of human milk averages 1.25 per cent (0.2 per cent nitrogen), the casein fraction comprising 0.50 per cent and the whey proteins (chiefly lactalbumin), 0.75 per cent. Corresponding values for cow's milk are 3.5 per cent protein (0.56 per cent nitrogen), 2.8 per cent casein, and 0.7 per cent whey proteins.
‡ Stare, F. J., and Hegsted, D. M.: The Nutritive Value of Wheat Germ, Corn Germ and Oat Proteins, Federation Proc. 3 : 120 (June) 1944.

and casein hydrolysates is for the present reserved for the treatment of abnormal states in which the ingestion or assimilation of natural proteins is difficult or detrimental.[11]

Fortunately, from the practical standpoint of feeding infants and children, the protein foodstuffs of animal origin in common usage (milk and milk products, meat, fish, eggs) supply all of the essential amino acids, and some of vegetable origin (whole grain cereals, bread, potato, legumes) supply most of them in varying but generally high concentrations.

Quantitative Considerations.—The quantity as well as the quality of dietary protein must be adequate to cover (a) maintenance needs[12]—the replacement or wear and tear quota and fecal loss—and (b) the growth quota. The wear and tear quota is a measure of metabolized protein. It varies with the caloric and protein intake and with the energy expenditure of the subject. It is estimated by analysis of the urinary nitrogen ($\times$ 6.25). The fecal loss is a measure of the coefficient of digestibility of ingested protein and it is determined by similar analysis of the stools. In the absence of diarrhea and with the types and amounts of protein foods commonly used by infants and children, fecal loss of protein averages 10 per cent of the intake at all ages. The difference between the intake and the combined excretion in urine and feces or the magnitude of the nitrogen balance ($\times$ 6.25) affords an estimate of the protein deposited in the body for physical growth and pre-

2. Kinsey, V. E., and Grant, W. M.: Adequacy of the Essential Amino Acids for Growth of the Rat, Science 99 : 303 (April 14) 1944. Almquist, H. J.: The Amino Acid Requirements and Protein Metabolism of the Avian Organism, Federation Proc. 1 : 269 (Sept.) 1942. Rose, W. C.; Hanes, W. J.; Johnson, J. E., and Warner, D. T.: Further Experiments on the Role of the Amino Acids in Human Nutrition, J. Biol. Chem. 148 : 457 (May) 1943. Holt, L. E., Jr.; Albanese, A. A.; Shettles, L. B.; Kadji, C., and Wangerin, D. M.: Studies of Experimental Amino Acid Deficiency in Man: I. Nitrogen Balance, Federation Proc. 1 (Pt. 2) : 116 (March 16) 1942.
3. Hier, S. W.; Graham, C. E., and Klein, D.: Inhibitory Effect of Certain Amino Acids on Growth of Young Male Rats, Proc. Soc. Exper. Biol. & Med. 56 : 187 (June) 1944. White, A., and Sayers, M. A.: Accelerated Rat Growth Rate on Dietary Nitrogen Obtained from Pancreas, ibid. 51 : 270 (Nov.) 1942.
4. Arginine is synthesized by the animal organism but not at a rate rapid enough to meet the demands for normal growth.
5. Rose, W. C.: The Nutritive Significance of Amino Acids, Physiol. Rev. 18 : 109 (Jan.) 1938. Rose, W. C., and Fierke, S. S.: The Relation of Aspartic Acid and Glucosamine to Growth, J. Biol. Chem. 143 : 115 (March) 1942.
6. Rose, W. C., and Rice, E. E.: The Significance of the Amino Acids in Canine Nutrition, Science 90 : 186 (Aug. 25) 1939.
7. Hartmann, A. F.; Meeker, C. S.; Perley, A. M., and McGinnis, H. G.: Studies of Amino Acid Administration; Utilization of Enzymatic Digest of Casein, J. Pediat. 20 : 308 (March) 1942. Shohl, A. T.; Butler, A. M.; Blackfan, K. D., and MacLachlan, E.: Nitrogen Metabolism During the Oral and Parenteral Administration of the Amino Acids of Hydrolyzed Casein, ibid. 15 : 469 (Oct.) 1939.
8. Albanese, A. A.; Holt, L. E., Jr.; Brumback, J. E., Jr.; Kadji, C., and Wangerin, D. M.: Nitrogen Balance in Experimental Lysine Deficiency in Man, Proc. Soc. Exper. Biol. & Med. 48 : 728 (Dec.) 1941. Holt, L. E., Jr.; Albanese, A. A.; Brumback, J. E., Jr.; Kadji, C., and Wangerin, D.: Nitrogen Balance in Experimental Tryptophan Deficiency in Man, ibid. 48 : 726 (Dec.) 1941. Rose, Hanes, Johnson and Warner.[5]
9. Beiling, C. A., and Lee, R. E.: Treatment of Hypoproteinemia by Oral Administration of Protein Hydrolysates, Arch. Surg. 43 : 735 (Nov.) 1941. Robscheit-Robbins, Frieda S.; Miller, L. L., and Whipple, G. H.: Hemoglobin and Plasma Protein: Simultaneous Production During Continued Bleeding as Influenced by Amino Acids, Plasma, Hemoglobin and Digests of Serum, Hemoglobin and Casein, J. Exper. Med. 77 : 375 (April) 1943. Madden, S. C.; Carter, J. R.; Kattus, A. A., Jr.; Miller, L. L., and Whipple, G. H.: Ten Amino Acids Essential for Plasma Protein Production Effective Orally or Intravenously, ibid. 77 : 277 (March) 1943. Elman, R., and Lischer, C.: The Occurrence and Correction of Hypoproteinemia (Hypoalbuminemia) in Surgical Patients, Surg., Gynec. & Obst. 76 : 503 (June) 1943.

10. Lewis, H. B.: Proteins in Nutrition, J. A. M. A. 120 : 198 (Sept. 19) 1942. Albanese, A. A. and Irby, V.: Observations on the Biological Value of a Mixture of Essential Amino Acids, Science 98 : 286 (Sept. 24) 1943. Bauer, C. D., and Berg, C. P.: The Amino Acids Required for Growth in Mice and the Availability of Their Optical Isomers, J. Nutrition 26 : 51 (July) 1943.
11. Elman, R.: Parenteral Replacement of Protein with the Amino Acids of Hydrolyzed Casein, Ann. Surg. 112 : 594 (Oct.) 1940. Farr, L. E.: Indications for the Therapeutic Use of Intravenous Amino Acids, Connecticut M. J. 5 : 24 (Jan.) 1941.
12. The specific dynamic action of protein is a by-product and not an intrinsic maintenance need for this foodstuff. On the usual milk diets of infants and mixed diets of children this effect produces a rise of between 5 and 10 per cent above basal metabolic levels. Similarly, exercise does not raise the protein requirement, provided the total dietary calories are adequate.

sumably for other anabolic functions such as the manufacture of serum proteins and formation of enzymes, hormones and antibodies above antecedent levels.

Besides measurements of nitrogen balance, adequacy of the protein intake for growth is also judged by the rate and composition of gain in body weight. The latter may be estimated from the creatinine output in the urine and from the ratio of nitrogen retained to total accretion of body weight. A total gain of body weight conforming to the normal growth curve for height and age as estimated from standard weight tables, with the concurrent deposition of protein per unit of weight gain in amounts approximating the nitrogen content of the body as chemically determined (from 2.0 per cent in the newborn to 2.6 per cent in adults).[13] presumably characterizes an optimal state of quantitative and qualitative growth and nutrition.

Based on such evidence, the Food and Nutrition Board of the National Research Council has recently proposed daily allowances which may be accepted as an approximate guide of the protein requirements during growth. For physicians having a special interest in children, these allowances will serve a more useful purpose if they are amplified to include premature infants and broken down into shorter age intervals for the infantile period.

Provided the dietary protein is chiefly of animal origin and in digestible form and the regimen is adequate in all the other known nutrients, these allowances afford a good margin of safety for healthy infants and children. If a child does not thrive on this regimen the fault probably rests with him, his parents or the environment and not with the diet per se. On the other hand, it should be stressed that all dietary regimens are subject to modification. A diet should conform to the needs of the individual child and not the child to the diet.

TABLE 2.—Recommended Daily Allowances for Protein, Expanded for the Growing Period

Subject	Age	Total 1	Per Kg. 2	Per Lb. 3	% of Dietary Calories Average
Premature †	1 week to 1 month		6.0-4.4	2.7-2.0	17
Premature ‡	1 week to 1 month	4.3	5.0-4.4	2.3-2.0	15
Premature	1 to 3 months	per	4.4-3.3	2.0-1.5	13
Full term	2 days to 3 months	Kg.	4.4-3.3	2.0-1.5	13
All infants	4 months to 1 year		4.0-3.0	1.8-1.4	13
Toddlers	1 through 3 years	40	(4.2-2.9)	(1.9-1.3)	(13)
Preschool	4 through 6 years	50	(3.3-2.5)	(1.5-1.1)	(13)
School	7 through 9 years	60	(2.6-2.1)	(1.2-1.0)	(12)
School	10 through 12 years	70	(2.2-1.8)	(1.0-0.8)	(11)
Youths, female	13 through 15 years	80	(1.8-1.5)	(0.8-0.7)	(11)
Youths, male	13 through 15 years	85	(2.0-1.7)	(0.9-0.8)	(11)
Youths, female	16 through 20 years	75	(1.6-1.4)	(0.7-0.6)	(13)
Youths, male	16 through 20 years	100	(2.1-1.7)	(1.0-0.8)	(11)

* Column 1 gives the allowances recommended by the Food and Nutrition Board, columns 2 and 3 the suggested modifications for infants. The figures in parentheses in these columns, beyond 1 year, represent the total allowances in the original recommendations (column 1) per unit of body weight on the basis of average weights for age groups derived from the tables of Baldwin and Wood.
† Premature infants weighing less than 2,000 Gm. (4 pounds 6 ounces).
‡ Premature infants weighing 2,000 Gm. and over.

The high level of protein intake advocated for young premature infants calls for an explanation. Many of these infants have difficulty in digesting and absorbing fat.[14] Their dietary calories are therefore preferentially derived from protein and carbohydrate. Human milk, when fed in the amounts needed to meet the high

13. Vierordt, H.: Anatomische, physiologische und physikalische Daten und Habellen, Jena, G. Fischer, 1906.
14. Gordon, H. H., and McNamara, H.: Fat Excretion of Premature Infants: I. Effect on Fecal Fat Decreasing Fat Intake, Am. J. Dis. Child. 62: 328 (Aug.) 1941.

requirements for maintenance and growth (120 calories per kilogram, 55 per pound), furnishes, per kilogram of body weight, 180 cc. of fluid (2.7 ounces per pound), 2.2 Gm. of protein (1 Gm. per pound), 6.7 Gm. of fat (3 Gm. per pound) and 13 Gm. of carbohydrate (6 Gm. per pound). Although this level of dietary protein in the form of human milk is compatible with

TABLE 3.—Formulas for Feeding Premature Infants per Kilogram of Body Weight and in Percentages of Dietary Calories

Milk Type	Amount, Cc.	Sugar, Gm.	Water, Cc.	Protein Gm.	Protein Per Cent	Fat Gm.	Fat Per Cent	Carbohydrate Gm.	Carbohydrate Per Cent	Calories
Human	180	..	0	2.2	7	6.7	50	12.9	43	120
Cow's Whole	100	13	50	3.5	13	3.5	27	17.8	60	120
Lactic acid	140	6	..	4.8	16	5.5	41	12.9	43	120
Evaporated	70	6	80	4.8	16	5.5	41	12.9	43	120
Powdered half skimmed (Alacta)	18	11	150	6.0	20	2.2	16	19.4	64	120

positive nitrogen balances of appreciable magnitude (between 0.2 and 0.25 Gm. per kilogram) the total fluid intake is excessive and the level of dietary fat frequently exceeds the fat tolerance of these subjects, especially of those weighing 1,500 Gm. (3 pounds 6 ounces) or less. For these and other reasons[15] heated cow's milk mixtures are preferred in the routine feeding of small and young premature infants.

In isocaloric amounts (120 calories per kilogram) cow's milk mixtures may be prepared to provide less total fluid and fat, higher protein, and equivalent or higher carbohydrate. Examples of such mixtures are given in table 3. Comparative studies of such mixtures of heated cow's milk and of unmodified human milk for the past ten years in the premature unit of the New York Hospital[16] favor the former feedings. The daily gain in total body weight is more constant and at higher levels (25 to 30 Gm. as against perhaps 15 to 20 Gm.), the nitrogen balances are of higher magnitude (0.3 Gm. or more per kilogram as against 0.25 Gm. or less) and the coefficient of digestibility of the more liberal protein intakes is not reduced (85 to 90 per cent at all levels of dietary protein). It may further be pointed out that intakes of human and heated cow's milk of equivalent but lower protein content (2 to 3 Gm. per kilogram) yield absolute and percentile retentions of nitrogen of similar magnitude (0.2 + Gm. per kilogram and above 50 per cent of the intake[17]). This parity of utilization above maintenance levels of the proteins of human and cow's milk for growth in premature infants, contrary to the findings in animals,[18] is in accord with expectation on the basis of the qualitative similarity of amino acid composition of the milk proteins, casein and lactalbumin, noted in table 1. For

15. Catherwood, R., and Stearns, G.: Creatine and Creatinine Excretion in Infancy, J. Biol. Ch. 119: 201 (June) 1937. Benjamin, H. R.; Gordon, H. H., and Marples, E.: Calcium and Phosphorus Requirements of Premature Infants, Am. J. Dis. Child. 65: 412 (March) 1943.
16. These studies have been carried out by Dr. H. H. Gordon with the aid of the Children's Bureau of the United States Department of Labor. The results have not yet been fully analyzed and tabulated.
17. Gordon, H. H.; Levine, S. Z.; Wheatley, M. A., and Marples, E.: Respiratory Metabolism in Infancy and in Childhood: XX. The Nitrogen Metabolism in Premature Infants—Comparative Studies of Human Milk and Cow's Milk, Am. J. Dis. Child. 54: 1030 (Nov.) 1937.
18. Kik, M. C.: Nutritive Value of Lactalbumin versus Casein, Proc. Soc. Exper. Biol. & Med. 37: 129 (Oct.) 1937.

heavier and older premature infants, better able to tolerate fat and high fluid intakes, human milk is as satisfactory as cow's milk mixtures of higher protein content.

As the absolute rate of growth decelerates in later infancy, the protein intake may be correspondingly reduced to the recommended daily levels of 3 to 4 Gm. per kilogram of body weight. Concomitant with this decline in total increment of daily weight gain, the absolute and percentile retentions of dietary protein at equivalent and adequate intakes has been found to decline from average levels of 0.3 Gm. of nitrogen per kilogram or above 50 per cent of the intake in premature infants and of 0.2 Gm. or less than 40 per cent in full term infants under 3 months of age to average levels of 0.15 Gm. or 15 per cent for infants 5 months of age and older.[19] Analysis of available data for infants under 1 year establishes that the recommended daily allowances of protein as modified in table 2 are compatible with a normal rate of total weight gain and a ratio of nitrogen retained to total increment of gain which approximates the rising nitrogen content of the body (from 2.0 per cent at birth to more than 2.5 per cent during the growing period[20]).

Protein intakes below 2.2 Gm. per kilogram (1 Gm. per pound) in infancy may lead to negative nitrogen balances; levels above those recommended are wasteful since there are no body depots for reserve protein, absorbed amino acids in excess of the needs for growth and maintenance entering interchangeably with fat and carbohydrate into the energy exchange; excess of dietary protein may tax the kidneys by increased excretion of nitrogenous end products, and some of the incoming amino acids may be incompletely metabolized by the young infant in the absence of added vitamins.[21]

With further deceleration in the growth curve with increasing age beyond infancy, lower levels of dietary protein per unit of body weight are required for nitrogen retention and protein deposition. The daily allowances recommended by the National Research Council are generally acceptable. Based on average weights for each group, these allowances progressively fall from a maximal level of 4 Gm. per kilogram at 1 year of age to 1.4 Gm. per kilogram for girls of 20 years. The percentage of dietary calories (at the recommended levels) derived from protein remains constant between 11 and 13 per cent for all ages. The bulk of available evidence indicates that the recommendations are compatible with normal qualitative and quantitative nutrition as judged by dietary surveys, nitrogen balance studies, urinary excretion of creatinine, growth curves and clinical appraisement.[22] Some observers report improvement in measurements of children of preschool and school age on higher protein intakes of 4 Gm. as against 3 Gm. per kilogram.[23] Whether such acceleration is desirable raises the perennial question of maximal versus optimal nutrition, a problem which awaits further study and clarification. It seems valid to state that in the presence of undernutrition from any cause the higher allowances are preferable.[24]

Dietary Prescription.—Human or cow's milk ordinarily comprises the sole protein-containing food in early infancy. The protein content of human milk averages 1.25 per cent (0.75 per cent whey proteins, 0.50 per cent casein), that of cow's milk, 3.5 per cent (0.7 per cent whey proteins, 2.8 per cent casein). Since both casein and the whey proteins of milk contain abundant and comparable amounts (per gram of protein) of all the amino acids (except leucine) essential for growth in young animals and presumably in infants (table 1), the protein needs for growth are automatically met by providing sufficient milk. The concept of a higher biologic value of human over cow's milk, erroneously postulated on the basis of a deficiency of cystine in the casein fraction, has been discarded since it has been shown[25] that methionine and not cystine is the sulfur-containing amino acid required for growth and that cow's milk contains the latter amino acid in concentrations as high as or higher than human milk. From the standpoint of protein alone, it seems fair to conclude on the basis of current information that in equivalent content of protein above maintenance levels the two milks are equally nutritious.

A daily allowance (from the first few days after birth) of 175 to 200 cc. of human milk per kilogram of body weight (2½ to 3 ounces per pound) or of 100 to 130 cc. of heated cow's milk (1½ to 2 ounces per pound) covers the protein needs of young full term infants. The daily allowance of cow's milk for young premature infants, as previously indicated, is better set at somewhat higher levels (130 to 140 cc. per kilogram). For older infants in both groups the lower levels are adequate.

When the infant is old enough to take additional foods, other proteins of animal origin (eggs, meat, cheese, fish) and some vegetable proteins (cereals, bread, potato, legumes) progressively replace milk as the sole source of protein. It is a good rule to limit the daily intake of milk in the infantile period to a maximum of 1 liter (quart) and to introduce solid foods in the diet at around 4 months. In children above infancy, from two thirds to three fourths of the total protein intake is preferably derived from animal sources, approximately 50 per cent of total dietary protein being supplied by milk (750 cc. or 1½ pints), 25 per cent by meat and eggs, 15 per cent by bread, cereals and potato, and the remaining 10 per cent by fruits, vegetables and other foods.[26] Dietary surveys reveal that the amounts and distribution of protein in the daily diets of growing children are below the

19. Levine, S. Z.; McEachern, T. H.; Wheatley, M. A.; Marples, E., and Kelly, M. D.: Respiratory Metabolism in Infancy and in Childhood: XV. Daily Energy Requirements of Normal Infants, Am. J. Dis. Child. 50: 596 (Sept.) 1935. Marples, E.: Creatinuria in Infancy and in Childhood: II. Creatinuria of Premature Infants, ibid. 64: 996 (Dec.) 1942. Gordon, Levine, Wheatley and Marples.[17] Gordon and McNamara.[14]
20. Stearns, G.: The Mineral Metabolism of Normal Infants, Physiol. Rev. 19: 415 (July) 1939. Moulton, C. R.: Age and Chemical Development in Mammals, J. Biol. Chem. 57: 79 (Aug.) 1923.
21. Levine, S. Z.; Dann, M., and Marples, E.: A Defect in the Metabolism of Tyrosine and Phenylalanine in Premature Infants: III. Demonstration of the Irreversible Conversion of Phenylalanine to Tyrosine in the Human Organism, J. Clin. Investigation 22: 551 (July) 1943; and earlier papers of series.
22. Koehne, M., and Morrell, E.: Food Requirement of Girls from 6 to 13 Years of Age, Am. J. Dis. Child. 47: 548 (March) 1934. Wait, B., and Roberts, L. J.: Studies in the Food Requirement of Adolescent Girls: III. The Protein Intake of Well Nourished Girls 10 to 16 Years of Age, J. Am. Dietet. A. 8: 403 (Jan.) 1933. Rose, M. S.: The Foundations of Nutrition, New York, Macmillan Company, 1933. Daniels, A. L.; Hutton, M. K.; Knott, E. M.; Wright, O. E.; Everson, G. J., and Schoular, F.: A Study of the Protein Needs of Preschool Children, J. Nutrition 9: 91 (Jan.) 1935. Maroney, J. W., and Johnstone, J. A.: Caloric and Protein Requirements and Basal Metabolism of Children from 4 to 14 Years, Am. J. Dis. Child. 54: 29 (July) 1937.

23. Hawks, J. E.; Bray, M. M., and Dye, M.: The Influence of Diet on the Nitrogen Balances of Preschool Children, J. Nutrition 15: 125 (Feb.) 1938.
24. Wang, C. C.; Kern, R., and Kaucher, M.: Metabolism of Undernourished Children: IX. A Study of the Basal Metabolism, Caloric Balance and Protein Metabolism During a Period of Gain in Weight. Am. J. Dis. Child. 38: 476 (Sept.) 1929.
25. Rose, W. C., and Wood, T. R.: The Synthesis of Cystine in Vivo, J. Biol. Chem. 141: 381 (Nov.) 1941. Womack, M.; Kemmerer, K. S., and Rose, W. C.: The Relation of Cystine and Methionine to Growth, ibid. 121: 403 (Nov.) 1937.
26. Butler, A. M.: Nutritional Requirements in Infancy and in Childhood, Am. J. Dis. Child. 64: 898 (Nov.) 1942. Boyd, J. D.: Prescribed Diets for Normal Children, J. Pediat. 24: 616 (June) 1944.

recommended levels in many parts of the country.[27] The quantities and sources of proteins in the common foodstuffs are reviewed in another paper of this series.[28]

PROTEINS IN DISEASE

The role of proteins and their constituent amino acids for growth in health is likewise important in such abnormal states as malnutrition, obesity treated, by reduction diets, epilepsy treated by ketogenic diets, diabetes mellitus, recovery from acute illness and in the course of chronic disease. Fever, starvation and malnutrition further deplete the already meager stores of body protein, which are of lower magnitude to begin with in children than in adults and in those whose rate of metabolism is higher. The heightened needs in these conditions require attention in planning dietary regimens.

Besides this generally increased demand for protein in illness, this foodstuff by virtue of its unique properties serves a specific role as a therapeutic agent in certain states. The roles of protein and amino acid therapy in pregnancy, lactation and disease are reviewed in other papers of this series.[29] This section presents a brief outline of the use of protein in some disorders common to infants and children.

Disorders of the Alimentary Tract.—In health the coefficient of digestibility of protein is high, only 10 per cent or so of the intake being lost in feces. This high tolerance for protein is least impaired of all the organic foodstuffs in most digestive disturbances of infants and children. This fact, doubtless ascribable to the high levels even in early infancy of gastric rennin and pepsin, pancreatic trypsin and chymotrypsin and intestinal peptidases, explains the usage of properly heated milk mixtures, relatively high in protein and low in fat and carbohydrate, as the common method of resumption of enteral feeding in the recovery period of epidemic diarrhea of the newborn and infantile diarrhea of enteral and parenteral origin. Such mixtures include protein milk, skimmed lactic acid milk and skimmed milk with or without added casein. For analogous reasons, diets of high protein content form the basis of regimens in such specific disturbances of the alimentary tract as pancreatic fibrosis, the celiac syndrome (chronic intestinal indigestion) and ulcerative colitis, in the absence of an allergic basis for the two latter conditions.

Since ample evidence is at hand to show that the minimal amounts of unaltered protein normally absorbed into the blood stream are increased in, digestive disturbances in early life.[30] predigested proteins in the form of enzymatic casein hydrolysates are gradually replacing native proteins in treatment during the acute stage of many of these conditions.[31] This form of ther-

apy has the advantage of minimizing the hazard of subsequent hypersensitiveness.

Conditions Associated with Edema.—The importance and explanation of action of the blood serum proteins in regulating oncotic pressure relationships and fluid balance in the body are well known. They rise normally from average levels of 5.5 Gm. per hundred cubic centimeters at birth (albumin 3.8 per cent, globulin 1.7 per cent) to 7.0 Gm. per hundred cubic centimeters (albumin 5.0 per cent, globulin 2.0 per cent) at 2 years. The specific property of the serum proteins, particularly the albumin fraction, of combating edema forms the basis for the abundant administration of this foodstuff in such conditions of infancy and childhood as nutritional edema, infectious colitis, lipoid nephrosis, extensive burns, other states inducing shock, and juvenile cirrhosis of the liver. The hypoproteinemia common to all these conditions is explained in the 6 instances respectively by inadequate intake, excess fecal loss, excessive urinary excretion, skin seepage, plasmapheresis or hemorrhage, and defective production within the body. Natural proteins by mouth, enzymatic casein hydrolysates enterally and parenterally, whole blood, plasma and serum transfusions have been used with varying effect. The reader is referred to the other papers of this series and to other articles [32] which review the relative efficacy and the amounts of these substances recommended for therapy.

Allergic States.—Food allergies are more common in infants and young children than in later life. This predilection is probably explained by the greater permeability of the intestinal tract of these subjects to unaltered protein.[33] The most commonly implicated protein foods are milk, egg, meat, fish and wheat. In order of increasing age, clinical sensitivity to protein is manifested by infantile eczema, angioneurotic edema, mucous colitis and bronchial asthma. Detection of the responsible protein or proteins is made preferably by therapeutic test (ingestion) or by skin tests. If possible, avoidance of the specific foodstuff with the substitution of other protein foods is the therapeutic method of choice. If this cannot be done, immunization (desensitization) may be attempted. Because of the biologic nonspecificity of amino acids, such mixtures, as they become more readily available, will undoubtedly serve an increasingly important therapeutic role in these conditions.[34]

An attempt has been made in this brief review to evaluate the specific role of protein in pediatrics. It should be emphasized, in closing, that many conditioning factors, both dietary and physiologic, influence the requirements for this foodstuff, and that they must be given consideration in the dietary prescription of protein for infants and children in health and in disease.

525 East Sixty-Eighth Street.

27. Inadequate Diets and Nutritional Deficiencies in the United States: Their Prevalence and Significance, Bulletin 109, National Research Council, November 1943.
28. Turner, D. F.: Selection of Protein Containing Foods to Meet Protein Requirements, J. A. M. A., to be published.
29. Williams, P. F.: Importance of Adequate Protein Nutrition in Pregnancy, J. A. M. A. 127: 1052 (April 21) 1945. Stare, F. J., and Thorn, G. W.: Protein Nutrition in Problems of Medical Interest, ibid. 127: 1120 (April 28) 1945. Lund, C. C., and Levenson, S. M.: Protein in Surgery, ibid. 128: 95 (May 12) 1945.
30. Anderson, A. F., and Schloss, O. M.: Allergy to Cow's Milk in Infants with Nutritional Disorders, Am. J. Dis. Child. 26: 451 (Nov.) 1923.
31. Hartmann, A. F.; Lawler, H. J., and Meeker, C. S.: Studies of Amino Acid Administration: II. Clinical Uses of an Enzymatic Digest of Casein, J. Pediat. 24: 37 (April) 1944. Shohl, A. T.; May, C. D., and Shwachman, H.: Studies of Nitrogen and Fat Metabolism of Infants and Children with Pancreatic Fibrosis, ibid. 23: 267 (Sept.) 1943. Shohl, A. T.: Nitrogen Storage Following Intravenous and Oral Administration of Casein Hydrolysate to Infants with Acute Gastrointestinal Disturbance, J. Clin. Investigation 22: 257 (March) 1943. Cook, M. M.: Diarrheal Diseases in the Newborn Infant, J. Missouri M. A. 40: 64 (March) 1943.

32. Weech, A. A.: Puzzles of Protein Privation: A Decade of Research into the Biologic Effects of Restricted Dietary Protein, J. Pediat. 19: 608 (Nov.) 1941. Best, C. H., and Ridout, J. H.: The Pancreas and the Deposition of Fat in the Liver, Am. J. Physiol. 122: 67 (April) 1938. Ravdin, I. S.: Protection of Liver from Injury, Surgery 8: 201 (Aug.) 1940. Farr, L. E.; Emerson, K., Jr., and Fritcher, P. H.: Comparative Efficiency of Intravenous Amino Acids and Dietary Protein in Children with Nephrotic Syndrome, J. Pediat. 17: 595 (Nov.) 1940. Also references in footnote 31.
33. Wilson, S. J., and Walzer, M.: Absorption of Undigested Protein in Human Beings: IV. Absorption of Unaltered Egg Proteins in Infants and Children, Am. J. Dis. Child. 50: 49 (July) 1935. Ratner, B., and Gruehl, H. L.: Passage of Native Proteins Through the Normal Gastrointestinal Wall, J. Clin. Investigation 13: 517 (July) 1934. Lippard, V. W.; Schloss, O. M., and Johnson, P. A.: Immune Reactions Induced in Infants by Intestinal Absorption of Incompletely Digested Cow's Milk Protein, Am. J. Dis. Child. 51: 562 (March) 1936.
34. Hill, L. W.: Amino Acids as a Source of Nitrogen for Allergic Infants, J. A. M. A. 116: 2135 (May 10) 1941.

STUDIES ON THE PROTEIN METABOLISM OF INFANTS[1]

II. Tryptophane Requirement of the Infant

ANTHONY A. ALBANESE, L. EMMETT HOLT, JR., VIRGINIA IRBY,
SELMA E. SNYDERMAN AND MARILYN LEIN

*From the Department of Pediatrics, New York University College of Medicine and the
Children's Medical Service, Bellevue Hospital, New York*

Although it has long been known that on a body weight basis the protein requirements of the infant are approximately five times greater than those of the adult (1), it is as yet not known whether the high nitrogen requirements of the infant are created by a proportionate increase in all of the amino acids or by a limiting effect caused by higher demands of the growing organism for one or several of the amino acids. The need for an answer to this question, which is of obvious importance to practical infant nutrition and the physiology of growth in general, prompted us to undertake investigations on the amino acid requirements of the infant. The studies reported here reveal that on the basis of nitrogen retention data, rate of weight gain and blood protein levels, the infant requires 5 times more tryptophane per kilo of body weight than does the adult (2). We were surprised to note that within 10 days the tryptophane deficient diet caused a marked hypoproteinemia in the infant whereas our previous studies had shown that the blood proteins of the adult were unaffected by administration of a tryptophane deficient diet for 6 weeks (3).

EXPERIMENTAL

Procedures. The observations reported here were made on 3 normal healthy white male infants. They were given the experimental diets in 5 feedings daily at the rate of about 100 calories per kilo of body weight which were supplemented with 50 mg. of ascorbic acid and 15 drops of oleum percomorpheum per diem. The diet periods were consecutive and varied in duration from 3 to 7 days, but collec-

[1] The work described in this report was supported by grants from the Rockefeller Foundation, National Live Stock and Meat Board and the Nutrition Foundation, Inc.

tions of the excreta were omitted on week ends to avoid complications which might arise from continued use of restraints. The subjects were immobilized by the use of abdominal restraints. 24-hour urine specimens were collected by means of adapters in bottles containing 10 cc. of 15 per cent (by volume) HCl and 1 cc. of 10 per cent alcoholic thymol and the feces collected in 19 cm. porcelain evaporating dishes held in place by a properly shaped excavation in the mattress and subsequently accumulated under refrigeration for the period in jars containing 200 cc. of 70 per cent alcohol. The infants were weighed daily during the course of the experiment.

The composition of the diets employed is shown in Table I. These were made to contain approximately 100 calories per 100 gm. and have the following percentile caloric distribution: protein, 14; fats, 36; carbohydrate, 50. The protein moiety of the tryptophane deficient diet (TH) was prepared by sulfuric acid hydrolysis of casein as previously described by us (4). In order to improve the cystine-poor characteristic of this preparation, the final product was reinforced with 1 per cent $l(-)$-cystine of the protein content estimated as N x 6.25. The protein component of the control diet (CTH) was similarly derived and then supplemented with 1.5 per cent of $l(-)$-tryptophane. In an attempt to ascertain the minimal tryptophane requirement under these dietary conditions, the tryptophane addition to the diet was made step wise, 0.5 and 1.0 per cent of the protein content and these diets are designated as $\frac{1}{3}$ CTH and $\frac{2}{3}$ CTH respectively. Owing to uncertainties regarding the complete human requirements of B complex vitamins, Brewers' yeast was employe' instead of a mixture of the synthetically available vitamins. The quantities of tryptophane derived from this source appear to be ~ roximately 6 mg. per gram (5). Thus the amount of tryptophane provided by the diets per kilogram of infant body weight can be roughly estimated (Table I). The final nitrogen content of each batch of diet was determined by micro-Kjeldahl analysis.

Data on the nitrogen retention were calculated from the results of micro-Kjeldahl analyses of the daily 24 hour urine collections, period pools of feces and daily N intake computed from the consumption record and nitrogen content of diet.

Pooled specimens of urines representative of each diet period were analyzed for 10 amino acids and other metabolites by methods described by others and ourselves. Since urinary tryptophane undergoes destruction on standing even at refrigerator temperatures, this amino acid was determined in the daily samples (6) and the daily values averaged for each period.

Blood samples (10 cc.) were collected over lithium oxalate on the last day of each period by vena puncture. The hemoglobin content of these specimens was determined colorimetrically in the Klett-

TABLE I

Composition of Diets

DIETS	TH	⅓ CTH	⅔ CTH	CTH
	gm.	*gm.*	*gm.*	*gm.*
Acid hydrolyzed casein*.................	3.5	3.5	3.4	3.4
$l(-)$-Tryptophane......................		0.017	0.034	0.053
$l(-)$-Cystine..........................	0.035	0.035	0.035	0.035
Brewers' yeast†........................	1.0	1.0	1.0	1.0
Olive oil..............................	4.0	4.0	4.0	4.0
Dextri-maltose #2†....................	9.6	9.6	9.6	9.6
Arrowroot starch......................	2.3	2.3	2.3	2.3
Salt mixture‡.........................	1.6	1.6	1.6	1.6
Water................................	78.0	78.0	78.0	78.0
Total................................	100.0	100.0	100.0	100.0
Estimated tryptophane content, mg.......	6	23	40	59

* N x 6.25 = gm. of protein.

† Kindly supplied by the Mead Johnson and Company.

‡ The salt mixture employed had the following composition (measured in gm.): $FeSO_4$ 0.9, NaCl 6, Ca gluconate 48, $Ca(OH)_2$ 12, KH_2PO_4 20, K_2HPO_4 7, KCl 6, MgO 0.1.

Summerson photoelectric colorimeter. The total plasma proteins, albumin and non-protein N were determined by the usual procedures (7). The globulin was estimated as the difference of total protein and albumin. The amino N content of the plasma was determined by the copper method (8).

RESULTS

The data collected in Table II show that in the absence of dietary tryptophane all three subjects underwent a marked decrease in the daily weight gain and a drop in nitrogen retention. Since the growing organism is normally in a state of high positive nitrogen balance a drop from the nitrogen retention values characteristic of the individual must be given the same interpretation as the inducement of a negative nitrogen balance in the adult, namely that tryptophane must be regarded as a dietary essential for the infant. This inference is corroborated by the concomitant decrease in body weight gain

TABLE II

Effect of Dietary Tryptophane on the Nitrogen Retention and Body Weight Gain of the Infant

INITIAL AGE AND WEIGHT OF SUBJECT	DIET	PERIOD	AVER- AGE DAILY WT. GAIN	INTAKE PER KG.		TOTAL NITROGEN INPUT	NITROGEN OUTPUT			NITROGEN RETEN- TION
				Vol- ume	Nitro- gen		Urine	Feces	Total	
		days	*gm.*	*cc.*	*gm.*	*gm.*	*gm.*	*gm.*	*gm.*	*mg./kg.*
R. D., male	CTH	7	16.0	102	0.69	5.01	3.33	0.63	3.96	145
6 mos.	TH	7	2.1	104	0.64	4.63	3.28	0.53	3.81	110
7.281 kg.	TH	4	−39	68	0.53	3.24	3.06	0.19	3.25	−1
	CTH	7	79	109	0.68	4.82	1.61	0.40	2.01	380
D. P., male	CTH	7	12.0	100.2	0.69	4.96	3.46	0.47	3.93	144
7 mos.	TH	7	2.1	103.2	0.64	4.57	3.45	0.28	3.73	101
7.136 kg.	TH	4	−32.0	77.5	0.53	3.77	3.37	0.37	3.74	4
	CTH	3	104.0	105.9	0.67	4.80	1.90	0.49	2.39	334
	CTH	4	50.6	102.1	0.67	4.92	3.35	0.55	3.90	135
S. A., male	CTH	7	19.9	103	0.65	6.65	4.43	0.88	5.31	130
12 mos.	TH	7	4.0	98	0.66	6.50	4.45	0.82	5.27	129
10.262 kg.	TH	7	−18.1	82	0.51	5.15	4.17	0.39	4.56	57
	⅓ CTH	4	−54.3	80	0.45	4.51	2.99	0.90	3.89	59
	⅔ CTH	3	66.0	98	0.52	5.29	2.97	0.36	3.33	169
	CTH	4	22.8	99	0.60	6.19	3.71	0.49	4.20	194

caused by the tryptophane deficient diet and the restoration of both growth functions to the norm on the CTH-diet. Incidentally, it is to be noted that in every instance the decrease in weight gain preceded the drop in nitrogen retention.

Attention is also called to the fact that due to the onset of a persistent anorexia in the second TH diet period, the total daily nitrogen intake fell about 1 gram in all three subjects. This anorexia disappeared dramatically with the addition of tryptophane to the diet.

It might therefore be inferred that the drop in nitrogen retention was associated by the decreased intake. However, this does not appear to be the case, since we and others before us (1) have observed that infants of this age are able to retain upwards of 120 mg. of nitrogen per kilogram on intakes of 3.0 gm. of nitrogen derived from milk protein preparations. Further evidence of this phenomenon is to be derived from the data on subject S. A., who retained 169 mg. of N per kilo on an intake of 5.29 gm. of N from $\frac{2}{3}$ CTH diet but retained only 57 mg. of N per kilo of 5.15 gm. of N from TH diet.

Further examination of these data reveals that feeding of CTH diet to subjects R. D. and D. P. following the 11 days of tryptophane poor diet causes an abnormally high nitrogen retention and weight gain which returned to normal levels in the second week of CTH diet (subject D. P.). Inasmuch as this did not occur in subject S. A. who was given the $\frac{1}{3}$ CTH and $\frac{2}{3}$ CTH diets prior to the CTH, suggests that a vigorous and compensatory resumption of growth under a limited tryptophane intake is only possible when the full complement was made available to the organism.

Inasmuch as diets TH and CTH furnish respectively about 6 and 59 mg. of tryptophane per kilo of body weight, the tryptophane requirement of the infant must lie between these two limits. In the single experiment (S. A.) in which the tryptophane content of the diet was increased stepwise, it was found that unlike the $\frac{1}{3}$ CTH diet, the $\frac{2}{3}$ CTH caused a return of both growth functions to the norm. This finding suggests that under the dietary conditions of these studies, the tryptophane requirement of the infant is between 23 and 40 mg. per kilo, or approximately 15 times the adult need.

The implications of the nitrogen balance measurements appear to be supported by variations in urinary tryptophane output induced by the various diets (Table III). Thus it will be noted that in all subjects the tryptophane output falls below the normal of each individual with the removal of tryptophane from the diet and returns to the norm on restoration of tryptophane to the diet. Interestingly enough, the upsurge in urinary tryptophane occurred during the $\frac{2}{3}$ CTH diet and not in the $\frac{1}{3}$ CTH diet period. These findings lend additional support to the notion that the tryptophane level of the urine may serve as a criterion for the estimation of the minimum dietary requirement of the amino acid.

Measurements of the blood proteins during the various regimens disclosed that within 10 days a tryptophane-poor diet caused an

TABLE III

Effect of Dietary Tryptophane on the Daily Urinary Tryptophane Output of the Infant*

R. D., MALE, 5 MO., 7.28 KG.			D. P., MALE, 7 MO., 7.14 KG.			S. A., MALE, 12 MO., 10.26 KG.		
Diet	Period	Tryptophane	Diet	Period	Tryptophane	Diet	Period	Tryptophane
	days	*gm.*		*days*	*mg.*		*days*	*mg.*
CTH	7	27	CTH	7	24	CTH	7	58
TH	7	20	TH	7	26	TH	7	47
TH	4	14	TH	4	12	TH	7	31
CTH	7	20	CTH	3	10	$\frac{1}{3}$ CTH	4	16
			CTH	4	32	$\frac{2}{3}$ CTH	3	31
						CTH	4	54

* Unlike the microbiological procedures the chemical procedure (6) employed in this work measures the total (free and bound) tryptophane output.

TABLE IV

Effect of Dietary Tryptophane on the Blood Proteins of the Infant

SUBJECT	DIET	PERIOD	TOTAL PLASMA PROTEINS	ALBUMIN	GLOBULIN	A/G RATIO	NON-PROTEIN NITROGEN	HEMOGLOBIN	AMINO NITROGEN
		days	*gm. %*	*gm. %*	*gm. %*		*mg. %*	*gm. %*	*mg. %*
R. D., male	CTH	7	5.88	3.78	2.10	1.80	30.3	9.7	7.7
5 mos.	TH	7	5.35	3.54	1.81	1.96	29.6	10.5	8.1
7,281 gm.	TH	4	4.88	3.32	1.56	2.13	24.3	10.4	8.1
	CTH	7	5.54	3.58	1.96	1.96	17.9	9.7	7.9
D. P., male	CTH	7	5.64	4.05	1.59	2.54	28.9	8.4	8.1
7 mos.	TH	7	4.68	2.92	1.76	1.66	25.7	9.1	9.4
7,136 gm.	TH	4	4.32	2.82	1.50	1.88	27.7	9.2	9.9
	CTH	3	—	—	—	—	—	—	—
	CTH	4	5.96	3.82	1.73	2.21	16.2	9.1	8.7
S. A., male	CTH	7	5.88	3.41	2.47	1.38	29.1	8.5	7.0
12 mos.	TH	7	5.13	3.03	2.10	1.44	29.8	8.5	8.5
10,262 gm.	TH	7	4.28	2.80	1.48	1.89	30.9	10.2	8.4
	$\frac{1}{3}$ CTH	4	5.69	3.02	2.67	1.13	17.8	10.0	8.1
	$\frac{2}{3}$ CTH	3	5.53	3.04	2.49	1.22	23.4	10.5	8.4
	CTH	4	5.93	2.99	2.94	1.02	20.6	10.7	8.1

appreciable hypoproteinemia which is reflected for the most part in a decreased albumin level (Table IV). Attention is called to the finding in subject S. A., where the nitrogen retention, weight change and urinary tryptophane values became normal during the $\frac{2}{3}$ CTH diet period, while the plasma proteins were returned to nearly normal levels by the $\frac{1}{3}$ CTH diet. This observation suggests to us that the blood proteins have a higher priority on the available nutrients than other body tissues. The hemoglobin concentration and amino N level of the blood do not appear to be influenced by the brief period of tryptophane deficiency. Cell counts remained within normal levels at all times during the course of the studies.

COMMENTS

We have previously reported that on the basis of nitrogen balance and urinary tryptophane data, the tryptophane requirement of the adult was approximately 6 mg. per kilogram of body weight (2). In the present study measurements of nitrogen retention, rate of body weight gain, urinary tryptophane output and plasma protein levels indicate that infants 5 to 12 months of age require about 30 mg. of $l(-)$-tryptophane per kilo of body weight for normal growth. It appears, therefore, that on a weight basis, the tryptophane, like the nitrogen needs of the infant are five times as great as those of the adult and that the high protein requirement of the infant is predicated in part by the tryptophane needs. In our studies on the effect of an experimental tryptophane deficient diet in the adult (3) we observed that the plasma proteins failed to reflect the dietary defect even after six weeks of the regimen. This result is to be contrasted with the rapid drop of plasma protein levels induced in the infant by the tryptophane poor diet. A reaction, indeed, more rapid than that observed in the immature or adult rat (4). This phenomenon cannot but impress one of the relatively greater biological sensitivity of the infant to dietary privations and of the desirability of measuring the nutritional requirements of the infant directly rather than upon inferences derived from results of adult human or rat experiments.

The pronounced anorexia which all three subjects developed to the tryptophane deficient diet and its disappearance on supplementation of the deficient diet with $l(-)$-tryptophane arouses considerable speculation as to its etiology. The infants' dislike for the deficient diet cannot reasonably be attributed to a difference in taste of the two preparations, since the addition of the necessary but small amount of tryptophane could not be expected to greatly improve the taste of the preparation; and indeed a change in taste could not be detected by us. Apparently, the symptom is caused by the same psycho-biological factors which regulate self-selection of diets in experimental animals (9) which have also been shown to function in the child (10).

SUMMARY

It has been found that the infant requires approximately 30 mg. of $l(-)$-tryptophane per kilogram of body weight per day for the maintenance of normal growth, nitrogen retention and plasma protein levels. The significance of these findings is discussed.

We wish to thank Mrs. Barbara Saur for some analyses performed in connection with this work.

BIBLIOGRAPHY

1. ALBANESE, A. A.: The amino acid requirements of the human, in Advances in Protein Chemistry. New York, Vol. III, pp. 227–268 (1946).
2. HOLT, L. E., ALBANESE, A. A., FRANKSTON, J. E., AND IRBY, V.: Bull. Johns Hopkins Hospital, **75**: 353 (1944).
3. HOLT, L. E. JR., ALBANESE, A. A., BRUMBACK, J. E., JR., KAJDI, C., AND WANGERIN, D. M.: Proc. Soc. Exp. Biol. and Med., **48**: 726 (1941).
4. ALBANESE, A. A., HOLT, L. E., JR., KAJDI, C. N., AND FRANKSTON, J. E.: Biol. Chem., **148**: 299 (1943).
5. CARTER, H. E., AND PHILLIPS, G. E.: Fed. Proc., **3**: 123 (1944).
6. ALBANESE, A. A., AND FRANKSTON, J. E.: J. Biol. Chem., **157**: 59 (1945).
7. ROBINSON, H. W., PRICE, J. W., AND HOGDEN, C. G.: J. Biol. Chem., **120**: 481 (1937).
8. ALBANESE, A. A., AND IRBY, V.: J. Biol. Chem., **153**: 583 (1944).
9. RICHTER, C. P.: The Self-Selection of Diets. Essays in Biology, 501–506 U. of Calif. press 1943.
10. SWEET, C.: J. A. M. A., **107**: 765 (1936).
    DAVIS, C. M.: Am. J. D. C., **36**: 651 (1928); **46**: 743 (1933).

8

Reprinted from *Pediatrics*, **26**(1), 51–61 (1960)

COMPARATIVE STUDY OF ADEQUACY OF PROTEIN FROM HUMAN MILK AND COW'S MILK IN PROMOTING NITROGEN RETENTION BY NORMAL FULL-TERM INFANTS

Samuel J. Fomon, M.D.

Department of Pediatrics, College of Medicine and University Hospitals, State University of Iowa

WHETHER the protein of cow's milk is equivalent to the protein of human milk in infant nutrition is not known. Nutritional equivalence would imply that infants receiving similar intakes of protein from the two sources would be similar with respect to objective indices of nutritional state. Such indices might include rate of growth, concentrations of certain constituents of the blood, performance in metabolic balance studies, body composition, and possibly other evidences of state of health such as susceptibility to infection. Ideally, long-term studies should be performed with two large groups of normal infants receiving similar intakes of protein from the two sources.

Thus far, only short-term studies of weight gain and retention of nitrogen have been reported. Gordon et al.[1] found no difference in rate of gain in weight or retention of nitrogen by premature infants while receiving human milk or a cow's milk formula with similar concentration of nitrogen. The authors call attention to the difficulty in drawing conclusions from studies of such short duration: "In longer periods of observation, differences in the retention of nitrogen or significant differences in health due to varied biologic properties might be demonstrated." In studies of full-term infants receiving similar intakes of nitrogen from human milk or cow's milk, Barness et al.[2] found less, but not significantly less, retention of nitrogen with the cow's milk formula.

Casein, the predominant protein of cow's milk, and lactalbumin, the predominant protein of human milk, have been shown[3] to be equally effective in promoting nitrogen retention by normal adults during short periods of observation. It was hoped that results of the present study would permit a more definite statement concerning whether or not the proteins from human milk and cow's milk are equivalent in infant nutrition, at least with respect to the ability to promote growth and retention of nitrogen. Data will be presented concerning relatively long-term studies with infants less than 6 months of age fed a formula containing protein from cow's milk at a concentration similar to that of human milk. These data are compared with data from a previous study[4] performed with infants fed pooled, pasteurized human milk.

SUBJECT MATERIAL

Eight normal full-term infants, five girls and three boys, were studied during the first 6 months of life. In contrast to the previous study with pasteurized human milk[4] in which all of the infants lived continuously in the Metabolism Ward, in the present study only two of the infants (G.Y. and T.Wi.) lived in the Metabolism Ward; the other infants were admitted to the Metabolism Ward only for performance of a 3-day metabolic balance study once in each 2-week period. Information about the families of the subjects is presented in Table I.

FEEDING

The formula under study (Formula 1257)

Supported by grants from Ross Laboratories and Mead Johnson and Company and by a grant from the National Dairy Council on behalf of the Milk Industry Foundation.

ADDRESS: Iowa City, Iowa.

TABLE I

INFORMATION ABOUT FAMILIES OF THE SUBJECTS

Subject	Father Height (cm)	Weight (kg)	Mother Height (cm)	Weight (kg)	Additional Information*
G.Y.	185	80	162	60	3 older siblings; parents unmarried; father in air force.
T.Wi.	170	68	164	70	Father undergraduate student; mother attending high school.
T.Wh.	192	81	172	60	Father graduate student, mother R.N.
S.H.	173	80	166	61	1 older sibling 2 years of age; father undergraduate student.
D.Ma.	179	90	176	66	3 older siblings aged $3\frac{1}{2}$, $2\frac{1}{2}$ and $1\frac{1}{2}$ years; 2 were subjects of previous metabolic studies; father dairy worker; mother had been under observation in sanatorium for possible active tuberculosis.
T.S.	170	66	162	54	1 older sibling 15 months of age, weight 10 kg; father undergraduate student.
P.L.	180	85	163	50	Father and mother undergraduate students.
D.D.	183	101	163	57	Father graduate student in physiotherapy.

* Mother a housewife unless otherwise stated.

was prepared° from cow's milk protein, vegetable oils (57.5% corn oil, 37.5% coconut oil, 5.0% olive oil) and lactose. The formula was supplied as a powder and, when diluted, had the following mean content in 100 ml: 60 calories, 1.03 gm protein, 3.4 gm fat and 6.5 gm lactose.

All infants received a vitamin supplement°° and, after 3 months of age, a preparation containing iron.°°°

Three infants (G.Y., T.Wh. and D.Ma.) received the formula under study (Formula 1257) as the sole source of calories from the first week of life until 4 to 6 months of age. Only two infants received Formula 1257 for less than 3 months (T.Wi., 85 to 151 days of age and 162 to 183 days of age; D.D., 68 to 156 days of age). Complete feeding histories are presented in Table II.

PROCEDURES AND METHODS

The operation of the Metabolism Ward has been described previously.[5] Procedures and methods in the present study were similar to those of other studies,[4-6] with the exception

---

° The formula was prepared by Ross Laboratories at the request of the author.

°° Deca-Vi-Sol®, 0.3 ml daily, supplied 2500 I.U. vitamin A, 500 I.U. vitamin D, 25 mg ascorbic acid, 0.5 mg thiamine, 0.75 mg riboflavin, 5 mg niacinamide, 0.5 mg pyridoxine hydrochloride, 1.5 mg panthenol, 0.5 μg crystalline vitamin B₁₂, 15 μg biotin.

°°° Fer-In-Sol®, 0.3 ml daily, supplied 7.5 mg elemental iron in the form of ferrous sulfate.

that separate urinary and fecal excretions of nitrogen were estimated for girls (see below), whereas in previous studies only total excretions were reported for girls.

Estimation of Urinary and Fecal Excretion of Nitrogen by Girls

In the present study, two containers were used for storage of urine from each infant, one for "uncontaminated urine" and one for urine contaminated with feces. By close observation of the infants and by transferring urine to the storage container in the refrigerator soon after each voiding, it was possible to obtain the greater portion of the 72-hour specimen of urine uncontaminated with feces. The volumes of uncontaminated and contaminated urine were then measured and the contaminated specimen added to the fecal collection.

The *total excretion* of nitrogen was determined from the volume and concentration of nitrogen of uncontaminated urine plus the volume and concentration of nitrogen of the fecal homogenate to which had been added the urine contaminated with feces.

The *urinary excretion* of nitrogen was estimated from the total volume of urine (contaminated with feces and uncontaminated) and the concentration of nitrogen in the uncontaminated urine. Fecal excretion of nitrogen was obtained by subtracting the estimated urinary excretion from the total.

It will be appreciated that the reported urinary and fecal excretions of nitrogen by girls lack the precision of these measurements in

TABLE II

Information About Infants Fed Formula 1257

Subject Hosp. No.	Sex Race Birth Wt.	Birth Date	Food* and Period When Fed	Remarks
G.Y. 58-7555	Female Negro 3,135 gm	6- 7-58	Formula 1257, 3–177 days	Lived on Metabolism Ward. Rhinorrhea without fever at 93 days of age. Small furuncle of head noted at 142 days of age, enlarged, incised at 157 days of age.
T.Wi. 58-11218	Male Negro 3,135 gm	8-20-58	WCM, 19–84 days; Formula 1257, 85–151 days and 162–183 days; Formula 223, 152–161 days	Lived on Metabolism Ward. Rhinorrhea without fever at 117 days of age; poor appetite and frequent stools at 145 days of age.
T.Wh. 59-4374	Male Negro 3,465 gm	4- 1-59	FHM, 0–6 days; Formula 1257, 7–127 days	
S.H. 59-6566	Female White 2,965 gm	5-14-59	Formula S, 0–4 days; Formula 1257, 5–90 days	
D.Ma. 58-8211	Male White 3,600 gm	6-11-58	Evaporated milk formula, 0–5 days; Formula 1257, 6–152 days	
T.S. 59-1905	Female White 3,625 gm	2- 8-59	Formula S, 0–12 days; Formula 1257, 13–123 days	Rhinorrhea without fever at 64 days of age.
P.L. 58-16246	Female Negro 3,365 gm	11-28-58	FHM, 0–78 days; Formula 1257, 79–181 days	
D.D. 58-4001	Female White 3,400 gm	3-22-58	FHM, 0–11 days; Formula 223, 12–67 days; Formula 1257, 68–156 days	Rhinorrhea without fever at 64 days of age. Fracture of skull without symptoms noted at 124 days of age.

* WCM = undiluted, homogenized whole cow's milk; Formula 223 = a formula with 7% of the calories from protein, concentration of lactalbumin similar to that of human milk: FHM = breast-fed; Formula S = Similac®, supplying 11% of calories as protein.

boys, from whom completely separate collections of urine and feces were made. However, the total excretion is equally accurate in each group.

RESULTS

Growth

Growth curves of the eight infants are presented on Iowa Growth Charts[7] in Figure 1. With one exception (D.D.) the growth curves progressed along or somewhat below the 50th percentile. The length and weight of one infant (T.Wi.) remained below the 16th percentile throughout the study. Length and weight of another infant (T.S.) were at the 50th percentile at 1 month of age but had decreased to the 16th percentile for length and to less than the 16th percentile for weight by 4 months of age.

Analysis of Blood

Concentrations of hemoglobin in the blood and of total nitrogen and urea nitrogen in the serum are presented in Table III.

Between 1 and 6 months of age the mean concentration of hemoglobin was 10.2 gm/

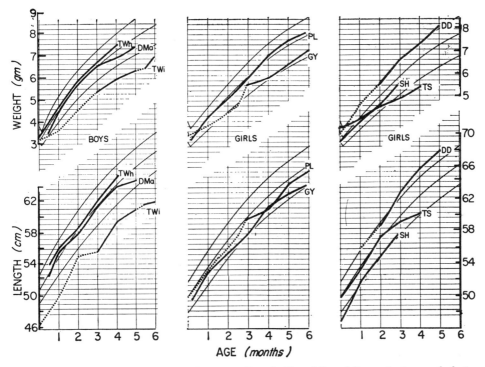

FIG. 1. Growth curves of infants plotted on Iowa Growth Charts.[7] Dotted lines refer to growth during periods of observation when the infants were not receiving Formula 1257 (Table II).

100 ml (standard deviation, 0.9), compared with a reported mean value of 12.2 gm/100 ml for normal infants 3 to 5 months of age.[8] The lower mean values in this study, as in previous studies in this Metabolism Ward,[1,6,9] are probably attributable primarily to the effect of periodic withdrawal of blood.

The mean concentration of total nitrogen in 19 determinations with serum of infants between 1 and 6 months of age was 9.1 gm/l. Assuming that 1 gm of nitrogen in serum corresponds to 6.25 gm of protein, the mean concentration of total protein during this age period was 5.7 gm/100 ml.

With one exception (D.Ma., 145 days of age) the concentration of urea nitrogen in the serum ranged between 2.7 and 8.1 mg/100 ml and the mean value (6.0 mg/100 ml) was similar to that of infants fed human milk.[4,9]

Metabolic Studies

Sixty metabolic balance studies were performed with the eight infants. Data from these studies are presented in Table IV and Figures 2 to 5.

VOLUME OF INTAKE: As in previous studies, the volume of intake with respect to body weight decreased with increasing age (Fig. 2). Mean daily volumes of intake during metabolic balance studies in the four age periods, 8 to 45 days, 46 to 90 days, 91 to 136 days and 137 to 182 days, were 200 (standard deviation, 24), 167 ± 21, 151 ± 27 and 141 ± 18 ml/kg, respectively. Corresponding mean volumes of intake by infants fed pasteurized human milk were 218 ± 22, 173 ± 24, 157 ± 20 and 140 ± 10 ml/kg.

Mean volumes of intake during metabolic balance studies with G.Y. and T.Wi., the two infants living continuously in the Me-

TABLE III

CONCENTRATION OF HEMOGLOBIN IN BLOOD AND
OF TOTAL NITROGEN, TOTAL PROTEIN AND
UREA NITROGEN IN SERUM

Subject	Age (days)	Hemoglobin (gm/100 ml)	Total Nitrogen (gm/l)	Urea Nitrogen (mg/100 ml)
G.Y.	16	14.1	8.9	3.3
	96	9.6	8.5	7.5
	121	10.4		7.9
	149	9.3		8.1
	177	11.4	9.7	6.9
T.Wi.	103	10.5	8.9	4.8
	131	11.3	8.5	
	160	11.0		3.8
	181	10.9	9.1	
T.Wh.	34			4.6
	63	9.6	8.8	4.5
	90	9.3	9.1	4.7
	126	9.3		
S.H.	12	13.2		2.7
	53	9.0	8.5	
	76	9.7	8.9	
D.Ma.	13	16.6	8.5	4.9
	47	9.2		
	73	10.7	9.1	
	105	11.1		6.8
	117	10.5	9.1	6.2
	145		9.5	10.4
T.S.	24	14.5	8.2	7.8
	66	9.7	8.6	5.8
	93	8.5		6.0
	121	9.2	9.8	7.0
P.L.	111	9.6	9.1	6.8
	138	10.6	9.3	5.4
	165	10.0	9.9	5.8
D.D.	110	11.4	9.4	6.7
	136	10.8	8.7	6.6

tabolism Ward, were almost identical to those of the six infants who lived at home during the intervals between metabolic balance studies.

INTAKE OF CALORIES: Because the formula supplied approximately 60 cal/100 ml, the mean daily caloric intakes in the four age periods may be calculated to have been approximately 120, 100, 91 and 84 cal/kg, respectively, compared with estimated intakes (assuming 67 cal/100 ml) from pasteurized human milk of 146, 114, 104 and 94 cal/kg, respectively.

INTAKE OF NITROGEN: Intakes of nitrogen were generally slightly less by infants fed Formula 1257 than by infants fed pasteurized human milk (Fig. 3). This difference was due jointly to the somewhat lower volumes of intake and lower mean concentrations of nitrogen in Formula 1257 than in the pasteurized human milk. The mean daily intakes of nitrogen by infants fed Formula 1257 in the various age periods were as follows: 320 (standard deviation, 52), 279 ± 41, 248 ± 41, 233 ± 29 mg/kg. Corresponding intakes of nitrogen by infants fed pasteurized human milk were 383 ± 45, 296 ± 49, 274 ± 29 and 240 ± 27 mg/kg, respectively.

RETENTION OF NITROGEN: Retentions of nitrogen by infants fed Formula 1257 may be compared with those by infants fed pasteurized human milk in Figure 4. Thirty-seven of 60 retentions of nitrogen in the study with Formula 1257 were below the regression line calculated from data pertaining to infants fed human milk. This result was, perhaps, to be anticipated since intakes of nitrogen were less in 44 of the 60 balance studies.

RELATION OF GAIN IN WEIGHT TO RETENTION OF NITROGEN: The relation of gain in weight to retention of nitrogen is shown in Figure 5. The gain in weight in most instances represented the mean daily gain during a 14-day interval from 7 days before to 7 days after the first day of a metabolic balance study. It was not always feasible to arrange for the six infants living at home to be weighed and measured according to this plan. Weight gain was estimated on the basis of a 14-day interval in 50 of the 60 metabolic balance studies, on the basis of a 10 to 13-day interval in three instances and on the basis of a 15 to 17-day interval in four instances. In three instances weight gain could not be calcu-

ADEQUACY OF PROTEIN

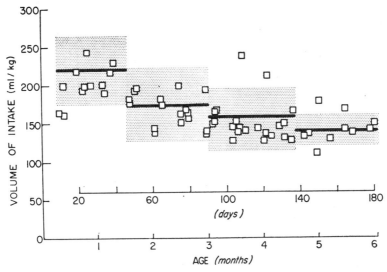

Fig. 2. Daily volume of intake in relation to age of infants fed Formula 1257. Each square refers to the mean volume of intake during the 3 days of a metabolic balance study. The horizontal lines indicate the mean volume of intake of infants fed pasteurized human milk[4] during the various age periods and each stippled area includes two standard deviations above and below the mean.

lated within the time intervals mentioned, and data concerning these metabolic balance studies are not included in Figure 5. It may be seen that the variability of gain in weight for a given retention of nitrogen is somewhat greater for infants fed Formula 1257 than for those fed pasteurized human milk but that the relation of

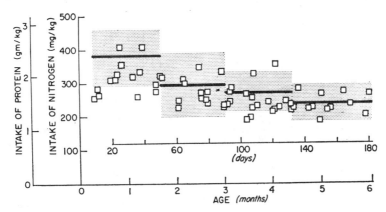

Fig. 3. Daily intake of nitrogen and calculated intake of protein in relation to age of infants fed Formula 1257. Each square refers to the mean intake of nitrogen during the 3 days of a metabolic balance study. The horizontal lines indicate the mean intakes of nitrogen by infants fed pasteurized human milk[4] during the various age periods and the stippled areas include two standard deviations above and below the mean. It may be seen that intakes of nitrogen in studies with Formula 1257 were generally in the lower portion of the range observed in studies with infants fed pasteurized human milk.

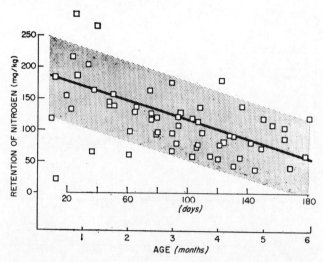

Fɪɢ. 4. Daily retention of nitrogen in relation to age of infants fed
Formula 1257. Each square refers to the mean retention of nitrogen
during the 3 days of a metabolic balance study. The regression line
applies to the data concerning infants fed pasteurized human milk[4]
and the stippled area includes two standard errors of the estimate
above and below the regression. Retentions of nitrogen by infants fed
Formula 1257 were below the regression in the majority of the balance studies (37 of 60 balance studies) as was to be anticipated
because intakes were generally also less (44 of 60 balance studies).

gain in weight to retention of nitrogen is
generally similar with the two groups.

DISCUSSION

The 50th percentile values of the Iowa
Growth Charts[7] not only fall distinctly
above the mean values for length and
weight of the infants serving as subjects in
the present study and those studied previously,[4, 6, 9] but also fall distinctly above
the mean values reported for 3 and 6-
month-old infants in several longitudinal
studies of growth of unselected normal infants.[10, 11]

The mean concentration of total protein
in the serum (5.7 gm/100 ml) is similar to
mean values reported by several investigators who have employed microKjeldahl digestion in determination of concentrations
of total protein in the serum. Poyner-Wall
and Finch[12] found a mean value of 5.66
gm/100 ml in 63 determinations with serum
of normal infants from 3 weeks to 6 months

of age. Dodd and Minot[13] reported a mean
value of 5.44 gm/100 ml in 16 determinations with serum of infants from birth to
3 months of age, and 6.19 gm/100 ml in
34 determinations with serum of infants
from 3 months to 2 years of age. Trevorrow
et al.[14] demonstrated a gradual rise in concentration of protein in the serum from a
mean value of 5.33 gm/100 ml at 1 month
of age to approximately 6.0 gm/100 ml at
6 months of age. Somewhat greater mean
concentrations of total protein in serum
were reported from study of normal full-
term infants by Levin et al.[15] The mean concentration between 4 weeks and 2 months of
age was 5.81 gm/100 ml, gradually increasing to 6.55 gm/100 ml between 5 and 6
months of age. Study of 308 slightly older
infants in Sweden[16] (90% were between 6
and 9 months of age), demonstrated a mean
concentration of 6.77 gm/100 ml.

Systematic procedural errors in metabolic balance studies are likely to summate

TABLE IV

DAILY METABOLIC BALANCES OF NITROGEN OF INFANTS FED FORMULA 1257

Subject	Age (days)	Weight (gm)	Length (cm)	Volume Intake (ml/kg)	Intake of Nitrogen (mg)	Intake of Nitrogen (mg/kg)	Excretion of Nitrogen Urine (mg)	Excretion of Nitrogen Feces (mg)	Excretion of Nitrogen Total (mg)	Retention of Nitrogen (mg)	Retention of Nitrogen (mg/kg)	Retention of Nitrogen (% of intake)
G.Y.	9	3,200	50.0	163	820	256			440	380	118	46
	23	3,660	52.1	197	1,202	328	270	137	407	795	217	66
	37	4,180	53.8	215	1,401	335	504	216	720	681	163	49
	51	4,525	54.6	195	1,423	314	580	212	792	631	139	44
	65	5,000	56.4	173	1,495	299	581	230	811	684	137	46
	79	5,425	57.7	162	1,483	273	612	210	822	661	121	44
	93	5,825	58.8	163	1,597	274	716	176	892	705	121	44
	107	6,250	60.2	152	1,414	226	762	171	933	481	77	34
	128	6,725	61.0	145	1,664	247	760	277	1,037	627	93	38
	142	6,985	63.4	130	1,536	220	810	196	1,006	530	76	34
	156	7,320	63.4	130	1,643	224	780	144	924	719	108	48
	168	7,580	63.6	138	1,807	238	866	626	1,492	315	41	17
T.Wi.	94	5,475	56.3	165	1,564	286	648	233	881	683	125	44
	110	5,950	58.4	140	1,372	231	553	246	799	573	97	42
	131	6,000	60.2	149	1,432	239	646	243	889	543	91	38
	164	6,300	61.6	157	1,734	275	792	276	1,068	666	105	38
	180	6,675	61.8	150	1,793	269	767	226	993	800	120	45
T.Wh.	19	4,155	54.0	217	1,290	310	486	157	643	647	155	50
	33	4,685	56.0	200	1,502	320	488	57	545	957	204	64
	47	5,275	57.3	175	1,452	275	519	166	685	767	145	53
	61	5,800	58.4	136	1,304	225	583	153	736	568	98	44
	75	6,060	60.8	161	1,650	272	697	183	880	770	127	47
	89	6,550	62.8	139	1,527	233	718	176	894	633	97	42
	103	6,725	63.4	144	1,793	267	753	240	993	800	119	44
	124	7,375	65.0	132	1,646	223	890	160	1,050	596	81	36
S.H.	11	3,205	49.2	199	909	284	202	122	324	585	183	64
	25	3,440	50.8	242	1,410	410	278	159	437	973	283	69
	39	3,785		229	1,548	409	376	169	545	1,003	265	65
	74	4,690	56.6	199	1,630	348	722	147	869	761	163	46
	88	5,045	56.6	192	1,747	346	732	117	849	898	178	51
D.Ma.	12	3,525	52.3	161	932	264	693	163	856	76	21	8
	26	4,200	55.0	199	1,489	355	498	209	707	782	186	52
	47	5,075	56.0	181	1,501	296	582	216	798	703	139	47
	61	5,625	57.5	143	1,394	248	597	453	1,050	344	61	24
	75	6,025	58.6	150	1,527	253	638	180	818	709	117	46
	89	6,360	61.2	136	1,457	229	780	250	1,030	427	67	29
	103	6,425	62.3	127	1,215	189	670	176	846	369	57	30
	117	6,525	64.0	141	1,592	244	982	223	1,205	387	59	24
	131	7,000	64.7	130	1,524	218	963	263	1,226	298	43	20
	145	7,270	64.7	135	1,654	228	1,079	306	1,385	269	38	17
T.S.	22	3,585	53.1	191	1,117	312	517	130	647	470	132	42
	36	3,860	53.3	189	1,008	261	598	149	747	261	68	26
	50	4,115	55.5	191	1,326	322	490	188	678	648	157	49
	64	4,350	57.5	180	1,352	311	554	242	796	556	128	41
	78	4,700	59.1	167	1,173	250	558	176	734	439	94	38
	92	4,815	59.1	149	1,131	235	587	164	751	380	79	34
	106	5,050	59.5	138	1,000	198	540	97	637	363	72	36
	120	5,210	59.8	127	1,124	216	703	134	837	287	55	25

57

TABLE IV (Continued)

Subject	Age (days)	Weight (gm)	Length (cm)	Volume Intake (ml/kg)	Intake of Nitrogen		Excretion of Nitrogen			Retention of Nitrogen		
					(mg)	(mg/kg)	Urine (mg)	Feces (mg)	Total (mg)	(mg)	(mg/kg)	(% of intake)
P.L.	108	4,935	59.6	236	1,622	328	717	226	943	679	137	42
	122	5,565	60.6	212	1,992	358	803	185	988	1,004	180	50
	136	5,955	62.3	165	1,689	284	737	118	855	834	140	49
	150	6,205	64.4	178	1,655	267	731	185	916	739	119	45
	164	6,550	64.4	141	1,449	221	699	174	873	576	88	40
	178	6,800	65.0	142	1,380	203	852	161	1,013	367	54	27
D.D.	79	6,175	60.7	155	1,486	241			880	606	98	41
	93	6,615	63.2	150	1,630	246	774	139	913	717	108	44
	107	6,915	65.2	144	1,772	256	800	190	990	782	113	44
	121	7,200	66.0	136	1,581	220	784	243	1,027	554	77	35
	135	7,675	66.6	127	1,709	223	1,106	168	1,274	435	57	26
	149	8,055	68.4	112	1,512	188	766	171	937	575	72	38

so as to result in apparent retentions of nitrogen that are falsely high and are proportionately greater in studies with feedings having high concentrations of protein. The nature of these errors is that volumes of intake are more likely to be overestimated than underestimated (a small amount of milk adheres to the sides of the

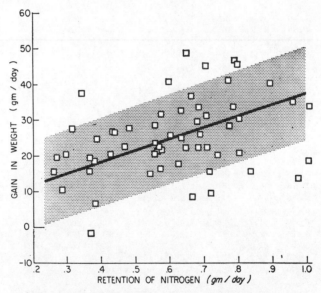

Fig. 5. Gain in weight in relation to retention of nitrogen by infants fed Formula 1257. Each square refers to the mean daily gain in weight during an interval of approximately 14 days (see text) and the mean daily retention of nitrogen during a metabolic balance study performed in this interval. The regression line applies to data concerning infants fed pasteurized human milk[4] and the stippled area includes two standard errors of the estimate above and below the regression.

bottle or is lost from the infant's mouth during feeding and is assumed to have been ingested and retained); conversely, the volume of urinary and fecal excretion is more likely to be underestimated than overestimated (a small amount of feces adheres to the infant's buttocks or a few drops of urine are lost). With suitable metabolic techniques, summated errors of this type are not great even in studies with feedings containing high concentrations of protein. However, in the present study in which concentrations of nitrogen in the two feedings were similar, systematic procedural errors should contribute approximately equally in the two groups.

Except in the last age period (137 to 182 days of age), intakes of nitrogen by infants fed Formula 1257 were less than those by infants fed pasteurized human milk. In 44 of 60 metabolic balance studies, intakes of nitrogen by infants fed Formula 1257 were less than the mean values for the various age groups of infants fed human milk (Fig. 3). Similarly, in 37 of the 60 metabolic balance studies with Formula 1257, retentions of nitrogen fell below the regression calculated from data concerning infants fed human milk (Fig. 4). It is therefore probably safe to conclude that Formula 1257 promoted retention of nitrogen as well as did pasteurized human milk.° In the final age period, when mean intakes of nitrogen with the two feedings were nearly identical, mean retentions of nitrogen were also nearly identical.

It seemed possible that the periodic change in environment from home to Metabolism Ward might be sufficiently upset-

---

° An abstract has been published[17] concerning preliminary results of studies with Formula 1257. Also mentioned in the abstract were studies with a nearly identical feeding, designated Formula 657, that was supplied as a concentrated liquid rather than as a powder. The studies suggested that Formula 657 was nutritionally inferior to human milk and to Formula 1257.

More recent studies (unpublished) with another lot of the same formula have failed to substantiate the initial impression of nutritional inferiority.

ting to those infants ordinarily living at home (all infants except G.Y. and T.Wi.) to interfere with nitrogen retention. If such interference with retention of nitrogen did occur, it was not sufficient to depress the retention of nitrogen below that anticipated with similar intakes of nitrogen from human milk.

There can be little doubt that breast feeding by a healthy woman receiving an adequate diet provides adequate nutrition for the normal full-term infant during the early months of life. The vagueness of the phrase, "the early months of life" calls attention to an uncertainty concerning whether breast feeding as a sole source of calories is adequate only during the first month or two of life or whether the duration of its adequacy is considerably longer. It has been demonstrated that after 4 or 5 months of age the breast-fed infant grows in length and weight less rapidly than does the infant receiving certain formulas of cow's milk.[15] However, greater rates of growth do not necessarily indicate superiority of feeding. As judged by nitrogen balance studies, it would appear that ad libitum ingestion of Formula 1257 (supplying 60 cal/100 ml and 7% of the calories as protein) would appear adequate as a sole food during the period that human milk is adequate.

SUMMARY

Eight normal full-term infants have been studied during ad libitum ingestion of a formula (Formula 1257) containing 60 calories/100 ml and providing 7% of the calories as protein from cow's milk, 50% from a mixture of vegetable oils and 43% from lactose. The mean concentration of nitrogen in this formula was slightly less than the mean concentration in human milk in a previous study.[4]

Growth of the infants is interpreted as within normal limits.

The mean concentration of urea nitrogen in the serum was 6.0 mg/100 ml. Between 1 and 6 months of age the mean concentration of total protein in the serum was 5.7 gm/100 ml.

Both the mean volume of intake and the mean concentration of nitrogen in the feeding were slightly less than those of the infants fed pasteurized human milk. Consequently, in 44 of 60 metabolic balance studies with infants receiving Formula 1257, intakes of nitrogen were less than the mean intakes of infants of similar age receiving pasteurized human milk (Fig. 3). Similarly, retentions of nitrogen in 37 of the 60 metabolic balance studies fell below the regression calculated for infants fed pasteurized human milk (Fig. 4). The retentions of nitrogen were generally in the range of those of infants fed pasteurized human milk and it is concluded that the two feedings have similar abilities to promote retention of nitrogen by infants.

Acknowledgment

The major contributions to this study made by Lora Thomas, R.N., and her staff of nurses and by Mr. Robert L. Jensen, who supervised the laboratory staff, are gratefully acknowledged.

REFERENCES

1. Gordon, H. H., et al.: Respiratory metabolism in infancy and childhood. II. The nitrogen metabolism in premature infants—comparative studies of human and cow's milk. Am. J. Dis. Child., 54:1030, 1937.
2. Barness, L. A., et al.: Nitrogen metabolism of infants fed human and cow's milk. J. Pediat., 51:29, 1957.
3. Mueller, A. J., and Cox, W. M., Jr.: Comparative nutritive value of casein and of lactalbumin for man. J. Nutrition, 34: 285, 1947.
4. Fomon, S. J., and May, C. D.: Metabolic studies of normal full-term infants fed pasteurized human milk. PEDIATRICS, 22: 101, 1958.
5. Fomon, S. J., Thomas, L. N., Jensen, R. L., and May, C. D.: Determination of nitrogen balance of infants less than 6 months of age. PEDIATRICS, 22:94, 1958.
6. Fomon, S. J., and May, C. D.: Metabolic studies of normal full-term infants fed a prepared formula providing intermediate amounts of protein. PEDIATRICS, 22:1134, 1958.
7. Jackson, R. L., and Kelly, H. G.: Growth charts for use in pediatric practice. J. Pediat., 27:215, 1945.
8. Wintrobe, M. M.: Clinical Hematology, 4th Ed. Philadelphia, Lea, 1956, p. 100.
9. Fomon, S. J., Thomas, L. N., and May, C. D.: Equivalence of pasteurized and fresh human milk in promoting nitrogen retention by normal full-term infants. PEDIATRICS, 22:935, 1958.
10. Stuart, H. C.: Standards of physical development for reference in clinical appraisement. Suggestions for their presentation and use. J. Pediat., 5:194, 1934.
11. Falkner, F., et al.: Some international comparisons of physical growth in the first two years of life. Courrier, 8:1, 1958.
12. Poyner-Wall, P., and Finch, E.: Protein requirements of infants. 4. Serum protein concentrations in normal full term infants. Arch. Dis. Childhood, 25:129, 1950.
13. Dodd, K., and Minot, A. S.: The occurrence of moderately reduced serum albumin in five hundred children in a southern clinic. J. Pediat., 8:452, 1936.
14. Trevorrow, V., et al.: Plasma albumin, globulin, and fibrinogen in healthy individuals from birth to adulthood. II. "Normal" values. J. Lab. & Clin. Med., 27:471, 1942.
15. Levin, B., et al.: Weight gains, serum protein levels, and health of breast fed and artificially fed infants. Medical Research Council, Special Report Series No. 296. London, H.M. Stationery Office, 1959, p. 123.
16. Mellander, O., et al.: Breast feeding and artificial feeding. A clinical, serological, and biochemical study of 402 infants, with a survey of the literature. The Norbotten study. Acta paediat., 48:Suppl. 116, 1959.
17. Fomon, S. J.: Equivalence of protein from human milk and cow's milk in promoting retention of nitrogen by infants (Abstract). A.M.A. J. Dis. Child., 98:584, 1959.

Part III

CARBOHYDRATES

Editor's Comments
on Papers 9 Through 12

The carbohydrate controversy, concerning the composition and amount of sugar to be added to the simple dilution of cow's milk formulas, polarized opinion as thoroughly as did the protein curd. The story of Finklestein's concept of the carbohydrate cause of gastrointestinal disorder, and the resultant professional furor, are nicely summarized in Porter and Dunn's article (Paper 9). Their basic concepts and straightforward conclusions permitted a practical, commonsense approach to the use of sugars. The question of which was the most appropriate carbohydrate additive remained unsolved and, indeed, perhaps not worthy of solution, in that the normal infant was shown by Greenwald and Pennell (Paper 10) to absorb well all the usual carbohydrate additives, with the best tolerance being for lactose. The advantage of lactose were positively propounded by Jarvis (Paper 11).

For those who remained unconvinced, there was the solution offered by McMahon (Paper 12), later substantiated in another series by McCulloch (1944). With the use of an evaporated milk formula, a simple dilution without any added carbohydrate also allowed normal infants to thrive when a sufficient quantity of milk was provided to satisfy the total caloric needs. His observations that fewer gastrointestinal disorders were manifest on this regimen repeated those of Finklestein but drew no heated retorts from those convinced of the protein-sparing effect of added carbohydrate. Indeed, in 1959 there were no less than 26 carbohydrate modifiers commercially available.

9

Reprinted from *Am. J. Dis. Child.*, **10**(2), 77–86 (1915)

SOME STUDIES ON SUGAR IN INFANT FEEDING *

LANGLEY PORTER, M.D.
SAN FRANCISCO

AND

CHARLES HUNTER DUNN, M.D.
BOSTON

Some years ago Finkelstein[1] caught the attention of the world by formulating a new conception of the underlying causes of what were then considered diseases of gastro-intestinal origin. He described them as purely nutritional disturbances, divorced them from any relationship with the bacterial invaders of the intestine, and laid the blame of their genesis on an element of diet that had heretofore been considered innocuous, namely, the sugar. Especially did he attribute that serious, acute form of infantile disease accompanied by stupor, mellituria, and fever to the sugars. The last two symptoms were, he taught, directly and proportionately due to its presence in the food. Later, he implicated the mineral salts of cows' milk, still later prepared his celebrated "Eiweissmilch" and offered it as a remedial food for sugar intoxications, apparently overlooking the fact that as this mixture contained 1.5 per cent. of the deadly lactose its use in practice contradicted his theory. Lactose was especially the sugar he feared, so much so that he stated that even minute doses of milk containing its natural carbohydrate were damaging. Babies were injured with lactose, dextrose, lactose salt mixtures, and dextrose alkali or lactose alkali mixtures, given in isotonic, hypertonic, or hypotonic proportions. The injury was considered always to express itself in mellituria and fever, and F. M. Schapps, Leopold and Von Reuss were one in thinking with Finkelstein that lactose was "exquisitely pyrogenic." This point was emphasized by the findings of Finkelstein and Meyer that 3 gm. of sodium chlorid in 100 c.c. of water given by mouth could produce fever in many healthy infants, while if nutritional disorders were present 1 gm. sufficed to produce pyrexia.

In the next few years the men of this school decided that sugar damage was not alone a simple sugar injury, but made itself felt as the result of the previous or coincident action of salts in improper

---

* Received for publication May 27, 1915.

* Read at the Annual Meeting of the American Pediatric Society, Lakewood, N. J., May 25-27, 1915.

proportions in the food, the presence of the chlorin ion combination with sodium being especially blamed. About four years ago the idea that fermentation of sugar in the intestine played some rôle in these disorders began to be emphasized in Finkelstein's writings, and Finkelstein and Meyer laid greater stress on the fermentation of lactose in the intestine and less on the toxicity of sugar acting parenterally. They even admitted that human milk, which of course is high in lactose, may be the optimum food for certain of the cases that occurred under their classification of intoxication, apparently thus abandoning the view that milk sugar is a fatal poison in such disorders. This inference from the writings of Finkelstein is confirmed by his pupil Schultz, whose experiments did not bear out the pyrogenic or intoxicating action of the sugars. The latest position of Finkelstein's school seems to be that fermenting lactose injures the permeability of the intestinal wall, permits the absorption of salts in abnormal kind or quantity, and that these salts, either alone or in combination with the sugar, produce the poisoning which is evidenced by the glycosuria.

As to fever, there was some reason to believe that when it occurs it is the result of tissue damage such as is often seen following injections of sterile water or salt solution when they break up the erythrocytes, analogous to the fever not at all infrequently seen in childhood that follows extensive bruising or the production of hematomata.

The most convincing work among the group of men that oppose the Finkelstein-Langstein view was done by Allen working in Rosenau's laboratory. In a long series of experiments with animals in the nursling stage the effects of sugars were tested when given both by mouth and subcutaneously. Experimental animals were used and the experiments ingeniously devised to meet all objections. The animals were given large doses and small doses, some were given repeated injections and some single large doses. Those animals which received their sugars by mouth, especially lactose, showed as effects vomiting and diarrhea, which undoubtedly were due to the fermentation of the sugars in the intestine. In no one of the animals was there any sign or symptom of an intoxicating action of sugar, nor was Allen able to produce any symptoms at all approaching the clinical picture of the sugar intoxications as outlined by the Germans. On the contrary, in spite of glycosuria, which occurred in all experimental animals, he was able to see that subcutaneous injections of glucose were very definitely beneficial to his kittens and puppies, especially to one group that was weaned early and doing very badly. This seems a more rational finding than the view that implicates sugar as a poison to metabolism, as every one has seen the apparent benefit of glucose injections in the case of very sick babies.

The study of the literature would make it seem that the origin of the idea of sugar damage went back to Grosz, and was later elaborated by Langstein and Steinitz in a paper, "Lactase und Zucker Ausscheidung," published in 1906, which seems to have turned Finkelstein's interest toward the sugars as agents of possible damage in infantile nutritional disturbances. These authors in fourteen cases of severe gastro-intestinal disorders proved to their own satisfaction that a part at least of the sugar excreted into the urine was lactose. In five cases they found a second sugar which they believed to be galactose. They conclude that there can be no doubt that infants with severe gastro-intestinal disease excrete milk sugar, and its split-off product, galactose, in the urine, and that this excretion is independent of the excretion of lactase in the stool. They further say that in severe cases of gastro-intestinal disease only part of the milk sugar is split by lactase into dextrose and galactose. These are then burned in the organism or the galactose is excreted if the oxidizing power of the tissues has suffered. The second portion is absorbed unsplit and excreted as lactose in the urine. They admit that the largest proportion may be split by fermentation in the intestine and may be lost to the organism.

The views of Kendall are that lactose, far from being an injurious food, is of essential importance in so maintaining the flora of the intestine that the fermentative processes will always be slightly dominant, and will prevent the putrefactive action on protein which produces soluble toxin of undoubted damage to the general metabolism. The work of Allen and the paper of Kendall are both worthy of very close study by any one who is interested in the subject. Raphael showed that many patients assimilate large doses of sugar better than small ones. Schlessinger says that the appearance of the traces of sugar in the urine are no indication that the sugar tolerance of the body has been passed. Naunyn says that small traces of sugar may be ignored in animals who may show a slight glycosuria, with small doses and none with large. Platenze says sugar is often to be found in urine of babies who show no sign of intoxication and who seem perfectly well.

The dosage usually given for pure dextrose as one that will exceed the sugar tolerance is between 100 and 250 gm. for the adult, but many individuals can assimilate more. After the subcutaneous injection of 100 gm. of glucose, glycosuria may last as long as eight hours. The single dose maximum seems to be from 2 to 4 gm. per kilo, by mouth, 10 gm. per kilo per day, and subcutaneously 1 to 1.5 gm. per kilo per dose.

The presence of traces or of even considerable amounts of reducing bodies in the urine does not mean that sugar is present. Schultz says that a reduction test which will exclusively demonstrate the presence of sugar is not known, and further, reducing substances such as uric acid, creatinin, albumen, coloring matter, acetone, glycuronic acid, all or any may be present. Fluckiger reports the presence in normal adult urines of non-fermentable reducing bodies which produce osazones of a value equal to 1/1500 to 1/2500 gm. of grape sugar in the twenty-four hours. Salkowski put it at 0.4 gm., Monk at 0.3 gm., and other observers at variable points. Creatinin has especially been dealt with by Sedgwick, Steinitz, Fluckiger, Amberg and Morris, so that it is clear that in infants' urines there may be considerable reducing power due to bodies other than carbohydrates, a fact well substantiated for the normal urine of adults.

This fact, together with the report by the Finkelstein school of the frequent presence of sugars in the urines of infants suffering with a less severe nutritional disturbance, made it seem desirable to test the urine of a group of infants in the Boston Infants' Hospital, who were suffering from what would be known in Europe as "balance disturbance," but which in the nomenclature of the Boston school is called "chronic indigestion." There were eighteen of these babies investigated; none of them were of the premature type such as Aschenheim found to have intestines more permeable to sugar than those of older nurslings. The first tests were all made while the children were receiving what was considered a normal amount of sugar advisable for their individual peculiarities. Later, attempts were made on a number of the cases to find the limit of physiologic tolerance for the sugars. The reagent used in the determinations was one recommended by Folin as the most sensitive to reducing bodies. It was made in two solutions, of which 3.5 c.c. of each were mixed at the time of using and from 1 to 3 c.c. of the urine added after boiling the mixture. The mixture was then centrifuged. Solution 1 contained copper sulphate 10 gm., glycerin 150 c.c., and water to make 500 c.c. Solution 2 contained 500 c.c. of a 50 per cent. solution of potassium carbonate. This reagent has shown definite amounts of reducing bodies in every adult urine tested with it. This is not true of infants' urines. Twelve per cent. showed no reduction whatever, and of the remainder, 50 per cent. gave no reduction on repetition of the test after saturation with picric acid and shaking through ten minutes to remove the creatinin which is present in appreciable quantities in nearly all infants' urines, and which reduces nearly all the copper reagents especially the more delicate. In none of the urines was it possible to measure the reduction quantitatively by Benedict's solution.

The fact having been determined that there was no measurable sugar in any of the urines tested, attempts were made to pass the sugar tolerance limit of 2 to 4 gm. per kilogram of body weight without the production of a measurable glycosuria. Such attempts

have been made before and have always failed to cause a glycosuria
except in those cases of deep intoxication such as were studied by
Finkelstein and his pupils.

A summary of the work done in this investigation is as follows:
Patients observed, 18; samples of urines tested, 105; number of tests
made, 235; signs double + and triple + are used as follows: + indicates on the addition of the urine to the heated reagent a few grains
of copper oxid; ++ indicates that on centrifuging definite layer of
copper oxid forms in the bottom of the tube; +++ that there is a
visible reduction in the tube before centrifuging. Sixteen of the
eighteen patients showed reducing bodies in some tests before the
treatment with picric acid. Eight showed a loss of reducing power
after shaking with picric acid. Three of the patients (+++) showed
appreciable amounts of reduction constantly in all samples of urine
after the picric acid treatment. One of these had an eczema corresponding in type to the exudative diathesis of the Czerny school, but
in spite of the fact that this patient received as much as 120 gm. of
lactose, 15 per cent. of his intake per day while he was receiving
4 per cent. of fat at the same time, there was never enough sugar in
the urine to be assured by any of the usual quantitative methods and
coincidently the skin condition improved steadily under local treatment. The other two patients of this group were suffering from rather
extreme malnutrition. Of the 105 samples of urine, 58 showed
reducing powers to our solution before shaking with picric acid. Of
these 58, 27 lost their reducing power after such treatment. Of the
eighteen patients, excepting the three referred to above, none showed
reducing bodies every day, and in no instance did there seem to be
any relation between the amounts of sugar ingested and the presence
of these bodies as they were found in the urine with minimum intake,
and were frequently absent following the highest ingestion.

The clinical results in these cases in which an effort was made to
surpass the supposed limits of sugar tolerance were very interesting.
Not knowing how severe the symptoms of intolerance might prove to
be, we did not wish to give large doses of sugar suddenly, but adopted
the method of a gradual increase in the amount of sugar given. The
percentage of sugar in the food was increased at the rate of 0.5 per
cent. a day until symptoms of intolerance developed. Lactose only
was used in nine cases, dextrimaltose only in 1 case, and the tolerance
for both lactose and dextrimaltose was tested in six cases.

None of the cases tested were of the severest type of malnutrition. One or two of the patients were babies having no gastro-intestinal disturbance. One presented a case of congenital obliteration of
the bile ducts. The majority were babies who had presented difficult

feeding cases in the Out-Patient Clinic, and had been sent in to the hospital to be straightened out. None showed any marked intolerance for any of the food elements. The majority were comparatively mild cases of fat intolerance, showing indigestion and excessive fat in the stools when the fat was increased. No case known to have a marked intolerance of carbohydrate was tried.

Symptoms of intolerance developed eventually in twelve of the sixteen cases. Three patients were taken home, and one patient died, before the experiment was completed.

TABLE 1.—MAXIMUM SUGAR TAKEN WITHOUT SYMPTOMS

Case	Percent. in Food	Gm. in 24 Hours	Gm. in 24 Hrs. per Kg. of Body Weight	Gm. in a Single Feeding per kg. of Body Weight
1	Lactose, 9.5	91	9	2.25
2	Lactose, 7	83	20	3.00
3	Lactose, 14.5	169	31	4.75
4	Lactose, 14	119	40	4.00
5	Lactose, 11.5	134	28	4.00
6	Lactose, 15.5	144	32	4.40
7	Lactose, 8.5	79	18	3.00
7	Maltose, 9.5	91	20	3.00
8	Lactose, 15.5	168	27	4.50
9	Lactose, 5	53	10	2.00
9	Maltose, 12.5	158	27	4.50
10	Lactose, 7.5	67	24	2.00
11	Lactose, 8.5	100	20	3.00
11	Maltose, 8.5	100	20	3.00
12	Lactose, 12	160	17	3.00
13	Maltose, 11.5	119	33	3.10
14	Lactose, 10.5	140	30	3.00
14	Maltose, 18.5	170	54	5.40
15	Lactose, 11.5	150	18	3.00
15	Maltose, 17.5	225	27	4.50
16	Lactose, 13	146	22	3.10
16	Maltose, 18	182	30	4.00

The symptoms of intolerance were very constant. The first symptom, showing the coming on of intolerance, was marked irritation of the skin of the buttocks, in spite of the most careful nursing. The symptoms which soon followed were loose green movements, usually about five or six daily, distention of the abdomen with gas, eructations of gas, and vomiting. Loss of weight was slight; on the development of distinct signs of intolerance, the sugar was at once cut down. In no case were seen any toxic symptoms, or any signs of sugar intoxication, or any fever, except that one case developed fever at about the time of the other signs of sugar intolerance, but at the same time this baby had an acute otitis media. The symptoms of sugar intolerance, therefore, judging from this series of cases, are in no way suggestive of intoxication, but are suggestive only of a fermental process localized within the intestinal canal.

The amount of carbohydrate taken without intolerance was surprising. The quantities of sugar given to the several cases are shown in the tables. Table 1 shows the maximum quantities of sugar taken

TABLE 2.—Amount of Sugar on Which Symptoms of Intolerance Developed

Case	Percent. in Food	Gm. in 24 Hours	Gm. in 24 Hrs. per Kg. of Body Weight	Gm. in a Single Feeding per kg. of Body Weight
1 *	....	...	...	...
2 †	....	...	...	...
3	Lactose, 15	141	26	4.0
4	Lactose, 14.5	113	40	4.0
5	Lactose, 12	144	30	4.25
6	Lactose, 16	146	32	4.40
7	Lactose, 9	76	17	3.00
7	Maltose, 10	105	32	3.20
8 †	....	...	...	...
9	Lactose, 6	53	10	2.00
9	Maltose, 13	150	26	4.60
10	Lactose, 8	72	26	2.00
11	Lactose, 9	105	20	3.00
11	Maltose, 9	105	20	3.00
12	Lactose, 12.5	172	18	3.00
13 †	....	...	...	...
14	Lactose, 11	145	30	3.00
14	Maltose, 19	170	55	5.40
15	Lactose, 12	152	18	3.00
15	Maltose, 18	227	19	4.50
16	Lactose, 13.5	148	22	3.10
16	Maltose, 18.5	186	31	4.00

* Patient died before intolerance developed.
† Patient discharged before intolerance developed.

without intolerance. These quantities were in general far above the supposed limit of 10 gm. daily per kilogram of body weight. The percentage of sugar taken without intolerance varied from 5 to 18.5 per cent., the grams in twenty-four hours varied from 53 to 225, the grams daily per kilogram of body weight varied from 9 to 54, and the grams of sugar at a feeding per kilogram of body weight varied from 2 to 5.40. The quantities on which intolerance eventually developed were slightly higher, and are shown in Table 2. Only one baby in

TABLE 3.—Periods of Increased Sugar, Quantity of Sugar Taken, and Gain or Loss in Body Weight

Case	Food	Period of Increased Sugar (Days)	Percent. of Sugar in Food at Beginning of Period	Percent. of Sugar in Food at End of Period	Sugar in 24 Hours per kg. of Body Weight at Beginning of Period gm.	Sugar in 24 Hours per kg. of Body Weight at End of Period gm.	Gain or Loss in Body Weight During Period gm.	Average Daily Gain or Loss in Body Weight During Period gm.
1	Lactose	8	9.5	9.5	9	9	— 500	— 63
2	Lactose	13	7.0	7.0	20	20	+ 290	+ 22
3	Lactose	20	7.0	15.0	16	31	+ 780	+ 36
4	Lactose	18	7.0	14.5	22	40	+ 120	+ 7
5	Lactose	18	6.5	12.0	18	28	+ 330	+ 13
6	Lactose	20	6.5	16.0	14	32	+ 670	+ 33
7	Lactose	8	5.5	9.0	13	18	+ 220	+ 27
7	Maltose	10	6.0	10.0	14	20	+ 260	+ 26
8	Lactose	19	6.5	15.5	12	27	+ 1,000	+ 52
9	Maltose	16	6.0	13.0	14	27	+ 500	+ 31
10	Lactose	4	6.5	8.0	21	26	+ 120	+ 30
11	Lactose	7	7.0	9.0	16	20	+ 30	+ 4
11	Maltose	7	7.0	9.0	16	20	+ 90	+ 13
12	Lactose	13	6.5	12.5	9	18	+ 210	+ 16
13	Lactose	20	6.5	16.5	11	33	+ 1,000	+ 50
14	Lactose	7	7.0	10.5	20	30	+ 200	+ 27
14	Maltose	22	7.0	18.5	20	55	+ 680	+ 30
15	Lactose	10	6.5	11.5	9	18	+ 220	+ 22
15	Lactose	22	6.5	17.5	9	28	+ 790	+ 36
16	Lactose	13	6.5	13.0	14	28	+ 250	+ 19
16	Maltose	22	6.5	18.0	14	36	+ 580	+ 26

the series showed inability to take more than 7 per cent. of sugar, or more than 10 gm. per kilogram of body weight in twenty-four hours.

In the six cases in which the comparative tolerance for maltose and lactose was tried, it was found to be about the same in two cases, but distinctly higher for maltose than for lactose in the other four cases. In no case was there the slightest evidence of any relation between the amount of sugar given and the presence of a positive sugar test in the urine. The sugar was just as likely to be absent as present in cases taking a maximum of sugar, or in cases showing symptoms of intolerance. The three cases showing the constant presence of sugar, showed the same reaction irrespective of the amount of sugar given. The other cases show positive and negative urinary tests at all stages. The last three cases, numbered 14, 15 and 16, showed sugar more often present with maltose than with lactose. Whether this is the rule requires further observation.

The effect of the increased quantity of sugar on the weight curves of the babies was most surprising, and is shown in Table 3. The majority of the cases not only gained weight, but gained weight very rapidly during the period of sugar increase. Also the gain, while less rapid after sugar intolerance developed and the sugar was cut down, was in all cases maintained. In some instances the gain was really enormous. Patients 8 and 13, both on lactose, gained 1,000 gm. in twenty days. Only one case, which afterward proved to be tuberculous, failed to gain. Excluding this case, the average daily gain for the whole series during the sugar period was 26 gm.

It seems to us that the idea of sugar injuries and sugar intoxication has possibly kept us from the use of large amounts of soluble carbohydrate in certain cases, particularly those unable to take a quantity of fat sufficient to meet their nutritive requirements. That many such babies have intolerance of sugar is indoubtedly true. But the danger of pushing the sugar to the limit of tolerance we believe to have been exaggerated. The signs of sugar indigestion are distinct and easily recognized, and do not appear to be in any way serious. In many cases great benefit appears to be obtainable by greatly increasing the carbohydrate content of the food, and therefore this proceeding may prove a valuable addition to our stock of resources in dealing with difficult feeding cases.

240 Stockton Street, San Francisco—178 Marlboro Street, Boston.

REFERENCES

Finkelstein, H.: Zur Aetiologie der Ernährungsstörungen der Säuglinge, Gesellsch. f. kinderh., 1906, xxiii, 117.
Schapps, F. M.: Salz und Zuckerinjektion beim Säugling, Gesellsch. f. Kinderh., 1907, xxiii, 153.

Leopold, J. S. and v. Reuss, A.: Experimentelle Untersuchungen über Milchzuckerausscheidung nach wiederholten subkutanen Injektionen, Monatschr. f. Kinderh., viii, 1 and 453.

Finkelstein, H. and Meyer, L. F.: (1A) Ueber Eiweissmilch, Jahrb. f. Kinderh., 1910, lxxi, 525.

Finkelstein, H. and Meyer, L. F.: Ueber Ernährung magendarmkranker Kinder mit Eiweissmilch, Berl. klin. Wchnschr., 1910, p. 1165.

Schlutz: Am. Jour. Dis. Child., February, 1912.

Allen, F. M.: Quoted in Glycosuria and Diabetes.

Grosz, J.: Beobachtungen über Glykosurie im Säuglingsalter nebst Versuchen über alimentäre Glykosurie, Jahrb. f. Kinderh., 1892, xxxiv, 83.

Langstein-Steinitz: Laktase und Zuckerausscheidung bei magendarmkranken Säuglingen, Beitr. z. chem. Phys. u. Path., 1906, vii, 575.

Kendall, A. L.,: Certain Fundamental Principles Relating to Activity of Bacteria in the Intestinal Tract; Their Relation to Therapeutics. Jour. Med. Research, 1911, xxv, 117.

Kendall, A. L. and Farmer, C. J.: Studies in Bacterial Metabolism, I, II, III, Jour. Biol. Chem., 1912, xii, 1, 19, 215.

Kendall, A. L. and Farmer, C. J.: Studies in Bacterial Metabolism, V, VI, VII, Jour. Biol. Chem., 1912, xii, 465; Ibid., 1912, xiii, 63.

Kendall, A. L., and Farmer, C. J., Bagg, E. P., and Day, A. A.: Studies in Bacterial Metabolism, IV, Jour. Biol. Chem., 1912, xii, 219-21.

Rapheal, F.: Untersuchungen über alimentäre Glykosurie, Ztschr. f. klin. Med., 1899, xxxvii, 19.

Schlesinger, W.: Zur Klinik und Pathogese des Lävulosediabetes, Arch. f. exper. Path. u. Pharm., 1903, l, 273.

Naunyn, B.: Diabetes Mellitus, Wien, 1906.

Platenza, B. P. B.: Finkelstein's Doctrine Concerning Disturbances of Nutrition in Children, Nederl. Tijdschr. v. Geneesk., 1910, xi, 1304; ref. in Maly's Jahresbericht, 1910, p. 625.

Schultz: Nebaurs des Harnes, p. 288.

Fluckiger: Ztschr. f. physiol. Chemie, 1885, ix, 322.

Sedgwick: Jour. Am. Med. Assn., 1910, lv, 1178.

Steinitz: Zentralbl. f. inn. Med., 1904, No. 3.

Fluckiger: Ztschr. f. physiol. Chemie, 1891, xxiv, 521.

Amberg and Morris: Jour. Biol. Chem., iii, 311.

Reprinted from Am. J. Dis. Child., 39, 493–503 (1930)

THE CARBOHYDRATE METABOLISM OF THE NORMAL NEW-BORN INFANT

II. THE EFFECT ON THE CONCENTRATION OF THE BLOOD SUGAR OF FEEDING VARIOUS SUGARS TO NEW-BORN INFANTS *

HARRY M. GREENWALD, M.D.

AND

SAMUEL PENNELL, M.D.

BROOKLYN

In a previous paper we reported observations on the blood sugar values during fasting in normal new-born infants.[1] In this paper we report the results of studies on the dextrose, saccharose, lactose and dextrimaltose tolerance in new-born infants. In addition, the blood sugar curve after a breast feeding was determined in eighteen infants. We found a number of reports [2] in the literature on carbohydrate tolerance in infants ranging in age from 1 month to 2 years, but a careful search failed to reveal any studies on new-born infants.

TECHNIC

In all the work done, the values of the blood sugar were estimated on blood from the great toe, according to the technic described in a previous paper.[1]

Three hours after a feeding, the blood was taken and the sugar content was determined. Immediately after the blood was taken, 2 Gm. of dextrose, saccharose, lactose or dextrimaltose per kilogram of body weight was given in a 20 per cent solution. No difficulty was encountered in getting the infants to take the solution. If vomitting occurred, the infant was excluded from the study. Two grams of carbohydrate per kilogram of body weight was decided on: first, because Rumpf [3] found that the smallest amount of dextrose that produced an alimentary glycemia in older infants was 1.3 Gm. per kilogram of body weight, and second

---

* Submitted for publication, Oct. 29, 1929.

* From the Pediatric Service of the United Israel Zion Hospital.

1. Greenwald, H. M., and Pennell, S.: The Carbohydrate Metabolism of the Normal New-Born Infant: I. Average Concentration of the Blood Sugar in Normal New-Born Infants During Fasting, Am. J. Dis. Child. 39:281 (Feb.) 1930.

2. Mogwitz: Monatschr. f. Kinderh. 12:569; 1914. Bergmark: Jahrb. f. Kinderh. 80:373, 1914. Nieman: Jahrb. f. Kinderh. 83:1, 1916. Frank, A., and Melhorn, L.: Jahrb. f. Kinderh. 91:313, 1920. Götzky: Ztschr. f. Kinderh. 9:44, 1913. Bing and Winderlow: Ztschr. f. Kinderh. 9: 64, 1913. Spence, J. C.: Quart. J. Med. 14:314, 1921. Mertz, A., and Rominger, E.: Arch. f. Kinderh. 69:81, 1921. Rumpf, F.: Jahrb. f. Kinderh. 105:321, 1924. Brown, M. J.: Quart. J. Med. 18:175, 1925. Tisdall, F. F.; Drake, T. Y. H., and Brown, A.: Carbohydrate Metabolism of Normal Infant, Am. J. Dis. Child. 30:675 (Nov.) 1925. MacLean, A. B., and Sullivan, R. C.: Dextrose Tolerance in Infants and in Young Children, Am. J. Dis. Child. 37:1146 (June) 1929.

3. Rumpf (footnote 2, ninth reference).

because this quantity closely approximates the amount of carbohydrate usually taken by a new-born infant under normal conditions after the secretion of milk in the mother has become established. For example, it has been fairly well established that an infant weighing from 6 to 7 pounds (2.7 to 3.2 Kg.) at the fifth or sixth day of life will take from 70 to 80 Gm. of breast milk per feeding, which contains approximately from 5 to 6 Gm. of lactose; this is about 2 Gm. of carbohydrate per kilogram of body weight.

Estimations were made of the blood sugar concentration during fasting and at one-half hour, one hour and two hours after the meal. Each sugar was administered to fifteen infants so that in all, sixty infants were studied. These infants ranged in age from 2 to 10 days.

RESULTS

Blood Sugar Values after Breast Feeding.—The blood sugar during fasting was determined and estimations were made one-half hour, one

TABLE 1.—*Increase in Blood Sugar Concentration After a Breast Feeding, During First Forty-Eight Hours of Life*

Infant No.	Age in Hrs.	Blood Sugar, Per Cent				
		Fasting	½ Hour	1 Hour	1½ Hours	2 Hours
1	2½	0.060	0.066	0.080	0.090	.....
2	9	0.074	0.083	0.074	0.074	0.069
3	14	0.074	0.073	0.074	0.069	0.071
4	16	0.062	0.071	0.071	0.064	0.066
5	16	0.069	0.066	0.067	.....	0.064
6	18	0.060	0.064	0.066	0.080	0.080
7	22	0.087	0.087	0.077	0.080	0.079
8	22	0.074	0.074	0.071	0.071	0.070
9	27	0.077	0.080	0.077	0.080	.....
10	30	0.087	0.080	0.083	0.077	.....
11	33	0.071	0.074	0.087	0.111	0.100
12	33	0.077	0.080	0.080	0.074	0.080
13	36	0.077	0.087	0.077	.....	0.077
14	40	0.069	0.083	0.091	0.087	0.083
15	40	0.062	0.062	0.062	.....	0.064
16	48	0.077	0.077	0.080	.....	0.105
17	50	0.087	0.082	0.076	0.077	0.087
18	52	0.082	0.064	0.063	0.066	0.069

hour, one and one-half hours and two hours after the breast feeding. In six infants the tolerance curve was followed from the first to the sixth day of life, estimations being made at the same time each morning.

In the eighteen infants studied after a breast feeding, no rise in the blood sugar concentration occurred after a breast feeding, during the first forty-eight hours of life, except in infants Nos. 11, 13 and 15 (table 1). This is undoubtedly due to the fact that the breasts secrete little or no milk, as a rule, during the first forty-eight hours after delivery. Colostrum, while it contains as much lactose as breast milk (6.8 to 7.59 per cent [4]), is secreted in but comparatively small amounts, and it is our opinion that not enough lactose is absorbed to produce a rise in the blood sugar curve during this period. Infants Nos. 11, 13 and 15 were born of multiparous mothers whose breasts secreted a fairly large

4. Abt, I. A.: Pediatrics, Philadelphia, W. B. Saunders Company, 1923, vol. 1, p. 616.

amount of milk as early as the second day post partum. In the eighteen infants studied, a rise occurred in one and no rise in eight infants on the first day of life; on the second day there was an equal number in which no rise and a rise occurred. On the third day, six did and two did not show a rise in the blood sugar curve; on the fourth day, the breast feeding was followed by a rise in three infants and in two it was not (chart 1).

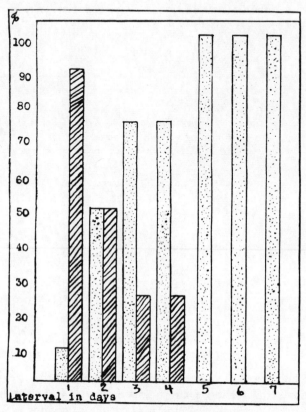

Chart 1.—Rise of blood sugar at intervals. The dotted columns indicate percentage of cases showing rise of blood sugar at various intervals; the lined columns, the percentage of cases showing no rise in blood sugar.

Table 2 is a summary of the blood sugar curves in the six breast-fed infants from the first to the sixth day of life. It will be seen that in only one infant a significant rise in the blood sugar concentration did not occur after a feeding until the fourth day of life (infant No. 4). In all the others, significant elevations occurred after the third day. In most instances the greatest value was usually reached one-half hour after the feeding. Exceptions were infants Nos. 12 and 16, in whom the peak was not reached until two hours after a feeding. Whether this delayed rise was due to imperfect or tardy absorption in the gastro-intestinal tract or to changes in the carbohydrate metabolism is impossible to say at this time. The maximum value obtained was 0.182 per cent, one hour after a breast feeding, in infant No. 17.

The average values obtained during the first forty-eight hours of life are shown in chart 2. The average values obtained in the six infants studied from the third to the sixth day of life are shown in chart 3.

TABLE 2.—*Blood Sugar Concentration After a Breast Feeding in Infants Aged from 1 to 6 Days*

Infant	Age	Weight. Lbs. Oz.	Blood Sugar Per Cent				
			Starving	½ Hour	1 Hour	1½ Hours	2 Hours
1	16 hours....	7 10	0.069	0.066	0.077	.....	0.064
	40 hours....	7 3	0.062	0.062	0.062	.....	0.064
	3 days.....	7 5	0.069	0.111	0.095	.....	0.095
	4 days.....	7 7	0.080	0.111	0.095	.....	0.087
	5 days.....	7 10	0.066	0.118	0.111	.....	0.111
2	3 days.....	7 15	0.074	0.111	0.100	.....	0.100
	5 days.....	.....	0.083	0.154	0.182	.....	0.125
	6 days.....	.....	0.087	0.144	0.133	.....	0.083
3	3 days.....	7 6	0.077	0.077	0.095	.....	0.133
	5 days.....	.....	0.087	0.133	0.118	.....	0.095
	6 days.....	.....	0.074	0.118	0.105	.....	0.095
4	9 hours....	7	0.074	0.083	0.074	0.074	0.069
	33 hours....	.....	0.077	0.080	0.080	0.074	0.080
	57 hours....	.....	0.080	0.060	0.057	0.060	0.069
	81 hours....	.....	0.066	0.069	0.087	0.087	0.083
	105 hours....	.....	0.083	0.095	0.087	0.087	0.083
5	16 hours....	.....	0.062	0.071	0.071	0.064	0.066
	40 hours....	.....	0.069	0.083	0.091	0.087	0.083
	64 hours....	.....	0.069	0.071	0.074	0.087	0.091
	88 hours....	.....	0.069	0.080	0.087	0.111	0.091
	112 hours....	.....	0.066	0.074	0.083	0.105	0.100
6	2 days.....	.....	0.077	0.077	0.080	.....	0.105
	3 days.....	.....	0.091	0.111	0.118	0.100	0.100
	4 days.....	.....	0.091	0.125	0.118	0.095	0.091
	5 days.....	.....	0.071	0.133	0.100	0.071	0.077
	6 days.....	.....	0.095	0.166	0.154	0.105	0.077

Dextrose Tolerance.—Fifteen normal new-born infants, ranging in age from 2 to 10 days, were fed 2 Gm. of dextrose per kilogram of body weight, and the blood sugar curve was determined. In all but one a prompt and definite rise occurred in from one-half to one hour after the feeding. The highest point was 0.150 per cent in three cases. In twelve infants the blood sugar level during fasting was reached at the end of two hours. In the remaining three infants there was a decided lag. In one, the blood sugar reached a higher level two hours after the ingestion of dextrose than it did one hour after ingestion. In two infants the blood sugar was exactly the same at the end of two hours as after one hour. Maximum absorption occurred at the end of one-half hour in seven infants and at the end of one hour in an

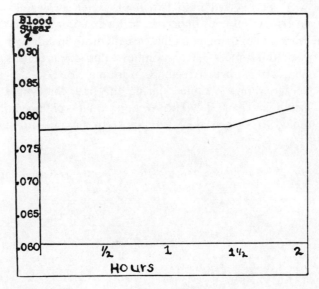

Chart 2.—Curve following breast feeding during first forty-eight hours of life.

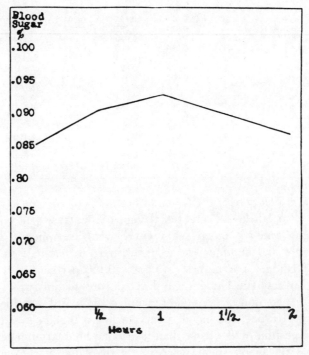

Chart 3.—Curve following breast feeding from the third to the sixth day of life.

equal number. The average value at the end of one-half hour was 112 mg.; at the end of one hour, 115 mg., and at the end of two hours, 90 mg. (table 3).

These blood sugar curves correspond closely to those obtained by MacLean and Sullivan [5] in their studies on the dextrose tolerance in infants varying in age from 5 weeks to 3 years. A comparison of the alimentary dextrose tolerance of children from 5 weeks to 3 years of age and new-born infants with that of adults is given in chart 4. The sugar tolerance curve in the new-born infant is essentially the same as in older infants and adults, except that the curve is at a lower level.

Cane Sugar Tolerance.—In only two infants were maximum values of 140 mg. or above obtained after the ingestion of cane sugar, as compared with the values obtained in three infants after the ingestion

TABLE 3.—*Dextrose Tolerance*

Infant	Age in Days	Weight	Blood Sugar Per Cent			
			Starving	½ Hour	1 Hour	2 Hours
1	7	7:4	0.069	0.111	0.133	0.157
2	7	7:5	0.077	0.080	0.091	0.091
3	6	6:15	0.080	0.111	0.125	0.125
4	7	8:0	0.062	0.091	0.133	0.154
5	6	8:8	0.069	0.144	0.144	0.083
6	6	7:10	0.083	0.125	0.144	0.105
7	5	8:6	0.062	0.118	0.154	0.069
8	5	7:13	0.062	0.111	0.095	0.095
9	4	7:13	0.069	0.100	0.125	0.105
10	9	6:2	0.077	0.154	0.118	0.100
11	9	7:10	0.074	0.111	0.091	0.077
12	5	7:13	0.087	0.100	0.118	0.077
12	8	7:13	0.071	0.111	0.080	0.086
14	5	5:12	0.071	0.111	0.091	0.069
15	4	6:7	0.069	0.095	0.083	0.077

of dextrose. In two infants the two hour level was higher than the one hour level, as compared with that obtained in one infant following the dextrose feeding. In eleven infants, the fasting blood sugar level was reached at the end of two hours; in the remaining two, the curve showed a definite downward trend at the end of this period. Maximum absorption occurred at the end of one-half hour in six infants, and at the end of one hour in seven infants. The average value at the end of one-half hour was 0.105 per cent; at the end of one hour, 0.112 per cent, and at the end of two hours, 0.080 per cent. The two hour value with cane sugar feeding was closer to the blood sugar level during fasting than that obtained after feeding any other sugar (table 4).

Lactose Tolerance.—In two infants a maximum value of 140 mg. was obtained. In only one infant was the two hour value higher than the one hour value. In two infants the two hour value was the same as

5. MacLean and Sullivan (footnote 2, twelfth reference).

the one hour value. The other curves were at a distinctly lower level than the curves obtained following the ingestion of dextrose or saccharose. In one, practically no rise occurred. The maximum value was obtained at the end of one-half hour in five infants and at the end

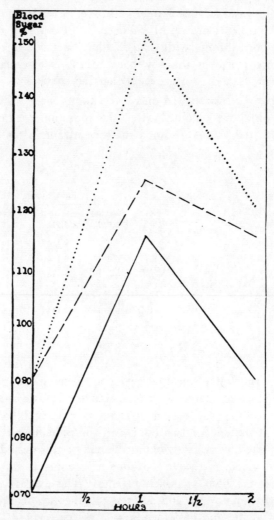

Chart 4.—Curves of blood sugar concentration of adults, infants aged from 5 weeks to 3 years and new-born infants, after the ingestion of dextrose. The dotted line indicates blood sugar concentration of adults; the dash line, the concentration of infants from 5 weeks to 3 years of age (MacLean and Sullivan), and the solid line, the concentration of new-born infants.

of one hour in nine. In nine infants the blood sugar level during fasting was reached at the end of two hours; in the remaining six, there was a definite lag. The average value at the end of one-half hour was 0.1

per cent; at the end of one hour, 0.114 per cent, and at the end of two hours, 0.09 per cent. Apparently, there is a slower rate of absorption for lactose than for dextrose or cane sugar (table 5).

Dextrimaltose Tolerance.—The most irregular curves were obtained following the feeding of dextrimaltose. In four infants practically flat curves were obtained. In one infant, no rise occurred. In three infants

TABLE 4.—*Cane Sugar Tolerance*

Infant	Age in Days	Weight	Blood Sugar Per Cent			
			Starving	½ Hour	1 Hour	2 Hours
1	6	7:1	0.060	0.100	0.111	0.091
2	4	6:1	0.064	0.083	0.091	0.111
3	10	7:6	0.071	0.111	0.118	0.077
4	4	5:1	0.069	0.133	0.125	0.069
5	4	7:0	0.066	0.133	0.154	0.071
6	3	6:15	0.069	0.125	0.133	0.074
7	7	6:12	0.066	0.111	0.111	0.066
8	7	6:6	0.064	0.087	0.111	0.087
9	7	7:2	0.052	0.071	0.080	0.080
10	5	8:1	0.071	0.074	0.133	0.095
11	8	7:14	0.077	0.125	0.100	0.077
12	3	...	0.059	0.125	0.111	0.077
13	2	7:8	0.077	0.111	0.166	0.083
14	5	9:0	0.059	0.118	0.057	0.053
15	3	7:5	0.071	0.091	0.100	0.080

TABLE 5.—*Lactose Tolerance*

Infant	Age in Days	Weight	Blood Sugar Per Cent			
			Starving	½ Hour	1 Hour	2 Hours
1	3	7:4	0.055	0.100	0.105	0.071
2	5	6:2	0.080	0.111	0.111	0.091
3	6	6:14	0.077	0.118	0.105	0.105
4	5	6:12	0.080	0.091	0.105	0.069
5	4	6:11	0.087	0.118	0.095	0.071
6	4	7:8	0.077	0.105	0.125	0.105
7	3	5:5	0.057	0.091	0.080	0.069
8	2	6:0	0.077	0.144	0.111	0.080
9	2	5:10	0.071	0.095	0.144	0.133
10	10	6:4	0.074	0.105	0.125	0.080
11	2	6:13	0.062	0.062	0.100	0.087
12	6	8:1	0.083	0.095	0.118	0.133
13	8	7:5	0.074	0.087	0.091	0.091
14	4	6:13	0.077	0.095	0.105	0.077
15	4	7:10	0.080	0.125	0.166	0.100

a high value of 0.14 per cent was found. The maximum rise occurred at the end of one-half hour in only three infants. In four infants the maximum rise occurred at the end of one hour; in five infants the two hour value was higher than the one-half hour or one hour value; in three infants the blood sugar level during fasting was reached at the end of two hours, and in three infants, although the curve showed a downward trend, the two hour value was still definitely above the blood sugar concentration during fasting. In other words, eight infants showed a definite lag with dextrimaltose, whereas only six showed it with lactose; only two with cane sugar and three with dextrose. The average value at the end of one-half hour was 0.095 per cent; at the end of one hour, 0.102 per cent, and at the end of two hours, 0.095 per cent (table 6).

The dextrimaltose curve closely parallels that for the breast-fed infants and is much flatter than the curve found in infants fed with other sugars. The amount of breast milk taken by each infant was not controlled, and it is therefore obviously incorrect to compare the curves obtained after a breast feeding with the curves obtained after feeding definite amounts of various sugars. If it is assumed that the breast-fed infants studied received adequate amounts of milk, it must be concluded that the best tolerance is for lactose, as it exists in breast milk. It is unlikely that the flatness of the curve is

TABLE 6.—*Dextrimaltose Tolerance*

Infant	Age in Days	Weight	Blood Sugar Per Cent			
			Starving	½ Hour	1 Hour	2 Hours
1	10	6:12	0.074	0.100	0.105	0.095
2	10	8:0	0.080	0.105	0.118	0.105
3	?	7:0	0.080	0.095	0.087	0.095
4	7	6:9	0.066	0.077	0.125	0.154
5	7	7:7	0.064	0.095	0.111	0.083
6	4	6:0	0.071	0.125	0.154	0.118
7	4	6:13	0.069	0.105	0.133	0.125
8	7	5:15	0.062	0.082	0.157	0.060
9	8	7:0	0.077	0.111	0.144	0.111
10	6	7:2	0.060	0.062	0.052	0.059
11	5	7:2	0.069	0.118	0.111	0.066
12	4	7:15	0.071	0.091	0.100	0.105
13	4	8:8	0.077	0.091	0.087	0.095
14	2	7:8	0.071	0.087	0.071	0.069
15	1	7:2	0.066	0.083	0.080	0.091

due to delayed absorption since it is generally conceded that breast milk is the ideal food, particularly for the new-born infant. In addition, the presence of protein, fat and salts in breast milk may be a factor in the absorption and assimilation of lactose. This phase of the problem is being studied at the present time, and the results will be reported in a subsequent paper.

It is questionable whether the flatness of the curve following the ingestion of dextrimaltose may be considered due to an increased tolerance for this sugar, as was the case with lactose present in breast milk. It is more likely that dextrimaltose is absorbed more slowly than the other sugars, since with no other sugar did we obtain as large a number of flat and lag curves.

Chart 5 gives the average values for cane sugar, dextrimaltose, lactose and saccharose. With all sugars, the maximum value was obtained at the end of one hour. The curves obtained following the feeding of lactose, cane sugar and dextrose closely parallel each other, except that the two hour period for cane sugar more closely approximated the blood sugar level during fasting. The average curve for dextrimaltose showed a decided lag. The best absorption occurred with dextrose. The curve obtained after feeding dextrose closely approximated the curves obtained in adults and older children after the ingestion of dextrose, except that it was at a definitely lower level, as is indicated by chart 4.

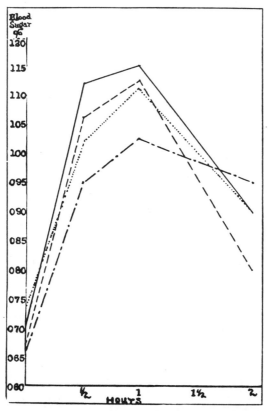

Chart 5.—Average curves for dextrose, saccharose, lactose and dextrimaltose. The solid line indicates course of dextrose; the dash line, saccharose; the dotted line, lactose, and the dot and dash line, dextrimaltose.

SUMMARY

In eighteen infants the blood sugar concentration was followed after a breast feeding during the first forty-eight hours of life; practically no increase in the blood sugar concentration occurred. This was most likely due to an insufficient secretion of breast milk during this period. In seven infants, the blood sugar curve after a breast feeding was studied from the first to the sixth day of life. A definite rise in the blood sugar concentration occurred in from one-half to one hour in practically all infants after the second day of life. From the curves obtained, it is concluded that the best tolerance is for lactose as it occurs in breast milk.

Sixty infants were fed definite amounts of dextrose, lactose, saccharose and dextrimaltose; each sugar was administered to fifteen infants. The blood sugar curve after a dextrose meal is at a definitely lower level during the neonatal period than at any other period in life. The best rate of absorption occurred after the ingestion of dextrose, saccharose, lactose and dextrimaltose in the order in which they are named. The most irregular curves were obtained with dextrimaltose; with dextrose, saccharose and lactose fairly uniform curves were obtained.

11

Reprinted from *Am. J. Dis. Child.*, **40**, 993–999 (1930)

MILK SUGAR IN INFANT FEEDING

A STUDY OF THE EFFECTS OF THE ROUTINE USE OF MILK SUGAR IN INFANT FEEDING *

B. WINSTON JARVIS, M.D.

NEW YORK

The object in this investigation was to observe the effects of the routine use of milk sugar (lactose) in infant feeding, approved methods being used for giving the other elements of the formulas the maximum digestibility.

The routine use of any given type of modified infant feeding has led to a kind of "faith dispute" among physicians. This is probably due to the fact that expert work with a given method always yields commendable results. Such results tend to confirm the belief of the general practitioner that there is no panacea in infant feeding. What he wants is a simple method for the average case.

The literature on infant feeding contains many opinions of the advantages of this or that sugar, but most of them lack any scientific proof of the conclusions drawn. These, combined with timely commercial propaganda, have given rise to a vast array of sugar preparations, for each of which unsurpassable advantages are claimed. As one result, the use of lactose in modified infant feeding has diminished. Many pediatricians dispute the identity of lactose of other mammalian milks with that of human milk. Others imply that lactose is no more meant for the infant than is cow's milk. These observers overlook, however, the chemical fact that regardless of the kind of mammal, lactose occurs in the milk of all. The statement "lactose is animal sugar and is meant for animal development" stands as a fact. Prior to the twentieth century, disturbances of nutrition giving rise to gastro-intestinal upsets were attributed to lactose per se, and some workers conducted clinical experiments from which it was concluded that lactose is a toxic substance. Apprehension at once arose regarding its use, and in a measure has not as yet been dispelled. Today it is known that many of its alleged evils are due to diminished digestibility of the other ingredients of the formulas, to say nothing of the large part played by actual infection within or without the gastro-intestinal tract proper. Hence, no attempt

---

* Submitted for publication, May 1, 1930.

* From the Department of Pediatrics, New York Post-Graduate Hospital and Medical School.

will be made to summarize the literature on this subject prior to the last two decades, and reference will be made only to work within this last period that seems scientifically pertinent.

While carbohydrates have a more or less uniform caloric value, their availability in metabolism varies greatly. Chapin,[1] in 1912, showed the fallacy of assuming that the best available sugar is of the greatest value to the infant's metabolism, that the energy expended in storing carbohydrate as glycogen in excess of body requirement detracts correspondingly from growth energy, and that excess water is bound in the tissues. This is not true in the case of milk sugar, as its slower rate of absorption precludes excessive glycogen formation. Weight for weight, infants fed on milk sugar possess correspondingly more living tissue than when an excess storage of glycogen exists as in the case of infants fed on vegetable sugar. Lactose, therefore, should be the sugar of choice for normal infants, as its digestion and assimilation occur more slowly than with vegetable carbohydrates and its molecule yields only one molecule of available dextrose. Talbot and Hill,[2] in 1914, showed that lactose facilitates assimilation of nitrogen within certain limits when administered in increasing amounts. Thierfelder,[3] in 1914, Mathews,[4] in 1921, and Kimmelstiel,[5] in 1929, identified and correlated lactose and galactose with cerebrosides and brain tissue and showed the rapid development of the brain tissue during the period of artificial feeding, indicating an ever increasing need for a source of galactose during this period.

Bergeim,[6] in 1926, demonstrated that lactose facilitated calcium and phosphorus absorption markedly as compared with any other sugar. This work has been confirmed by Killian, whose paper is to be published shortly. In 1928, Steuber and Seifert [7] demonstrated that the infant is unable to transform lactose into fat and cannot substitute it biologically. Therefore, illusions about growth and development in the form of fat storage will not exist when this sugar is used.

1. Chapin, H. D.: The Properties, Uses and Indications of Various Carbohydrates Used in Infant Feeding, J. A. M. A. **59**:2221 (Dec. 21) 1912.

2. Talbot and Hill: Influence of Lactose on Metabolism of Infants. Am. J. Dis. Child. **8**:218 (Sept.) 1914.

3. Thierfelder, H.: Ztschr. f. physiol. Chem. **85**:35, 1913; **89**:248, 1914; **91**:107, 1914.

4. Mathews, A. P.: Textbook of Physiological Chemistry, ed. 3, New York, William Wood & Company, 1921, pp. 56 and 310.

5. Kimmelstiel, P.: Biochem. Ztschr. **212**:359, 1929; Chem. Abstr. **24**:386, 1930.

6. Bergeim, C.: J. Biol. Chem. **62**:45 and 49, 1924-1925; **70**:29, 1926.

7. Steuber and Seifert: Arch. f. Kinderh. **85**:12, 1928.

In 1928, Gerstley, Wang, Boyden and Wood [8] showed that the stool of a breast-fed infant is rather constant regarding weight, volatile acid output and total titratable acidity, and that it varies in the infant fed on cow's milk. They [9] also demonstrated that excess lactose feeding to the breast-fed infant causes little change in the feces while in the infant fed on cow's milk an increase of free acid occurs, and the frequency and weight of the stools are affected. When the lactose was increased to 12 per cent, the relationship existing between total titratable acidity and total volatile acidity approached that observed in the breast-fed infant. No alimentary disturbance resulted from excess lactose feeding. When an intercurrent parenteral infection took place, it was a potent agent in producing a tremendous increase in weight and acidity of stools which lasted for weeks after clinical symptoms had disappeared. Furthermore, although the same dosage of lactose was continued, no increase of symptoms and no changes in the stools were noted. These authors concluded that intestinal fermentation is not a primary dietary disturbance. Randoin and Lecoq [10] and L. Knudson [11] showed that neither lactose nor galactose is toxic to the animal organism, but that galactose must be assimilated in a strict equilibrium with dextrose, i. e., in the relationship existing in lactose during digestion and assimilation.

EXPERIMENTAL WORK

Killian,[12] who collaborated with me in this investigation, but who will report separately in the near future, studied the effect of lactose as the only carbohydrate of the diet on the composition of the soft tissues of the bodies of rats:

Thirty-six albino rats of known ancestry, twenty-eight days after birth, were weaned and divided into three groups of twelve each. McCollum's control diet was used for one group; the remaining two groups were given diets containing only sucrose and lactose, respectively, as the source of exogenous carbohydrate. All diets were maintained over a period of sixty days, and weights were determined every seven days. McCollum's diet being adopted as the standard for

8. Gerstley, J. R.; Wang, C. C.; Boyden, R. E., and Wood, A. A.: Influence of Feeding on Certain Acids in Feces of Infants, Am. J. Dis. Child. **36**:289 (Aug.) 1928.

9. Gerstley, J. R.; Wang, C. C.; Boyden, R. E., and Wood, A. A.: Influence of Feeding on Certain Acids in Feces of Infants, Am. J. Dis. Child. **35**:580 (April) 1928.

10. Randoin, L., and Lecoq: Compt. rend. Acad. d. sc. **184**:1347, 1927; **185**: 1068, 1927; **189**:1188, 1929.

11. Knudson, L.: Ann. Missouri Bot. Garden **2**:659, 1915.

12. Killian, John A.: A Study of the Effects of Lactose Feeding, as the Only Source of Carbohydrate in the Diet of Rats, upon the Composition of the Soft Tissues, to be published.

comparison of weight curves the sucrose-fed rats averaged 11 per cent above the control curve, while the lactose-fed rats averaged 5 per cent below the control curve and 16 per cent below the sucrose curve. Six rats from each group were ashed in toto, after which the following determinations were made: The ash was 3.73 per cent of the body weight in the control rats, 3.27 per cent in those fed sucrose and 3.87 per cent in those fed lactose. It is evident that the greater weight of the sucrose-fed rats is not due to mineral salt content. It is also evident that lactose facilitates the absorption of mineral salts, as has been previously mentioned in reference to Bergeim and Killian—the fixation of calcium and phosphorus.

The tissue of the remaining six rats of each group were removed, desiccated to a constant weight and analyzed, with the following results:

	Control Rats, Gm.	Rats Fed Sucrose, Gm.	Rats Fed Lactose, Gm.
Water	72.0	78.1	70.7
Total solids	28.0	22.9	29.3
Protein	18.3	14.7	19.1
Ether extract (Lipoids)	3.5	3.7	2.8
Ash	5.2	4.2	5.9
Glycogen	0.17	0.29	0.24

The very significant observations were the greater amount of total solids (i. e., less water) in the tissues of the lactose-fed rats. It is also noteworthy that the lipin content of lactose-fed rats is less than that of either the control or sucrose-fed rats. The lower water content of the lactose-fed rats is partially due to the lower glycogen and lipoid content of their tissues and also probably due to the slight diuretic and laxative action of the lactose per se. However, of greatest importance is the fact that more living tissue is present in the lactose-fed rat than in either the control or the sucrose-fed rat, weight for weight.

I used lactose for longer or shorter periods in over 1,000 consecutive cases and observed 100 cases critically over a two year period of routine feeding with modified formulas containing lactose, in order to determine the tolerance of the infant to lactose during both the winter and the summer months and to note any clinical values of this type of feeding. Routine formulas were composed of whole cow's milk, water and lactose. Careful attention was given to adequate vitamin prophylaxis. Specified amounts of milk, water and lactose were mixed together cold and boiled for three minutes, stirring continuously, thereby rendering the protein and fat more available for digestion. Cereals and vegetables were added between the ages of 5 and 8 months depending on development and dentition, and all cases were observed weekly. Ten grams of lactose were first added and increased by an equal amount every third day to percentages varying between 5 and 9, depending on the clinical progress and indications. During the first few days following the beginning of lactose administration slight tympanitis was frequently noted when the sugar had been of vegetable origin previously. This, however, subsided with the appearance of normal stools. The cases observed were average and not selected; the periods of observation included failures to gain or actual losses of weight due to intercurrent infections as they appeared.

This group comprised sixty-four infants under 6 months of age, including five immature infants (table 1) and ten malnourished infants, and thirty-six infants over 6 months. The progress of the immature and malnourished infants is shown in table 2. The average age at the beginning of the experiment was 2½ months for the infants under 6 months of age; their average weight was 10¾ pounds (4.8 Kg.) and average birth weight 7¾ pounds (3.5 Kg.). The average time of the experiment was 13¾ weeks, and the average gain per week 5¾ ounces (163 Gm.). The average weight of the infants over 6 months of age was 15 pounds (6.7 Kg.) at the beginning of the experiment. Their average birth weight was 7¼ pounds (3.3 Kg.). The average gain was 4½ ounces (127 Gm.) per week, and the average time of the experiment was 14¼ weeks.

TABLE 1.—*Weekly Gain in Weight in Immature Infants*

Age at Start, Months	Birth Weight		Weight at Start		Weekly Gains, Ounces	Time, Weeks
	Pounds	Ounces	Pounds	Ounces		
1	6	..	5	7	4	21
2	4	4	7	11	10½	14
2	4	8	6	11	6¾	17
2	7	1	6	13	6½	24
2	6	4	6	11	5½	24

TABLE 2.—*Weekly Gain in Weight in Cases of Malnutrition*

Age at Start, Months	Birth Weight		Weight at Start		Weekly, Gains, Ounces	Time, Weeks
	Pounds	Ounces	Pounds	Ounces		
1	8	8	8	..	6	19
1	8	14	9	15	5	6
1½	6	8	7	6	6¼	18
1½	7	..	8	14	5½	20
1½	12	..	10	9	9¼	19
2	8	5	9	5	5	18
2	8	..	7	3	5	13
3	9	..	10	9	12	14
4	8	8	8	11	4½	9
4½	10	..	13	12	5¼	12

RESULTS

1. No intolerance toward lactose was noted in clinical manifestations. In no instance was a given percentage of lactose reduced. It is interesting to note that over 1,000 infants received lactose, inclusive of complementary and supplementary formulas, without evidence of intolerance.

2. Gains in weight varied, but averaged the amount previously noted. So many factors affect the growth impetus, such as environment, prenatal health of the mother, heredity, etc., that little need be said but that the average environment was poor, most of these children coming from New York's tenement districts.

3. The tissues of these children seemed more firm than that of the average infant receiving vegetable sugar and resembled that of the breast-fed infant. Fat babies were rarely observed.

89

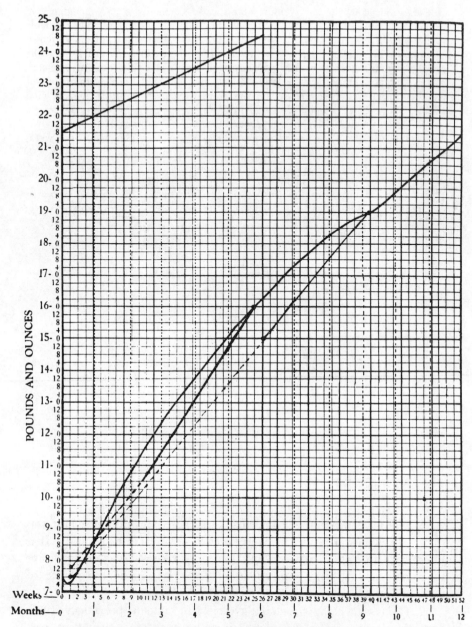

The upper curve shows the gain in weight of sixty-four infants under 6 months of age. The average age at the beginning of the investigation was 2½ months; the average birth weight, 7¾ pounds; the average weight at the start, 10¾ pounds, and the average gain, 5¾ ounces a week for thirteen and three-fourths weeks. The lower curves show the gain in weight of thirty-six infants over 6 months of age. The average age at the start was 6 months; the average birth weight, 7½ pounds; the average weight at the start, 15 pounds, and the average gain, 4¼ ounces a week for fourteen weeks.

4. These children, with rare exceptions, did not lose weight during the course of an intercurrent infection, but simply failed to gain properly. No clinical dehydration developed even in the presence of parenteral gastro-intestinal upsets with acidosis.

5. No protracted nutritional disturbances developed.

6. There was no complaint of habitual anorexia by the mother.

7. There was no complaint of habitual constipation. The average number of stools varied from one to two per day.

8. No infantile eczemas developed.

9. The general nervous and mental status was placid.

10. When lactose was used in complementary and supplementary diet, both breast and bottle feedings were taken well on the average throughout the period of infant feeding.

CONCLUSIONS

I urge a more common use of lactose in infant feeding, based on the following observations:

1. Lactose is well tolerated by the infant when the other elements of formulas are rendered more available for digestion; and it may be increased to amounts of the eventual formula in 10 Gm. doses (i. e., 1 level tablespoon) at three-day intervals with safety.

2. Boiling and stirring the formula for three minutes renders the protein and fat of cow's milk more available for digestion by making it a more favorable medium for the administration of lactose than unboiled milk.

3. The lactose-fed infant resembles but does not equal the breast-fed infant in firmness of tissues and resistance toward infections.

4. The danger of sudden dehydration with acidosis in the presence of parenteral infection is less acute in lactose-fed infants than, as is well known, in infants fed on vegetable sugar. This is probably due to tissues of less water content normally.

5. Age-weight for age-weight, the lactose-fed infant possesses more living tissue than does the infant fed on vegetable sugar. This is due to the lower water content as well as to the lower fat content of the tissues of the infant fed on milk sugar.

6. Lactose formulas facilitate complementary and supplementary feedings with less danger of refusal by either the breast-fed or bottle-fed infant.

7. Lactose formulas lessen the dangers of the development of habitual anorexia or constipation.

8. As a source of galactose for the development of the central nervous system, lactose is especially desirable as a sugar for modified feeding in an optimal amount.

12

Reprinted from *Wisconsin Med. J.*, **38**, 874–876 (1939)

A Simplified Infant Feeding Formula

A Report of the Use of Irradiated Evaporated Milk and Water in 2,004 Cases*

By HENRY O. McMAHON, M. D.

Milwaukee

BASED on a long experience in private practice with feeding infants on milk mixtures containing no additional carbohydrate, some observations were made at the Milwaukee County Hospital to test the suitability of this type of feeding for normal infants under controlled conditions.

Previously, in this hospital, there had been considerable latitude in the construction of infant feeding formulas. This was particularly true with respect to carboydrate additions. Various types of carbohydrate were in use. Carbohydrate was routinely added to all formulas. The infants received additional carbohydrate in their prelacteal feedings in the form of lactose water. In these procedures the hospital was following common practices. Digestive upsets, diarrheas and rashes were frequent among the infants and for their correction protein milk, barley water and other special formulas were prescribed. Occasionally there was disagreement or lack of cooperation on the nursery staff.

In an effort to improve the condition a system was started whereby accurate and detailed records were kept on the progress of all babies from birth to discharge from the hospital. Feeding mixtures were standardized as to type of milk and carbohydrate, but essentially the same proportions of these substances were used as formerly. At the end of a year (November, 1936) the records showed that little progress had been made in reducing gastrointestinal disturbances.

At this point, carbohydrate was omitted entirely from infant feeding formulas. Standard mixtures were installed. The mixtures consisted of irradiated evaporated milk and water. They were standardized at four dilutions (see table 1) and graduated

* From the Department of Pediatrics, Marquette University, and the Pediatric Clinic, Milwaukee County Hospital.

in milk content in proportion to the average infant's needs for growth.

TABLE 1.—*Standard Feeding Mixtures at Milwaukee County Hospital*

Mixture	No. 1	No. 2	No. 3	No. 4
Irradiated evaporated milk	5 parts	7 parts	8½ parts	10 parts
Water	10 parts	10 parts	10 parts	10 parts

Mixture 1 is the standard complementary feeding mixture for newborns and also is used as the entire feeding for the newborn where breast feeding is contraindicated. At the fifth day the formula is raised to mixture 2, which in most cases is continued during the balance of the lying-in period. At the time of discharge the mother is given instructions for preparing mixture 3, which is used until the infant is one month old, at which time mixture 4 is started. Mixture 4 has the strength of whole milk. No further modifications are necessary.

Each normal infant weighing six pounds or over at birth goes to the breast every eight hours from birth to forty-eight hours after birth. Only sterile water is used during the prelacteal period. On the third day the infant goes to the breast every four hours if *over* six and one-half pounds in weight, and every three hours if *under* six and one-half pounds in weight. If by the end of the fourth day the baby's hunger is unsatisfied, complementary feeding with mixture 1 is started. Complementary feedings are poured in two ounce quantities.

If the infant comes off the breast, three ounces of total fluid per pound of body weight are given. A seven pound infant, for example, receives two and one-half ounces of mixture 1 seven times, plus two bottles of water in twenty-four hours. Such an infant receives thirty-six calories per pound of body weight, which corresponds closely to

TABLE 2.—*Record of Feedings Prepared Before and After November, 1936, When Standard Mixtures Containing No Additional Carbohydrate Were Adopted*

Date	Barley Water	Protein Milk	Special Formulas	Lactose Water	Old Standard Mixtures (With Sugar)	Sterile Water	New Standard Mixtures 1 and 2 (Without Sugar)
1936 (Jan. 1–Nov. 15)	492	3,050	1,507	25,571	26,660		
1936 (Nov. 15–Dec. 31)		364	222			5,440	3,331
1937		210	292			24,440	35,904
1938 (Jan. 1–Nov. 1)						31,595	32,658

the number of calories in the diet of the breast-fed infant at this early age. At the same time the infant receives ample protein and calcium for optimal development.

With the installation of the new feeding plan, stools were carefully checked and found to be within average limits of frequency and normal in appearance. Repeated analyses indicated that fat was being metabolized satisfactorily. Routine blood sugar analyses showed normal blood sugar despite the lower carbohydrate intake. For a period of a year and a half from the beginning of the study, several home calls were made on every baby to check its progress and assure continuation of the feeding regimen. In June, 1938, an outpatient clinic was set up to follow the progress of the children systematically.

Results

There was a striking reduction in the occurrence of such symptoms as loose stools, sore buttocks, rashes, and excess regurgitation. This improvement followed the standardization in the hospital of infant feeding mixtures consisting of irradiated evaporated milk and water without carbohydrate. In table 2 the records of the hospital's milk laboratory are set forth.

It is noteworthy that the use of preparations for the management of digestive disturbances such as barley water, protein milk and special formulas decreased abruptly

with the installation of the new schedule and disappeared from the milk laboratory's records in 1938.

There occurred a marked increase in the percentage of infants who had regained or were above birth weight at the time of discharge from the hospital. Table 3 shows the percentages for each year of the study.

From a "low" of 38.4 per cent discharged at or above birth weight during the year when carbohydrate was included in the feedings, this percentage rose to 72.4 during the first year of the "no sugar" regime and to 75.6 during the second year.

Discussion

Smith[1] has demonstrated the importance of avoiding overfeeding during the neonatal period. The caloric intake of the infant who is wholly or partially bottle-fed should correspond throughout infancy to that of the breast-fed infant. Especially is this important during the early weeks of life. House formulas in many hospitals supply more food than the infant needs, particularly as regards caloric value. This results frequently in symptoms such as loose stools, vomiting, colic, or rashes, and may lead, later on, to failing appetite or other feeding problems.

In this study the milk mixtures were reduced in caloric value by omitting carbohydrate. The amount of milk in the formula

TABLE 3.—*Record of Weight of 2,004 Normal Newborn Infants on Discharge from Hospital, Before and After November, 1936, When "No Sugar" Formulas Were Adopted**

	Nov., 1935–Nov., 1936 (Sugar Formulas Used)		Nov., 1936–Nov., 1937 ("No Sugar" Regime)		Nov., 1937–Nov., 1938 ("No Sugar" Regime)	
	Number	Per cent	Number	Per cent	Number	Per cent
Number discharged at or above birth weight	331	38.4	567	72.4	923	75.6
Number discharged below birth weight	531	61.6	216	27.6	298	24.4
	862		783		1,221	

* Average weight of infants, five and one-half to eleven and one-half pounds; average age at time of discharge, ten days.

was increased slightly but remained within the accepted limits of one and one-half to two ounces of milk per pound (three-fourths to one ounce of evaporated milk), thus complying with the optimal requirements for protein and calcium. Obviously the sum of the fat, carbohydrate and protein occurring naturally in the milk satisfied the caloric needs of the infants. In view of the lower carbohydrate intake, it is probable that the diet more nearly met the infants' vitamin B_1 requirements than would a diet high in carbohydrate, since, as pointed out by Elvehjem,[2] and Williams and Spies,[3] vitamin B_1 (thiamin) is concerned quantitatively with carbohydrate metabolism.

Irradiated evaporated milks were used exclusively throughout the last two years of study. It was felt that the infants benefited from the vitamin D which was thus provided in the early days of life. Formulas were uniformly well tolerated. Also irradiated evaporated milks were prescribed for infants in the outpatient clinic since it seemed desirable for them to have this additional and automatic protection against rickets.

Summary

Accurate records were kept for three years of all normal newborn infants in a large hospital.

During the first year various types of feeding formulas were used, all containing carbohydrate. During the second and third years, standard mixtures of irradiated evaporated milk and water with no carbohydrate were used.

The infants given feedings without additional carbohydrate had, to a marked extent, fewer gastrointestinal symptoms.

During 1937 and 1938 when the "no sugar" formulas were used, more infants were discharged at or above birth weight than in the period when sugar formulas were used.

The new standard milk mixtures simplified hospital routine.

BIBLIOGRAPHY

1. Smith, C. H.: The diet of the infant. Maine M. J. 28: 89–100 (May) 1937.
2. Elvehjem, C. A.: The vitamin B complex in practical nutrition. J. Am. Dietet. A. 15: 6–12 (Jan.) 1939.
3. Williams, R. R., and Spies, T. D.: Vitamin B_1 (thiamin) and its use in medicine. New York: The Macmillan Company, 1938.

Part IV

FATS

Editor's Comments
on Papers 13 Through 16

13 BRENNEMANN
Nutritional Disturbances in Infancy Due to Overfeeding

14 TALBOT
Physiology and Pathology of the Digestion of Fat in Infancy: Their Application to Infant-Feeding

15 GERSTENBERGER, HASKINS, McGREGOR, and RUH
Studies in the Adaptation of an Artificial Food to Human Milk

16 HANSEN, WIESE, BOELSCHE, HAGGARD, ADAM, and DAVIS
Role of Linoleic Acid in Infant Nutrition: Clinical and Chemical Study of 428 Infants Fed on Milk Mixtures Varying in Kind and Amount of Fat

As early as 1907, Brennemann was singling out fat as the disturbing element in the condition of overfeeding in infancy (Paper 13). The difference in quantity of fat in human and cow's milk is extremely slight. Yet, Brennemann points out, while human milk fat causes very little trouble, cow's milk fat is probably the most difficult element for the child to digest, for no entirely clear reason. He postulated that a major cause was the longer amount of time that the fat lay in the infant's stomach, being approximately two hours in a breast-fed child and four hours in the artificially fed infant. In any event, since the sole means of modifying the fat content in human milk is dilution of cow's milk or use of a base that is less rich in cream, he questioned the wisdom of using top milk or cream in the preparation of infant formulas.

Paper 14, by Talbot, not only establishes the physiology of the digestion of fat in the infant but also details vividly the techniques for examining the stool which, at the time, obsessed both pediatricians and parents. The absence of curds in the stools was a much sought-after goal.

Homogenization, now taken for granted, was first introduced as applicable to the infant formula by Gerstenberger in 1915. Paper 15 is unique in that it not only discusses homogenization of fats in the milk but also attempts to show the influence of substituting vegetable for animal fats in providing a more human-like fat mixture.

A specific scaling condition of the skin developed in rats when fed on a fat-free diet had been observed by Burr and Burr in the early 1930s. In 1933, in a brief report in the proceedings of the Society for Experimental Biology and Medicine, Hansen correlated these facts with the therapeutic effect of various oils and serum lipid changes in infantile eczema. Paper 16 is a classic summation by Hansen et al. of the role of linoleic acid in infant nutrition.

The benchmark article on the value of the use of polyunsaturates in infant feeding and/or skimmed milk instead of whole milk awaits the collection of sufficient data through a generation or more of use.

13

Reprinted from JAMA, 48(16), 1338–1344 (1907)

NUTRITIONAL DISTURBANCES IN INFANCY DUE TO OVERFEEDING

Joseph Brennemann, M.D.
Northwestern University Medical School

That overfeeding in infancy is apt to be followed by indigestion is a universally recognized fact. The term, however, usually suggests the giving to an infant of a food that is too rich in one or more food elements, or that is unsuitable to age and conditions, or that is given in too great variety and at too short and irregular intervals. We have not been sufficiently impressed with the fact that even an appropriate artificial food and one properly adapted to the individual case, can give rise to the profoundest nutritional disturbances when given in quantities that exceed the actual economic needs of the infant. In this discussion the term overfeeding will be used in this restricted sense, the giving to an infant of too great a total quantity of good, clean, fresh, unexceptionable, properly modified cow's milk, usually, but not necessarily, at too short intervals.

Continental writers have emphasized the danger of overfeeding in this sense for many years. Biedert was among the first to teach a doctrine of minimum feeding (*Minimalnahrung*), which called for the smallest amount of food necessary to insure perfect development with normal increase in weight. This most desirable minimum daily amount of food he placed at from 150 to 200 grams of fluid per kilogram of body weight, this amount to contain about 80 calories.

Heubner determined along metabolic lines the number of calories, per day, per kilogram of body weight, necessary to insure proper development in normal breast-fed babies. This so-called energy quotient he found to be about 100 from the third week to the end of the sixth month; a gradually diminishing amount after that time to about 80 or 85 at the end of the first year. He established 70 as the approximate energy quotient necessary to maintain a weight equilibrium.

Clinical observations, each extending over many months, have been made on breast-fed infants by Feer, Beutner, Budin, Schlossman, Nordheim, Czerny and Keller, Reyer and others, that have all confirmed rather closely the figures set down by Heubner, so that these can be used as a standard.

Budin of Paris uses a simpler measure. He feeds all of his babies "especially after the fifth or sixth month, or better, weighing 6 or 7 kg., one-tenth of their body weight daily of pure, sterilized, undiluted milk," and claims to have no symptoms of the overfeeding against which he warns so emphatically.

In this country, through the teachings of Rotch, Holt and their followers, we have come to think of nutritional needs and overfeeding rather in terms of percentage than of amount. Certain standards are set up as guides to the strength of food a child should receive, and these naturally find expression in more or less elastic tables of percentages of different food elements adapted to average healthy infants at various ages. Weight is given comparatively little significance, and for conditions other than normal we have most indefinite data.

To Czerny and Keller we are indebted for a symptomatology of overfeeding that, in its totality, is new and original, and is so clean cut and palpable that it alone can serve as a real guide to determine when proper amounts are beginning to be exceeded. Their exhaustive and truly scientific work[1] that has appeared only in part

* Read before the Chicago Medical Society, Nov. 28, 1906.
1. Des Kindes Ernährung, Ernährungsstörungen und Ernährungstherapie.

has placed the whole subject of infant feeding on as firm a foundation in reason and scientific investigation as that on which any other department of medicine stands. Finkelstein has put it none too strongly when he says: "When in the future we shall speak of the attainments of scientific pediatrics, Czerny and Keller's work will be placed first, and everyone who wishes to occupy himself in a scientific manner with the problems of infant feeding must find his foundations there." I wish to acknowledge that this paper and our own recent work in infant feeding has been, in a large measure, inspired by this work, and especially by the chapter on *Milchnährschaden*, a term perhaps most briefly and fully translated by the title of the present paper; a chapter in which they picture a definite and convincing symptom-complex resulting from overfeeding.

For some time we have recognized and studied this clinical picture; we have also, during that time, calculated energy quotients in all of our feedings and have been much impressed by the results. It seemed to me additionally instructive to study our old cases in this light. I have, therefore, recently gone over the histories of our old cases at the Northwestern University Medical School, as well as over my own private cases, to see what our past habits have been with reference to overfeeding, both from a calorimetric and a clinical or symptomatic standpoint, and from this, if possible, to make a deduction as to the prevalence of overfeeding under present conditions in this country.

Our conditions have been rather favorable for such a study. In practically all of these cases we have a complete history of the exact amount of certified milk or cream, of definite strength, that was used, together with the exact weighed amounts of other ingredients used in the mixture. Our weight record, on our own scales, is quite complete, and the rest of the history as to bowel movements, disposition, etc., sufficiently so for this purpose. In nearly all cases the foods were prepared at the diet kitchen—always individually for each case. We have, then, all the necessary data for calculating approximate energy quotients. We have considered the caloric value of 1 ounce of 4 per cent. milk at 21; 1 ounce of 16 per cent. cream at 54; 1 ounce of skimmed milk at 10; 1 ounce of sugar at 120; 1 ounce of cereal water at about 3. It is a simple matter, then, to multiply the number of ounces of each ingredient in the twenty-four-hour food by its caloric value, to add the products, divide by the number of pounds the baby weighs, and multiply the result by 2 1/5 to reduce from pounds to kilos. The end product is the energy quotient. By caloric value is meant the number of large calories, the latter being the universally recognized unit of measure of food value as expressed in terms of heat production and representing the amount of heat required to raise 1 kilogram of water from 0 C. to 1 C.

The dispensary babies were fed by a number of different instructors connected with the department of pediatrics. Until recently we all used the percentage method. We have, however, gradually come to look on fats with that feeling of caution that pervades our own literature (Holt, Southworth, Jacobi, etc.), and I believe that all of us fed considerably under the usual amounts rather than above them, especially of fat. In the last year most of us have stopped using cream altogether and have used only milk dilutions with the addition of carbohydrates. I believe, then, that I can assume that our conditions were representative, or at least not an exaggeration, of what is being done in this country by those who use these methods only.

I was convinced before looking over our records that overfeeding was a factor in our results, but after studying them, *I am positive that, in our past, overfeeding has been a factor in the production and maintaining of nutritional disturbances in infants that towers above all others.*

It seemed impossible to tabulate these cases and have the results of any more value than are general statements, so I have not attempted it. As far as calorimetric overfeeding is concerned, according to Heubner's standard, it can safely be stated that all of our cases were overfed ultimately, except those that were, at the time, suffering from some acute disorder. By overfeeding is not meant simply the exceeding of Heubner's energy quotient of 100, but rather using energy quotients of 120, to 150, to 200—in one case, fed by a physician not connected with the dispensary, who had had peculiarly valuable experience in infant feeding by the percentage method, an energy quotient of 330 was given for two weeks.

SYMPTOMS OF OVERFEEDING.

As to symptoms due to overfeeding, it can be said with equal certainty that they were present in the great majority of our babies, at some time, during the period that they were under our care. So typical and uniform are these symptoms that we associate with overfeeding that they form a clean-cut, easily recognized clinical entity. Individual cases differ from the well-marked type only in the number and the degree, rather than in the character of the symptoms, that make up this symptom-complex. Many of our cases gave only a few slight manifestations of trouble that had little or no bearing on the general condition of the child; in others there was every evidence of the profoundest nutritional disturbance.

An infant that is overfed becomes restless, often most strikingly shown by broken and restless sleep at night. At the same time it becomes constipated in a very characteristic manner; the bowel movements that were yellow in color and were soft and moist, become pale gray, hard and dry, will not mix with water, and are of the color and consistency of putty—so that they will roll from the diaper without leaving it soiled. The odor is strong and suggests decomposition. The urine has commonly a strong ammoniacal odor and easily produces irritation of the skin.

At the same time it is noticed that the child gives evidence of a fundamental disturbance of nutrition. It becomes pale, its tissues lose their tone, the abdomen becomes soft and moderately distended with gas. The child becomes less active; it plays less. A striking symptom, often the only one that gives any concern to one not familiar with this picture, is a failure to gain in weight on the same food, or a greater quantity of food, that up to this time has produced normal or even abnormal gain in weight. Still more striking is the fact that a continuation of the same amount of food, or of an increased amount, will regularly produce, not only a stationary weight, but after a time, a steady loss in weight. A further increase in food may again produce a temporary gain, often a large one, but it only makes surer and quicker the ultimate loss in weight.

OTHER RESULTS OF OVERFEEDING.

If this course is persisted in one of two results will follow: The child finally presents the picture of atrophy or marasmus. This we see, not rarely, in the pale, constipated, marantic baby that gives the history of having had a stationary weight, or steady loss in weight, for months, in spite of the fact that it has taken enormous quantities of cow's milk and has had no diarrhea or evident digestive disturbance.

The other result is the acute gastrointestinal catastrophe that may occur at any time in this course, and that is characterized by vomiting, diarrhea, prostration, loss in weight, often by fever, and, usually, by the inability to take more than the smallest amounts of cow's milk, sometimes for many weeks. This condition we have seen more commonly in weaker children, with poorer digestion, especially in those who were rapidly or excessively overfed; while in more robust children, with better digestion, in whom the overfeeding was a more gradual process, though excessive, there has been more of a tendency to the typical chronic course outlined above. In weaker children one often sees one catastrophe follow another, especially in hospital cases, the only progress being made during the period of low feeding generally recognized as necessary after such an upheaval; while in the stronger children the severest symptoms of overfeeding may be present for months before such a catastrophe occurs, if it occurs at all.

In many of these more chronic cases there is evidence of rickets, with the train of nervous symptoms that accompanies that disease. Two other symptoms very frequently appear at some time during the period of overfeeding. One of these, eczema, has been very frequent in those of our cases that have shown other well-marked symptoms of overfeeding, especially the characteristic constipation. It varies from the small, rough, reddish spots in the cheeks that are so well known, to the most extensive and intractable involvement of the cheeks, forehead, scalp, chest and back, and other parts of the body.

The other symptom alluded to is anorexia. Loss of the normal keen appetite of infancy, so that the child needs to be coaxed to finish its bottle, is very common in these cases that are well marked, but a refusal to take more than an ounce, or even less, at a time, is characteristic only of the graver cases, and then often forebodes a catastrophe. We have come to look on this symptom as due to overfeeding in practically all cases in infancy in which there is not some other evident acute, or chronic disorder. There is at present at Wesley Hospital a child of 17 months weighing 16 pounds in whom an increase of food from 26 ounces of milk, 10 ounces of barley water, 1 oz. of cane sugar, to 30 oz. of milk, and 6 oz. of barley water produced in one day a florid eczema of chest and back, spreading later to the cheeks and scalp, and within five days, loss of appetite, restlessness at night, fever and constipation, with hard, dry, gray bowel movements.

While most of our babies gave some evidence of overfeeding, and many of them had well-marked manifestations, such as constipation, pallor, restlessness, eczema, stationary weight, etc., there were very few in whom the final outcome was wholly bad. The ultimate picture of marasmus, of course, came to us in its finished state and was never produced by us. Some of our cases showed undoubted rickets, although under satisfactory control throughout. In general, we considered our results excellent. In some cases this was due not so much to our methods as to the fact that these cases can often stand a surprising amount of overfeeding. While many of our cases did well for weeks and months on energy quotients of 150, many gave evidence of serious trouble on those of from 110 to 120 or even less. Since calculating energy quotients in all of our cases we have seen few, if any, cases that required over 100, and we have usually regretted it if we have exceeded that "unsurpassable amount" (Heubner). In general, we have found the energy quotients of from 100, at the beginning, to 80, or less, at the end of the first year, as a wholly satisfactory working basis as to the approximate amount of food a child should get.

FAT THE DISTURBING ELEMENT.

There seems little doubt that the disturbing element in this condition is the fat of cow's milk, and that its non-digestion, non-assimilation and the resulting disturbed intermediary metabolism are the cause of this train of symptoms. Outside of the negative evidence that proteids and carbohydrate and salts can not produce this picture, there is very positive evidence that fat does. The characteristic dry, hard, pale bowel movement has been found to consist largely of the insoluble salts of the fatty acids (*Seifenstuhl*). If the amount of fat is increased all symptoms are increased. If the fat is sufficiently diminished, and the other food elements are left undisturbed, or increased, there will be rapid improvement. No other result in infant feeding is more striking than the mathematical certainty with which the dry, gray bowel movements of these infants, no matter what their ages, are replaced by characteristic smooth, nearly odorless, curdless, brown, salve-like bowel movements, when they are fed straight, undiluted skimmed milk—a food that is nearly fat free, but contains the maximum amount of proteids and carbohydrates. Nor is the general improvement less certain than that of this one symptom.

The immediate cause of this condition is probably an acidosis (Czerny and Keller), as shown by increased excretion of ammonia in the urine. This is due to the fact that alkalies are withdrawn from the body by the fatty acids produced in the intestines and to satisfy the normal acid products of metabolism ammonia is called on.

The following three cases may be cited as typical cases of overfeeding, in which the percentage method was used:

CASE 1.—Baby F., well developed, strong, healthy baby. Birth weight, 9 pounds 12 ounces. Maternal nursing alone for three weeks, with severe indigestion and considerable loss in weight. After the first month fed artificially on cream and whey mixtures; later on cream and milk. At four months weighed 13 pounds 8 ounces. At five months weighed 13 pounds, a loss of 8 ounces in one month. During this month the child had received a food mixture containing fats 3.6, proteid 2.0, sugar 7.0. Seven feedings of 5 ounces each were given at three-hour intervals. The energy quotient here was about 116. It did not take the food well and would often leave one or two ounces of a 5 ounce bottle. Child was rather pale and thin, but muscular and active. Cranio-tabes well marked. Bowel movements were pale yellow and somewhat dry and offensive. During the fifth month a sudden severe diarrhea occurred, with from twelve to fifteen green bowel movements a day. It was put on barley water for a short time and milk, later cream, was slowly added. Baby now took food eagerly and after the initial loss due to diarrhea and hunger diet, gained one pound in two weeks. Soon began again to refuse to take all of the 5 ounces of food, so the food was made more concentrated: Fat 4, proteid 2, sugar 7.5; the number of feedings was kept the same, as also was the frequency and the amount. The energy quotient now was about 137. Child became rather constipated, the bowel movements were pale, greenish yellow, and offensive, but it gained 20 ounces in eighteen days on this stronger food.

Two weeks later there was no gain in weight, the bowel movements were dry, pale and offensive, the baby was pale, and refused food more and more. Finally it would take only an ounce or two at a time, and was losing in weight. In three months it had gained only 1½ pounds. The mother then, on her own initiative, fed the child potato, bread and gravy, porridge, cracker, soup, etc., and stopped coaxing her to drink milk, the child soon taking less than a pint a day. There was immediate improvement. The child was happier and slept better, bowel movements became normal, and the child gained a little over a pound a month for four months. At eleven months the child weighed 19 pounds. Still rather thin and pale, but marked improvement over former condition. Only very slight evidence of rickets.

In this case the most serious results of overfeeding were avoided by the mother unconsciously meeting the two therapeutic indications, decreasing the milk and increasing the carbohydrates.

CASE 2.—Baby B., weight 11 pounds at birth; maternal nursing insufficient. Was rather underfed for two months, with stationary weight; for the next four months it gained steadily about 6 ounces a week on cream and milk mixtures. During the last two months of this time the child was badly constipated, one or two hard, dry, smooth, pale yellow bowel movements a day, offensive in odor. Eczema was first noticed about this time on cheeks, and later about the ears, then on the forehead and scalp, with one or two small spots on the body; it was variable in intensity. Child always rather pale, but very active and a good baby. During this time the food had a percentage never stronger than, fat 3.6, proteid 2.0, and sugar 6.5, but the energy quotient was from 160 to 165. The cream was diminished and the milk increased so that at nine or ten months the child was practically on about 40 ounces of whole milk, with the energy quotient under 100. Weighed 19 pounds at nine months, and the general condition was excellent. The eczema, which in this case was the chief symptom, had slowly disappeared, and was practically gone at nine months.

CASE 3.—Baby O., a typical case with all the classical symptoms, weighed 7 pounds at birth, was wet-nursed five months, when it weighed 16 pounds 4 ounces. Had been on milk and cream mixtures since then. At seven months the food mixture consisted of fat 3.0, proteid 1.5, and sugar 6.0, with an energy quotient of 86.

At eight months the child weighed 18 pounds and the food mixture was: Fat 4.0, proteid 2.0, and sugar 7.0; the energy quotient being 128.

At nine months: Fat 4.0, proteid 2.8, sugar 6.0, with energy quotient 130.

At ten months: Fat 4.0, proteid 3.0, and sugar 6.0; energy quotient 130.

At eleven months the child weighed 18 pounds 14 ounces—a gain of 14 ounces in three months; the energy quotient was 128.

When one year old the child weighed 19 pounds 8 ounces. The food was milk 40 ounces, sugar 1 ounce, with an energy quotient of 108. During the last few months this child has had no acute illness. Has been out of doors almost constantly. Bowel movements have generally been rather dry, grayish, often nearly white and offensive, typical *Seifenstuhl*. Has had slight eczema for some months, especially recently; is rather pale, does not drink well, and often leaves an ounce or two of food. When thirteen months old, had for several days refused bottle more and more, and finally would not take it at all. The eczema was well marked, and vomiting and diarrhea now set in. Baby was put on barley water for eight days, then milk was added slowly to 40 ounces. At sixteen months of age the child weighed 20 pounds 10 ounces, a gain of 10 ounces in two months. In the last few months the child had taken a daily mixture of milk 40 ounces, sugar 1 ounce, in addition to some carbohydrate food, granos, flaked wheat, etc. During the greater part of this time the stools had been hard, light-colored, and dry.

The child at sixteen and one-half months was rather pale, the anterior fontanelle measured 1 inch across, the head was rather large and square, and the tissues soft. The ribs were slightly beaded and the costal borders somewhat flared; the abdomen was soft and moderately distended.

This child lived under very favorable hygienic conditions, was out of doors nearly all of the time, was only moderately, but persistently, overfed, and yet developed mild rickets and gained only 24 ounces from the eighth to the eleventh month, or 2 pounds 10 ounces from the eighth to the sixteenth month.

TOO LARGE AMOUNTS VERSUS TOO LARGE PERCENTAGE.

So far cases have been cited in all of which high percentages of fat have been used—only once a little above 4 per cent., in the rest 4 per cent. or under. In a paper read before the American Pediatric Society in May, 1901.[2] Holt cites five cases resulting from too high percentages of fat (5 to 7+ per cent.). These he details under the following headings:

HOLT'S SERIES.—CASE 1.—Overfeeding with high fat, rapid increase in weight and progress in development till 8 months old; then general convulsions followed later by tetany, laryngismus, fatty liver (?). Recovery after three months' illness.

CASE 2.—Prolonged feeding with high fat, notwithstanding which constipation and the development of moderate rickets followed by acute disturbances of digestion with repeated convulsions.

CASE 3.—Overfeeding with high fat; convulsions.

CASE 4.—Habitual vomiting aggravated by high fat; serious gastric catarrh produced; finally cured by stomach washing.

CASE 5.—Feeding with high fat; eczema, habitual constipation and finally habitual vomiting.

So striking is the similarity of this symptomatology to that of the cases I have just cited that there can be no reasonable doubt as to an identical cause, i. e., too much fat. This excess Holt repeatedly states in terms of percentages as if the essential point were too high a percentage of fat—not too great an amount. It may seem a trivial matter to point out this difference of viewpoint—and yet right here is the very kernel of the matter—the essential difference between feeding by a percentage method and a method that determines the amount of food that should be given. That these digestive disturbances are not due to too high percentages of fat *per se,* can be demonstrated with the ease and certainty of a laboratory experiment by any one who will feed a number of babies on low milk dilutions in excessive amounts; they will get the identical symptoms that Holt has described and that are undoubtedly due to too much fat.

A year ago I started about a dozen babies on simple milk and water, or milk and cereal water dilutions (1 to 3, to 1 to 0), with about 5 to 7 per cent. sugar. Most of these babies were sick and required a preliminary one or two days' hunger diet. Such immediate results in the form of smooth, rich yellow, well-digested bowel movements I had never seen before. Gradually all those assisters in proteid digestion from alkalies to peptonization were dropped without any appreciable difference, except, in some cases, a beneficial one. These babies were not constipated, they gained rapidly in weight from the start—there was not that long anxious wait in the sicker cases that we were accustomed to in those we fed on whey and cream and cereal water mixtures. One after the other, however, these babies did become constipated, often very much so, with pale, hard, dry bowel movements. Some failed to gain after the first rapid gain. They became restless and did not sleep well at night. Many had eczema and some would not take all of their

2. Disturbances of Digestion in Infants Resulting from the Use of Too High Fat Percentages.

food. Some of them gained steadily and well and seemed in good condition. Practically, all were ultimately constipated except those in whom sudden severe attacks of diarrhea broke out, often without any apparent reason. We had been taught, and had ourselves taught, that simple milk dilutions would "invariably cause constipation," so this result was not unexpected, and the other symptoms were considered secondary to it. In certain cases I added cream and found, to my astonishment, that the condition was not only not relieved, but often made much worse.

I then began to estimate energy quotients in all cases, and found that all of these cases had been overfed, being given usually energy quotients from 120 to 170 during the period of eczema and maximum constipation, or just before the catastrophe. Since we have calculated energy quotients in every case constipation has given us comparatively little trouble and the other symptoms of overfeeding no longer occur. We have heard much of "fat diarrhea" in the last few years. Fat constipation deserves at least an equal place in our nomenclature. We have come to look on fat as the constipator—and the one condition in which we have never seen constipation is the use of straight, skimmed milk, the maximum proteid and minimum fat food. A single case from this series will illustrate what has been said:

CASE 4.—Baby E., born March 14. Weight 10 pounds (?) and was wet nursed one month, but lost in weight; so was then fed on modified milk. Was first seen May 12, when it weighed 8 pounds 12 ounces. Had had a good deal of colic, with three to four bowel movements daily, but was now constipated. Started the child on barley water for twenty-four hours, then 5 ounces of milk was added daily until it received the following: Milk, 15 ounces; barley water, 25 ounces; sugar, 2 ounces. The energy quotient was 154. The composition of the food was: Fat, 1.5; proteid, 1.5; and sugar 6.0. Eight 5-ounce feedings were given daily at three-hour intervals.

May 5: Weighed 9 pounds 12 ounces, a gain of 1 pound in one week! The baby was well in every way, so the food was continued. *This enormous gain in weight is characteristic of early rapid overfeeding, and we now consider such a gain an imperative indication for reduction in the amount of milk unless the energy quotient is very low.*

May 30: Weighed 10 pounds 3 ounces; had two or three bowel movements a day; yellow, not offensive, but a little too hard and pale, so that baby grunts a great deal in passing them. Slight eczema. The same food was continued.

June 9: Weighed 10 pounds 13 ounces. Food the same; energy quotient, 123. Two bowel movements daily, which were whitish, dry, formed and offensive. Eczema increased, spreading to chest and back as well as face. On account of the small gain of 2 ounces in one week, 2 ounces of milk was added, and three days later 2 ounces more. The food mixture was: Milk, 19 ounces; barley water, 21 ounces; milk sugar, 1½ ounces, giving an energy quotient of 126. The food strength was: Fat, 1.9; proteid, 1.9, and sugar, 6.0. The number of feedings, quantity and intervals remained as before.

June 30: Weighed 11 pounds 11 ounces, a gain of 14 ounces in fourteen days.

The increase in food, as often happens, even when there was no previous gain, increased the weight, but brought on the catastrophe: a diarrhea for ten days. For a time there were bowel movements every ten to fifteen minutes of a pale, yellow, curdled, cheesy, sour and offensive character. Child was restless, slept little and cried much.

July 3: Baby was put on barley water for two days and the crying stopped, and it slept well. Five ounces of milk were added, with six to eight bowel movements daily resulting, so child was put on barley water for four days longer.

July 7: Weighed 11 pounds 6 ounces. The addition of milk produced the same bowel condition as before. After several attempts to relieve conditions, including trying buttermilk (?) (not fat free), the mother decided to take the baby to the country and the further history is unknown. The child never had 2 per cent. of fat, although 3½ months old when the food disagreed, and was typically overfed on 1½ per cent. of fat.

The following case had less than 3 per cent. of fat at 19 months, but had severe symptoms of overfeeding on an energy quotient of 140 from which she recovered at an incredible rate on less milk—later skimmed milk with very low energy quotient; gaining 5 pounds 14 ounces in 51 days, nearly 13 ounces a week for over seven weeks.

CASE 5.—Baby McGuire (see chart).

August 20: Entered Wesley Hospital, 18 months old; had an enteritis of three weeks' standing; was thin, pale, haggard and

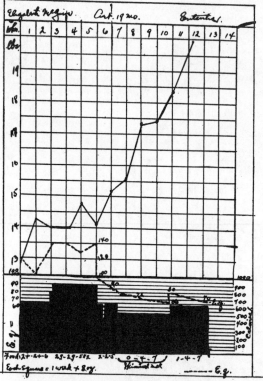

Case 5.—Baby McGuire. Rapid gain on e. q. of 120 followed by loss. No gain for 3 weeks on e. q. of 140. Enormous gain on e. q. of 66 to 80. In general as e. q. is lowered gain is increased, and vice versa. Maximum gain of 1 lb. 11 oz. in one week on e. q. of about 70. Food at this time: Skimmed milk 40 oz., cane sugar 1 oz.

listless, with eyes sunken and a temperature of 101 F. Frequent green, curdy, slimy bowel movements. She was given stimulation and placed on cereal water for four days, then milk was added, three ounces a day.

August 29: Weighed 12 pounds 13 ounces; bowel movements had been normal for several days, but had been losing to this time. Energy quotient was slowly raised to about 120. Food mixture consisted of: Milk, 25 ounces; cereal flour, malt, water, 23 ounces; cane sugar, 1½ ounces. Six 8-ounce feedings were given daily at three-hour intervals.

September 5: Weighed 14 pounds 4 ounces, a gain of 23 ounces in seven days. Food was the same, with an energy quotient of about 100.

September 14: Weighed 14 pounds, with food as before;

bowel movements were normal. On account of loss, the food was increased to milk, 35 ounces, barley water, 13 ounces, cane sugar, 1 ounce, fed as before, with the energy quotient 140.

September 21: Weighed 14 pounds on same food. One bowel movement daily; several days none; dry, pale, gray and hard. Child had not slept as well as before and showed eczema about the chest.

September 26: Weighed 14 pounds 12 ounces. Had gone home. The bowel movements were hard and dry, so that the child played with one, as with blocks; the eczema was worse. The same food mixture was given in five 10-ounce feedings at four-hour intervals.

October 3: Weighed 14 pounds 1 ounce. Child had not taken food well since she went home and will only take a few ounces at a time. Had five or six bowel movements daily, always gray or whitish; these were at times hard and formed, again soft and cheesy. Never green. Child was cross and peevish and restless at night, but had no fever. The milk was cut down to 20 ounces; barley water, 20 ounces; cane sugar, 1½ ounces, giving an energy quotient of 98.

October 10: Weighed 15 pounds 3 ounces, a gain of 1 pound 2 ounces in eight days. Had not been cross since the food was changed and took it well almost at once. Slept well and the diarrhea had stopped, but bowel movements are still a mass of whitish curds; the rest pale and yellow.

October 13: On account of the curds was put on straight skimmed (centrifuged) milk, 40 ounces; sugar, 1 ounce. Energy quotient of 75.

October 24: Weighed 15 pounds 10 ounces. Two good, yellow, normal bowel movements daily; no curds two days after being put on skimmed milk; the same food continued.

October 31: Weighed 17 pounds 5 ounces, a gain of 1 pound 11 ounces in one week. Energy quotient 66. Bowel movements normal.

November 7: Weighed 17 pounds 7 ounces. Still on the same food. On account of the small gain child was put on whole milk, 10 ounces; skimmed milk, 30 ounces; cane sugar, 1 ounce. Energy quotient, 80.

November 14: Weighed 18 pounds 5 ounces, a gain of 11 ounces in one week. Child had perfect digestion, good color, good disposition and slept well. Is getting solid; laughs and plays.

November 23: Weighed 19 pounds 15 ounces, a gain of 1 pound 10 ounces in nine days, on the same food. Energy quotient, 70. General condition excellent. Since this child went home it has received a small amount of additional food. I asked the mother many times as to just what this consisted of. She always stated positively that the child had one thin slice of bread about 2 inches square and a half cup of beef soup daily, and, every other day, she chewed a piece of meat the size of one-half a finger. This child had been so sick that the mother had given her up; the latter had been cautioned so often and so hard against giving too much food, and her faith in the last milk was so implicit that I believe her statement is accurate. To make doubly sure I asked the nurse in charge of the diet kitchen to go to the home and investigate the matter. She was equally convinced that the child was getting no more than the mother stated. For a study in actual, rather than relative energy quotients, the caloric value of these could be added to the milk.

Such enormous gains are not so alarming nor do they carry the same therapeutic indication, as when whole milk is given, especially in excessive amounts. The offending fat is not present in sufficient amount to cause trouble.

From all that has been said I believe the inference is justifiable that overfeeding to the point of producing well-marked symptoms is not only widely prevalent in this country, but the rule. Our present methods, especially the percentage method, must then be inadequate to prevent this. If by one method—that of using simple milk dilutions with the addition of carbohydrates, and with no definite check on the total amount to be given, a 7 months' old child among our cases, whose food is increased from 10 to 15 ounces of milk can develop extensive eczema, restlessness, typical constipation, later diarrhea, fever and loss in weight, then this method alone is not so accurate as it would be if combined with a procedure that would tell us in advance that that child's energy quotient was being sent up from a dangerous height of 130 to a disastrous one of 152. And if a schedule for an average healthy infant (Holt) of 6 months calls for a fat 4, proteid 2, sugar 7 mixture of 30 to 48 oz. then that schedule is not even approximately safe in itself when it permits us to go from a proper energy quotient of 90 to a decidedly dangerous one of 115 if our healthy child weighs 16 pounds, as it ought to. These tables uniformly recommend excessive amounts and too short intervals that must lead to overfeeding unless we are familiar with the above picture of overfeeding and have had an unusual experience. The percentage alone is an unreliable and irrational check even in the healthy child. If we could have our cases under ideal control at all times we might be satisfied with recognizing symptoms of overfeeding as they arise. But with our conditions, especially in those of limited experience, something safer and more tangible is necessary—something that will forestall symptoms rather than permit us to recognize them. We have become convinced that in our feeding cases determination of energy quotient is simply indispensable. Those of us who have adopted it have become enthusiastic over it as we have over no other procedure in infant feeding. It is this point that I wish to emphasize especially, that this determination of energy quotient is not merely an interesting study in physiology, but an intensely practical procedure of the greatest value not alone to the scientific pediatrician, but to any man who feeds babies and wants to be sure of results. It alone enables him to tell approximately how much food his baby really needs, and by keeping this in mind, and departing from it only when clearly indicated, he will avoid on the one hand a prolonged underfeeding that is by no means uncommon and, on the other hand, a still more disastrous overfeeding.

It is true that caloric value represents only one function of food, that of heat production. It is equally true that in our overfeeding we have to do with a real milk overfeeding and that the amount of milk, and not the caloric value, would perhaps be the surest guide to the prevention of this symptom-complex. In a child at Wesley of 17 months and weighing 16 pounds that has been mentioned before, a change of milk from 26 oz. to 30 oz., but with an actual lowering of energy quotient from 96 to 90, due to lessening of sugar and barley water, produced nearly all of the symptoms of overfeeding within a few days. And yet these symptoms would doubtless have arisen with less increase of milk if the higher energy quotient had been maintained. These are theoretical considerations. For practical purposes the method advocated is amply sufficient, and the most desirable one so long as we are all using well balanced but widely different food mixtures and need a common measure.

It need hardly be mentioned that this method is not to be used to the exclusion of other things. To feed a baby one needs all the help obtainable from every source. The baby itself must be weighed regularly and accurately, its disposition must be inquired into, its bowel movements must be seen, not alone described by the mother, the actual preparation of the food must be supervised. Nor is this method applicable only to the simpler milk dilutions, plus carbohydrates, that we use. Its use is indicated nowhere so much as in the use of high fats in the conventional percentage method, for obvious reasons. Such indications for increase of food as apparent hunger, restlessness, failure to gain or loss in weight, or mere lapse of time, need hardly be discussed after what has been said.

The treatment of this condition, after it is present, is more or less evident from its pathogenesis. In general the fat must be reduced and the carbohydrates increased to take its place. In milder cases it is enough to do only the former, together with lengthening the interval to at least four hours. In severer cases the milk must be greatly reduced and a gruel or flour water added. If this is not sufficient to produce normal bowel movements and gain in weight, more sugar must be added, either as cane sugar, or preferably, according to Czerny and Keller, as maltose. Milk sugar has not shown itself serviceable clinically. To meet this one indication of overfeeding with milk Keller's *Malzsuppe*[2] is intended. This or another combination of milk, flour and cane sugar or maltose, modified to meet the individual conditions, is best kept up for a number of weeks because these children are not readily lead back again to normal amounts of milk. The milk is then gradually increased and the carbohydrate diminished until the usual milk modification is again reached. Rapid improvement and ultimate cure are the rule.

We are handicapped in not having a desirable maltose, or a serviceable malt preparation, in this country. The ordinary malt extracts can not be used in large amounts on account of their laxative action, and the use of maltose itself is not feasible. In some cases we have used for this purpose a well-known "baby food" that is composed largely of maltose, with excellent results.

In all of these cases, but especially in the severer ones, the most rapid and certain *immediate* improvement is produced by the use of a fat-free milk, as we would expect. I believe it is a matter of indifference whether this fat-free milk is sweet, i. e., skimmed milk, or whether it is buttermilk. So uniformly certain is the action of buttermilk in these cases, as in nearly all other digestive disturbances of infancy, that its well-deserved popularity is easily understood, and we can see why Baginski considers its use in dyspepsia, for example, as "almost a specific, like antitoxin in diphtheria." After a considerable experience in the use of skimmed milk I am convinced that its action is the same as that of buttermilk, and that in both cases the striking results are due to the fact that we have a nearly fat-free food. If this is true then the use of skimmed milk has obvious advantages over that of buttermilk. It can be used in practically any strength, and is, of course, best prepared with the addition of sugar, and often also of flour, or a gruel, so that the absence of fat is compensated by the greater amount of carbohydrate in its place. The only objections to the use of skimmed milk in these cases of overfeeding are that it is rarely necessary to eliminate the fat so completely, and, secondly, it is often difficult to return from a fat-free to a fat-rich food in a reasonable length of time. Constipation and curds in the bowel movements quite regularly follow the addition of even a small amount of whole milk, i. e., of fat, and the change must usually be made very gradually.

2. Wheat flour, 50 g., are stirred up in 333 l. of cow's milk and run through a sieve. In a separate vessel 100 g. of Loefund's Malzsuppen extract is dissolved in 66 l. of lukewarm water. The two mixtures are then poured together and under constant stirring are brought to a boil.

Just what part food intervals play in the production of overfeeding is difficult to estimate. Of the therapeutic value of longer intervals than the customary two or three hours there can be doubt only in the minds of those who have not tried it. If cow's milk does not leave the healthy baby's stomach before the end of 2½ to 3 hours, and much later in the case of the sick one, then it would certainly seem indicated theoretically that the minimum interval should be 3 hours in health and 4 hours in pathologic conditions. A considerable and remarkably uniform experience has convinced us that the 4-hour interval is indicated in all pathologic cases and is preferable in all normal cases. Besides giving the stomach more rest and making the baby more comfortable, this long interval is a potent factor in preventing overfeeding, for it is manifestly more difficult to put enough food into a baby's stomach to overfeed it if that organ is filled only five or six times a day than if that process is repeated eight or ten times a day.

A word as to the ultimate results from feeding less fat. This consideration naturally limits itself to rickets and to the prevalent teaching as to its etiology, i. e., that these children get too little fat. There certainly is at the present time no real evidence that too small an amount of fat is an important factor in the causation of rickets, and there is an ever-increasing conviction that rickets can, and does, develop under our very eyes in spite of the fact that our cases are fed much fat—yes, often because of that fact (Holt and see babies O and F). Moreover, it is far from any one to recommend a small amount of fat. The child needs proportionately more of it early in the first year than at any other time in life, but that amount need never exceed an equal amount of proteid that the child can take with ease.

CONCLUSIONS.

1. Overfeeding is so prevalent in this country that it is the rule.

2. Overfeeding is second to no other factor in the pathogenesis of infant feeding.

3. Overfeeding presents an easily recognizable, definite symptom-complex.

4. The percentage method is inadequate to prevent overfeeding, the well-known feeding "schedules for an average healthy infant" of a given age fostering it by recommending excessive amounts; and, moreover, mere percentage leaves undetermined the amount of food the baby gets.

5. To feed rationally and especially to prevent overfeeding it is necessary to know how much food the baby is getting in proportion to its body weight, best expressed in terms of energy quotient.

6. The disturbing element in overfeeding with cow's milk is the fat.

7. Fat in excessive amounts regularly produces constipation—proteids never do so.

8. It is never necessary to give more fat than proteids of cow's milk.

9. The interval between feedings should be 4 hours.

6857 Wentworth Avenue.

14

PHYSIOLOGY AND PATHOLOGY OF THE DIGESTION OF FAT IN INFANCY

THEIR APPLICATION TO INFANT-FEEDING *

FRITZ B. TALBOT, M.D.

BOSTON

The food of infants comes in the main from two sources, human milk and cows' milk, the former being the natural food and the latter the best substitute we have when the former supply fails us. A brief description of these two milks is necessary for a clear conception of the subject.

The percentage of fat in cows' milk varies with the individual cow and the species. The milk of the ordinary grade cow, the Holstein or Ayrshire, contains 4 per cent. or less of fat, and that of the Jersey or Guernsey 4 per cent., or more, of fat. The fat is held in a coarser emulsion and separates more easily than that of human milk. There are other differences in the chemical and physical composition of the two milk-fats, but these will not be taken up in this paper.

Human milk normally contains, in round numbers, about 4 per cent. of fat; this percentage, however, may vary considerably in pathologic conditions, the extremes being 0.1 per cent.[1] and 13.7 per cent.[2] Every woman has a certain amount of fat to secrete in her milk, and, under like conditions, gives the same total day by day. The percentage of fat in the milk gradually increases in a certain definite curve from the beginning to the end of each nursing, the smallest percentages coming at the beginning and the highest at the end.[3] For example, the first part of the milk usually contains 2 per cent. of fat, and the last part 6 per cent. of fat; and the mixture of the whole amount of milk secreted in a single breast contains 4 per cent. of fat. The amount of milk secreted does not influence this curve otherwise than by making the ascent rapid or

---

* Read in the Section on Diseases of Children of the American Medical Association, at the Sixty-first Annual Session, held at St. Louis, June, 1910.

1. Moll: Ueber Fettvermehrung der Frauenmilch durch Fettzufuhr, nebst einem Beitrag für die Bedeutung der quantitativen Fettunterschiede für das Gedeihen der Brustkinder, Arch. f. Kinderh., xlviii, 161.

2. Forrest, M.: Ueber die Schwankungen im Fettgehalte der Frauenmilch und die Methodik der Milchentnahme zu Fettbestimmung, Arch. f. Kinderh., xlii, 1.

3. Engel: Ueber die quellen des Milch und Colostralfettes und über die bei der Milchsekretion wirkenden Kräfte, Arch. f. Kinderh., xliii, 194 and 204.

gradual.[4] Occasionally there is more fat in the first part of the milk than in the last part and the curve is just the reverse of the one just described.[5]

It is probable that the body-fat as well as the food-fat may be the source of milk-fat,[6] but it is not clear how the fat can be obtained from this source. Thiemich examined the literature on the influence of food on the quantity of fat secreted in the milk and came to the conclusion that a fat-free diet not only changed the quality of the fat, but also caused at the same time a diminution in the amount of fat in the milk. When a person is underfed, an increase in the fat in the food results in an increase in the fat in the milk,[7] but when large amounts of fat are added to a normal diet there is only a temporary increase in the amount of fat in the milk despite the excess of fat in the diet.[8] Ebstein[9] found in his clinic that many women with a fat-poor breast-milk would secrete more fat if they were given more fat in the food.

The amount of fat ingested by infants naturally depends on the amount in the milk, the amount of milk taken, and the part of the milk given. In asylums where one wet-nurse feeds two or more babies, the baby nursed first gets a milk relatively low in fat and the last one a milk relatively high in fat (possibly 6 per cent.). This fact is of great practical importance in feeding very delicate or sick babies, which are unable to digest large amounts of fat of any sort. Such babies may be given the first part of the milk which comes from the breast, or if desired skimmed drawn breast-milk. The wet-nurse is always instructed to nurse the sick baby first, and her own baby last; one of the reasons is that the sick baby does better on the weaker milk. In general, the amount of milk which

4. Aurnhammer: Ueber die Beziehungen zwischen Milch production und Fettgehalt der Milch, Arch. f. Kinderh., 1909, li, 160.

5. Engel: Zur Methodik der Fettbestimmung in der Frauenmilch und die Methodik der Milchentnahme zu Fettbestimmungen, Arch. f. Kinderh., 1906, xliii, 181.

6. Bendix: Ueber den Uebergang von Nahrungsfetten in die Frauenmilch. Deutsch. med. Wchnschr., 1888, No. 14; Thiemich: Ueber den Einfluss der Ernährung und Lebensweise auf die Zusammensetzung der Frauenmilch, Monatschr. f. Geburtsch. u. Gynäk., 1899, ix, No. 4; Gogitidse: Vom Uebergang des Nahrungsfettes in die Milch, Ztschr. f. Biol., xlv, 353; ibid., xlv, 403; Caspari: Ein Beitrag zur Frage nach der quelle des Milchfettes, Arch. f. Anat. u. Physiol. (Suppl.), 1899, 267; Engel: Ueber das Milchfett Stillender Frauen bei der Ernährung mit spezifischen Fetten, Wien. klin. Wchnschr., 1906, No. 29, p. 898.

7. Johannessen: Studien zur Sekretionsphysiologie der Frauenmilch, Jahrb. f. Kinderh., xxxix, 380.

8. Albert, F.: Ueber den Einfluss von Fettfütterung auf die Milchmenge und den Fettgehalt der Milch, Ref. Malys Jahresbr. f. Tierchemie, xxix, 253; Henriques and Hansen: Untersuchungen über die Fettbildung im Tierorganismus nach intensiver Fettfütterung, Malys Jahresbr. f. Tierchemie, xxix, 68.

9. Ebstein: Die Verdauungsstörungen im Säuglingsalter, Ebstein-Schwalbes Handb. d. prakt. Med., 1900, ii, 299.

a baby will take decreases, the richer it is in fat.[10] This, however, does not usually hold true of sick babies, because the amount of milk they take in twenty-four hours does not increase with the lowered percentage of fat, but only with the return to health.[1] Therefore, when a baby has an acute infection, such as pneumonia, the milk mixture should be diluted as a whole; the fat should not be removed entirely from the mixture, because it has twice as much food value as either the sugar or protein, and because in such cases the presence or absence of fat does not influence the amount of milk taken. If, on the other hand, a healthy infant is given 5 per cent. or more of fat in its food, it will usually take less and less, and if the amount of fat is diminished it will eat more. Many babies get 6, 10 and even 12 per cent. of fat in the food because the milk mixtures are prescribed ignorantly or made improperly. This could be avoided by estimating the amount of fat in the milk by the Babcock method. When normal babies are upset by fat, it is the rule rather than the exception to find that they are receiving more than 5 per cent. in the food.

PHYSIOLOGY

The physiology of the digestion of fat is not simple, but certain facts have been established which throw some light on what is happening to the fat in the gastro-intestinal canal.

STOMACH DIGESTION

The motility of the stomach is influenced by many things, such as the concentration and the character of the food.[11] Nothing has so much influence on the time required to empty the stomach as variations in the amounts of fat, which delay or hasten the evacuation of food into the duodenum. When there is a large amount of fat in the food, the food is kept in the stomach longer, and when a small amount, a shorter time.[12] According to some writers,[13] the stagnation of fat has a connection with the pathologic condition of pyloric stenosis. It has been demonstrated in animals that fat delays the secretion of hydrochloric acid. Cannon has shown that the cardiac orifice remains open as long as the reaction of the cardia is alkaline; as soon as the reaction becomes acid, the cardiac orifice closes and remains so until the neighboring food components become alkaline. The pyloric valve acts in a manner directly

10. Gregor: Der Fettgehalt der Frauenmilch und die Bedeutung der physiologischen Schwankungen desselben in bezug auf das gedeihen der Kinder, Samml. klin. Vort. von Volkmann, 1901, No. 302.

11. Clark: Am. Jour. Med. Sc., May and June, 1909.

12. Tobler and Bogen: Ueber die Dauer der Magenverdauung der Milch und ihre Beeinflussung durch verschiedene Factoren, Monatschr. f. Kinderh., vii, 12.

13. Tobler: Beobachtungen über die Zusammensetzung des Mageninhalts bei kongenitaler Pylorusstenose, Verhandl. d. Gesellsch. f. Kinderh., 1907, p. 411.

opposed to that at the cardia. When the material in the antrum pylori is acid, the valve opens and *vice versa.*[14]

These two facts may be applied clinically in explaining regurgitation due to too much fat in the food. Fat delays or inhibits the secretion of hydrochloric acid, and the cardiac sphincter, or lid to the stomach, remains open so that milk can be pushed back into the esophagus by the peristaltic movements of the stomach. If the amount of fat in the food is diminished, regurgitation stops, presumably because the normal amount of hydrochloric acid is again secreted, causing the entrance to the stomach to close and the outlet to open at the proper time.

It has been assumed until recently that only the pancreatic juices contain fat splitting ferments. Sedgewick[15] found a ferment in the stomach contents of infants which is capable of splitting in the test-tube one-fourth of the fat, and in the body about 12 per cent. of the fat ingested. Ibrahim[16] found this same ferment in the mucous membrane of the stomach of both the fetus and the new-born baby, and proved conclusively that there is a very powerful fat-splitting ferment which in a 9-months old baby that had died from pneumonia split in twenty-four hours over 40 per cent. of the fat in the yolk of an egg.

Nature, however, provides that too much fat shall not be set free in the stomach at one time. This is brought about in the following manner: When the casein of milk is coagulated in the stomach, practically all the fat is entangled in its meshes. The casein surrounding it must be digested before any more fat can be reached by the digestive juices, and thus only as much fat is set free as the progress of digestion warrants.

INTESTINAL DIGESTION

When the stomach digestion is complete, the food is discharged into the duodenum accompanied by organic or inorganic acids which start the secretion of the pancreatic juice and bile.[17] Ibrahim[18] substantiated Zweifel's[19] findings that the pancreas of the fetus contains a fat-splitting ferment and that the action of this ferment is increased materially by the

14. Cannon: Am. Jour. Physiol., 1908, xxiii, 105.

15: Sedgewick: Die Fettspaltung im Magen des Säuglings, Jahrb. f. Kinderh., 1906, lxiv, 194.

16. Ibrahim, J., and Kopec, T.: Die Magenlipase beim menschlichen Neugeborenen und Embryo, Ztschr. f. Biol., München., 1909, liii, 201.

17. Baylies and Starling: Jour. Physiol., 1902, xxviii, 325; 1903, p. 174.

Laqueux: Sur la présence et la localisation de la sécrétine dans l'intestin du nouveau-né et du fœtus humain, Compt. rend. Soc. de biol., 1896, lxi, 33.

Ibrahim and Gross: Zur Verdauungsphysiologie des Neugeborenen, Ref. in Deutsch. med. Wchnschr., 1908, No. 25, p. 1128.

18. Ibrahim: Neuere Forschungen über die Verdauungsphysiologie des Säuglingsalters. Verhandl. d. Gesellsch. f. Kinderh., 1908, p. 25.

19. Quoted by Ibrahim (see note 18).

addition of bile,[20] just as it is in the adult. Ibrahim was unable to find any fat-splitting ferment in the mucous membrane of the small intestine or large intestine.

ABSORPTION

There is considerable evidence that neutral fat (unsplit fat) is not absorbed as such into the intestinal wall: for example, hydrous wool fat and paraffin, which may be made into emulsions and cannot be split, are not absorbed.[21] It has also been shown by animal experimentation that the amount of fat in the chyme is directly proportional to the amount of fat split.[22] It is also taught by some that fat is absorbed both in the form of an emulsion and in the form of water-soluble soaps, neither view excluding the other. This latter view has been strengthened by the investigations of Kastle and Loevenhart[23] who demonstrated the almost universal presence of lipase in the tissues, and showed that this ferment could reverse its action. That is to say, it can synthesize or change soaps back into neutral fats as well as split neutral fats and form soaps. It is, therefore, possible that the soaps, which have been formed during digestion, may be changed during their passage through the intestinal epithelium by the reversible action of lipase back into neutral fat, because one finds neutral fat almost exclusively in the lymph-stream. Whitehead's[24] experiments on cats seem to strengthen this statement, because he found that butter-fat stained with Sudan III lost the stain during absorption (soaps will not stain with Sudan III): Sudan-staining fat was seen in the lumen of the intestine; none was seen in the intestinal epithelium and a Sudan-staining fat was again found in the lacteals of the villi.

A large part of the fat absorbed goes through the portal veins to the liver,[25] and the rest of it is carried by the lymphatics through the thoracic duct to the blood-stream, where it may be demonstrated by the ultra-microscope. It is called digestion lipemia and commences two to three hours after meals and disappears after seven to eight hours.[26] The

20. Uffenheimer: Physiologie des Magendarmkanals beim Säugling, Ergebn. d. inn. Med. u. Kinderh. 1908, No. 2, 321.

21. Connstein, W.: Arch. f. Anat. u. Physiol., 1899, p. 30; Henriques and Hansen: Zentralbl. f. Physiol., 1900, xiv, 313.

22. Levites: Ueber die Verdauung der Fette im tierischen Organismus, Ztschr. f. physiol. Chem., xlix, 273; liii, 349.

23. Kastle and Loevenhart: Am. Chem. Jour., 1900, xxiv, 491.

24. Whitehead, R. H.: A Note on the Absorption of Fat, Am. Jour. Physiol., 1909, xxiv, 294.

25. Weinland: Physiologie der Leber, Nagel's Handb. d. Physiol., ii, Part 2, 456

26. Ueber ultramikroskopische Blutuntersuchungen zur Zeit der Fettresorption bei Gesunden und Kranken, Wien. klin. Wchnschr., 1907, p. 851; Schelble: Untersuchungen über die Fettresorption des Säuglings, München. med. Wchnschr., 1908, No. 10; Bahrdt: Demonstration zur Untersuchung der Lipämie beim Säugling, Breslauer Tagung der Freien Vereinigung für wissenschaftliche Pädiatrie, 1908, Monatschr. f. Kinderh., vii, 107.

height of the curve is dependent on the amount of fat in the food, and the age and condition of the infant.

The absorption of fat is extraordinarily good in health in babies fed on cow's milk as well as in those fed on human milk; it is usually over 90 per cent. and may be as high as 98 per cent. of the fat ingested.[27] Eight per cent. to 11 per cent. of the ingested fat is absorbed in the upper part of the small intestine[22] and the absorption of fat is nearly complete at the ileocecal valve.[22] The large intestine is capable of absorbing fat in large amounts under special favorable conditions[28] but under ordinary circumstances absorption here is probably very little.

Estimation of the amount of fat in the stools of babies in starvation and in health makes it probable that the greater part of the fecal fat comes from the food and not from the intestinal secretions.[27] It is evident, therefore, that microscopic fat that is found in the stools gives us valuable information about the digestion. It is necessary first to know how much fat may normally be found in a stool. There is a comparatively large amount of fat present in the first days of life, and this amount gradually becomes less[29] as the babies grow older, decreasing from 50 per cent. of the dried stools to between 14 and 25 per cent. There is so much fat passed in the stools during the early weeks that it is practically impossible to ascertain by simple microscopic examination whether there is an excess or not. In later infancy less fat is present and therefore, microscopic examinations are of more value. In normal and in many pathologic conditions the greater part of the fat, 75 per cent. or more, is split by the digestive juices and bacteria into fatty acids and soaps.

A recapitulation of the facts given above is in brief as follows: most of the fat in cows' milk or human milk is in the form of neutral fat; in normal digestion this is partially split in the stomach by the gastric lipase. When the food is emptied into the duodenum, the remainder of the fat is presumably split by the pancreatic juice and saponified by the alkalies surrounding it. This digested fat is absorbed in the small intestine between the duodenum and the ileocecal valve and only the overflow fat goes into the large intestine with the intestinal secretions and bacteria. There the fecal remains are desiccated and eventually evacuated. The normal appearance of stools varies according to the food which the infant

27. Czerny-Keller: Der Kinder Ernährung, Ernährungsstörungen und Ernährungstherapie, Leipzig u. Wien, 1906, p. 263; Freund: Physiologie und Pathologie des Fettstoffwechsels im Kindesalter, Ergebn. d. inn. Med. u. Kinderh., 1909, ii, 139.

28. Hamburger, H. J.: Ueber die Resorption von Fette und Seife im Dickdarm, Engelmann's Arch., 1900, 433.

29. Talbot, F. B.: The Composition of Small Curds in Infants' Stools, Boston Med. and Surg. Jour., Jan. 7, 1909.

is taking. An excellent description of these stools may be found in a paper by Morse.[30]

STOOLS: MICROSCOPIC EXAMINATION

Much valuable information concerning the digestion of the various food components may be obtained from careful gross and microscopic examinations of the stools. This evidence is definite and accurate and is not misleading like the symptoms obtained from mothers and nurses. There are several quick methods of estimating the fat in the stool under the microscope.

1. The first consists in staining a bit of stool with saturated alcoholic solution of Sudan III. Neutral fat drops stain red. Fatty acids may be in the form of drops or crystals; the former always stain and the latter sometimes stain. Soap splinters and crystals never stain. The total fat in the slide may be estimated by adding a drop of glacial acetic acid to the already stained preparation, and warming it gently until it begins to bubble. This changes soaps into fatty acids which are red drops as long as they remain hot and often when they become cold. The error in this method comes from the fact that it is impossible to differentiate neutral fat and fatty acid drops. I have used this stain nearly three years.

2. The second method consists[31] in staining a scrap of stool with carbol-fuchsin and examining under the microscope. With this, neutral fat remains unstained, fatty acids stain a brilliant red and soaps a dull rose-red. Recently, I have used both stains, one on each of two cover-glass preparations, and thus obtained an estimate of the total amount of fat present, and the relative amounts of neutral fat, fatty acids, and soaps. Preparations from several parts of each stool should be examined in this way because the picture is apt to vary in stools which are not uniform.

The following terms are based on innumerable microscopic examinations of stools many of which were controlled by quantitative chemical analyses:

1. *Entire Digestion of Fat.*—Microscope, No. 7 objective, No. 3 eyepiece. Stain. alcoholic Sudan III. No fat in freshly stained specimen. One to three drops in field after acetic acid and heat.

2. *Normal Digestion.*—No fat or five to eight neutral fat-drops in the entire cover-glass in freshly stained specimen. Five to eight drops in a field after addition of acetic acid and heat. No change in amount of fecal residue.

3. *Slight Excess of Fat.*—No fat or two to four neutral fat-drops in a field. Eight to a dozen drops in a field after acetic acid and heat. No change in amount of fecal matter.

4. *Moderate Excess of Fat.*—No fat or six to eight neutral fat-drops in a field. More than twelve large drops after addition of acetic acid and heat. Considerable fecal material remains unchanged.

30. Morse, J. L.: The Stools in Infancy, New Orleans Med. and Surg. Jour., August, 1910.

31. Jacobson: Sur une réaction colorante des acides gras, Presse méd., 1906, No. 19, p. 147.

5. *Large Excess of Fat.*—No fat, or many fat-drops in a field. Practically the whole slide turns into fat-drops after acetic acid and heat, leaving very little fecal matter unchanged.

If there are any fat-drops in the original preparation it should always be stained with carbol-fuchsin to differentiate neutral fat from fatty acids. The entire cover-glass should be examined and it is usually better to examine preparations from several parts of the stool.

The following deductions can be drawn from these findings:

1. *Entire Digestion of Fat.*—It is always safe to increase the amount of fat in the food if so desired.

2. *Normal Digestion.*—It is usually safe to give more fat if necessary.

3. *Slight Excess of Fat.*—It is difficult to say how much significance should be attached to this. Probably very little.

4. *Moderate Excess of Fat.*—Without symptoms of indigestion it warns the observer to watch the fat more carefully. Yet, curiously enough, the percentage of fat may be increased without causing symptoms of indigestion and subsequently the stool may show "normal digestion." In case there are symptoms of indigestion, however, the microscope confirms our suspicions, and indicates the cause of the symptoms.

5. *Large Excess of Fat.*—This always means too much fat in the food and even if there are no symptoms, it is safer to decrease the amount of fat and examine the stool again. Usually there are symptoms of indigestion with this microscopic picture.

Fat is usually found in a normal stool in some form or other. Neutral fat appears as drops of different size and shape and sometimes as irregular flakes. When there is a very large amount it may be seen with the naked eye; it may be colorless, yellowish or slightly bile stained.

Free fatty acids may be indistinguishable from neutral fat drops except by staining with carbol-fuchsin. Neutral fat drops do not stain, while fatty acids stain; the more intense red the more acid they contain. When they are in the form of crystals, gentle warming will cause them to become drops, which recrystallize on cooling. Soaps may be amorphous or in the form of crystals. They are less shiny than fatty acids and may be stained yellow with bile coloring matter. The bushel-stained soap crystals may be in clumps and are shorter and thicker than fatty acids.

The microscopic examination of the stools of babies only occasionally gives information that the gross examination does not give, but it is a valuable control to inspection. In a few instances, the information is very surprising. It is important to bear in mind that even with considerable microscopic fat, a baby can remain perfectly happy, continue to gain and have no symptoms. This information, therefore, should be taken with reserve. In childhood, when foods other than milk are taken, small amounts of microscopic fat are of more significance. During the third year there should be only a few fat-drops on the whole slide in a normal digestion. More means a disturbance in the digestion of fat.

The closer a child comes to the adult type of diet, the more significance can be attached to information given by the microscope.

MACROSCOPIC EXAMINATION

The gross examination of the stool is the more important because it gives the most valuable information. The commonest abnormal constituents in a stool are soft, fatty curds. Soft curds are either flat white flakes (which look like undigested milk particles) or pin-head elevations; both may be present in the same stool and they are always associated with more or less mucus, which is stained green or yellow. About 60 per cent. of their dried substance is fat. These curds are usually present at one time or other in the stools of all nursing babies and are of no significance even with slight symptoms of indigestion. They are more important in the stools of bottle-fed babies. If there are no symptoms of indigestion and the baby is gaining and happy, the percentage of fat should not be changed, but the significance of these curds should be remembered. If there are symptoms of indigestion, loss of weight, and soft, fatty curds in the stools, there is too much fat in the food. When it is diminished, the curds disappear, the baby becomes happy and gains weight.[32]

These curds should not be confused with tough casein curds, which are white or bile-stained, bean-like masses of varying size and shape. They may be easily differentiated from the fat curd by their physical characteristics. The latter will smooth out on a napkin while the former will not; casein hardens in liquor formaldehydi (formalin) while fat does not. I recently proved [32] by the precipitin reaction that the protein in these curds is cow-casein. They contain varying amounts of neutral fat which is entangled in the meshes of the casein when it coagulates in the stomach. This fat has not been acted on by the digestive juices because it is protected by a coating of casein. It is present in larger or smaller amounts, according to the percentage of fat in the milk and may, therefore, be considered accidental.[33]

Soap stools are very light yellow or white, usually smooth, sometimes salve-like, at other times dry and brittle. The shiny appearance of the fresh surface suggests fat. They are composed almost entirely of soap. Fifty per cent. to 70 per cent. of their dried substance may be fat. They often occur in constipation due to too much fat in the food and disappear when the fat is replaced by other food components. They may be the precursors of a fat diarrhea and if their full significance is not appreciated, they may eventually become part of the clinical picture of infantile atrophy.

---

32. Talbot, F. B.: Casein Curds in Infants' Stools. Biological Proof of Their Casein Origin, Arch. Pediat., June, 1910.

33. Talbot: The Composition of Large Curds in Infants' Stools. Boston Med. and Surg. Jour., June 11, 1908.

Fat stools are very bright yellow (like Indian meal), oily and soft. They are composed of large amounts of fats, a good proportion of which is in the form of neutral fat or fatty acid. When one of these stools is placed on paper and then removed, there remains behind a grease-spot which will not absorb water (oiled paper). They are usually accompanied by very severe symptoms. Fat should be removed entirely from the milk for a time and very frequently these babies cannot be saved without human milk.

METABOLISM

Most of the figures offered us by metabolism experiments are obtained by the Rosenfeld method of extracting fat, and very recently by the Kumagawa and Suto method. These and other modern methods of fat extraction have been given in more or less detail in the appendix of this paper. Despite the fact that the figures so obtained may not be absolutely correct, I believe that they are of great relative value and help to clear up many of the cases of perverted digestion. While they do not say the final word on the subject, they lead to a more intelligent grasp of the pathology of digestion. This paper does not pretend to consider the rôle of the intestinal flora in normal and abnormal digestion, but I believe that they are of great significance in certain conditions and that they will be found to influence metabolism. For example, Kendall[34] has shown that two factors are necessary for fermentation: a carbohydrate food, and fermentative bacteria; in like manner putrefaction cannot take place without protein plus putrefactive bacteria. Fermentative bacteria cannot act on protein, and putrefactive bacteria cannot act on carbohydrate. It is very difficult, therefore, to draw any conclusions in a subject which is complicated by so many factors. The problems of digestion depend on the balance of all the factors concerned and when the normal balance is upset by any one or many factors, we have a pathologic condition.

The significance of fatty acids and soaps is as yet unknown; probably they are of very little significance in the questions of absorption. Freund (quoted above) has shown that an acid dyspeptic stool can be changed in many instances to a formed "soap stool" by a relative increase in the amount of casein, while an alkaline soap stool can be changed into an acid stool by a relative increase in the amount of carbohydrates. Coincident with the change from an acid to an alkaline stool (according to Kendall) there is a change of the intestinal flora; the acid-forming bacteria which previously predominated are replaced by the putrefactive group of bacteria. When an alkaline stool is made acid the reverse takes

---

34. Kendall: Boston Med. and Surg. Jour., 1911, clxiv (to appear in March). Read before Suffolk District Medical Society.

place. Bahrdt[35] has recently shown that babies passing "soap stools" have diminished powers of absorption and that they lose more fat than was formerly taught. He found the absorption of fat (Kumagawa and Suto method) as follows:

Name of Baby.	Age, Months.	Weight, Gm.	Fat absorbed. Per cent.	Character of Stools.
Schröder, 7 days	9	7470	82.4	Soap stools
Schüler, 7 days	2	3945	83.2	Mostly soap stools
Weiss, Ia, 5 days....	9/10	3750	81.9	Soap stool
Weiss, Ib	9/10	3750	86.0	Soap stool
Weiss II, 8 days.....	10	3900	93.0	Normal stools
Breast and skim milk.				

The fat absorption in these babies with soap stools is, therefore, considerably less than that of normal infants. There is, however, not such a loss of fat as in diarrhea. There is a loss of magnesium and calcium[36] in these soap stools and there is no loss of sodium and potassium. If the stools become acid and change into soft fatty curds there is no longer a loss of calcium and magnesium, but there is a loss of sodium and potassium. With this change comes an increased loss of fat from the body.[36] If this condition becomes more pronounced with diarrhea, there is a considerable loss of fat with the alkalies; the baby loses weight and takes on the appearance of "infantile atrophy."[37] Such babies can only be saved by human milk.[38]

Biedert[39] and Demme[40] designated severe chronic disturbances of digestion in which the stools contained very large amounts of fat as "fat diarrhea." The latter had one such case which came to autopsy and was found to have disease of the pancreas. Hecht[41] and Reuss[42] have reported cases of congenital obliteration of the bile-duct with normal pancreas, in which only one-half of the fat was split. I examined the stools

---

35. Bahrdt, H.: Untersuchungen über das Symptom der Seifenbildung und die Ausscheidung der Basen im Darm des Säuglings, Jahrb. f. Kinderh., 1910, lxxi, 249.

36. Meyer, L. F.: Jahrb. f. Kinderh., April, 1910, p. 379.

37. Finkelstein: Ueber Alimentäre Intoxikation III, Jahrb. f. Kinderh., 1908, lxviii, 521 and 692.

38. Finkelstein's so-called alimentary intoxication will not be considered in this paper because I believe that the majority of cases which clinically come under this category are not diseases of metabolism, but are bacterial infections of the gastro-intestinal canal, and that the physiologic powers of digestion are so lowered by the disease that the various food components are not digested.

39. Biedert: Jahrb. f. Kinderh., 1879, xiv, 336; ibid. 1888, xxviii, p. 21.

40. Demme: Jahrb. über die Tätigkeit des Jennerschen Kinderspitals in Berlin, 1874 and 1877; quoted from Hecht, Die Faeces des Säuglings, etc., p. 128.

41. Hecht: Die Faeces des Säuglings und Kindes, Berlin-Wien, 1910, p. 128.

42. Reuss: Case of Obliterated Bile Duct (congenital) Reported in Discussion, Jahrb. f. Kinderh., December, 1908, 729.

of a baby, the autopsy on which showed biliary cirrhosis[43] and a patent bile-duct, and found a similar type of stool.

Tuberculous peritonitis in babies is primarily a disease of the lymphatic system and when the mesenteric glands become caseous they form a dam beyond which the fat cannot pass. It has been shown earlier in this paper that part of the fat is normally carried by the lymphatics to the blood stream. If this road is blocked with tuberculous tissue, it is reasonable that some of the fat should be lost from the body. I have found large amounts of fat in the stools of such babies. Hecht believes that 80 per cent. of the fat in the stool should be split, and considers that great divergence from this amount means either trouble with the bile or pancreatic juice. He reports a seven months, premature baby which was only able to split 53 per cent. of the fat, and considers this to be due to weak action of the pancreatic fat-splitting enzyme, which presumably is not completely developed. Finizio[44] explains a large amount of fat in the stool of an 11-months-old baby with mumps by probable trouble in the pancreas.

Czerny[45] believes that babies with an exudative diathesis can be harmed by fat. He finds that an increase in the amount of fat in the food will bring eruptions out on the skin. Steinitz and Weigert[46] have apparently proved the correctness of this assumption by a metabolism experiment.

There is no doubt that large amounts of fat can do a great deal of harm to most babies. Such babies come under two classes—those which have a normal digestion and are unable to digest excessive amounts of fat, and those which have diminished powers of digestion and are unable to digest normal amounts of fat. So much attention has been paid to the few babies that are unable to digest fat that we are apt to forget that most babies can digest fat within reasonable limits. L. F. Meyer[47] has recently shown in Finkelstein's clinic that when fat is increased in the food of normal healthy babies there is no loss of fat, or salts from the body. This dispels, in a very convincing way, the false impression that normal babies are unable to digest fat. John Howland of New York showed in a recent investigation (not yet published) that a baby could be fed on large quantities of fat without symptoms of indigestion and without acidosis. In my experience, it has been safe to increase the

43. Morse, J. L.: Jaundice in the New-Born, Boston Med. and Surg. Jour., Feb. 24, 1910.

44. Finizio: A Case of Fat Diarrhea Following Mumps, Pediat., September, 1909; Rev. in Jahrb. f. Kinderh., 1910, lxxi, 205.

45. Czerny: Zur Kenntnis der exudative Diathese, Part 1, Monatschr. f. Kinderh., 1906, iv, 1; ibid. Part 2, 1908, vi, 1; ibid. Part 3, 1909, vii, 1.

46. Steinitz and Weigert: Monatsch. f. Kinderh., 1910, ix, 385.

47. Meyer, L. F.: Jahrb. f. Kinderh., April, 1910, p. 379.

percentage of fat gradually up to 4 per cent. in most normal babies whose digestive powers have not previously been lowered by gross errors in feeding or by infection, and that they develop normally without any of the signs or symptoms of fat indigestion so long as their hygiene is perfect and they have no intercurrent infection.

APPENDIX

METHODS OF ESTIMATION OF FAT IN FECES

There is no such thing as a theoretically perfect method of estimating fat in the feces. The methods employed may be grouped under two heads: 1. Extraction methods which attempt to obtain all the substances soluble in ether. 2. Saponification methods, in which the higher fatty acids are set free by saponification from the various combinations in which they occur, separated as far as possible from the other products of the action of alkali used, and weighed as fatty acids.

EXTRACTION METHODS

These methods estimate all the substances soluble in ether without considering what form the fat was in. The criterion in determining the value of the particular method under consideration has been the gross yield of substance soluble in ether. The method which has been taken as a standard in recent years is that of Rosenfeld, because it gave higher yields than other methods of substances soluble in ether. This method has been criticized because the substances weighed contain nitrogen and phosphorus and a low percentage of fatty acid. I used a modification of this method[48] as follows:

The feces are weighed, thoroughly mixed with 95 per cent. alcohol and dried at 43-45 C., transferred to a desiccator, and dried to constant weight. A weighed portion of the dried feces is placed in a paper capsule and boiled in absolute alcohol for one-half hour. The capsule is then transferred to a Soxhlet tube and extracted eighteen hours with chloroform. The combined absolute alcohol and chloroform extracts are evaporated to dryness, and the residue from each extracted with petroleum ether. The petroleum ether is then filtered and the filter paper thoroughly washed with warm petroleum ether until the wash ether shows no trace of fat, by evaporation on a watch glass. The filtrate is evaporated to constant weight. This weight is recorded as representing the quantity of neutral fat and fatty acid in the weighed portion of dry stool.

The dishes used for the evaporation of the alcohol and chloroform extracts from the first extraction are washed with hot 3 per cent. hydrochloric acid alcohol. The filter paper, used for filtering the petroleum ether in the first step, is added to the capsule from which the neutral fat and fatty acid have been extracted and boiled one-half hour under a reflux condenser in 3 per cent. hydrochloric alcohol to which the HCl alcohol washings from the dishes, mentioned in the first step, are added. Next, it is boiled one-half hour with absolute alcohol; the combined capsule and filter paper are then transferred to a Soxhlet tube and extracted for eighteen hours. The hydrochloric acid absolute alcohol and chloroform extracts are evaporated separately, the residue in each is taken up in petroleum ether and the combined petroleum ether extract is filtered. The filtrate is evaporated to constant weight; this represents soaps.

The neutral fat and fatty acids (the fat first weighed) are dissolved in equal parts of absolute alcohol and sulphuric ether and the acidity determined by titrating against decinormal alcoholic sodium hydrate solution, using phenolphthalein as an indicator.

Kumagawa and Suto[49] found that the solvent which gave the largest yield of substances soluble in ether was alcohol used near its boiling point in a continu-

48. Boston Med. and Surg. Jour., Jan. 11, 1908.

49. Kumagawa and Suto: Ein neues Verfahren zur quantitativen Bestimmung des Fettes und der unverseifbaren Substanzen im tierischen Material nebst der Kritik einiger gebräuchlichen Methoden, I, Biochem. Ztschr. 1908, viii, 212.

ous extraction apparatus. This explains why the Rosenfeld method and its modifications obtain higher yields of fat than other methods. The Rosenfeld method, however, is the best one yet devised to estimate the relative proportion of neutral fat, fatty acids and soaps.

Folin and Wentworth[50] criticize this method because they have observed that prolonged chloroform extraction brings away materials with a distinct fecal odor, and they say that the best method for extraction is that which takes out the smallest amount and not that which extracts the largest amount. They have devised a method which apparently has many advantages over the Rosenfeld method. It is briefly as follows:

One gram of very finely powdered feces is weighed into a fat-free paper capsule, placed in an extraction apparatus and boiled twenty hours with an ethereal hydrochloric acid solution. The ether is then distilled off and with it goes the hydrochloric acid. A low boiling petroleum ether (Ligroin) is added and allowed to stand over night. This solution is filtered the next day into a weighed beaker and dried at a temperature of 95 C. for five hours. It is then dried and weighed as neutral fat and fatty acids. The next step is a new departure in chemistry, according to Folin and Wentworth, and is very important. The fat is dissolved in benzol, .5 per cent. alcoholic phenolphthalein added and it is heated almost to boiling. It is then immediately titrated against N/10 sodium alcoholate (made by dissolving 2.3 gm. metallic sodium in one liter absolute alcohol and standardized); 1 c.c. of this=28.4 m.gm. stearic acid. This method of titration undoubtedly has a great advantage over all that have been devised thus far.

SAPONIFICATION METHOD

Lieberman-Szekely described a method of determining the fat in the stool by first saponifying it and then splitting with acid and extracting with ether. This extract was purified with petroleum ether. This method does not estimate the fat in the stool, but all the higher non-volatile fatty acids in various combinations: and according to Kumagawa-Suto the fat may be reckoned from this by multiplying by the factor 1.046.

Kumagawa and Suto's[49] method gives the highest results of all methods and has been controlled by very accurate and painstaking experiments. It is as follows:

Two to 5 gm. of powdered feces are mixed in a beaker with 25 c.c. 5 per cent. NaOH(20NaOH in 100 c.c.) and heated two hours over a water bath. The beaker should be covered with a watch glass during this process. During the saponification the mixture is stirred now and then with a glass rod. After about ten minutes the powder dissolves and there are small flocculi left behind. After about two hours, the solution is transferred, still hot, into a hermetically closed separating funnel with a capacity of 250 c.c. The beaker is washed two or three times with about 5 c.c. warm water. Next the solution is acidified with 30 c.c. 20 per cent. H_2SO_4. After cooling well 70 to 100 c.c. ether is added and shaken well. A precipitate remains between the layers of solution. The clear water is decanted after separation. Then the brown colored ether is carefully decanted into a beaker. The funnel with the precipitate is washed twice with ether; it is then dissolved and shaken again with 30 to 50 c.c. ether and to that is added the strongly acid water of the first shaking, and it is again well shaken. The reaction is then acid and the remaining fatty acid is dissolved in the ether. These ether extracts are united, evaporated and again taken up with absolute ether, filtered through asbestos and evaporated. This extract, which contains coloring matter, fatty acid, lactic acid and other components, is heated at 50 C. first and extracted with petroleum ether. If this solution is milky it is allowed to stand one hour and then filtered through asbestos, dried at 50 C. and weighed. More detail concerning this method may be obtained by referring to Kumagawa and Suto's original article in which there is a vast amount of experimental data and criticism of other methods. In it the bibliography concerning the extraction of

50. Folin and Wentworth: Determination of Fat and Fatty Acid, Jour. Biol. Chem., June, 1910.

fat from the animal tissue is very complete. These findings have been substantiated by Inaba.[51]

Bahrdt, Edelstein, Langstein and Welde[52] have used a new method for the quantitative estimation of the free volatile fatty acids in the feces. This method is based on a method by W. Steinkpf which used vacuum distillation and steam for extraction. The method in brief is as follows:

A weighed amount of fresh feces was distilled in a temperature of 60 C. for two hours, with steam drawn through on the one side by a vacuum on the other. The distillate is titrated against N/10 sodium hydrate, with phenolphthalein as an indicator. The amount of acid present is estimated in terms of decinormal acid. The temperature of the water bath during the whole distillation should be 60 C. Generally the distillation goes well if there are 600 to 900 c.c. distillate in one hour. The original article should be consulted for detail of the method and the apparatus necessary.

This brief description of the newer methods of fat and fatty acid extraction has been added so that those who have a desire to commence metabolism work on babies will be able to choose for themselves and go back to the original sources. I feel that the last word has not been said, and that it is necessary to extract all feces, both by the Kumagawa and Suto method, and by some modification of the Rosenfeld method. The method offered by Folin and Wentworth is still in the experimental stage and the writers are "now working to perfect it."

311 Beacon Street.

BIBLIOGRAPHY

The following additional references cover as many of the important works on this subject as possible, without making it unwieldy. An attempt has been made to give only those references which are up to date and have stood the test of time.

Abderhalden, E., and Brahm, D.: Ist das am Aufbau der Körperzellen beteiligte Fett in seiner zusammensetzung von der Art des aufgenommenen Nahrungsfettes abhängig? Ztschr. f. physiol. Chem. Strass., 1910, lxv, 330.

Adler, Max: Contributions to the Question of Fat Absorption under Pathological Conditions in Men and Animals, Ztschr. f. klin. Med., 66, p. 302.

Amberg, S., and Morrill, P.: A Study of the Metabolism of a Breast-fed Infant with Special Reference to the Ammonia Co-efficient. Proc. Am. Soc. Biol. Chem., 1908, p. 35.

Ballantyne: Quoted by Savonnat, Arch. de Méd. des Enf., 1906, xi, No. 1.

Bendix: Ein Stoffwechselversuch beim atrophischen Säugling, Engelmann's Arch., 1899 (Suppl.), p. 206.

von Bergmann, S., and Reicher, K.: Zur Pary'schen Hypothese der Fettbildung in der Darmwand, Ztschr. f. exp. Path. u. Therap., Berl., 1908-1909, v, 742.

Biedert: Kinderernährung im Säuglingsalter, ed. 4, Stuttgart, 1900.

Biernatzki: Ueber den Einfluss der überfetteten Nahrung auf den Magendarmkanal und den Stoffwechsel, Zentralbl. f. Physiol. u. Path., 1907, N. F. 2, p. 401.

Birk: Ueber den Magnesiumumsatz des Säuglings, Jahr. f. Kinderh., 1907, lxvi, 300; Untersuchungen über den Einfluss des Phosphorlebertrans auf den Mineralstoffwechsel gesunder und rachitischer Säuglinge, Monatschr. f. Kinderh., 1908, vii, 450.

Blauberg: Experimentelle und kritische Studien über Säuglings feces, Berlin. Hirschwald, 1897.

Boldyreff: Ueber den selbständigen und künstlich hervorgerufenen Uebergang von Pancreassaft in den magen und über die Bedeutung dieser Erscheinung für die praktische Medizin, Zentralbl. f. Physiol. u. Path., 1908, N. F. 3, p. 209.

Budin: The Nursling, Caxton Pub. Co., London, 1907.

51. Inaba: Biochem. Ztschr., 1908, viii, 352.

52. Bahrdt, Edelstein, Langstein and Welde: Untersuchung über die Pathogenese der Verdauungsstörungen im' Säuglingsalter, Ztschr. f. Kinderh., 1910, i, No. 2, 139.

Camerer, Sen.: Das Energiegesetz in der Menschlichen Physiologie, Jahrb. f. Kinderh., 1907, lxvi, 129.

Camerer, jun.: Untersuchung über die Ausscheidung des Milchfettes, Verhandl. d. Gesellsch. f. Kinderh., 1906, p. 135.

Camus, J., and Nicloux: Contribution à l'étude de la digestion des graisses dans les differentes segments du tube digestif, Compt. rend. Soc. de biol., 1910, lxviii, 619; Abstr. in Chem. Abstracts, 1910, iv, No. 17; Digestion intra-gastrique des graisses sans l'influence de la lipaséidine. Compt. rend. Soc. de biol., 1910, lxviii, 680.

Chacuet: Recherches sur l'absorption des graisses, etc., Thèse de Paris.

Cohnheim: Physiologie der Verdauung, in Nagel's Handb. d. Physiol., ii, 516.

Cohnheim, O., and Dreyfuss, S. L.: Zur Physiologie und Pathologie der Magenverdauung, Ztschr. f. physiol. Chem., 1908, lviii, 50.

Connstein: Ueber fermentative Fettspaltung. Asher-Spiro, Ergebn. d. Physiol., 1904, i, 194.

Croner, W.: Versuche über Resorption von Fetten im Dünndarm, Biochem. Ztschr., 1910, xxiii, 97.

Czerny: Ueber die Beziehungen zwischen Mästung und skrofulösen Hautaffectionen, Monatschr. f. Kinderh., 1904, ii, 57; Die Exudative Diathese, Jahrb. f. Kinderh., 1905, lxi, 198.

Dormeyer, C.: Die quantitative Bestimmung von Fetten, seifen und Fettsäuren in thierischen Organen, Pflüger's Arch., 1897, lxv, 90.

Emmett: The Determination of Fatty Matter in Normal Feces by Ether and Carbon. Tetrachlorid. Jour. Am. Chem. Soc., June, 1909, p. 693.

Engel: Ueber das Fett der Frauenmilch, Ztschr. f. phys. Chem., 1905, xliv, 354; Zur Secretions physiologie des Milchfettes, Med. Klinik, 1905, No. 24.

Engel: Nahrungsfett und Milchfett. Verhandl. d. Gesellsch. f. Kinderh. in Meran, 1906, No. 22.

Engel: Zur Kenntnis der Magensaftsekretion beim Säugling, Arch. f. Kinderh., 1908, xlix, 16.

Engel and Plauth: Art und Menge des Fettes in der Nahrung Stillender Frauen und die Wirkung seiner Entziehung auf das Milchfett, München. med. Wchnschr., 1906, p. 1158.

Faust and Talquist: Ueber die Ursachen der Bothryocephalusanämie. Schmiedeberg's Arch., 1907, lvii, 380.

Faust and Schmincke: Ueber chronische ölsäurevergiftung, Schmiedeberg's Arch., 1908, p. 171; Festschrift für Schmiedeberg.

Finizio, S.: Sulla digestione gastrica dei grassi nel lattante. Pediat., Napoli. 1910, q. s., viii, 1-24; Rev. in Jahrb. f. Kinderh., April, 1910, 503.

Finkelstein: Zur diatetischen Behandlung des konstitutionellen Säuglingsekzms, Med. Klinik, 1907, 1098.

Frank: Zur Lehre von der Fettresorption, Ztschr. f. Biol., 1898, xxxvi, 568.

Freund, W.: Bemerkungen zu der Arbeit von P. Reyler über den Fettgehalt der Frauenmilch. Jahrb. f. Kinderh., 1905, lxi, 900; Zur Wirkung der Fettdarreichung auf den Säuglingsstoffwechsel, Jahrb. f. Kinderh., 1905, N.F., lxi, 36; Milchnährschaden und Fettresorption. Vortrag auf der Dresdner Tagung der freien Verseining für wissenschaftliche Pädiatrie, Ref. Monatsch. f. Kinderh., 1908, vi, 54; Säuren und Basen im Urin kranker Säuglinge. Monatschr. f. Kinderh., 1903, i, 230; Zur Kenntnis des Fet und Kalkstoffwechsels im Säuglingsalter, Biochem. Ztschr., 1909, xvi, 453.

Friedenthal: Ueber die Permeabilität der Darmwandung, etc., Engelmann's Arch., 1902, 149 and Supp., 449.

Gilkin, W.: Untersuchungen zur Methode der Fettbestimmung im thierischen Material, Pflüger's Arch., 1903, xcv, 107.

Gillet: Le trouble de la sécrétion pankreatigue chez les enfants. Quoted by Czerny-Steinitz in Von Noorden's Handbook, Pathology of Metabolism, iii, 833. W. T. Keener & Co., Chicago, 1909.

Glaessner and Singer: The Liver in Respect to Absorption of Fat, Med. Klin., 1909, No. 51, 1917.

Grosser: Der Chemismus bei Pylorusstenose, Monatschr. f. Kinderh., vii, 106.

Hall, Walker: Examination of Fat in Feces, Canadian Pract. and Rev., March, 1908.

Hamburger, H. J.: Sind es ausschliesslich die Chylusgefässe welche die Fettresorption besorgen, Engelmann's Arch., 1900, 554.

Hamsik, A.: Reversible Wirkung der Darmlipase, Ztschr. f. physiol. Chem., 1909, ix, 1.

Hartley, P.: On the Nature of Fat Contained in the Liver, Kidney and Heart, Jour. Physiol., 1907, xxxvi, 17; Jour. Physiol., 1909, xxxviii, 353.

Hartley and Mavrogordato: Fat in Normal and Pathological Livers, Jour. Path. Bact., 1908, xii, 371.

Hecht: Ueber das Verhalten der Eiweiss und Fett Spaltenden Fermente im Säuglingsalter, Wien. klin. Wchnschr., 1908, 1551; Untersuchungen über die Fettresorption auf Grund der chemischen Zusammensetzung der Fette, Jahrb. f. Kinderh., 1905, lxii, 612; Vorschlag einer klinischen Prüfung der Fettresorption, Wien. klin. Wchnschr., 1907, No. 17; Ueber die Bedeutung der Seifenstühle im Säuglingsalter. München. med. Wchnschr., 1908, 1010; Das Verhalten der Fettsäurebildung im Darminhalt des Säuglings, München. med. Wchnschr., 1910, lvii, 62.

Heinsheimer: Experimentelle Untersuchungen über fermentative fettspaltung im Magen. Deutsche med. Wchnschr., 1906, p. 1194.

Heubner and Rubner: Die natürliche Ernährung eines Säuglings, Ztschr. f. Biol., 1898, xxxvi, p. 1; Die künstliche Ernährung eines normalen und eines atrophischen Säuglings, Ztschr. f. Biol., 1899, xxxviii, p. 315.

Hoffmann, E.: Ueber mikroskopische Fäcesuntersuchungen, Monatschr. f. Kinderh., 1907, vi, p. 662; Fermentuntersuchungen und Fettresorption beim Säugling, Jahrb. f. Kinderh., 1910, xxii, 280.

Howland: Fat Incapacity in Infants and Children, Arch. Pediat., 1908, xxv, 225.

Hüssy: Zur Kenntniss der Acidosis im Kindesalter, Zentralbl. f. d. ges. Physiol. u. Path. d. Stoffwechsels, N. F., 1906, p. 1.

Ibrahim, J.: Zur Verdauungsphysiologie des menschlichen Neugeborenen, Ztschr. f. physiol. Chem., 1910, lxiv, 95.

Jakobson, G.: Graisses neutres et acides gras dans les selles des nourissons, Compt. rend. Soc. de biol., 1909, lxvii, 145.

Jäckle: Ueber die Zusammensetzung der menschlichen Fette, Ztschr. f. physiol. Chem., 1902, xxxvi, 52.

Joannovies and Pick: Rôle of the Liver in Resorption of Fat, Wien. klin. Wchnschr., xxiii, 673.

Johannessen and Wang: Studien über die Ernährungs physiologie des Säuglings, Ztschr. f. physiol. Chem., 1898, xxiv, 482.

Loevenhart: On the Relation of Lipase to Fat Metabolism Lipogenesis. Am. Jour. Phys., 1902, vi, 331.

Keller: Phosphor und Stickstoff im Säuglingsorganismus, Arch. f. Kinderh., 1900, xxix, 1; Fettunsatz und Acidose, Monatschr. f. Kinderh., 1903, i, 234; Zur Kenntnis der Gastroenteritis im Säuglingsalter, II Mitt. Ammionakausscheidung, Jahrb. f. Kinderh., N. F., xliv, 25.

Knöpfelmacher: Untersuchungen über das Fett im Säuglingsalter und über das Fettsklerem, Wien. klin. Wchnschr., 1897, 228; Die Ausscheidung flüssiger Fette die Faeces und die Resorption des Milchfettes bei Kindern, Wien. klin. Wchnschr., 1897, 695.

Knöpfelmacher and Lehndorf: Das Hautfett im Säuglingsalter, Ztschr. f. Exper. Path. u. Therap., 1906, ii, 133.

Krause, P.: Lipämie im Coma diabeticum, Verhandl. d. Kongresses f. inn. Med., München, 1906, xxiii, 521.

Lange and Berend: Stoffwechselversuche an dyspeptischen Säuglingen, Jahrb. f. Kinderh., 1897, xliv, 339.

Langstein and Lempp: Die Bedeutung des Fettes für die Verdauung der Milcheiweisskörper, Monatsch. f. Kinderh., 1907-8, vi, 55.

Langstein and Meyer: Die Acidose im Kindesalter, Part I, Jahrb. f. Kinderh., 1905, lxi, 454; Part II, Jahrb. f. Kinderh., 1906, lxiii, 30; Säuglingsernährung und Säuglingsstoffwechsel, Ein Grundriss für den praktischen Arzt, Wiesbaden, 1910.

Langstein and Steinitz: Zucker und Lactaseausscheidung beim magendarmkranken Säugling, Hofm. Beitr., 1905, vii, 575.

Langstein and Niemann: Ein Beitrag zur Kenntniss der Stoffwechselvorgänge in den ersten vierzehn Lebenstagen normaler und frühgeborener Säuglinge, Jahrb. f. Kinderh., 1910, lxxi, 604.

Laves: Untersuchung des Fettes der Frauenmilch, Ztschr. f. physiol. Chem., 1894, xix, 369.

Leathes, J. B.: Functions of the Liver in Relation to Metabolism of Fats, Lancet, London, 1909, clxxvi, 594.

Leathes and Wedell: Desaturation of Fatty Acids in the Liver, Jour. of Physiol., 1909, 38 Proc., xxxviii and xl.

Lehndorf: Ueber das Magenfellpolster der Säuglinge, Jahrb. f. Kinderh., 1907, lxvi, 286.

Lewinsky: Die gewinnung des Pankreassekretes aus dem Magen und ihre diagnostische Verwertbarkeit, Deutsch. med. Wchnschr., 1908, 1582.'

Liebermann and Székely: Eine neue Methode der Fettbestimmung in Futtermitteln, Fleisch, Koth, etc., Pflüger's Arch., 1898, lxxii, 360.

Litmanowicz and Müller: Ueber das Verhalten des Ptyalins unter normalen und krankhaften Bedingungen, Zentralbl. f. d. gesamte Phys. u. Path. d. Stoffwechsels, 1909, No. 3.

London: Zum Chemismus der Verdauung im tierischen Körper VII Mitteil. Ein reiner Pylorusfistelhunde und die Frage über gastrolipase. Ztschr. f. physiol. Chem., 1906-1907, l, 125; ibid. 1909, lx, 191; Zum Studium der allmählichen Fortbewegung Verdauung und Resorption der Eiweisstoffe, Fette, und Kohlenhydrate bei einzelner Darreichung und bei der Darreichung in verschiedenen Kombinationen, Ztschr. f. physiol. Chem., 1909, lx, 194.

Magnus-Levy: Die Acetonkörper. Argebn. d. inn. Med. und Kinderh., 1908, i, 352.

Meyer, L. F.: Beitrag zur Kentness der Unterschiede zwischen natürlicher und künstlicher Ernährung, Verhand. d. Gesellsch. f. Kinderh., 1906, 122; Zur Kenntniss des Mineralstoffwechsels im Säuglingsalter, Biochem. Ztschr., 1908, xii, 422; Zur Kenntniss des Stoffwechsels bei der alimentären Intoxikation, Jahrb. f. Kinderh., 1907, lxv, 585; Zur Kenntniss der Acetonurie bei den Infectionskrankheiten der Kinder, Jahrb. f. Kinderh., 1905, lxi, 438; Saltzstoffwechsel beim normalen und ekzematösen Säugling, Monatschr. f. Kinderh., 1908-9, vii, 104; Die Bedeutung der Mineralsalze bei den Ernährungs Störungen des Säuglings, Jahrb. f. Kinderh., 1910, lxxi, 1.

Moll: Fat Content of the Mucus Membrane of the Small Intestine During Absorption of Fat, Zentralbl. f. Physiol., 1909, xxiii, 290.

Monges, J.: Soap in Feces, Compt. rend. soc. de biol., 1909, lxvii, 596.

Mottram, V. H.: Fatty Infiltration of the Liver in Hunger, Jour. Physiol., 1909, xxxviii, 281; A Method of Fatty Acid Extraction, Jour. Physiol., 1910, xl, 122.

Müller, Erich: Beitrag zur Frage der natürlichen Nutzstoffe der Frauenmilch, Berl. klin. Wchnschr., 1908, No. 22.

Munk, I.: Ueber Darmresorption nach Beobachtungen an einer Lymphfistel Menschen, Arch. Anat. Physiol. (Physiol. Abth.), 1890, 376; Zur Lehre von der Spaltung und Resorption der Fette, Arch. Anat. Physiol. (Physiol. Abth.), 1890, 581.

Neumann, Julius: Ueber Beeinflussung der tryptischen Verdauung durch Fettstoffe, Berl. klin. Wchnschr., 1908, No. 46, 2066.

Neisser and Bräuning: Ueber Verdauungslipämie, Ztschr. f. exp. Path. u. Therap., 1907, iv, 747.

Neumann, J.: Zur Theorie der Schädigung magendarmkranker Säuglinge durch fetthaltige Ernährung, Arch. f. Kinderh., 1909, 1, 45; Ueber Beeinflussung der tryptischen Verdauung durch Fettstoffe; Berl. klin. Wchnschr., 1908, xlv, 2066.

Noll, A.: Ueber Fettsynthese im Darmepithel des Frosches bei der Fettresorption, Arch. f. Physiol., 1908, Suppl., 145.

Von Noorden: Handbook of Pathology of Metabolism, Eng. Ed. published by W. T. Keener & Co., Chicago, 1907.

Oppel, A.: Lehrbuch der vergleichenden mikroskopischen Anatomie, 1897, ii; Verdauungs-Apparat, Ergebn. d. Anat. u. d. Entwick., 1902, xii, 61.

Orgler: Der Eiweissstoffwechsel des Säuglings, Ergebn. der inn. Med. u. Kinderh., 1908, ii, 464; Beiträge zur Lehre von Stickstoffwechsel im Säuglingsalter, Monatschr. f. Kinderh., 1908, x, 135; Ueber Entfettungskuren im Kindesalter, Jahrb. f. Kinderh., 1905, lxi, 106.

Overton: Ueber den Mechanismus der Resorption und Sekretion, Nagel's Handbuch der Physiol. II, 890.

Pflüger: Die Resorption der Fette vollzieht sich dadurch, das sie in wässerige Lösung gebracht werden, Pflüger's Arch., lxxxvi, 1.

Philips, F.: Dextrinisiertes und nicht dextrinisiertes Mehl in der Säuglingsnährung, Monatschr. f. Kinderh., 6, 1908, vi, 26.

Plant, O. H.: Absorption of Fat from an Isolated Loop of Small Intestine in Healthy Dogs, Am. Jour. Physiol., 1908, xxiii, 65.

Raczynski: Die saure Dyspepsie der Brustkinder, Przeglad lekarski, 1902, Nos. 26-29; Ref. in Monatschr. f. Kinderh., 1903, i, 30; Dyspepsia Intestinalis Acida Lactorum, Wien. klin. Wchnschr., 1903, 342.

Radnitz: Sammelreferat über die Arbeiten aus der Milchchemie, Monatschr. f. Kinderh., 1903-4, ii, 422; ibid. 1905-6, iv, 258.

Reyber: Ueber den Fettgehalt der Frauenmilch, Jahrb. f. Kinderh., 1905, lxi, 601; Beitrag zur Frage nach dem Nahrungs- und Energiebedürfniss des natürlich ernährten Säuglings, Jahrb. f. Kinderh., 1905, lxi, 553.

Rietschel: Ueber die Lipase im Magensaft des Säugenden Tieres, Monatschr. f. Kinderh., 1907-8, vi, 333.

Rosenberg: Zur Physiologie der Fettverdauung, Arch. f. Physiol., 1901, lxxxv, 152.

Rosenfelt: Zu den Grundlagen der Entfettungsmethoden, Berl. klin. Wchnschr., 1899, 665; Fettbildung bei Asher-Spiro, Ergebn. d. Physiol. 1902, ii, I Abteil., 651; Fettbildung bei Asher-Spiro, Ergebn. d. Physiol., 1903, iii, 50 Abteil.; Zur Methodik der Fettbestimmung, Centr. f. Inn. Med., 1900, xxi, 833.

Rothberg: Ueber den Einfluss organischer Nahrungskomponenten (Eiweiss, Fett, Kolehydrate) auf den Kalkumsatz künstlich genährter Säuglinge, Jahrb. f. Kinderh., 1906, lxvi, 69.

Rousselet: Intestinal Chemism of the Alimentary Fats. Jour. Pharm. Chem., xxx, 60.

Rubner: Die Gesetze des Energieverbrauchs bei der Ernährung, Leipzig and Wien, 1902; Beiträge zur Ernährung im Knabenalter, Berlin, 1902.

Salge: Ein Beitrag zur Bakteriologie des Enterokatarrh, Jahrb. f. Kinderh., 1904, lix, 399.

Sarvonnat: Etude chimique et histologique du sclérème du nouveau-né. La Tribune méd., Sept. 21, 1907; Sur un cas de Sclérème des Nouveau-nés. Arch. de Méd. des Enf., 1906, ix, No. 1.

Schkarin: Beiträge zur Kenntnis des Säuglingsstoffwechsels bei Infectionskrankheiten, Arch. f. Kinderh., 1901, xli, Parts 1 and 2.

Schlossman: Weiteres zur Frage der Natürlichen Säuglingsernährung, Arch. f. Kinderh., 1902, xxxiii, 338.

Selter: Nahrungsreste in den Säuglings fäces, Zentralbl. f. Physiol. u. Path., 1907, N. F. ii,, 609.

Schelbe: Absorption of Fat by Infants, München. med. Wchnschr., 1908, 489.

Schlesinger: Disturbance of Fat Absorption and Its Relation to the Excretion of Calcium, Magnesium and Ammonia, Ztschr. f. klin. Med., 1904, lv, 214.

Schlossmann, A.: Beiträge zur Physiologie der Ernährung des Säuglings, Verhandl. d. Versamml. d. Gesellsch. f. Kinderh., deutsch. Naturf. u. Aerzte (1909), Wiesb., 1910, 67.

Shaw and Gilday: A Study of the Absorption of Fats in Infants, Brit. Med. Jour., 1906, No. 2, 932.

Siegert: Ueber das Verhalten der festen und flüssigen Fettsäuren im Fett des Neugeborenen und des Säuglings, Hofm. Beitr., i, 183.

Sommerfield: Zur Kenntnis der Magensaftsekretion nebst einigen Bemerkungen über Speichelsekretion, Arch. f. Kinderh., 1908-9, xlix, 1.

Soxhlet: Die Erzeugung fettreicher milch, Ref. Malys Jahresb. d. Tierschemie, 1896, No. 2.

Steinitz: Zur Kenntnis der chronischen Ernährungsstörungen der Säuglunge. Jahrb. f. Kinderh., 1902, lvii, 689; Ueber den alimentären Einfluss des Fettes auf die renale ammoniakausscheidung, Zentralbl. f. inn. Med., 1904, No. 3.

Steinitz and Weigert: Ueber den Einfluss einseitiger Ernährung mit Kolehydraten auf die chemische, Zusammensetzung des Säuglingskörpers, Hofm. Beitr., vi, 206; Ueber die chemische Zusammensetzung eines ein Jahr alten atrophischen und rachitischen Kindes, Monatschr. f. Kinderh., 1905-6, iv, 1.

Teireira de Mattos: Die Buttermilch als Säuglingsnahrung, Jahrb. f. Kinderh., 1902, lv, 1.

Terrione, E. F.: Zur Kenntniss der Fettspaltung durch Pankreassaft, Biochem. Ztschr., 1910, xxiii, 404.

Thiemich: Ueber die Herkunft des fötalen Fettes, Zentralbl. f. Physiol., xiii, 850; Jahrb. f. Kinderh., lx, 174; Zur Kenntnis der Fette im Säuglingsalter und der Fettleber bei Gastroenteritis, Ztschr. f. physiol. Chem., 1898-9, xxvi, 189.

Tobler: Ueber die Verdauung der Milch im Magen, Ergebn. d. inn. Med. u. Kinderh., 1908, i, 288.

Tschernoff: Ueber sogenannte Fettdiarrhoea nach Demme und Dr. Biedert, Jahrb. f. Kinderh., 1885, xxii, 1.

Uffelmann: Ueber den Fettgehalt der Faeces gesunder Kinder des ersten Lebensjahres und über die Ausnutzung des Fettes Seitens derselben bei Verschiedener Ernährung, Arch. f. Kinderh., 1881, ii, 1.

Uffenheimer: Die arbeiten des Finkelsteinschen Schule über Ernährungspathologie und Ernährungs therapie des Säuglings, Monatschr. f. Kinderh., 1910, ix. No. 7, 265.

Usuki: Das Schicksal des Fettes im Darm des Säuglings unter normalen und pathologischen Verhältnissen, Jahrb. f. Kinderh., July, 1910, 19.

Volhard: Ueber Resorption und Fettspaltung im Magen, München. med. Wchnschr., 1900, p. 141; Ueber die Untersuchung des Pankreassaftes beim Menschen und eine Methode der quantitativen Trypsin bestimmung, München. med. Wchnschr., 1907, p. 403.

Wegscheider: Ueber die normale Verdauung bei Säuglingen, In-Dissert., Berlin, 1875.

Weigert: Ueber den Einfluss der Ernährung auf die chemische Zusammensetzung des organismus, Jahrb. f. Kinderh., 1905, lxi, 178; Ueber den Einfluss der Ernährung auf die Tuberculose, Berl. klin. Wchnschr., 1907, No. 38.

Wells, John W.: The Digestibility of Fats and Oils, with Especial Reference to Emulsions, Brit. Med. Jour., 1902, x, 18.

Wentworth: Utilization of Milk Fat by an Atrophic Infant, Arch. Int. Med., Oct. 15, 1910.

Wilson, G. E.: Absorption of Fat in the Intestines, Tr. Canadian Inst., 1900, viii, 241.

15

Copyright © 1915 by the American Medical Association
Reprinted from, Am. J. Dis. Child., **10**, 249–265 (1915)

STUDIES IN THE ADAPTATION OF AN ARTIFICIAL FOOD TO HUMAN MILK *

H. J. GERSTENBERGER, M.D., H. D. HASKINS, M.D.
H. H. McGREGOR, Ph.D., AND H. O. RUH, M.D.
CLEVELAND, O.

INTRODUCTION BY H. J. GERSTENBERGER

In 1910, the physiologist, Friedenthal[1] again picked up the threads which led to the ideal set up by the pediatrist Biedert a generation ago; namely, to the production of an artificial milk similar in all its important characteristics to the best food for the human infant, namely, breast milk. By not getting the results that it had expected from mixtures which took into consideration the quantities of protein, lactose, and fat in human milk, the pediatric world became discouraged and considered the production of an artificial human milk that would give good practical results a hopeless task. Friedenthal gathered courage for another attempt for the solution of this important and interesting problem from the fact that the salt content and the physical-chemical characteristics of human milk had been entirely neglected, and also from the conviction that these were important, if not the most important individual factors to be considered in the making of an artificial food that was to be similar to breast milk and which would give satisfactory results. Müller and Schloss,[2,4] and Helbich[3] had also independently of Friedenthal begun with the attempt to come closer to the composition of breast milk. They received their stimulus from Finkelstein's theory of the injuriousness of the whey of cow's milk. Their first object, therefore, was to modify by reduction the deleterious

---

* Submitted for publication July 15, 1915.

* From the Babies' Dispensary and Hospital, the Departments of Pediatrics, Chemistry and Biochemistry of Western Reserve University, and from the Walker-Gordon Laboratory, Cleveland, Ohio.

* For the apparatus, the materials and help used in making G-R milk, we are indebted to the Walker-Gordon Laboratory, Cleveland, Ohio.

* Presented at the Annual Meeting of the American Pediatric Society, Lakewood, N. J., May 24, 1915.

1. Friedenthal, H.: Ueber die Eigenschaften künstlicher Milchsera und ueber die Herstellung eines künstlichen Menschenmilchersatzes, Zentralbl. f. Physiol., 1910, xxiv, 687.

2. Müller, Erich, and Schloss, Ernst: Die Versuche zur Anpassung der Kuhmilch an die Frauenmilch zu Zwecken der Säuglingsernährung, Jahrb. f. Kinderh., 1914, lxxx, 42.

3. Helbich, H.: Die Bedeutung der Molkenreduktion für die Ernährung junger Säuglinge, Jahrb. f. Kinderh., 1910, lxxi, 655.

4. Schloss, E.: Ueber Säuglingsernährung, Berlin, 1912, S. Karger.

whey of cow's milk.   They, however, encouraged by the favorable results that they had had in their institution with high fat milks, also attempted to simulate more accurately than heretofore the composition of breast milk.   Schloss stated in his address at the Königsberger meeting of the Gesellschaft für Kinderheilkunde in 1910, that he and his co-workers were convinced that the road that they were following would ultimately lead to the solution of the problem of the producton of an adequate artificial food.   So while they had visions of accomplishments along this direction, Friedenthal[1] had already, from theoretical grounds, worked out a plan according to which a more complete adaptation of an artificial food to breast milk could be obtained. In his article Friedenthal states that artificial woman's milk ought to contain 0.7 per cent. casein, 0.8 per cent. albumin and globulin, 7 to 8 per cent. milk sugar, $3\frac{1}{2}$ per cent. fat, ash, a freezing point of —0.56, degrees electrical conductivity of 23×10^{-4} at 18 degrees, neutral reaction (H Ion Content 5×10^{-8}) besides traces of nuclein, lecithin and albuminoids, and have the proper energy content.   Friedenthal further states in a later contribution (note 20) that the correlation of the salt components is of greater importance than is the total ash content.

Schloss[2, 4] then tried out Friedenthal's milk but did not get satistory results and, therefore, again modified this product.   Schloss, in order to have more accurate data as to the ash composition of human and cow's milk, himself made analysis.   The analyses on breast milk made by Schloss are of great value because he was the first to use samples of twenty-four hour quantities of breast milk for his determinations.   In addition, he took samples of a mixed milk composed of full twenty-four hour specimens of eight women.   The analyses that he got differed from those accepted up to that time.   His further work, therefore, was based on the more dependable, analytical figures obtained by himself in this manner.   Schloss,[4] however, felt that the poor results that he had obtained with Friedenthal's milk were due mainly to the lactose content, and he therefore replaced this with the preparation containing maltose and dextrin, and oftentimes in addition cornstarch.   He also added a proprietary preparation of sodium caseinate to bring up the protein content.

By making these changes Schloss really left the road that leads to the complete adaptation of an artificial food to woman's milk, and, therefore, Friedenthal's milk, although based on less accurate analytical data, comes closer to the accomplishment of this ideal than does Schloss' milk.

Bahrdt[5] reports favorably his experience with the feeding of this milk in eighty-one cases.   He states that at least among the children

5. Bahrdt, H., Bamberg, Edelstein, Hornemann: Ernährungsversuche mit Friedenthalscher Milch, Ztschr. f. Kinderh., Orig., 1914, x, 303.

of the Kaiserin Augusta Victoria-Haus, Friedenthal's milk promises better results than those obtained with mixtures of simple dilutions with carbohydrate additions.   Although the analytical and the metabolism work presented in his article has been seemingly justly criticized by Müller and Schloss,[2] this fact does not necessarily disprove the good clinical results obtained by Bahrdt.   It was the writer's impression when he in 1913 personally conversed with Bahrdt regarding his results with Friedenthal's milk that this food did really give good results and did mean a distinct addition to our means.   Both in the personal conversation and in the article which Bahrdt published later, he emphasized the nearly universal presence of vomiting and marked spitting and of dyspeptic stools in most of the infants fed with this food.

This fact, together with the interesting and important experimental data obtained by Huldschinsky,[6] namely, (1) that the stomach of infants fed with human milk contains very small amounts of the low volatile fatty acids; (2) that the stomach of infants fed with cow's milk contains three to six times as much; (3) that the amount of the low volatile fatty acids found in the stomach of babies fed with cow's milk corresponds to the amount of fat in the milk; and (4) that the formation of these free low volatile fatty acids in the stomach of a healthy infant fed on cow's milk is caused by the splitting of the glycerids of these acids by a ferment, and that the type of the former low volatile fatty acids found in the stomach corresponds to the type existing in a preformed state in the milk fat, led me to believe that probably the qualitative differences between cow's milk fat and breast milk fat were to blame, in a large measure at least, for the excessive spitting, vomiting, and dyspeptic stools.

It is a recognized fact that cow's milk fat contains many more of the low volatile fatty acids than does breast milk fat (10 per cent. to 1.6 per cent. Langstein and Meyer[7]), and there are those—Bokai,[8] Bahrdt,[9] Czerny,[10] and others—who believe that the low volatile fatty acids play an important part in the production of acute nutritional dis-

6. Huldschinsky, K.: Untersuchungen über die Pathogenese der Verdauungsstörungen im Säuglingsalter; Mitteilung, V.: Ztschr. f. Kinderh., Orig., 1912, III, 366.

7. Langstein-Meyer: Säuglingsernährung und Säuglingsstoffwechsel, Ed. 2 and 3, pp. 22, 23, 29 and 133.

8. Bokai, A.: Experimentelle Beiträge zur Kenntniss der Darmbewegungen. C. Ueber die Wirkung einiger Bestandteile der Fäces auf die Darmbewegungen, Arch. f. exper. Path. u. Pharmokol., 1888, xxiv, 153.

9. Bahrdt, H., and McLean, Stafford: Untersuchungen über die Pathogenese der Verdauungsstörungen im Säuglingsalter; VIII. Mitteilung, Ztschr. f. Kinderh., Orig., 1914, xi, 143.

10. Czerny-Keller: Des Kindes Ernährung Ernährungsstörungen und Ernährungstherapie, Abt. 7, p. 137, Franz Deuticke, Wien, 1909.

turbances in infants. While Bahrdt[11] states that Huldschinsky's findings of the abscence of an increase in the low volatile fatty acid content in the stomach of infants ill with acute nutritional disturbances speak against the importance of the low fatty acid content of infants' stomachs, on the other hand, he does believe that a disturbance of the motor and secretory powers of the stomach might alter conditions in the stomach and upper intestine in a manner that would permit the low fatty acids of the stomach contents to play an important etiologic rôle. It seemed plausible to the writer to imagine that if, for instance, the function of the pylorus could be disturbed in a manner that would permit larger quantities of food to enter the duodenum than it would under normal circumstances, that then the actual per cent. of low volatile fatty acids in the stomach contents at the time might be an important factor in the production of an acute nutritional disturbance and in the determining of the severity of the same, and that, therefore, the relatively large per cent. of low volatile fatty acids in cow's milk fat might be of decided etiologic importance. He therefore decided to attempt to obtain a fat, vegetable or animal, or a combination of such fats, that would give the same per cent. of the low volatile fatty acids as found in the fat of breast milk. In the first conference which I had, during December, 1913, with Dr. H. D. Haskins, Assistant Professor of Biological Chemistry at Western Reserve University, regarding this plan, the practical question of mixing such a fat with Friedenthal's milk was considered. It was immediately realized that the only hope lay in the use of an homogenizer, in which I had become interested a few years previously in an attempt at the Walker-Gordon Laboratory to make a very fine curd for casein milk. It was then learned that the Belle Vernon-Mapes Dairy Company was planning to put an homogenizer in the new plant which they were building, and it was therefore decided to wait with the practical work until the homogenizer had arrived, and in the meantime finish, if possible, our theoretical plans. In the literature I came across Arnold's[12] work, "*Ueber Frauenmilchfett*," in which he makes a statement that it is possible to make out of a mixture of 14 per cent. cocoanut oil and 86 per cent. lard, of the following characteristics:

	Cocoanut Oil	Lard
Refraction	35.1	47.7
Saponification number	259.0	197.5
Reichert-Meissl number	9.0	0.4
Iodin number	8.5	53.0
Polenske number	15.8	0.15

11. Bahrdt, II., Edelstein, F., Hanssen, P., Welde, E. F.: Untersuchungen ueber die Pathogenese der Verdauungsstörungen im Säuglingsalter; X. Mitteilung, Ztschr. f. Kinderh., Orig., 1914, xi, 416.

12. Arnold, W.: Ueber Frauenmilchfett, Ztsch. f. Untersuch. d. Nahrungsu. Genussmittel, 1912, xxiii, 433.

a fat that would give a refraction, saponification number, Reichert-Meissl number, iodin number, and Polenske number, very close to that of the fat of breast milk. It was decided, therefore, to use these data in the experimental and clinical work as soon as the homogenizer had arrived. While we were waiting, Niemann's[12] article on "Ueber die Möglichkeit einer Fettanerreichung der Säuglingsnahrung," appeared. He evidently had in mind the same goal as I, but had decided to reach it over another route, namely, over that of washed butter. Inasmuch as he claimed in his article to get an adequate removal of the low fatty acids from the butter by washing it with water, and also by vigorous stirring of a heated mixture an adequate and permanent emulsion of fat, together with Drs. Haskins and Ruh, I set myself at work to carry out Niemann's suggestion regarding the freeing of butter from the low volatile fatty acids with the idea of adding this fat to Friedenthal's milk. We hoped that by heating and vigorous stirring we were to accomplish the same permanent emulsification that Niemann[13] had obtained, with what results will be stated later.

The work of Funk[14] regarding vitamines, and his theory on the etiology of rickets, the work of Osborne and Mendel,[15] Peiser[16] and Bruning[17] on the growth value of the various food substances, especially fats, the work of Hess[18] on scurvy, the findings of Bahrdt,[7] Edelstein and Csonka[19] regarding the iron content of human and cow's

13. Niemann, Albert: Ueber die Möglichkeit einer Fettanreicherung der Säuglingsnahrung, Jahrb. f. Kinderh., 1914, lxxix, 274.

14. Funk, Casimir: The Nitrogenous Constitutents of Lime-Juice, Biochem. Jour., vii, 81; Forschritte der experimentellen Beriberiforschung in den Jahren 1911 bis 1913, München. med. Wchnschr., 1913, lx, 1997; An Attempt to Estimate the Vitamine-Fraction in Milk, Biochem. Jour., 1913, vii, 211; Studien ueber das Wachstum, Mitteilung 1. Das Wachstum auf vitaminhaltiger und vitaminfreier Nahrung, Hoppe-Seylers Ztschr. f. physiol. Chem., 1913, lxxxviii, 352; Ueber die physiologische Bedeutung gewisser bisher unbekannter Nahrungsbestandteile der Vitamine, Ergebn. d. Physiol., 1913, xiii, 124.

15. Osborne, Thos. B., and Mendel, Lafayette B.: Mendel, Lafayette V.: Viewpoints in the Study of Growth, Biochem. Bull., 1914, iii; The Nutritive Significance of Different Kinds of Foodstuffs, Med. Rec., New York, 1914, lxxxv, 737. Osborne, Thos. B., and Mendel, Lafayette B.: The Influence of Butter-Fat on Growth, Jour. Biol. Chem., 1913, xvi, 423; The Influence of Codliver Oil and Some Other Fats on Growth, Jour. Biol. Chem., 1914, xvii, 401; Feeding Experiments with Fat-Free Food Mixtures, Jour. Biol. Chem., 1912, xii, 81; Further Observations on the Influence of Natural Fats Upon Growth, Jour. Biol. Chem., 1915, xx, 379.

16. Peiser, J.: Ueber Fettaustausch in der Säuglingsernährung, Berl. klin. Wchnschr., 1914, li, 1165.

17. Brüning, Hermann: Untersuchungen ueber das Wachstum von Tieren jenseits der Säuglingsperiode bei verschiedenartiger künstlicher Ernährung, Jahrb. f. Kinderh., 1914, lxxix, 305.

18. Hess, Alfred F., and Fish, Mildred: Infantile Scurvy: The Blood, the Blood Vessels, and the Diet, Am. Jour. Dis. Child., 1914, viii, 385.

19. Edelstein, F., and Csonka, F. v.: Ueber den Eisengehalt der Kuhmilch, Biochem. Ztschr., 1912, xxxviii, 14.

milk, the theories of Friedenthal[20] regarding the need of sufficient "*Bausteine der Kernstoffe*," are all of the greatest importance to the solution of the problem of a more perfect and complete adaptation of an artificial food to human breast milk, and must receive full consideration. While various mixtures have been prepared with the object of taking into account the work of some of the authors just mentioned, the present presentation aims to confine itself mainly to the analytical, bacteriologic, physical, mechanical, practical and few clinical data obtained in the work with the preparation of our so-called G-R milk No. 2, which represents nothing more or less than Friedenthal's milk in which butter fat has been replaced with another fat having about the same per cent. of low volatile fatty acids as breast milk has, and having in addition other characteristics more similar to breast milk fat than to cow milk's fat. Some analytical data regarding the fats of G-R milk Nos. 3, 4, and 5 will also be presented as well as the experience of the authors with butter washed according to Niemann.

PART I

Homogenization

A. Homogenizer.—The machine procured for us by the Walker-Gordon Laboratory was a Manton-Gaulin machine with a pressure capacity for 500 kilograms. Its liquid capacity was found by us to be about 200 c.c. The pressure used by us was 250 kilograms.

B. Technic Carried Out in the Homogenization of Various Mixtures.—(*a*) Fats — butter fat, lard, cocoanut oil, cocoa butter, codliver oil: The various fats were weighed out in sterile granite dishes. The dishes with the fats were put into a steam jacketed kettle of hot to boiling water until the contents became liquid. The pans containing the fat were then emptied and drained into a larger steam jacketed kettle into which all the other ingredients of the food had been mixed. The amount of fat remaining in the pans after thorough draining was so small as to be negligible.

(*b*) Sugar: The lactose was at first added in the form of a sugar solution of 19 to 21 per cent. Later on it was found more convenient and more accurate to simply weigh the lactose in the sterile granite pan and dump it into the common mixing kettle.

(*c*) Salts: The salts were accurately weighed in a glass receptacle. The contents of the receptacle were dumped into the mixing vat and the particles adhering to the inside of the dish rinsed out with distilled water. This amount, of course, was deducted from the batch of distilled water measured for the entire quantity.

(*d*) Skimmed milk: The amount of required skimmed milk was added to the mixture in cubic centimeters. To save time different granite pitchers were carefully marked for definite amounts.

(*e*) Water: The amount of required distilled water, less 200 c.c. for the capacity of the machine, was measured in cubic centimeters and added to the

20. Friedenthal, H.: Ueber Säuglingsernährung nach physiologischen Grundsätzen mit Friedenthal'scher Kindermilch und Gemüsepulvern, Berl. klin. Wchnschr., 1914, li, 727.

mixture. To save time different granite pitchers were carefully marked for definite amounts.

(*f*) Quantity: The amount most frequently used by us for an individual batch was 30 liters.

(*g*) Mixing: 1, mixing before homogenization: Inasmuch as the largest steam jacketed kettle at our disposal could comfortably hold but 20 liters, the fat, salt, sugar, skimmed milk, and enough water to make about a total of 20 liters were put into the vat, stirred vigorously, and brought by steam heat to a temperature of 150 F. In order to avoid an excessive loss of the fat, which would occur if the mixture were allowed to go through the homogenizer undisturbed, it was necessary to keep up a constant stirring. Soon it was possible to develop a special technic in this respect that enabled a constant mixture of the fat with the other parts of the batch. At a time when nearly all of the 20 liters had passed through the homogenizer, the remaining water was poured into the vat and run through the machine.

Recently another larger receptacle has been used for mixing all of the milk and water at one time. Out of this receptacle the milk and water mixture is run in desired amounts into the steam jacketed kettle containing the sugar, the fat, and salts. The use of this extra receptacle has lessened the time and made the practical part of the work more simple.

2. Mixing after homogenization: From the above, it will be recognized that the first part of the mixture going through the homogenizer is much more concentrated than the second part. Therefore, it is essential that a mixture of all these parts be brought about before bottling. This was managed by pouring from one can to another.

Recently we have been pouring all of the homogenized milk into the same receptacle in which the water and skimmed milk had been mixed before homogenization. This also is more simple and saves time.

(*h*) Temperature: The temperature of the mixture is brought to 150 F. before it is allowed to go through the homogenizer. It is easy to keep the batch at this temperature by regulating the steam going through the kettle and the cold skimmed milk and water coming out of the large mixing receptacle. The temperature of the milk rises about 8 to 10 degrees in the process of homogenization. During the filling, bottling, capping, etc., it drops again to about 145 to 135, and it usually enters the ice box at this temperature.

(*i*) Bottling: From the large mixing vat the milk is run into a small enamel bottling machine and filled into bottles sterilized in an autoclave. The bottles are then capped with a simple cap and with a cover cap and placed in the ice box.

(*j*) Cleanliness: All of the bottles, dishes, and utensils are sterilized in the autoclave. The mixing vat is sterilized by allowing the water to boil in it. The homogenizer is cleansed and, in all probability, sterilized by running this boiling water through it just before the homogenization of the milk is to take place. This procedure also gives one the opportunity of testing the machine for any leaks.

No more than the usual precautions are taken with the packing, shipping, etc., of the fats, sugar, skimmed milk and water.

The hands of the individuals making the milk are simply cleaned with soap and water.

The authors are aware that Friedenthal requires that the skimmed milk be not heated. They have, however, felt that for their present work, at least, it would be better and safer practically to pasteurize the finished product. In all probability there will be no difficulty when the time comes to add at least a big part of the skimmed milk in a raw state to the finished product.

PART II

Butter Fat

A. Creamery Butter.—(*a*) · Cold water washing: Fresh, sweet creamery butter, in packed and in granular form, was vigorously and thoroughly rubbed and washed with some eight to ten changes of cold water. The acidity of the wash water was determined by the use of phenolphthalein and a tenth-normal sodium hydroxid solution. The amount of acids washed out was so small as to be insignificant.

(*b*) Hot water washing: Assuming that hot water might give better results, the butter was melted and the fat separated from the curd by passing through a cheesecloth. The filtered liquid was poured, together with hot distilled water, into a large bottle. The mixture was kept hot by placing the bottle in a water-bath. After thorough shaking the bottle was replaced in the water-bath and the fat allowed to separate from the wash water, which was then siphoned off for determination of its acidity. Four washings were carried out with each batch. Records of the amounts of tenth-normal sodium hydroxid required to neutral-ize the acids of the combined wash waters have been lost, but it can be stated that the amounts were so small as to be absolutely insignificant, and were, in all probability, due to the presence of a small amount of free acids and also caseinogen, which was being dissolved out. Burr and Weise[21] report that fresh butter fat always has a small amount of free fatty acids in amounts that require for 10 gm. of butter 0.6 to 1.4 c.c. tenth-normal sodium hydroxid solution. The best proof that the reduction in the low volatile fatty acid content of the butter was very insignificant is the finding for the same of a Reichert-Meissl number of 28, practically the same obtained in ordinary unwashed butter.

Grimmer[22] in his abstract of Niemann's article, criticizes Niemann's pro-cedure and states that it is impossible to wash the low volatile fatty acids out of the butter because they are present in it in the form of glycerids, just as the higher acids are, and are, therefore, not free. In other words, Grimmer's statement corresponds with our findings.

(*c*) Alcohol washing: 263 gm. of clear butter fat were removed from one pound of fresh creamery butter, 255 c.c. of redistilled alcohol were added and the materials brought to boiling under thorough mixing. The mixture was then cooled to a low temperature and the alcoholic liquid decanted from the solid fat. The solid fat was then heated until the alcohol in it had evaporated. The residue weighed 252 gm. The Reichert-Meissl value of this residue fat was 4.0, and the iodin value 38.9. The addition of 10 gm. of sesame oil to 100 gm. to this alcohol washed fat gave an iodin value of 44.3. In other words, it is possible to remove the glycerids of the low volatile fatty acids from butter fat by washing with hot alcohol. The same plan has been carried out by Hunziger and Spitzer.[23]

(*d*) Emulsification according to Niemann: Both the cold water and the hot water washed butter fat were added to Friedenthal's milk in amounts to bring the fat content up to 4.5 per cent. The mixture was brought to the boiling point and was vigorously stirred, as directed by Niemann. The results were not the same as those obtained by Niemann, for the fat on standing and cool-ing rose to the surface. Niemann, however, used an entirely different mixture,

21. Burr, A., and Weise, H.: Ueber den Gehalt frischen Butterfettes an freien Fettsäuren und flüchtigen Fettsäuren, Molkereizeitung, Hildesheim, 1914, No. 16.

22. Grimmer, W.: Die Arbeiten auf dem Gebiete der Milchwissenschraft und Molkereipraxis im Jahre, 1914, I Semester, Monatschr. f. Kinderh., Referate, 1915, xiv, 81.

23. Hunziker, O. F., and Spitzer, G.: A Study of the Chemical Composition of Butterfat, and its Relation to the Composition of Butter, Proc. Indiana Acad. Sc., xxv, 15.

which contained 50 gm. of mondamin (cornstarch) to each liter of milk, and this addition to his milk mixture was, in all probability, responsible for the difference in our results.

(*e*) Clinical data: Owing to the fact that the homogenizer was a very large machine used for the homogenization of large quantities of cream and was too large and unhandy for our work, and owing also to the climatic conditions that existed at that time — heat, August, 1914 — only a few older, well babies were put on the milk simply to get a rough idea how the children would take it and react to it; that is, whether there would be an improvement over Bahrdt's[5] experiences or not. Only three older infants were put on Friedenthal's milk with cold water washed butter and two on Friedenthal's milk with hot water washed butter. Two of the former reacted with thin, yellow stools in increased numbers and one vomited severely. One of the latter reacted in the same manner. The mothers of these children were not enthusiastic about our giving their babies this "new milk" under such conditions, and we, therefore, because of this and the further reasons for limiting the number of babies in the first place, decided to discontinue our clinical investigations until the arrival of cooler weather and of the smaller homogenizer, which the Walker-Gordon Company was having made for our use. The impression that we gained from this very meager experience with Friedenthal's milk and water washed butter was that there was no improvement over the results obtained by Bahrdt with the regular Friedenthal's milk.

B. Process Butter.—Process butter was considered by us because of its cheapness and also because of the fact that it surely had ample chance to decompose and so have many of the low volatile fatty acids in a free state, which condition would enable us to remove the latter by washing the butter with water. The work with this material was soon dropped because of our inability to rid it from the very disagreeable odor.

PART III

Mixed Fats, Animal and Vegetable

A. General Statement.—As stated in the introduction, our main object was to find a fat or combination of fats that would be more similar to breast milk fat than cow's milk fat, especially regarding the low fatty acid content, and to see whether a substitution of such a fat for the cow's milk fat in Friedenthal's milk might not improve this milk and represent a further step in the more complete adaptation of artificial food to human milk.

B. Experimental Data.—The accompanying table by Arnold[12] (Table 1) directed our attention to the use of lard and cocoanut oil:

TABLE 1

FROM ARNOLD'S WORK, "UEBER FRAUENMILCHFETT"

	Cocoanut Oil	Lard	Mixture	Woman's Milk Fat, I
Refraction	35.1	47.7	47.65	47.6
Saponification number	259.0	197.5	206.1	206.08
Reichert-Meissl number	9.0	0.4	3.0	2.65
Iodin number	8.5	53.0	46.77	46.25
Polenske number	15.8	0.15	1.65	1.65

For many reasons it seemed worth while to try to make cod-liver oil a part of this fat combination. In order to make such a mixture more palatable cocoa butter was added. We, therefore, prepared four batches of fats in the following manner:

No. 2. Lard 86.00 per cent., cocoanut oil 14 per cent.

No. 3. Lard 74.88 per cent., cocoanut oil 14 per cent., codliver oil 11.11 per cent.

No. 4. Lard 63.78 per cent., cocoanut oil 14 per cent., codliver oil 11.11 per cent., cocoa butter 11.11 per cent.

No. 5. Lard 74.88 per cent., cocoanut oil 14 per cent., cocoa butter 11.11 per cent.

It was our intention to use all four of these, but for practical reasons, after having found out that infants would take any one of them, we decided to limit our experiences for the beginning to G-R milk No. 2.

Table 2 gives first, the character numbers of the individual fats; second, the character numbers of the fats of G-R milk Nos. 2, 3, 4, and 5, obtained by calculation on the basis of the character numbers actually found for the individual fats (the individual fats were mixed by heating at 60); third, the character numbers of the fats mixed in the same proportion as they were mixed in the milk; fourth, the character numbers for the mixture of lard and cocoanut oil in the proportion as they were used in G-R milk No. 2, and heated for the same period of time as required to extract the fat from G-R milk No. 2; and fifth, the character numbers of the fat extracted from G-R milk No. 2.

TABLE 2.—DATA CONCERNING VARIOUS FATS USED

	Reichert-Meissl	Polenske	Iodin	Saponification
Lard	0.08	0.49	63.07	195.5
Cocoanut oil	6.436	13.69	8.836	259.5
Cocoa butter	0.34	0.30	36.35	196.4
Codliver oil	0.27	0.315	170.0	189.9
Mixed fats:				
(Same proportions)				
As Milk II (calculated).	0.9698	2.337	55.45	204.5
As Milk II found	1.638	1.231	55.46	206.8
As Milk II found *	2.524	1.22	.....	.....
Fat from Milk II.......	2.72	1.2	55.0	206.0
(Same proportions)				
As Milk III (calculated)	0.9914	2.318	66.24	203.8
As Milk III found	2.09	1.288	67.5	205.1
(Same proportions)				
As Milk IV (calculated)	1.188	2.297	63.14	204.0
As Milk IV found	2.127	1.498	64.49	205.4
(Same proportions)				
As Milk V (calculated).	0.8128	2.318	52.52	204.6
As Milk V found	1.971	1.301	52.75	206.3

* Fats in same proportion as in Milk II heated with ether for same period of time as required to extract fat from milk.

Table 2 reveals the fact that it is possible to calculate the iodin and the saponification values of mixtures of fats before or after homogenization in milk, from a consideration of these values in the individual fats. The data with equal clearness show that the Reichert-Meissl and Polenske numbers may not be so calculated, but that the mixing of the fats produces a change in the relative amounts of soluble and insoluble fatty acids that will volatilize with steam in the time required for the determination. It is noteworthy that the total amount of the volatile fatty acids is not greatly changed, for the sum of Reichert-Meissl and Polenske numbers as found is in each case approximately the same as the sum of the calculated values. This variation is not now understood and further work will be done to determine the cause of the change in value.

The slight increase of 0.2 in the Reichert-Meissl number of the fat from G-R milk No. 2 over the mixture of the same fats in the same proportions and heated for the same period of time as required to extract the fat from G-R milk, is probably due to the 0.4 per cent. of butter fat present in the skimmed milk, as can be seen from Table 5.

By comparing the character numbers as given in Table 2 for G-R milk No. 2 with Arnold's figures for his mixture and for his woman's milk fat No. 1, it will be seen that the Reichert-Meissl and saponification numbers are nearly identical; that there is a slight difference between the Polenske numbers, and a decided difference between the iodin numbers. The difference between the iodin numbers is due to the high iodin value of the batch of lard used in our work (G-R milk, lard 63.07; Arnold, lard 53.0). By rearranging the mixture we could have procured an iodin value for the G-R milk fat which would have been closer to Arnold's figures for woman's milk fat, but by doing so we would have changed the Reichert-Meissl and the saponification numbers; but as the Reichert-Miessl value seems of first importance to us, we decided to continue to use this mixture without any further change, and it is, of course, probable that a fair increase in the iodin number above that found in woman's milk fat is of no great importance.

The following figures given by Arnold[12] for his analysis of another woman's milk fat (*Frauenmilchfett No. 2*).

```
Refraction .......................... 48.75
Saponification ...................... 205.0
Reichert-Meissl ..................... 1.5
Iodin ............................... 45.65
Polenske ............................ 1.45
```

show, as one, of course, would expect, that fat from milk coming from different women will show variances in the character numbers of their respective fats.

Merkel[24] reports the following as character numbers of a butter made from the cream of a four-day quantity of milk from a wetnurse:

```
Saponification number ............... 209.3
Reichert-Meissl number .............. 1.5
Polenske number ..................... 2.2
Iodin number ........................ 46.8
Refraction at 40° ................... 46.3
```

Table 3 shows that by making use of tallow—which one might imagine from Osborne and Mendel's[15] work, might even have an added value over lard—in the fat mixture, a greater resemblance as regards iodin numbers can be obtained.

_____

24. Merkel, Eduard: Zur Kenntnis des Frauenmilchfettes, Pharm. Zentralhalle, 1912, liii, 495.

TABLE 3.—CHARACTER NUMBERS OF INDIVIDUAL FATS

	Saponification	Reichert-Meissl	Iodin
Lard	195.29	0.08	63.1
Tallow	196.6	0.5	41.4
Cocoanut oil	259.5	6.43	8.8
Cocoa butter	196.4	0.34	36.3
Codliver oil	189.9	0.27	170.0

MIXTURE WITHOUT CODLIVER OIL

	Per Cent.	Saponification	Reichert-Meissl	Iodin
Lard	50			
Tallow	35	205.48	1.07	47.36
Cocoanut oil	15			

MIXTURE WITH CODLIVER OIL

	Per Cent.	Saponification	Reichert-Meissl	Iodin
Tallow	45			
Lard	15			
Cocoanut oil	15	205.46	1.285	45.17
Cocoa butter	20			
Codliver oil	5			

Table 4 shows the materials used for a typical batch of G-R milk No. 2. The table is analyzed to show the origin of the various contributing substances:

TABLE 4.—MATERIALS FOR G-R MILK No. 2

	Total gm.	Water	Salt	Protein	Fat	Lactose
Skimmed milk ...	9,890	27.23	0.2184	0.96	0.132	1.463
Water	19,800	60.07	......	....	.....	....
KCl	27	....	0.0819	....	.....	....
K₂HPO₄	13.5	....	0.0409	....	.....	....
KH₂PO₄	13.5	....	0.0409	....	.....	....
Lard	1,274.5	....	......	....	3.867	....
Cocoanut oil	207.5	....	......	....	0.629	....
Lactose	1,740	0.0425	......	....	.....	5.235
Totals	32,966	87.34	0.382	0.96	4.628	6.698

The distribution of the substances from the skimmed milk shown in Table 4 is based on the analysis of the milk used, shown in Table 5.

TABLE 5.—DISTRIBUTION OF SUBSTANCES FROM SKIMMED MILK

SKIMMED MILK JUNE 18

Water	90.51
Ash	0.728
Protein	3.2
Fat	0.44
Lactose	4.87

The composition and characters of the G-R milk No. 2 prepared from the batch given in Table 4, as determined by analysis, are summarized in Table 6.

TABLE 6.—COMPOSITION AND CHARACTER OF G-R MILK No. 2

ANALYSIS

Water	87.21
Ash	0.378
Protein	0.93
Fat	4.617
Lactose	6.65

General characters: Specific gravity 15.5 °, 1.032; specific conductivity 20 °, 3.41 × 10^{-3} recip. ohms; freezing point depression 0.618°; caloric value per kg., 739.6 cal.

Characteristics of fat content: Size fat globules, 0.2-1 micron; brownian movement vigorous; Reichert-Meissl value, 2.72; Polenske number, 1.2; iodin number, 55.0; saponification number, 206.0.

That the milk maintained the same general composition may be judged from the accompanying analyses made at different periods (Table 7).

TABLE 7.—ANALYSIS OF G-R MILK NO. 2, AT DIFFERENT PERIODS

	May 18	May 20	June 5	June 18
Water	86.8	87.14	87.44	87.21
Ash	0.43	0.37	0.37	0.378
Protein	1.1	0.97	0.91	0.93
Fat	4.52	4.58	4.6	4.617
Lactose	7.07	6.63	6.51	6.65

The somewhat low protein and lactose content is due, in a part at least, to the fact that the milk was added as grams instead of c.c.

TABLE 8.—BACTERIAL COUNTS FOR SKIMMED AND FINISHED MILKS

Date			Count	Skim, Count
May 6	No. 2	II	Sterile	......
May 6	No. 2	III	Sterile	......
May 6	No. 2	IV	Sterile	......
May 6	No. 2	V	Sterile	......
May 12	No. 2	II	3,100	......
May 12	No. 2	III	5,000	......
May 12	No. 2	IV	16,100	9,850
May 19	No. 2		1,850	......
May 20	No. 2		4,500	55,300 *
May 21	No. 2		6,000	91,000 *
May 22	No. 2		Sterile	11,300 *
May 24	No. 2		Sterile	19,700 *
May 25	No. 2		Sterile	......
May 26	No. 2		Sterile	39,000 *
May 27	No. 2		Sterile	5,500 *
May 31	No. 2		Sterile	......
May 29	No. 2		4,900	......
June 2	No. 2		1,000	2,400
June 4	No. 2		Sterile	7,200
June 5	No. 2		300	8,400
June 7	No. 2		Sterile	157,200
June 9	No. 2		Sterile	6,800
June 11	No. 2		1,700	4,500
June 12	No. 2		9,000	2,000
June 14	No. 2		3,100	42,000
June 16	No. 2		Sterile	70,000
June 19	No. 2		200	3,200
June 20	No. 2		700	400
June 25	No. 2		200	300
June 26	No. 2		300	2,700

* Not certified skim.

Table 8 gives the bacteriological counts for the skimmed milk and for the finished milks, and shows on the whole very low bacterial counts for the prepared milk. These excellent results are, in all probability, due to the fact that, unknowingly, practically the same technic and conditions were established by us as advocated by Ayers and Johnson.[25]

Analytical Methods.—Water, Ash, Protein: The methods used for determining water, ash and protein are those of the A. O. A. C. described in Bulletin 107 of the Department of Agriculture.

Fat: The usual methods for fat extraction and estimation are completely unreliable with homogenized milk of this type. When the Babcock centrifugal method is used a definite separation of fatty from acid layer cannot be obtained. Various determinations were made by the Adams paper coil method, and the following figures obtained on milk that by more accurate analysis was shown to contain 4.5 per cent. of fat: 3.75, 3.69, 3.34, 2.24 per cent. A modification of the Werner-Schmidt acid method yielded fairly close results, but very great difficulty was experienced in securing a separation of the acid and ether layers. The Roese-Gottlieb process was then employed, and it was found that excellent results can be obtained when low-boiling petroleum ether (35 C.) is used, and the second and third extractions accomplished by inversion, without shaking, of the mixture. The above recorded analyses substantiate the accuracy of this method.

Method of Fat Extraction from Milk: 150 c.c. of milk were diluted with 250 c.c. water, and 9 c.c. of 1 per cent. sulphuric acid added, with constant stirring. A cylindrical cup made from fat-free filter paper was fitted closely into a Buchner funnel and after moistening the paper the acidified mixture was filtered. After normal filtering had ceased, the filtrate was discarded and suction applied until most of the water was removed. This final filtrate was shaken with ether, and the ether subsequently used for the extraction of the fat from the precipitate. The filter paper with precipitate was transferred to a mortar and ground with about 20 gm. anhydrous sodium sulphate, when a dry, somewhat waxy porous powder resulted. This powder was placed in a Soxhlet apparatus, where extraction was complete in two hours. The ether was then driven off, or in some cases the ether solution was transferred by pipet to the vessel in which a determination was to be made.

Reichert-Meissl Value: Leffmann and Beam's saponification method was used, and the distillation continued thirty minutes.

Polenske Number: Glycerol saponification was used, and the condenser tubes washed three times with water, then three times with alcohol.

Iodin Number: The Wjis method was used.

Saponification Number: One gm. of the fat was saponified with 5 per cent. potassium hydroxid in specially purified alcohol. It is of importance that the blank determination be heated on the water bath for the same period of time as the regular determinations.

Size of Fat Globules: The value of 0.2 to 1 microns was roughly approximated by the use of Thoma's hemacytometer. The fat globules exhibit remarkable uniformity of size, and all show vigorous brownian movement.

Lactose: The solid lactose used was examined both polarimetrically and by reduction, and found to be 99.2 per cent., $C_{12}H_{22}O_{11}.H_2O$. Lactose in milk was determined in each case by the polarimeter, using acid mercuric nitrate for precipitation, and estimating the solids by the method of double dilution. To check the polarimetric method, the milk analyzed on June 18 was determined also by the reduction method, using Soxhlet's modification of Fehling's solution, weighing the copper as cupric oxid, and calculating lactose from the

---

25. Ayers, S. H., and Johnson, W. T., Jr.: Pasteurization in Bottles and the Process of Bottling Hot Pasteurized Milk, Jour. Infect. Dis., 1914, xiv, 217.

Soxhlet-Wein tables. The results show the absence of any substances in the milk that would vitiate the accuracy of the polarimetric method.

Per cent. lactose by polariscope 6.51
Per cent. lactose by reduction 6.537

Specific Gravity: Quevenne's lactodensimeter was used at 15.5 C.

Conductivity: Conductivity was measured by the Kohlrausch method, using a cell with electrodes about 1 cm. apart and 2.5 cm. in diameter.

Depression of Freezing Point.—The determination was made by the usual method. It is highly important that the temperature of the freezing mixture be not lower than about −1.5 C. as the concentration of the solution by the settling out of ice changes the f. p. significantly.

Calorimetry: To determine the heating value, 2 c.c. of milk were accurately weighed in a small combustion cup. This was placed in a desiccator equipped with shelves holding dishes filled with calcium chlorid. Evacuation was accomplished by a water pump, and in twenty-four hours the material had dried and showed no evidence of loss by spattering. The dried milk was then burned in a Parr bomb with 20 atmospheres oxygen pressure. The calculation of heating value from the analysis of milk reported in Table 7 (June 18) closely agrees with the direct calorimetric determination.

CALCULATION FROM ANALYSIS

Protein   0.93 × 5.85   5.44 C.
Fat   4.617 × 9.1   42.02 C.
Lactose   6.65 × 3.96   26.33 C.
_____

73.79 C. per 100 gm. milk
Obtained from calorimeter 73.96 C. per 100 gm. milk

C. Clinical Data.—(*a*) Vomiting: The clinical experience until now has not been sufficient to be considered worthy of report. It is hoped at a later time to present the clinical results. A statement, however, can be made regarding the degree of vomiting and dyspeptic stools met with so frequently by Bahrdt in his patients fed with Friedenthal's milk prepared with unchanged cow's fat. Of a list of twenty babies, from 1 week to 7 months of age, there was spitting up or slight vomiting in five. In two of these this has disappeared; in a third, the vomiting continues once a day; and in the other two there still exists a slight vomiting. Two other children showed marked vomiting before they were put on the food; the one gradually improved while on the milk, and now does not vomit at all, and the other is a case of pylorospasm which continues to vomit, but which has begun to gain in weight since it has been getting the food.

(*b*) Stools: Of the twenty children only two showed dyspeptic stools. Two were constipated and passed rather firm, somewhat formed, fatty soap stools. The remainder had what we termed normal stools. These varied in color from a lemon-yellow to an orange-yellow, were of a lard-like, pasty consistency, and contained, in most instances, smaller or larger masses of soft, fatty soaps. Many of the stools changed from a yellow to an olive-green in the diaper.

These few data suffice to prove that the vomiting has been decidedly less and the stools decidedly more normal in our children than they were in Bahrdt's, and we believe that this is due to the removal of the low volatile fatty acids. Whether the fact that the milk was homogenized has anything to do with these better results is impossible to say at the present time. Birk, according to Grulee,[26] could find no improve-

_____

26. Grulee, Clifford G.: Infant Feeding, W. B. Saunders Co., 1912.

ment in the children by homogenizing their foods. On the other hand, Lavialle[27] believes that the homogenization greatly enhances the digestibility of a milk because it offers to the digestive ferments a much larger action surface, and because it causes, by reason of the marked brownian movement, the formation of currents, which are responsible for an active mixing of ferments and foods. Inasmuch as the fat in human milk does not exist in such a fine emulsion as the fat of homogenized milk, it can at least be assumed that a finer division than is present in human milk is not necessary; on the other hand, there is, at present, no reason to believe that any harm is done to the fat or any other constituent of the milk by homogenization, excepting, of course, the effect of the raised temperature on some of the constituents of skimmed milk; and it may be found that homogenization is of greater value in the production of artificial human milk than the mere mixing for which it has been used by us.

(c) Weight: The following figures are given to show that normal or slightly below normal infants made good gains in weight. Eighteen infants, from 1 week to 7 months of age, for a total period of seventy-three weeks, made a total gain of 10,630 gm., or an average of 145 + gm. per week.

D. *Economical Data.*—Friedenthal's milk made up with a mixture of fats like lard, tallow, cocoa butter, cocoanut oil, cod-liver oil, olive oil, cottonseed oil, sesame oil, and the like, can be produced at a price decidedly lower than when butter freed from a large per cent. of its low fatty acid glycerids is used. The cost of the fat per liter of various combinations with various fats, is as follows:

```
For a mixture of tallow 40 per cent., lard 10 per cent., cocoanut
    oil 20 per cent., cocoanut butter 20 per cent., codliver oil 10
    per cent. ............................................................1.30 cents
G-R Milk No. 2 .........................................................1.43 cents
G-R Milk No. 3 .........................................................1.60 cents
G-R Milk No. 5 .........-...............................................1.70 cents
G-R Milk No. 4 .........................................................1.80 cents
Friedenthal's milk with cow's butter fat, without considering the
    cost of washing the butter with alcohol......................3.70 cents
```

While the production cost of a milk for infants is not of the first importance, yet it is, nevertheless, true that there are many families who cannot get for their infants what they should have simply because of the price, and, therefore, if an adequate food can be prepared at a low cost it is an advantage that is important when it is desired that all families whose infants require it should get it. It is also interesting to think of the economy that would result in a general way by the reduction in the use of the more expensive butter and the increase in the use of fats that are distinctly cheaper.

27. Lavialle, P.: Le mouvement brownien dans le lait homogeneise, Clin. infant., 1913, xi, 490.

SUMMARY

1. By mixing varying proportions of different animal and vegetable fats, it is possible to get a fat that in its Reichert-Meissl number (small per cent. of low volatile fatty acid glycerids), saponification number, iodin number, and other characters, is nearly identical with the fat of human milk, as has previously been shown by Arnold.

2. By replacing in an artificial milk cow's-milk fat with the fat of the above description in an emulsified state (homogenized), a distinct step in advance towards the more complete adaptation of an artificial food to breast milk is made.

3. It is also possible to take into consideration the "growth factors," "vitamine factors," and the like, in choosing the individual fats for an acceptable mixture. This represents a further step in the more complete adaptation of an artificial milk to human milk.

4. The homogenizer represents the important means by which the mixing and emulsification of the fat in the artificial milk is possible. The homogenizer also changes the physical condition of the fat (smaller globules, brownian movement), which may be of advantage.

5. The meager clinical data suffice to show that the infants fed with Friedenthal's milk in which the cow's-milk fat has been replaced by a fat with a low volatile fatty acid glycerid content, similar to that of human milk fat, vomit less and have more normal stools than the children reported by Bahrdt, and fed with Friedenthal's milk containing unchanged cow's-milk fat.

6. Washing butter with cold or hot water does not remove the low volatile fatty acids from butter, except in an insignificant degree.

7. Washing butter with hot alcohol does remove the low fatty acid glycerids to a decided degree.

8. The manufacture of a food like G-R milk can be arranged to give a very low bacteriologic count.

9. The production of milk like G-R milk can be made at a reasonable cost.

16

Reprinted from *Pediatrics*, **31**, Pt. 2 (Suppl.), 171–192 (Jan. 1963)

ROLE OF LINOLEIC ACID IN INFANT NUTRITION

Clinical and Chemical Study of 428 Infants Fed on Milk Mixtures Varying in Kind and Amount of Fat

Arild E. Hansen, M.D., Ph.D.,* Hilda F. Wiese, Ph.D., Arr Nell Boelsche, M.D.,
Mary Ellen Haggard, M.D., Doris J. D. Adam, M.D., and Helen Davis, M.D.

*Department of Pediatrics, University of Texas School of Medicine, Galveston, Texas, and
Bruce Lyon Memorial Research Laboratory, Children's Hospital of the East Bay,
Oakland, California*

INTRODUCTION

THE STUDY reported here attempts to evaluate the role of fat and to determine the relative importance of the kind and amount of fat included in the diet of infants. Clinical and chemical findings are presented concerning more than 400 infants maintained on diets without fat and with fat having different fatty acid compositions. The study embraced a 4-year period.

Many attempts have been made to develop milk mixtures that emulate human breast milk in composition. One of the recognized differences between human and cow's milk concerns the nature of the fat. Significant in this regard is the fact that the linoleic acid content of human mother's milk is four to five times greater than that in cow's milk. Previous studies from this laboratory[1-3] strongly support the hypothesis that linoleic acid is an essential nutrient for infants. The results of the present study provide further confirmation of this concept.

MATERIALS AND METHODS

Milk Preparations Used

The original plan of study was to feed each of four groups of 100 babies on one of four different milk formulas for the first 6 months to 1 year of life. Three formulas contained the same total amount of fat but variable amounts of linoleic acid obtained from appropriate mixtures of vegetable oils and from butterfat. The fourth preparation was a skimmed-milk formula which contained almost no fat, hence, only traces of linoleic acid. The pediatricians did not know the specifications regarding the nature of the fat in the different formulas. Relatively early in the study, because of evidences of fat deficiency in the infants fed the low fat milk, a fifth formula was substituted which was equal in fat content to the other three mixtures, but was composed of saturated fatty acids, a small amount of oleic acid, and only traces of linoleic acid. The composition of the five different formulas after dilution with equal parts of water is presented in Table I.

The milk mixtures were sterilized in cans containing 13 fluid ounces and labeled "Infant Formula #1, #2, #3, #4, or #5." Each label was a different color and contained the statement, "Prepared especially for the Department of Pediatrics, University of Texas School of Medicine."* The same chemist and plant superintendent

---

* Dr. Hansen died on October 16, 1962.

* Kindly supplied by The Baker Laboratories, Inc., Cleveland, Ohio.

Supported by grants-in-aid from The Baker Laboratories, Inc., Cleveland, Ohio, and Gerber Products Company, Fremont, Michigan.

Material supplementary to this article has been deposited as Document number 7344 with the ADI Auxiliary Publications Project, Photoduplication Service, Library of Congress, Washington 25, D.C. A copy may be secured by citing the Document number and by remitting $7.50 for photoprints, or $2.75 for 35-mm microfilm. Advance payment is required. Make checks or money orders payable to: Chief, Photoduplication Service, Library of Congress.

ADDRESS: (H.F.W.) Bruce Lyon Memorial Research Laboratory, Children's Hospital of East Bay, Grove and 51st Streets, Oakland 9, California.

TABLE I

COMPOSITION OF MILK FORMULAS AT FEEDING
DILUTION

Components*	Formula Number				
	1	2	3	4	5
Fat (%)	3.0†	3.0†	3.0‡	0.1‡	3.0§
Protein (%)	2.5	2.6	2.3	2.4	2.5
Carbohydrate (%)	7.4	7.3	7.5	13.5	7.0
Ash (%)	0.7	0.7	0.7	0.7	0.7
Water (%)	86.4	86.4	86.5	83.3	86.8
Calories/oz‖	20	20	20	19	20
Linoleic acid (% cal)	2.8	7.3	1.3	0.04	0.07
Total fat (% cal)	41	41	41	1	42
Protein (% cal)	15	15	14	15	15
Carbohydrate (% cal)	44	44	45	84	53

* Vitamin Content: vitamin A, 2500 U.S.P. units;
vitamin D, 800 U.S.P. units; ascorbic acid, 50 mg;
thiamine, 0.6 mg; niacin, 5 mg; riboflavin, 1.1 mg; and
vitamin B₆, 0.18 mg. Iron ammonium citrate was
added to supply 7.5 mg elemental iron per quart.
† Blend of corn and coconut oils.
‡ Butterfat.
§ Hydrogenated coconut oil.
‖ Carbohydrate (corn syrup) was added to equalize
the caloric value of the mixtures.

supervised the preparation of all the mixtures. Supplies were shipped at monthly intervals in order to prevent the possibility of age thickening.

The infants were given solid foods according to the schedule in Table II. An adequate supply of the different products was prepared at one time,° so each type of solid food had the same composition throughout the study. The composition of the solid foods is shown in Table III.

Subjects of Study

Before any infant was placed on a diet of one of the milk mixtures, the nature of the study was explained to the mother by one of the staff physicians participating in the co-operative venture. The members of the staff had agreed to provide, as private physicians, all pediatric care for the first year of life, including periodic examinations

° Kindly supplied by Gerber Products Company, Fremont, Michigan.

and routine immunizations. The pediatricians also answered calls for emergency conditions. The milk and solid foods were provided gratis for the duration of participation in the study.

The subjects were infants seen in the well baby clinics under the supervision of members of the pediatric staff and included children of members of the staff, of medical students, of nurses, and of technicians. In 1956, 132 were introduced to the study; 174 were added in 1957, 106 in 1958, and 16 in 1959. The distribution between premature and full-term infants was 109 and 319 respectively. The birthweights of five of the premature infants were so close to being marginal (2,500 gm) they were included with the full-term group because they had been started on the special milk mixtures relatively late compared to most of the infants and had gained very well. Eighty-six per cent of the premature infants and nearly 50% of the full-term infants were started on the special milk mixtures while still in the hospital nurseries. There were 355 infants who began the special formula within the first 3 weeks of age, 64 between 3 and 6 weeks, 9 between 6 and 12 weeks. The distribution of 20, 108, and 300, respectively, among Latin American, white, and Negro infants was approximately the same as seen in the outpatient service. There were 202 males and 226 females. The study included observations on 10 sets of twins. In order to prevent confusion for

TABLE II

SCHEDULE OF SOLID FOODS

Age of Infant (mo.)	Type of Food Added
2–3	Cereals: rice, oatmeal, mixed
4–5	Vegetables: peas, green beans, mixed vegetables, carrots, beets, squash
	Fruits: prunes, pears, bananas, applesauce, pears-pineapple, applesauce-apricots, plums-tapioca, fruit-dessert
6	Meats: veal, beef, lamb
	Breads: teething biscuits

TABLE III

Composition of Infant Foods per 100 Grams

| Type | Calories | Protein | CHO | Fat | | Linoleic Acid | | Crude Fiber | Ash | Total Solids | Average Serving, 3–6 months (gm) † |
				Total	% Cal.	Total	% Cal.				
Cereals											
Oatmeal	400	15.3	64.6	7.8*	18.1	2.9	6.7	1.2	4.3	93.2	10–12
Rice	381	6.6	75.1	5.1*	12.1	1.7	4.1	0.8	5.4	93.0	10–12
Mixed	388	13.8	69.4	5.1*	11.9	2.2	5.2	1.1	4.3	93.7	10–12
Vegetables											
Peas	52	4.0	8.3	0.3	5.3	..	..	0.4	0.8	13.8	67
Green beans	24	1.4	4.3	0.1	3.9	..	..	0.8	0.9	7.5	67
Mixed vegetables	37	2.4	6.3	0.2	5.0	..	..	0.7	1.0	10.6	67
Carrots	24	0.7	5.1	0.1	3.7	..	..	0.5	1.0	7.4	67
Beets	38	1.1	8.1	0.1	2.4	..	..	0.6	1.2	11.1	67
Squash	24	0.7	5.0	0.1	3.9	..	..	0.7	0.9	7.4	67
Fruits											
Prunes	86	0.6	20.2	0.3	3.2	..	..	0.8	0.6	22.5	47–67
Pears	59	0.2	14.2	0.1	1.5	..	..	1.2	0.2	15.9	47–67
Bananas	92	0.5	22.0	0.2	2.0	..	..	0.2	0.3	23.2	47–67
Applesauce	85	0.2	20.8	0.1	1.1	..	..	0.6	0.2	21.9	47–67
Pears/pineapple	73	0.4	17.6	0.1	1.3	..	..	1.3	0.3	19.7	47–67
Applesauce/apricot	97	0.4	23.2	0.3	2.9	..	..	0.6	0.5	25.0	47–67
Plums/tapioca	98	0.4	23.8	0.1	0.9	..	..	0.3	0.2	24.8	47–67
Meats											
Veal	98	16.6	..	3.5	33.0	0.09	0.8	..	1.1	21.2	50
Beef	94	14.4	..	4.0	40.0	0.10	1.0	..	1.0	19.4	50
Lamb	99	16.3	..	3.7	35.0	0.15	1.4	..	0.8	20.8	50

* Determined by Acid Hydrolysis.

† ½ can = 67 gm; ⅓–½ can = 47–67 gm; ½ can = 50 gm.

the mother, both twins were assigned the same milk mixture.

Each subject was given a case number to facilitate record keeping. During the first year of the study, random sample procedures determined assignment of one of the four original milk formulas to the individual infant. Because of the necessity of change in the formulas, only 32 subjects were started on formula 4 and 65 subjects on formula 5, instead of the 100 or more as for the other three formulas. In 26 instances because of intercurrent illness, clinical judgment, death, parental complications, or failure to keep appointments, the infant was dropped from the study before any significant clinical or chemical observations could be made. In other words, of 454 infants given a case number, there were 428 on whom clinical evaluations were made

for an average period of 9½ months. Approximately 60% were followed through the first year of life. Throughout the study, careful attention was given to the maintenance of a continued healthy state of all the infants. Each of the pediatricians followed the semi-demand basis in regard to the timing and amount of milk offered. Solid foods were usually withheld for the first 3 months in order to evaluate better the effect of the particular milk mixture. However, if the physician deemed the earlier use of solid food advantageous to the infant's progress, the necessary additions were made. No pediatrician had more than 60 patients under supervision at any one time.

Clinical Observations

The plan of study called for outpatient visits to a special clinic at 3-week intervals for the first 12 weeks, then at monthly intervals. The same personnel were in charge of the clinic throughout. The following clinical features were given careful attention, and the observations were recorded on charts, with special attention to skin (moist and soft, scaly and dry, irritated or infected), stools (soft and regular, frequent, copious and foul, hard but regular, hard and infrequent), intercurrent illness (coryza, upper respiratory infection, otitis media, pneumonia), general features, (vomiting, regurgitation), and satiety (happy, content, placid, fretful, irritable). Measurements of weight, length, and head circumference were made, and, when indicated, temperatures were taken. The body measurements were plotted on Wetzel grids.

The mother was requested to record the dietary intake of the infant for a 4-day period between visits to the special clinic. Mimeographed forms "Mother's Record of Feeding," were provided. These showed subjects' name, formula number and dilution, and the date. Most infants were seen on Friday, and it was recommended that the dietary intake be recorded for the 4 days immediately preceding the visit. Spaces on the charts were delineated for noting the feeding time, the number of ounces taken at each feeding and the ounces of water given in addition. The usual household measures (teaspoonful, tablespoonful, cup or can) were used for recording the intake of cereals (dry), vegetables, fruits, and meat. In order to calculate the average daily weight gain, the gain between each visit was divided by the number of days in the interval.

When the mother and/or the physician felt that an infant was not thriving satisfactorily, one of the alternate milk mixtures was substituted. In a number of instances, when symptomatology of fat deficiency was suspected, a specific fatty acid (linoleic, palmitic, oleic, or arachidonic) was given either in the form of an ester or as the triglyceride. This was mixed with a small amount of food or placed directly in the mouth with a dropper at the time of feeding. More often, however, when manifest signs of linoleic acid deficiency appeared, they were corrected by switching the infant to one of the mixtures containing liberal amounts of linoleic acid.

Laboratory Procedures

Determinations of the serum lipids were made at 3-month intervals beginning with the third month, or before changing formulas. Mothers were instructed to withhold feedings from midnight on, prior to these tests, allowing water ad libitum, however. The method of Wiese and Hansen[4] was used for determination of the total fatty acids in the blood serum, employing the alkaline isomerization technique for the distribution of the dienoic, trienoic, and tetraenoic acids. Total proteins of the serum were measured by nesslerization. Hemoglobin and total and differential leukocyte counts were made at the same time. Other laboratory studies (such as urinalysis, serum electrolytes, roentgenographic and bacteriologic procedures) were made when indicated.

RESULTS

Clinical Features

Information is deposited with the American Documentation Institute Auxiliary Publications Project as Table C (see footnote on title page) concerning each individual infant, including birth date, sex, race, birthweight, age started on milk mixture, duration on the study, data regarding changes to other milk mixtures, and serum lipid values. Summary comments concerning significant observations made by staff physicians also are given.

GENERAL CONSIDERATIONS: Data on the number of infants started on each mixture and the number changed to other mixtures during each 3-month period are summarized in Table IV. The percentage of infants requiring a change in formula were: #1, 2.6; #2, 0.0; #3, 3.8; #4, 50; and #5, 41.5%. Detailed data of formula changes for full-term infants are given in Table V-A, and for premature infants in Table V-B. The percentage of full-term infants remaining on the study in each of the five groups at the end of each 3-month period (Table V-A) was greater for the mixtures containing linoleic acid than for those lacking linoleic acid. For premature babies, the parallel data (Table V-B) reveal a similar, although less clear-cut, pattern. In both groups, the percentage of infants who remained on formulas 4 and 5 increased somewhat after the first quartile. The relative stability with aging may be attributed, at least in part, to the addition of solid foods or, in several instances, to dietary supplementation with linoleic acid.

SATIETY: The mothers' periodic descriptions of satiety (happy, content, placid, fretful, irritable) showed no significant group differences in the reactions of the babies to any of the five formulas.

GROWTH AND DEVLOPMENT RECORDS: Most of the subjects had satisfactory growth patterns as indicated by chartings on the Wetzel grid. Inspection of data for head circumference and body length revealed no particular trends.

At the completion of the investigation, the participating pediatricians jointly studied the growth curve for each subject and selected those showing marked deviation from the normative channels. These deviations presumably represent exceptionally poor or exceptionally favorable growth trends. The findings are summarized in Table VI. Although the numbers involved are small, the higher proportions of greater-than-anticipated growth rates in groups 1, 2, and 3, and of lower-than-anticipated growth rates is groups 4 and 5 are significant.

Since the values for the average gain in weight per day, at 6, 9, and 12 weeks were almost identical for groups 1 and 2, they were combined for statistical comparison with groups 3 and 5. The data for group 4 were too few for consideration. The statistical summary of weight gains is given in Table VII. There was no difference in mean weight gain between groups 1 and 2 combined and group 3. As indicated in the P values the differences were significant for

TABLE IV
MILK FORMULA CHANGES

Subjects	Formula Number				
	1	2	3	4	5
Total started	116	112	103	32	65
>2,500 gm	93	86	74	20	46
<2,500 gm	23	26	29	12	19
Changed to other mixtures					
During 0–3 months					
Total	3	0	2	12	13
>2,500 gm	3	0	2	5	9
<2,500 gm	0	0	0	7	4
During 4–6 months					
Total	0	0	1	4	6
>2,500 gm	0	0	1	3	4
<2,500 gm	0	0	0	1	2
During 7–9 months					
Total	0	0	0	0	6
>2,500 gm	0	0	0	0	4
<2,500 gm	0	0	0	0	2
During 10–12 months					
Total	0	0	1	0	2
>2,500 gm	0	0	0	0	2
<2,500 gm	0	0	1	0	0
Total changes for year	3	0	4	16	27

groups 1 plus 2 versus 5, and for group 3 versus 5.

CALORIC CONSUMPTION: Because of the many variabilities in the feeding of premature infants, data regarding food consumption are presented only for the full-term infants.

The staff physicians individually evaluated the social and personal factors which were believed to influence the reliability of the records made by the mothers. The physicians then collectively performed further screening. After results of serum lipid de-

TABLE V-A

DATA REGARDING NUMBER OF FULL-TERM INFANTS GIVEN DIFFERENT MILK MIXTURES, WITH CHANGES MADE

Changes	Formula Numbers				
	1	2	3	4	5
1st 3 months					
Started (no.)	93	86	74	20	46
Shifted to (no.)	+6	+9	+1	+1	+2
Shifted from (no.)	−3	0	−2	−5	−9
Dropped (no.)	−1	−1	−1	−6	−3
Remaining (no.)	95	94	72	10	36
Completing quartile (%)	96	99	97	48	75
Remaining at 3 months (%)	96	99	97	48	75
4–6 Months					
At end of 3 months (no.)	95	94	72	10	36
Shifted to (no.)	+3	+1	+2	0	+2
Shifted from (no.)	0	0	−1	−3	−4
Dropped (no.)	−10	−8	−4	−2	−3
Remaining (no.)	88	87	69	5	31
Completing quartile (%)	90	92	93	50	82
Remaining at 6 months (%)	86	91	91	24	62
7–9 months					
At end of 6 months (no.)	88	87	69	5	31
Shifted to (no.)	0	+3	+1	0	0
Shifted from (no.)	0	0	0	0	−4
Dropped (no.)	−5	−10	−14	0	−3
Remaining (no.)	83	80	56	5	24
Completing quartile (%)	94	89	80	100	77
Remaining at 9 months (%)	81	81	73	24	48
10–12 months					
At end of 9 months (no.)	83	80	56	5	24
Shifted to (no.)	0	+2	0	0	0
Shifted from (no.)	0	0	0	0	−2
Dropped (no.)	−13	−17	−4	−1	−1
Remaining (no.)	70	65	52	4	21
Completing quartile (%)	84	79	93	80	88
Remaining at 12 months (%)	69	64	68	19	42
Total full-term infants receiving formula	102	101	78	21	50

terminations had been ascertained, each case was again evaluated by the staff physicians and the biochemist. In several instances the results of serum lipid values were such as to arouse suspicion that strict adherence to the special formula had not been maintained. Caloric intake data for these cases were eliminated. This step

TABLE V-B

DATA REGARDING NUMBER OF PREMATURE INFANTS GIVEN DIFFERENT MIXTURES, WITH CHANGES MADE

Changes	Formula Number				
	1	2	3	4	5
1st 3 months					
Started (no.)	23	26	29	12	19
Shifted to (no.)	+2	+5	+3	0	+1
Shifted from (no.)	0	0	0	−7	−4
Droppped (no.)	−9	−12	−12	−2	−7
	—	—	—	—	—
Remaining (no.)	16	19	20	3	9
Completing quartile (%)	64	58	61	25	45
Remaining at 3 months (%)	64	58	61	25	45
4–6 months					
At end of 3 months (no.)	16	19	20	3	9
Shifted to (no.)	+1	+1	0	0	+1
Shifted from (no.)	0	0	0	−1	−2
dropped (no.)	−2	0	−2	0	−1
	—	—	—	—	—
Remaining (no.)	15	20	18	2	7
Completing quartile (%)	88	100	90	67	70
Remaining at 6 months (%)	58	61	55	17	33
7–9 months					
At end of 6 months (no.)	15	20	18	2	7
Shifted to (no.)	0	+1	+1	0	0
Shifted from (no.)	0	0	0	0	−2
Dropped (no.)	−1	−3	−2	0	0
	—	—	—	—	—
Remaining (no.)	14	18	17	2	5
Completing quartile (%)	93	85	89	100	71
Remaining at 9 months (%)	54	55	50	17	24
10–12 months					
At end of 9 months (no.)	14	18	17	2	5
Shifted to (no.)	0	+1	0	0	0
Shifted from (no.)	0	0	−1	0	0
Dropped (no.)	−3	−2	−3	0	−1
	—	—	—	—	—
Remaining (no.)	11	17	13	2	4
Completing quartile	79	94	76	100	80
Remaining at 12 months	42	50	38	17	19
Total premature infants receiving formula	26	34	33	12	21

proved to be necessary in surprisingly few cases. Such eliminations were made, however, if a period of recording intake coincided with an acute illness or some questionable episode.

In considering the caloric intake, per se, the high standard deviations in the individual groups made differences in the mean values not statistically significant. However, when the caloric intake was related to

TABLE VI

INTERPRETATION OF GROWTH AND DEVELOPMENT
RECORDS

Records	Formula Number				
	1	2	3	4	5
Full-term infants	93	86	74	20	46
Exceptionally favorable	7	9	8	1	0
Exceptionally poor	4	2	4	6	20
Premature infants	23	26	29	12	19
Exceptionally favorable	1	1	0	0	0
Exceptionally poor	2	1	2	2	10
Totals	116	112	103	32	65
Exceptionally favorable	8	10	8	1	0
Exceptionally poor	6	3	6	8	30

weight gain, significant differences were noted (Table VIII).

INTERCURRENT ILLNESS: Infections of the respiratory tract were recorded quite frequently, but the incidence did not appear to be influenced by the character of the diet. The frequency of vomiting, regurgitation, unusual feeding problems, or uncommon behavioral characteristics revealed no trends that appeared to be related to the diet.

Twenty-six infants were hospitalized during the study: five with pneumonia; three, bronchitis; four, skin infections; seven, diarrhea; two, hernia; one, slow weight gain; one, pyloric stenosis; one, meningitis; one, burn; and one, otitis media. Hospitalization occurred more frequently with infants receiving milk mixtures 4 and 5 (four of the five with pneumonia, three of the four with skin infections, and six of the seven with diarrhea) than with the other formulas. The incidence of staphylococcal skin infections, with or without severe complications was not influenced by the type of diet. The response to therapy likewise was not different whether or not linoleic acid was in the diet. Among the 454 infants started on the study there were 7 deaths, including 4 prematures. Three died within the first week of life, hence, could not be included in the final tabulation. The fourth (Case 443) died at 41 days of age of bronchopneumonia. He had been placed on formula 5 at 2 days of age and developed diarrhea at 14 days and again 2 weeks later. All three deaths in the full-term infants were associated with staphylococcal infections which coincided with an epidemic due to hemolytic Micrococcus aureus, multiple antibiotic resistant organisms of phage types 80-81, 42B and 44A, which occurred in the hospital newborn nursery.[5-7]

CONDITION OF STOOLS: The most notable feature in regard to bowel movements was the prevalence of loose stools among infants on the formulas lacking linoleic acid, particularly during the first quartile, and

TABLE VII

MEAN VALUES WITH STANDARD DEVIATIONS FOR DAILY WEIGHT GAIN AT 6, 9, AND 12 WEEKS FOR INFANTS
GIVEN FORMULAS 1 AND 2 COMPARED WITH FORMULA 3 AND WITH FORMULA 5

Formula Number	6 Weeks		9 Weeks		12 Weeks	
	Infants (no.)	Mean weight gain/day (gm)	Infants (no.)	Mean weight gain/day (gm)	Infants (no.)	Mean weight gain/day −gm)
#1+#2	113	35.4±11.8	119	32.7±10.6	125	28.0±8.2
#3	48	33.6± 9.9	52	31.5± 9.9	51	29.2±7.9
#5	23	25.9± 8.4	23	22.1± 6.6	20	22.9±8.2
Probability	#1+2 vs #5 P<0.001		#1+2 vs #5 P <0.001		#1+2 vs #5 P <0.01	
Probability	#3 vs #5 P <0.01		#3 vs #5 P <0.001		#3 vs #5 P <0.01	

TABLE VIII

MEAN VALUES WITH STANDARD DEVIATION FOR CALORIES CONSUMED PER KILOGRAM PER DAY FOR EACH
GRAM GAIN IN WEIGHT, AT 6, 9, AND 12 WEEKS FOR INFANTS ON FORMULAS 1+2 COMPARED
WITH FORMULA 3 AND WITH FORMULA 5

Formula Number	6 Weeks		9 Weeks		12 Weeks	
	Infants (no.)	Cal/kg/gm/day	Infants (no.)	Cal/kg/gm/day	Infants (no.)	Cal/kg/gm/day
#1+#2	113	3.82 ± 1.80	119	3.93 ± 1.64	125	4.47 ± 1.80
#3	48	4.50 ± 2.49	52	4.71 ± 2.05	51	4.50 ± 1.77
#5	23	5.32 ± 2.41	23	6.33 ± 2.28	20	6.63 ± 2.74
Probability	#1+2 vs #5 $P < 0.001$		#1+2 vs #3 $P < 0.01$		#1+2 vs #5 $P < 0.001$	
			#1+2 vs #5 $P < 0.001$		#3 vs #5 $P < 0.001$	
			#3 vs #5 $P < 0.01$			

especially among those on formula 4 (Table
IX). The stools were watery and sometimes
sirupy in character. The extremely high
carbohydrate intake undoubtedly was a factor in producing loose stools in infants on
formula 4; however, the incidence was
greater in infants receiving formula 5 than
1, 2, or 3. Hard stools were rarely noted
except for term infants in groups 2 and 3
during the early months of life. In the first
quartile, attacks of diarrhea were slightly
more common for infants on formulas 3 and
4 than for those on 1, 2, or 5.

CONDITION OF SKIN: The occurrence of
dry and scaly skin with thickening was by
far the most striking and significant abnormality observed among infants receiving
formulas low in linoleic acid. This feature
was most easily discernible in the Negro
infants because of the contrast of the white
scales against the dark background (Figs.
1 & 2). During the first 3 months, dryness
of the skin with desquamation, redness, and
oozing in the intertriginous folds was observed in all full-term infants receiving formulas 4 (no fat) and in 40% receiving formula 5 (saturated fat) (Table X-A). During
the second quartile only five full-term infants were still on formula 4, and all five
manifested the typical skin signs. Of the

31 infants on formula 5, 55% showed the
dry and scaly skin. During the third quartile, in a large proportion of the infants receiving milk mixtures 4 and 5, clearing of
the skin was gradual but continuous. During the first and second quartiles, dryness

TABLE IX

CONDITION OF STOOLS

Condition of Stool	Formula Number				
	1	2	3	4	5
	Number of Infants				
1st 3 months					
Full-term infants	93	86	74	20	46
Loose	5	8	4	14	23
Hard	5	16	14	1	2
Premature infants	23	26	29	12	19
Loose	2	1	3	7	6
Hard	1	0	0	0	0
4–6 months (all infants)	111	112	92	13	45
Loose	1	3	0	6	10
Hard	2	3	3	0	1
7–9 months (all infants)	103	106	87	7	38
Loose	1	1	0	0	1
Hard	0	4	3	0	2
10–12 months (all infants)	97	97	73	7	29
Loose	0	2	0	0	0
Hard	1	1	1	0	0
Total Infants	116	112	103	32	65

TABLE X-A

FULL-TERM INFANTS WITH SYMPTOMS REFERABLE TO THE SKIN AT VARIOUS AGES

Symptoms	Formula Number									
	1		2		3		4		5	
	No.	Visits	No.	Visits	No.	Visits	No.	Visits	No.	Visits
3–6 weeks	93	93	86	86	73	73	17	17	40	40
Total with skin symptoms	4		6		6		8		11	
Dry and scaly	1		2		3		7		10	
Perianal irritation	0		2		0		4		2	
Bacterial skin infection	3		2		3		0		2	
6–9 weeks	95	95	91	91	72	72	13	13	35	35
Total with skin symptoms	6		5		9		8		11	
Dry and scaly	5		2		6		7		9	
Perianal irritation	0		0		0		1		1	
Bacterial infection	1		3		3		0		1	
9–12 weeks	95	95	94	94	72	72	10	10	36	36
Total with skin symptoms	2		7		2		10		15	
Dry and scaly	1		3		2		10		14	
Perianal irritation	0		0		0		1		0	
Bacterial infection	1		4		0		1		1	
4–6 months	88	264	87	261	69	207	5	15	31	93
Total with skin symptoms	11		9		9		5		17	
Dry and scaly	4		3		4		5		17	
Perianal irritation	0		0		0		1		0	
Bacterial infection	8		6		5		0		0	
7–9 months	83	249	80	240	56	168	5	15	24	72
Total with skin symptoms	8		6		2		1		10	
Dry and scaly	2		2		0		1		9	
Perianal irritation	0		0		0		0		0	
Bacterial infection	6		4		2		0		2	
10–12 months	70	210	65	195	52	156	4	12	21	63
Total with skin symptoms	6		4		3		1		3	
Dry and scaly	1		2		2		1		2	
Perianal irritation	0		0		0		0		0	
Bacterial infection	5		2		1		0		1	
Total symptoms	102	1,082	101	1,041	78	812	21	99	50	375
Total with skin symptoms	24		26		24		14		34	

of the skin as a transient episode was noted in 14 of the infants receiving formulas 1, 2, and 3. In the premature infants, dry scaly skin was recorded infrequently on formulas 1, 2, and 3 and in nearly all receiving mixtures 4 and 5 (Table X-B). At 4 to 5 months in the premature infants receiving mixtures 4 and 5, the incidence of skin abnormalities was high but became less severe with increasing age.

Perianal irritation also tended to occur somewhat more frequently among infants on diets low in linoleic acid, but the incidence was not so great as with the dry, scaly skin syndrome. Perianal irritation disappeared after the first 3 months.

TABLE X-B

Premature Infants with Symptoms Referable to the Skin at Various Ages

Symptoms	Formula Number									
	1		2		3		4		5	
	No.	Visits	No.	Visits	No.	Visits	No.	Visits	No.	Visits
3–6 weeks	18	18	21	21	21	21	6	6	12	12
Total with skin symptoms	2		0		2		6		6	
Dry and scaly	0		0		0		5		3	
Perianal irritation	2		0		0		1		2	
Bacterial infection	0		0		2		2		2	
6–9 weeks	17	17	19	19	20	20	5	5	10	10
Total with skin symptoms	1		1		1		3		6	
Dry and scaly	1		0		0		3		6	
Perianal irritation	0		1		0		0		0	
Bacterial infection	0		0		1		0		0	
9–12 weeks	16	16	19	19	20	20	3	3	9	9
Total with skin symptoms	1		0		1		3		7	
Dry and scaly	1		0		1		3		7	
Perianal irritation	0		0		0		0		0	
Bacterial infection	0		0		0		0		1	
4–6 months	15	45	20	60	18	54	2	6	7	21
Total with skin symptoms	1		0		2		2		7	
Dry and scaly	1		0		0		2		7	
Perianal irritation	0		0		0		0		7	
Bacterial infection	0		0		1		0		0	
7–9 months	14	42	18	54	17	51	2	6	5	15
Total with skin symptoms	2		2		1		0		2	
Dry and scaly	1		1		0		0		2	
Perianal irritation	0		0		0		0		0	
Bacterial infection	1		1		1		0		0	
10–12 months	11	33	17	51	13	39	2	6	4	12
Total with skin symptoms	1		1		2		0		1	
Dry and scaly	0		0		0		0		1	
Perianal irritation	0		0		0		0		0	
Bacterial infection	1		1		2		0		0	
Total symptoms	26	192	34	244	33	226	12	44	21	94
Total with skin symptoms	7		6		9		8		10	

Laboratory Data

SERUM LIPIDS: In Table XI are summarized quartile data for the total fatty acids as well as diene, triene, and tetraene fatty acids in the blood serum of infants on the various milk mixtures. The mean, standard deviation, and standard error of the mean are presented for each group of subjects. When the diet was very low in linoleic acid content, the total fatty acids in the serum tended to be high. This is especially true for infants receiving formula 4 (no fat). In Figure 3 the inverse relationship between the amount of linoleic acid in the diet as well as the dienoic acid in the blood serum and the level of total

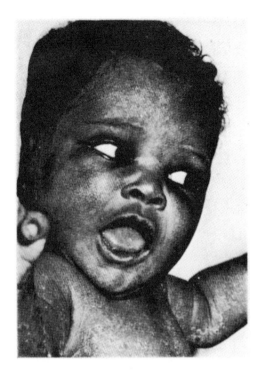

FIG. 1. At one week of age this female infant (Case 269) was started on a milk mixture (Formula 5) containing 42% of the calories as fat, but no linoleic acid. At 3 weeks a scaly dry skin was definitely discernible, becoming more pronounced with time (age in photograph, 10 weeks). At 2 months, pustules containing staphylococcus aureus developed; the child was referred to the hospital. Response to antibiotic therapy was satisfactory. At 2½ months, linoleic acid (trilinolein) was given in an amount equivalent to 2% of the caloric intake. Within 2 weeks there was great improvement in the skin, which soon became entirely clear. The linoleic acid supplement was discontinued after 32 days, and within 6 weeks the skin again became red and scaly, which condition gradually cleared. Solid foods were started at 3 months, and, as indicated from the serum lipid findings, there was an increase in dienoic acid level of the serum.

FIG. 2. Typical skin changes developed in a premature infant (Case 447) who received milk mixture 5. In an attempt to evaluate the role of oleic acid, triolein was given in an amount equal to 2% of the caloric intake, but no improvement occurred during a 2-week period, at which time the photograph was taken. No change in the serum lipid values followed the addition of oleic acid to the diet. Linoleic acid, as trilinolein, in an amount equal to 2% of the caloric intake was then added to the diet, and within 2 weeks the skin returned to normal.

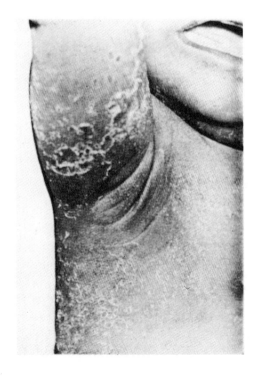

153

TABLE XI

MEAN, STANDARD DEVIATION, AND STANDARD ERROR FOR BLOOD SERUM TOTAL FATTY ACIDS (TFA) (IN MG/100 ML), WITH DIENE, TRIENE, AND TETRAENE ACIDS AS A PERCENTAGE OF THE TOTAL FATTY ACIDS, FOR ALL INFANTS

	Formula Number				
	1	*2*	*3*	*4*	*5*
3 months					
TFA (no. of determinations)	66	58	60	11	30
Mean	237	231	269	306	263
S. D.	45.5	37.8	48.0	79.2	66.6
SE$_m$	5.6	5.0	6.4	25.1	12.4
Di (no. of determinations)	66	58	60	11	30
Mean	28.97	35.40	12.87	2.80	5.55
S. D.	3.41	5.16	2.59	1.29	1.75
SE$_m$	0.42	0.68	0.34	0.41	0.32
Tri (no. of determinations)	66	58	60	11	30
Mean	1.77	1.39	2.50	5.54	3.74
S. D.	0.61	0.75	0.66	1.62	1.05
SE$_m$	0.08	0.10	0.09	0.51	0.19
Tetra (no. of determinations)	66	58	60	11	30
Mean	9.07	10.81	8.01	2.56	2.69
S. D.	2.17	2.14	1.37	1.00	1.45
SE$_m$	0.27	0.28	0.18	0.32	0.27
6 months					
TFA (no. of determinations)	60	62	52	4	27
Mean	245	235	282	301	265
S. D.	44.2	38.8	48.6	32.9	54.0
SE$_m$	5.8	5.0	6.8	19.0	10.6
Di (no. of determinations)	60	62	53	4	27
Mean	30.53	37.64	15.67	7.88	10.89
S. D.	3.79	3.48	2.05	1.95	3.89
SE$_m$	0.49	0.45	0.28	1.13	0.76
Tri (no. of determinations)	61	62	53	4	27
Mean	1.67	1.35	2.23	4.40	3.54
S. D.	0.79	0.80	0.73	0.68	0.61
SE$_m$	0.10	0.10	0.10	0.39	0.12
Tetra (no. of determinations)	61	62	53	4	27
Mean	9.81	10.50	8.63	3.30	3.92
S. D.	2.08	1.91	1.45	1.35	1.76
SE$_m$	0.27	0.25	0.20	0.78	0.35
9 months					
TFA (no. of determinations)	53	51	51	5	22
Mean	248	236	288	345	255
S. D.	39.1	35.7	32.9	94.8	43.9
SE$_m$	5.4	5.1	4.7	47.4	9.6
Di (no. of determinations)	53	51	52	5	23
Mean	30.77	36.87	17.65	9.18	17.13
S. D.	3.85	3.53	3.51	2.65	4.53
SE$_m$	0.53	0.50	0.49	1.33	0.97
Tri (no. of determinations)	53	51	52	5	23
Mean	1.82	1.38	2.28	3.10	3.39
S. D.	0.85	0.83	0.88	0.75	0.80
SE$_m$	0.12	0.12	0.12	1.37	0.17
Tetra (no. of determinations)	53	51	52	5	23
Mean	10.48	11.60	9.14	4.60	5.93
S. D.	2.05	2.05	1.28	1.24	2.15
SE$_m$	0.29	0.29	0.18	0.62	0.46

TABLE XI—(*Continued*)

| | Formula Number | | | | |
	1	*2*	*3*	*4*	*5*
12 months					
TFA (no. of determinations)	60	57	52	5	17
Mean	254	251	275	309	264
S. D.	37.4	42.5	37.7	60.7	59.7
SE_m	4.9	5.7	5.3	30.4	14.9
Di (no. of determinations)	60	57	53	5	16
Mean	30.58	36.46	20.89	12.48	19.94
S. D.	3.40	3.16	3.55	3.28	4.15
SE_m	0.44	0.42	0.49	1.64	1.07
Tri (no. of determinations)	60	57	53	5	17
Mean	1.83	1.80	1.99	3.14	2.48
S. D.	0.88	0.89	0.85	0.91	0.82
SE_m	0.12	0.12	0.12	0.46	0.21
Tetra (no. of determinations)	60	57	53	5	17
Mean	10.73	11.17	10.13	6.46	8.35
S. D.	1.78	1.80	1.20	1.71	2.32
SE_m	0.23	0.24	0.17	0.85	0.58

fatty acids in the blood serum is shown graphically for the infants at 3 months of age.

Of special interest are the diene fatty acid levels, which reflect so remarkably the linoleic acid content of the diet. The blood serum values for diene fatty acids were much higher for infants receiving formulas 1 and 2 than for the others. Although the serum values were much lower in groups 4 and 5, the lowest values were found in infants receiving formula 4. Intermediate values were found for the infants receiving milk mixture 3 (linoleic acid about 1.3% of the calories). The dienoic acid level of the blood serum changed very little at 6, 9, and 12 months for infants receiving formulas 1 and 2, but it increased markedly with increasing age for infants on the other formulas. Figure 4 portrays graphically the changes occurring with time for the infants on formula 5. The increase in the dienoic acid level of the blood serum coincided with the clinical improvement of the skin condition.

The level of trienoic acid in the blood serum varied inversely with the dienoic acid. Summary data are presented in Figure 5. The level of tetraenoic acid in the

blood serum tended to follow the pattern of the dienoic acid, although the change was not so great proportionately. Not shown in the compilation of serum lipid data (Table XI) were the results obtained from 24 premature infants in whom the serum lipids were determined before the age of 7 weeks. These infants were evenly distributed among the five dietary groups, and the 7-week values for total fatty acids, and dienoic, trienoic, and tetraenoic acids agreed very closely with the results obtained at 3 months of age.

Statistical comparisons of the serum lipid

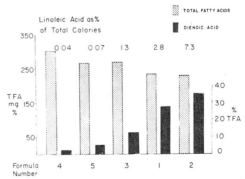

FIG. 3. Mean values for total fatty acids and dienoic acid levels in blood serum of infants 3 months of age in relation to dietary intake of linoleic acid as percentage of calories.

values were made between various subgroups such as full term and premature, white, Negro and Latin American, and males and females, in all possible combinations. There was no evidence that length of gestation, race, or sex had any influence on serum lipid values.

Serum Proteins: The values for the total proteins of the serum as well as albumin and globulin were summarized. (This information has been deposited with the American Documentation Institute. See footnote on title page.) Consideration of mean values, standard deviations, and probable errors of the means revealed no significant differences among the infants on the different formulas at the various age levels.

Routine Blood Counts: The mean values, standard deviations, and standard errors of the means for hemoglobin, total leukocyte count, and polymorphonuclear and mononuclear cells showed no relationship to the kind or amount of fat in the diet. (These data are deposited with the American Documentation Institute. See footnote on title page.)

Histologic Features: No attempt was made to examine skin biopsy specimens routinely. However, on several occasions, it was possible to obtain slivers of skin for histologic study. Sections of skin were obtained from eight infants, but in only one case was a biopsy specimen obtained from

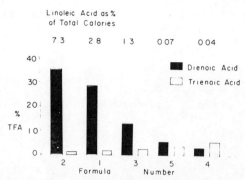

Fig. 5. Mean values for dienoic and trienoic acids as per cent of total fatty acids of the serum for infants at age 3 months fed on milk mixtures containing negligible amounts (< 0.1%) to 7.3% of the calories as linoleic acid.

an infant on a diet containing liberal quantities of linoleic acid. In order to make a more careful evaluation, sections of skin were obtained from an additional eight infants who formed the basis for the control histology. The usual methods of preparation and staining procedures (hematoxylin and eosin) were used.* The findings for control infants and those receiving milk mixtures low in linoleic acid content were remarkably similar to the histologic features demonstrated in previous studies with dogs,[8, 9] as well as with rats on control and low fat diets.[10-12]

Typical histologic sections of skin are illustrated in Figures 6 and 7. Figure 6 is for an infant (Case 177) who had received formula 5 (low in linoleic acid) for 3 months. Figure 7 is one of the 8 infants who served as control.

COMMENT

Published results of comparable infant feeding studies are not available; hence, it is not possible to interpret our findings in the light of previous investigative work. Moreover, in this type of study it is admittedly difficult to control such features as environment, social and economic conditions, psychological and emotional reac-

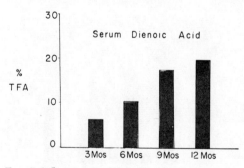

Fig. 4. Influence of solid food with increasing age on the mean dienoic acid levels of the blood serum of infants receiving a milk mixture having 42% of the calories as fat but extremely low in linoleic acid content (Formula 5).

* Prepared and interpreted by Dr. John G. Sinclair, Professor of Histology, University of Texas School of Medicine, Galveston, Texas.

tions, or to make consistently accurate objective observations for prolonged periods on a large number of infants.

In persuing the literature regarding the subject of infant feeding it is evident that numerous attempts have been made to compare the adequacy of feeding many types and kinds of milk with that of breast milk. In a comprehensive review, Aitken and Hytten[13] cited data comparing the relative effectiveness of breast and artificial feeding. In an extensive prospective study, Mellander *et al.*[14] in Sweden evaluated certain clinical and chemical features in breast and in artificially fed infants. It is surprising to note, however, that, insofar as we could discover, no long-term controlled studies have been carried out wherein an evaluation was made concerning the nature

of the fat in the milk, especially in relation to its linoleic acid content. Although it is recognized that there is a marked difference in the amount of linoleic acid in human and cow's milk, the distinct differences in the protein, mineral, and vitamin composition of the two milks may profoundly influence the results of comparative studies. In the study reported here the attempt was made, therefore, to vary the linoleic acid intake of the infants while holding other nutrients constant among the several groups. It should be pointed out, however, that it is difficult to evaluate completely the specific nutritional role of linoleic acid, because when the linoleic acid content of a fat is changed it must be replaced by fatty acids having different chain lengths and degrees of unsaturation. In our studies, inas-

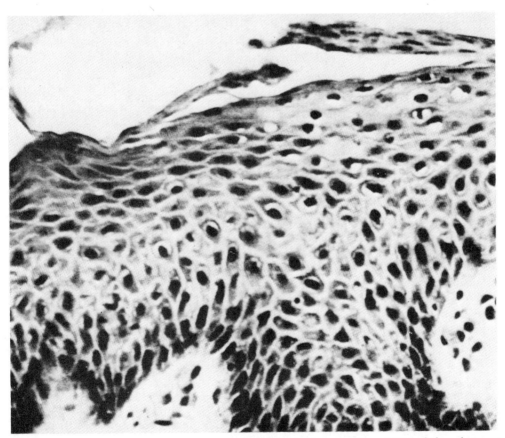

Fig. 6 Photomicrograph of histologic sections of skin from infant receiving < 0.1% of the calories as linoleic acid (Formula 5). (×600).

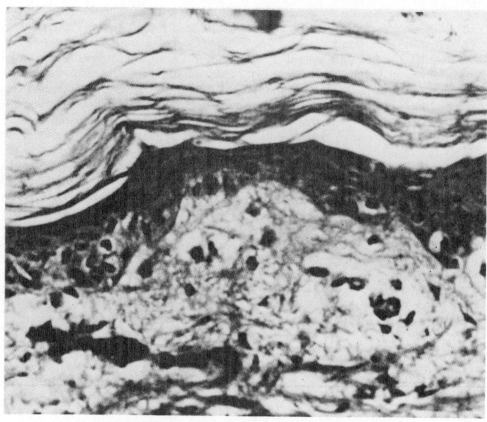

Fig. 7. Photomicrograph of skin from a newborn infant. (×600).

much as different fats were used to effect variations in the linoleic acid content, it was necessary to change to some extent the proportion of other fatty acids in the fat; nevertheless, the other nutrients (protein, minerals, and vitamins) remained the same in all the formulas. In one mixture carbohydrate was substituted isocalorically for fat. By and large, the clinical and chemical observations appear significant particularly when interpreted in the light of findings from studies with experimental animals. Data from the literature have been summarized by several authorities.[15][17] A recent review is that of Aaes-Jørgensen.[18]

The development of a dry and scaly skin with thickening as a persistent symptom in the very young, rapidly growing infant points to this phenomenon as a typical manifestation of linoleic acid deficiency.

The relative incidence of the occurrence of skin changes suggestive of fat deficiency for the infants receiving the different milk mixtures is presented graphically in Figure 8. In compiling these data only those subjects have been considered who were started on a particular milk mixture before the age of 6 weeks and remained on the same mixture for at least 3 months or until development of skin changes occurred. It is felt by the observers that if an infant is started on a diet lacking linoleic acid at a very young age, it would be suprising if he did not develop definitive skin changes within the matter of 2 to 3 months. On the basis of recent findings by Wiese et al.[19] with young puppies, rate of growth is important in the development of skin abnormalities in linoleic acid deficiency states.

Infants who received the milk mixture

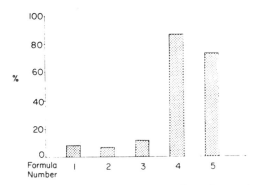

FIG. 8. Schematic representation of incidence of the occurrence of skin changes suggestive of fat deficiency in infants who were given the different milk mixtures before the age of 6 weeks and who were given the same mixture for a 3-month period or until dry scaly skin with thickening was definite.

containing saturated fat to equal 42% of the calories developed skin changes more slowly than the infants who received the skimmed milk mixture. This observation suggests either that linoleic acid even in small amounts such as in formula 5 delays the development of skin manifestations or that dietary fat per se has a protective effect on the skin. Also, the finding that the addition of solid foods to the diets was associated with a gradual amelioration of the skin abnormalities indicates that the linoleic acid provided by solid foods is effective in curing skin manifestations. The changes in serum lipid values with increasing age support this conclusion (Table XI). Particularly significant is the fact that the administration of linoleic acid per se effected not only clinical improvement in the skin condition, but also an increase of dienoic acid in the blood serum.

The incidence of bacterial infections of the skin was not significantly different among the various groups of infants (Tables X-A and X-B). Serious complications, however, occurred in several infants receiving the milk mixtures low in linoleic acid content, but by no means were they confined to this group, and the episodes did not occur concurrently. Experience in our own laboratories with experimental animals indicates increased susceptibility to bacterial infections resulting from fat deficiency.

The dermatologic evidences of fat deficiency which have been demonstrated in a great variety of experimental animals were emphasized in the original contributions of Burr and Burr[20,21] in their studies with rats. Adult animals on fat-free diets are known not to develop classical signs of fat deficiency readily. On the other hand, Barki et al.[22] showed that if severely depleted adult rats (reduced to half their starting weight) are given fat-free diets ad libitum, they manifest classical fat deficiency symptoms along with the gain in weight.

In 1919 von Gröer[23] and in 1937 von Chwalibogowski[24] maintained two infants each on low fat diets for prolonged periods. Skin changes were not observed in these four subjects. However, from their data it is not clear to what extent fat had been removed from the diet. All four infants were given solid foods early, especially cereals, and it may well be that there was sufficient linoleic acid in the diet to prevent skin manifestations. In 1935, Holt and co-workers[25] maintained three infants, 4 to 6½ months of age, on diets low in fat for periods of 2 to 7 days. One infant developed eczema. The eruption disappeared when fat was added to the diet again, only to recur when the low fat diet was resumed. The longest period of time an infant has been known to remain on a diet very low in fat was the patient reported in 1944 by Hansen and Wiese.[26] The special diet was given for its possible effectiveness in the management of his chylous ascites. As a young infant he developed impetigo, which was very resistant to treatment, compared with the results obtained with the other infants in the same ward. Likewise, with the occurrence of prickly heat during the hot weather season, a distinct dermatitis developed which persisted for months after the onset of cool weather and long after the skin of other children similarly affected had cleared. When the child was about 6 months of age, eczematous patches developed on the cheeks, scalp, and various parts of the body; however, the lesions responded readily to local therapy. Recently Warwick and co-workers[27] reported the development of abnormal skin symptoms in a child with chylous ascites, and lymphedema. This 4½-year-old girl had been maintained on a low fat diet, and the ectodermal changes were suggestive of a deficiency of unsaturated fatty acids.

As indicated from the work of Burr and Burr and confirmed by subsequent workers, impairment of growth appears to be a characteristic feature of fat deficiency in experimental animals. It cannot be concluded from the findings of von Gröer and von Chwalibogowski relative to the poor growth of their infants that this resulted from a deficiency of linoleic acid. In fact, it is difficult to ascertain from the information available to what extent other possible nutritional factors were lacking in the diets of their infants. Inasmuch as in our studies the diets were complete other than for fat and linoleic acid, there seems to be little doubt that the rate of gain in weight was related to the linoleic acid intake.

The finding of a greater caloric intake in relation to gain in body weight in infants lacking linoleic acid in the diet as compared to infants receiving dietary linoleic acid confirms not only earlier observations[28] on human subjects, but also early studies with rats by Wesson and Burr[29] and Burr and Beber.[30] This phase of the linoleic acid problem has been pursued more recently by Panos and co-workers.[31] They demonstrated increased basal oxygen consumption in rats reared on diets deficient in linoleic acid. Actually these authors observed that this was the earliest of all aberrations to appear in the fat deficient state.[32] By paired feeding of rats, Naismith[33] found food consumption of linoleic acid deficient animals to be 40 to 60% greater than that of the controls receiving 7.5% of their calories as linoleic acid. Combes et al.,[34] in studies with premature infants, found a lesser caloric consumption for each gram gain in body weight when the milk contained liberal quantities of linoleic acid than when this fatty acid was not provided. In recent studies by Panos[35] differences in insensible weight loss have not been demonstrable in infants with and without linoleic acid in the diets. On the other hand, determination of respiratory quotients on an adult subject maintained on a diet extremely low in linoleic acid for a period of 6 months revealed that the human being reacted metabolically in the same manner as the rat.[36]

It is quite obvious from the present study as well as previous observations both with experimental animals and human subjects that the serum lipid pattern readily reflects nutritional status regarding linoleic acid. Unfortunately, no attempt was made by von Gröer or von Chwalibogowski to determine the iodine number of the blood fat in the infants studied by them. Early work in our laboratories had demonstrated conclusively that the iodine number of the fat in the blood serum reflects the degree of unsaturation of the fat in the diet. The true magnitude of the change in specific fatty acids was not appreciated, however. It was some years later that Wiese et al.[37] showed that the diene and tetraene fatty acids in the blood serum varied directly with linoleic acid in the diet while the triene fatty acids varied inversely. This observation was found to hold true not only for young puppies but also for the human infant.[38] Study of the serum lipids appears to give quite conclusive evidence that rather liberal quantities of linoleic acid may be contributed by the addition of solid foods to the diet. This is particularly significant for the infants receiving milk mixtures low in linoleic acid. For example, in Figure 4 one may note the marked increase in the dienoic acid level of the blood serum with the passage of time, resulting no doubt from the addition of cereals and meats to the diets. Equally significant is the fact that the alterations in serum lipid findings are in keeping with the clinical improvement noted in these patients.

SPECIFICITY OF LINOLEIC ACID: It is quite apparent from the results of this study that young human infants do not thrive when placed on diets lacking linoleic acid. The inadequacy of the milk mixture containing 42% of the calories as fat, yet extremely low in linoleic acid content, speaks for the specificity of dietary linoleic acid, rather than for fat per se. Especially significant, of course, is the observation that the administration of linoleic acid, given as an ester or as trilinolein or as present in the formula or in solid foods, restored to normal the skin of infants who had received diets deficient in linoleic acid.

REQUIREMENT FOR LINOLEIC ACID: Before the recognition of specific requirements for many nutrients, it was generally believed that fat served only as a concentrated source of energy and had no other function. A later concept was that fat acted as a carrier for certain vitamins, but since fat per se is readily synthesized from carbohydrate and protein, it was thought to serve no other purpose. However, in 1918, Aron[39] reported that in rats, growth was unsatisfactory when the animals were deprived of fat (butter). It was this observation that prompted the studies by von Gröer employing human infants. In 1927 Evans and Burr,[40, 41] also found that rats failed to thrive when given a diet low in fat in spite of the addition of vitamin E to the diet. These authors[42] suggested that a gap be left in the developing vitamin nomenclature, namely "F," for an unknown nutrient. Although McAmis et al.[43] in 1929 reported unsatisfactory progress of rats on diets low in fat, it remained for Burr and Burr[20, 21] to prove the dietary essentiality of linoleic acid.

In estimating the requirement for linoleic acid in experimental animals, the criteria used have been growth and changes in the skin, hair and tail. Although rate of weight gain has been a valuable tool for the laboratory animal, it would be difficult, indeed, to depend upon this criterion alone for the human infant. As previously stated the serum levels of certain unsaturated fatty acids reflect to a remarkable degree the dietary intake of linoleic acid, both for the young infant and the puppy and are of particular significance in view of the excellent

correlations with clinical and histologic findings.[37, 38] Various studies carried on by the authors suggest that the requirement for linoleic acid by the human infant depends on the rate of growth as well as the composition of the diet. On the basis of observations regarding ectodermal changes and serum lipids as reported here, young rapidly growing infants developed evidences of deficiency when receiving less than 0.1% of their calories as linoleic acid and did not show these signs when receiving 1.0% or more of the calories as this fatty acid. The optimum dietary level is yet to be determined. That mother's milk supplies about 4 to 5% of the calories as linoleic acid bears special consideration in relation to establishment of nutritional requirements.

SUMMARY AND CONCLUSIONS

Four hundred and twenty-eight infants over a 4-year period were studied for approximately 4,000 patient-months of observation while receiving five different milk mixtures varying in linoleic acid content from less than 0.1 to 7.3% of the calories. It was found that linoleic acid is a required nutrient for the young human infant. The following pertinent observations were made. (1) Evidences of linoleic acid deficiency developed in young infants who received either a diet practically devoid of fat or one providing 42% of the calories as fat but extremely low in linoleic acid (less than 0.1% of the calories). (2) Manifestations of the deficiency state disappeared promptly when linoleic acid was given as the ester or triglyceride or in a milk mixture providing 1% or more of the calories as linoleic acid. (3) The most characteristic feature of the deficiency state was dryness of the skin with desquamation, thickening and later intertrigo. (4) The incidence of bacterial skin infections was the same in the different groups. It was noted that young infants receiving diets very low in linoleic acid seemed to react severely when outbreaks of staphylococcal infection developed in the hospital environment. (5) Records for rate of growth showed unsatisfactory progress for many of the infants on low linoleic acid intakes, whereas the course of events was satisfactory in almost all of the infants who received 1.3 to 7.3% of the calories as linoleic acid. (6) Blood serum levels for dienoic acid of $5.6 \pm 1.8\%$ of the total fatty acids were indicative of the deficiency state, whereas values of $12.9 \pm 2.6\%$ of the total fatty acids represented the minimal normal. 7) Histologic alterations in the skin of infants on diets low in linoleic acid showed the same characteristics as seen in experimental animals. (8) Infants given milk mixtures extremely low in linoleic acid had a gradual amelioration of fat deficiency manifestations as well as increasing levels of dienoic acid in the blood serum following the introduction of cereals to their diet.

REFERENCES

1. Hansen, A. E., et al.: Manifestations of fat deficiency in infants (Abstract). Fed. Proc., 16:387, 1957.
2. Hansen, A. E. et al.: Intake of linoleic acid in relation to serum unsaturated fatty acids and fat-deficiency symptoms in infants. Transactions of the American Pediatric Society (Abstract). J. Dis. Child., 94:398, 1957.
3. Hansen, A. E., et al.: Essential fatty acids in infant nutrition. III. Clinical manifestations of linoleic acid deficiency. J. Nutr., 66:565, 1958.
4. Wiese, H. F., and Hansen, A. E.: Semimicromethod for unsaturated fatty acids of blood serum. J. Biol. Chem., 202:417, 1953.
5. Bass, J. A., et al.: Epidemiologic study of a hospital outbreak of micrococcic infections. J. A. M. A., 166:731, 1958.
6. Bass, J. A., and Felton, H. M.: Utilization of laboratory findings in diagnosis and control of hospital staphylococcal infections. Amer. J. Pub. Health, 49:1512, 1959.
7. Felton, H. M., Willard, C., and Bass, J. A.: Management of an outbreak of staphylococcal infection in a nursery for the newborn and the results of an intensive control program. South. Med. J., 52:387, 1959.
8. Hansen, A. E., Holmes, S. G., and Wiese, H. F.: Fat in the diet in relation to nutrition of the dog: IV. Histologic features of skin from animals fed diets with and without fat. Tex. Rep. Biol. Med., 9:555, 1951.
9. Hansen, A. E., Sinclair, J. G., and Wiese, H. F.: Sequence of histologic changes in skin of dogs in relation to dietary fat. J. Nutr., 52:541, 1954.
10. Williamson, R.: A note on the epidermis of rat on fat-free diet. Biochem. J., 35:1003, 1941.
11. Ramlingaswami, V., and Sinclair, H. M.: The relation of deficiencies of vitamin A and of essential fatty acids to follicular hyperkeratosis in the rat. Brit. J. Dermat., 65:1, 1953.
12. Alfin-Slater, R., and Bernick, S.: Changes in tissue lipids and tissue histology resulting from essential fatty acid deficiency in rats. Amer. J. Clin. Nutr., 6:613, 1958.
13. Aitken, F. C., and Hytten, F. E.: Infant feeding: comparison of breast and artificial feeding. Nutr. Abstr. Rev., 30:341, 1960.
14. Mellander, O., Vahlquist, B., and Mellbin, T.: Breast feeding and artificial feeding: A clinical, serological and biochemical study in 402 infants, with a survey of the literature. Acta Paediat., 48 (Suppl. 116), 1959.
15. Sebrell, W. H., Jr., and Harris, R. S.: The Vitamins, Vol. 2. New York, Academic Press, 1954, pp. 267-319.
16. Deuel, H. J., Jr.: The Lipids, Vol. 3. New York, Interscience Publishers, 1957, pp. 783-834.
17. Sinclair, H. M.: International Conference on Biochemical Problems of Lipids—Essential Fatty Acids. Proceedings of the 4th Conference held at Oxford, 1957. London, W. C. 2, Butterworths and Company, 1958.
18. Aaes-Jørgensen, E.: Essential fatty acids, Physiol. Rev., 41: No. 1, 1961.
19. Wiese, H. F., Hansen, A. E., and Coon, E.: Effect of high and low caloric intakes on fat deficiency of dogs. J. Nutr., 76:73, 1962.
20. Burr, G. O., and Burr, M. M.: A new deficiency disease produced by the rigid exclusion of fat from the diet. J. Biol. Chem., 82:345, 1929.
21. Burr, G. O., and Burr, M. M.: On the nature and role of the fatty acids essential in nutrition. J. Biol. Chem., 86:587, 1930.
22. Barki, V. H., et al.: Production of essential fatty acid deficiency symptoms in the mature rat. Proc. Soc. Exp. Biol. Med., 66:474, 1947.
23. von Gröer, F.: Zur Frage der praktischen Bedeutung des Nähr Wertbegriffes nebst einigen Bemerkungen über das Fett minimum des menschlichen Säuglings. Biochem. Z., 93:311, 1919.
24. von Chwalibogowski, A.: Experimentaluntersuchungen über kalorisch ausreichende, qualitativ einseitige Ernährung des Säuglings. Acta Paediat., 22:110, 1937.
25. Holt, L. E., Jr., et al.: Studies in fat metabolism: fat absorption in normal infants. J. Pediat., 6:427, 1935.
26. Hansen, A. E., and Wiese, H. F.: Clinical and blood lipid studies in a child with

chylous ascites. Proceedings of the American Pediatric Society, Amer. J. Dis. Child., 68:351, 1944.

27. Warwick, W. J., et al.: Chylous ascites and lymphedema. Amer. J. Dis. Child., 98:317, 1959.

28. Adam, D. J. D., Hansen, A. E., and Wiese, H. F.: Essential fatty acids in infant nutrition: II. Effect of linoleic acid on caloric intake. J. Nutr., 66:555, 1958.

29. Wesson, L. G., and Burr, G. O.: The metabolic rate and respiratory quotients of rats on a fat-deficient diet. J. Biol. Chem., 91:525, 1931.

30. Burr, G. O., and Beber, A. J.: Metabolism studies with rats suffering from fat deficiency. J. Nutr., 14:553, 1937.

31. Panos, T. C., Finerty, J. C., and Wall, R. L.: Increased metabolism in fat-deficiency: relation to dietary fat. Proc. Soc. Exp. Biol. Med., 93:581, 1956.

32. Morris, D. M., et al.: Relation of thyroid activity to increased metabolism induced by fat deficiency. J. Nutr., 62:119, 1957.

33. Naismith, D. J.: The role of dietary fat in the utilization of protein: II. The essential fatty acids. J. Nutr., 77:381, 1962.

34. Combes, M., Pratt, E. L., and Wiese, H. F.: Essential fatty acids in premature infant feeding. PEDIATRICS, 30:136, 1962.

35. Panos, T. C., et al.: Metabolic effects of low fat feeding in premature infants (Abstract). Fed. Proc., 20:366, 1961.

36. Brown, W. R., et al.: Effects of prolonged use of extremely low-fat diet on an adult human subject. J. Nutr., 16:511, 1938.

37. Wiese, H. F., Hansen, A. E., and Baughan, M. A.: Effect of fat on diet on unsaturated fatty acids in phospholipid, cholesterol ester and glyceride fractions in serum of dogs. J. Nutr., 63:523, 1957.

38. Wiese, H. F., Hansen, A. E., and Adam, D. J. D.: Essential fatty acids in infant nutrition: I. Linoleic acid requirement in terms of serum di- tri- and tetraenoic acid levels. J. Nutr., 66:345, 1958.

39. Aron, H.: Über den Nährwert. Biochem. Z., 92:211, 1918.

40. Evans, H. M., and Burr, G. O.: A new dietary deficiency with highly purified diets. Proc. Soc. Exp. Biol. Med., 24:740, 1927.

41. Evans, H. M., and Burr, G. O.: New dietary deficiency with highly purified diets: II. Supplementary requirement of diet of pure casein, sucrose and salt. Proc. Soc. Exp. Biol. Med., 25:41, 1927.

42. A new dietary deficiency with highly purified diets. III. The beneficial effect of fat in the diet. Proc. Soc. Exp. Biol. Med. 25:390, 1928.

43. McAmis, A. J., Anderson, W. E., and Mendel, L. B.: Growth of rats on "fat-free" diets. J. Biol. Chem., 82:247, 1929.

Acknowledgment

The authors wish to express their appreciation for the helpfulness of Mrs. Charles Plyler in carrying on the activities of the special infant feeding clinic, of Miss Billie Rekoff and Dr. Michael G. Rekoff, Jr., for technical assistance, of Mrs. T. C. Mather and Dr. Lillian Lockhart for compilation of records, and of Miss Barbara Hirschler and Mr. Malcolm Roemer for preparation of the data. We are grateful to Dr. John Sinclair for his help with the histological studies. We feel especially indebted to Dr. Walter L. Thompson of The Baker Laboratories, Inc., and to Dr. Robert A. Stewart of Gerber Products Company for their complete cooperation in the maintenance of supplies and assistance in obtaining data regarding the food analyses. We are grateful to Dr. George M. Briggs of the Department of Nutrition, University of California, Berkeley, for suggestions regarding the manuscript. Special thanks are due to members of the pediatric resident staff at the University of Texas for their assistance in obtaining blood samples and to the many mothers for their excellent co-operation in making this study possible.

Part V

MINERALS AND WATER

Editor's Comments
on Papers 17 Through 20

Little attention was paid to the mineral salts in the diet of the infant. The earliest concerns were related to the roles of fat, protein, and carbohydrate. When appropriate balances among these three elements were managed successfully, it was concluded that the mineral salts would be attended to by the kidney. Hoobler (Paper 17) was the first to pay serious attention to the value of mineral salts, although other researchers were hotly contending the place of calcium in the diet. Hoobler reviews the literature with crisp clarity and reports the results of his own work. His presentation and discussion of the calcium and phosphorus phenomenon are almost totally without bias, a major accomplishment considering the temper of the times. The literature of the 1918 era is remarkable for the heated exchange between Bosworth and Bowditch in Boston, and Holt in New York, over the precise role of calcium and phosphorus and their relationship to each other and to other elements, primarily fat, in the diet.

Interestingly enough, it was L. E. Holt, Jr., who, years later in Baltimore, with advantages of time and technology, was able, together with other workers, to extend his father's studies and also to confirm certain of the Bowditch and Bosworth results (Paper 18).

166

The fundamental requirement for other ions and minerals has been less extensively studied. The obvious exception is the need for iron in the infant fed solely on the breast or modified milk formula. The original studies by Waddell et al. (1928) established without question that a profound nutritional anemia could be produced in young rats placed solely on a diet of cow's whole milk. These researchers also demonstrated the most efficient reversal of this phenomenon when ashed residues from dried beef liver, dried lettuce, and yellow corn were introduced into the diet. Although it had been shown by Stearns and Stinger (1937) that babies reared solely on breast milk were never actually in negative iron balance, they also showed that babies restricted to cow's milk did indeed lose an average of 0.05 microgram of iron daily. Based on these observations, a variety of iron preparations in a variety of doses were recommended with and without the addition of copper. Niccum et al. (Paper 19) provided the studies to show that 5 milligrams of ferrous iron administered daily to infants between the ages of three and six months would prevent the development of hypochromic anemia and, furthermore, that ferrous sulfate could be added to milk without destroying its absorptive qualities.

Trace metal needs have been described for copper, zinc, manganese, and magnesium in regard to hemoglobin and to synthesis of a variety of enzymes. At present, it would appear that specific milk formula supplements for trace metals are indicated only when the infant is known to have an underlying order of metabolism which mandates its use.

The Davis et al. article describing neonatal fits due to hypomagnesemia is listed in the Selected Bibliography.

The hydrolability of the infant and the importance of adequate water intake have long been accepted facts. Early estimates of daily fluid requirements, however, were based largely on gross measurements of the volume of milk voluntarily consumed. Levine et al. (Paper 20), in an attempt to validate such rough estimates, studied daily water exchange, taking all sources of incoming and outgoing water into account. Their results established that insensible water loss in infants accounted for 45 percent of the total available water, urine for 43 percent, and stool for 9 percent, under normal conditions of environment and diet. They also proved that additional fluid intake resulted almost entirely in an increase of urinary water, while fever enhanced elimination through the skin at the expense of urinary water—concepts that recognizably form the basis of rational fluid intake and therapy.

17

Reprinted from *Am. J. Dis. Child.*, **11**, 107–140 (1911)

THE RÔLE OF MINERAL SALTS IN THE METABOLISM OF INFANTS *

B. RAYMOND HOOBLER, M.D.

NEW YORK

It is the purpose of this paper to present, in rather broad outlines, the part which mineral salts play in carrying on the physiologic functions of the body, and in what manner they contribute to the various pathologic processes to which the infant and young child are subjected.

This field of metabolic research has been the last to be undertaken, and just now we are coming to realize its vast importance, not only in connection with their own functions, but in connection with the influence they have on the metabolism of fat, protein and carbohydrate. The chief reason for having failed to realize the importance of the mineral salts in metabolism is that it has long been thought that the salts contributed in no way to the nourishment of the child. It has been only recently that they have taken their rightful place as indirect energy producers.

HISTORICAL

The first investigator to concern himself with the value of mineral salts was von Liebig,[1] who, as early as 1840, studied the action of mineral salts both in animal and vegetable life, and many of his early deductions have become firmly fixed as laws in the field of mineral salts metabolism. C. Voit[2] is another investigator whose work on the action of sodium chlorid, as early as 1860, first gave to that salt its prominence above all others in the human economy. Vierordt was also an indefatigable worker, and as early as 1877, from meager data then present, had calculated absolute and relative heat and estimated child's metabolism. J. Forster,[3] in 1873, added his convincing experiments on the necessity of the mineral salts to the continuance of life, and these were further reinforced by the work of Lunin[4] in 1881. As time advanced, the roster of those who worked in the field of mineral metabolism contains the names of many

---

*Read, by invitation, before the meeting of the American Pediatric Society, Lake Mohonk, N. Y., June, 1911.

*From the laboratories of the Presbyterian Hospital and Cornell University Medical College.

1. Von Liebig, J.: Chemie in ihrer Anwendung auf Agrikultur und Physiologie, 1876, p. 332.

2. Voit, C.: Ueber den Einfluss des Kochsalzes auf den Stoffwechsel. München. 1860.

3. Forster, J.: Ztschr. f. Biol., 1873, ix.

4. Lunin, N.: Ztschr. f. physiol. Chem., 1881, v.

notable investigators, as G. v. Bunge, Michel, Keller, Loeb, Muller, Schlossman, Blauberg, Rubner, Huebner, Freund, v. Noorden, and in these latter days the work is being carried on enthusiastically by L. Langstein, L. F. Meyer, E. Schloss, J. A. Schabad and others abroad, and by Howland, Schwartz, Talbot, Veeder, and others in this country.

A GENERAL VIEW

In undertaking a problem of this kind, it is well at the beginning to take a general view, first of the physiologic action of the mineral salts as a whole, and then to study what has been definitely determined as to the action and influence of each of the mineral constituents. Then by inquiring into the mineral constituents of the new-born and of older children, one will be in position to learn the mineral needs of the growing organism, and, knowing them, to ascertain how best to supply them, and to study the factors which enter into the proper utilization of the salts ingested in the food and to determine whether or not this utilization is sufficient to meet the demands of the growing infant.

First, then, a general view of the physiologic action of the mineral salts as a whole. Physiologists are generally agreed, and their findings confirmed by physiologic chemists, that the important functions of the mineral salts are as follows:

1. They maintain the osmotic pressure in tissue cells, blood, and body fluids; controlling the flow of water to and from tissues; any deviation from normal causing a shrinking or swelling of tissue cells.

2. They regulate the reaction of the blood and tissue fluids. A deviation from this reaction inhibits the action of the various ferments, delays chemical processes, and if such reaction suffers much variation, death results.

3. Their presence in tissues and fluids gives rise to irritability of muscle and excitability of nerve through the action of their respective *ions*. Through this function the rhythmical contractions of the heart are maintained.

4. They act as catalysts for a large series of chemical reactions which take place during the processes of absorption, retention, utilization, and form combinations with waste products of metabolism in order to effect their elimination; for example, they act as carriers of excess acid materials in oxidation processes.

5. They share in the upbuilding and growth of the body, since they are a constituent of every cell; particularly do they take part in the changes which go on in the albumin bodies as they become intimately bound with the body proteins.

6. Their function in the intermediary metabolism of the ductless glands is very apparent from the large quantities of mineral salts found in these glandular organs.

7. Through a most excellent self-regulation, they protect against the acid poisons which the body is constantly producing.

8. Through the work of the various *ions*, electrically charged, some positively, some negatively, many important functions are being assigned to them, such as controlling body-weight, temperature, regulating the pulse, increasing leukocytes, etc. These and many more functions, not clearly defined, depend on the presence of the mineral salts in the body, and not on their presence alone, but their presence in definite relationships to one another.

169

ABSOLUTE NECESSITY OF SALTS

While physiologists have been busy defining the various functions of salts, other investigators have determined the absolute necessity to the maintenance of life of a certain quantity of mineral salts, and not only a certain quantity, but they have found that these salts must be in certain organic combination, as the following experiments will show:

Forster,[3] in 1873, fed pigeons on approximately ash-free diet, and found their bones brittle, and they all died within a month. He also fed dogs on salt-poor diet, and they lived from twenty-six to thirty-six days.

Lunin[4] showed by his classic experiment that the salts must be in organic combination to be available. He found that mice thrived well on dried whole milk, but that if the salts were extracted from the milk, and they were fed only the protein, fat and carbohydrate, they shortly died, and further, after abstracting the salts, if he substituted the same quantity of other mineral salts, adding them to the protein, fat and carbohydrate, the mice died. Furthermore, mice fed on ash-free food, plus sufficient sodium carbonate to take the place of the usual salts, lived twice as long as mice fed only on ash-free diet; nevertheless, they succumbed, demonstrating that even with the necessary amount of bases carbonates cannot supply the salt needed.

Rohmann[5] added further confirmation to the value of salts. He fed mice a mixture of simple organic and inorganic food-stuffs. These mice lived and were able to produce young, but the latter could not be raised on artificial food, nor could they be made to produce living young.

It is evident from this latter experiment that artificial foods may be sufficient for the adult, whose supply of minerals is well established, but it is not sufficient to produce healthy offspring.

Abderhalden[6] believes that the same physiologic importance of salts exists for the animal kingdom as has been shown by von Liebig and others to exist for the vegetable kingdom.

The salts have a very important bearing on the absorption and retention of other food constituents, e. g., in a large nitrogen retention there is usually a large ash retention, and when ash is eliminated in large quantities there is usually an accompanying loss of nitrogen.

T. B. Robertson[7] points out how intimately the precipitation and coagulation of protein depends on the salts present in the solution as *ions*. Indeed it is becoming more and more to be appreciated that the various food constituents have a very intimate influence, the one on the other, and it is along this particular line that metabolism studies are directing themselves.

Recognizing, then, that the mineral salts are necessary to life, let us inquire what salts, and in what proportion in the body, Nature has stored

5. Rohmann: Klin.-therap. Wchnschr., 1902, No. 40.
6. Abderhalden: Physiological Chemistry, p. 356.
7. Robertson, T. B.: Jour. Biol. Chem., May, 1911.

them, by the action of which not only life is maintained, but energy developed and growth permitted. We are indebted to a number of investigators for information on the ash-content of the human organism both during fetal life and later.

Fehling[8] gives us the following figures of the ash-content at different periods of fetal life:

Period of Life.	Ash Content; Per Cent. of Total Weight.
Fetus, 6 weeks	.001
Fetus, 4 months	.98
Fetus, 5th month, first half	1.4
Fetus, 5th month, second half	1.43
Fetus, 6th month	1.94
Fetus, 7th month	2.94
Fetus, 8th month	2.82
Fetus, 9th month	3.3
In the new-born	2.7
In the adult	4.4

It will be noted, therefore, that from the earliest observation of fetal life to those on adult bodies, there is a gradual increase of the ash-content. This increase is most rapid in terms of percentage of body weight during the fetal period, and thereafter the increase is much slower.

Let us now ask ourselves the question as to the mineral constituents contained in the total ash-content and study their relative amounts. Hugounencq[9] has given us this information for fetal life, and Soldner[10] for the new-born. Soldner found that there was 75 gm. of ash in a new-born child which was equal to 2.7 per cent. of its body weight, or 9.4 per cent. of the dry residue.

Total Ash in Parts Per 100

Period of Life.	Cl	P₂O₅	SO₃	CaO	MgO	K₂O	Na₂O	Fe₂O₃
	Cl	P_2O_5	SO_3	CaO	MgO	K_2O	Na_2O	Fe_2O_3
Fetus, 5 months	8.59	34.36	1.8	32.5	1.58	8.28	12.62	.4
Fetus, 6 months	7.75	34.94	1.78	34.6	....	7.21	10.62	.39
Fetus, 7 months	8.53	35.39	1.46	34.13	1.17	8.45	10.95	.398
New-born (Soldner), average of 6	6.61	....	2.02	38.08	1.43	7.06	7.67	.83

Soldner, arguing from the average ash content of six new-born infants, concluded that there was a daily need of 1.4 gm. of mineral ash, and an infant should retain of the intake, chlorin 14 per cent., potassium 11 per cent., sodium 35 per cent., CaO, MgO and P₂O₅ at least 65 per cent. of the intake.

It will be noted that phosphorus and calcium make up considerably over half; sodium about an eighth, and potassium and chlorin about a twelfth of the total ash-content, and that sulphur, magnesium and iron make up but a small part of the total.

---

8. Fehling: Cited by Freund, in Pfaundler and Schlossman, i, 363.
9. Hugounencq: Compt. rend. Soc. de biol., li, 537.
10. Camerer and Soldner: Ztschr. f. Biol., 1900-3, xxxix, xl, xliii, and xliv.

Bunge,[11] after a careful study of the mineral contents of the milk of lower animals and estimating the daily requirements of their offspring, attempted to show that the ash-content of the body was in correct proportion to the ash-content of the various animals. But when this was applied to the nursing infant his analogy failed, and the problem did not solve itself as readily as this hypothesis would indicate. It is evident that the main metallic elements are calcium, sodium, potassium and magnesium; the main acid salts being phosphoric, hydrochloric, carbonic and sulphuric, calcium phosphate being the most abundant of all the salts.

It should be further noted that the phosphorus and calcium content of the body increases in percentage, and that the other elements remain at the same or less percentage, but of course their absolute amount gradually increases.

The difference between the ash-content of a new-born and the ash-content of a 4-months' old child represents the change which must take place in the mineral salt storing. In actual figures the child must add to his weight, during the first four months, the following quantities of the various minerals:

	Gm.
K_2O	2.0
Na_2O	2.57
CaO	11.75
MgO	.31
Fe_2O_3	....
P_2O_5	10.48
Cl	1.12
S	....

It will be noted what really small quantities of the mineral salts are added to the body—extremely small when we consider the large quantity which a child during the first year must ingest. It is estimated that only about 4 per cent. of intake goes to growth in early months and later only half that amount. It is evident that a large quantity must be worked over. Taking mother's milk as a basis, during the first twelve months of life there is approximately 800 gm. of total ash ingested. This is divided among the various mineral salts as follows:

	Gm.
K_2O	276.
Na_2O	19.6
CaO	157.6
MgO	27.2
Fe_2O_3	8.0
P_2O_5	117.6
Cl	117.6
SO_3	57.4
Total	791.0

If we take cow's milk as a basis, the picture is entirely different. Taking the average amount fed as outlined in Dr. Holt's text-book, an

---

11. Bunge: Cited by Freund, Pfaundler and Schlossman, Vol. i.

infant would ingest approximately 1,500 gm. of total ash during the first year of life, which would be divided among the various mineral constituents as follows:

		Gm.
K_2O	....	377.0
Na_2O	....	93.0
CaO	....	344.0
MgO	....	41.0
Fe_2O_3	....	4.2
P_2O_5	....	487.4
Cl	....	84.0
S	....	69.4
Total	....	1,500.0

This naturally leads us to a two-fold conception of the use which the body makes of the salts. First, a certain small per cent. is firmly bound with the tissues of the body and only escapes when such tissues are destroyed in oxidation; and a second group which are simply held in solution in the body fluids ready to be excreted, or to act as bases or alkalies to take up the products of cell destruction, or combine with acids set free in the processes of catabolism, or in the form of *ions* to subserve definite physiologic functions. It should be borne in mind that only a small part of the mineral salt intake in any day's feeding is added as an integral part of the tissue, and that by far the largest part is simply held in solution awaiting its excretion, either through the skin, urine or back into the intestinal canal. With sulphur and phosphorus the problem is a little more complicated, as these two substances are in exceedingly close chemical relationship with albumin, and before they can be set free the foreign albumin molecule must be torn down before it can be again rebuilded into the tissue substance and fluids of the host.

Having noted just what minerals and acids are present in the body at the end of fetal life, it behooves us to inquire into the method by which we can continue to supply the needs of the infant as relates to its mineral constituents so as best to foster its normal growth and aid in supplying its daily energy requirement. Nature has supplied us with a most excellent criterion by which we may reach a solution of this problem, viz., in normal mother's milk. Let us, therefore, address ourselves to a study of Nature's method of supplying the need of the growing infant by carefully considering the mineral constituents and their relative proportions in mother's milk.

In early mother's milk, i. e., colostrum, according to Camerer,[12] we have a marked increase from the first to the seventh day in the ash-content as follows:

Day after delivery	1	2	3	4	5	6	7
Ash content in per cents	0.1	0.5	0.7	0.9	1.0	1.1	1.3

12. Camerer: Cited by Freund in Pfaundler and Schlossman, i. 386.

Thus Nature provides in the early nursing period for a very rapid increase in the mineral constituents of the food. In mother's milk there is about 2.0 gm. of total ash to 1,000 gm. of milk. This 2 gm. of ash is divided among the various mineral constituents according to various authors, as follows:

In 1,000 gm. of mother's milk, there is, according to

	Bunge 1[15] Gm.	Bunge 2[15] Gm.	Camerer[13] and Soldner	Blauberg[14] Gm.
K_2O	0.780	0.703	0.884	0.69
Na_2O	0.232	0.257	0.357	0.049
CaO	0.328	0.343	0.378	0.394
MgO	0.064	0.065	0.053	0.068
Fe_2O_3	0.004	0.006	0.002	0.02
P_2O_5	0.473	0.469	0.310	0.294
Cl	0.438	0.445	0.591	0.294
SO_3	....	.....	.....	0.143

The ash-content of mother's milk does not remain constant, as is shown by Soldner[16] in his examinations of mother's milk on the eighth and seventieth days. In 1,000 gm. of mother's milk on the eighth day, there was 3 gm. of total ash, and in the same quantity on the seventieth day there was 2 gm. of total ash divided as follows:

	Eighth day Gm.	Seventieth day Gm.
K_2O	1.008	.259
Na_2O	.448	.176
CaO	.376	.381
MgO	.054	.052
Fe_2O_3	.0022	.00125
P_2O_5	.320	.288
SO_3	.096	.063
Cl	.716	.342

From the above, it would seem that the fixed alkalies K and Na diminish greatly as does also the chlorin content of the milk, while the bone-forming constituents, viz., calcium, phosphorus and magnesium, remain nearly constant. In cow's milk the relations are entirely different as is shown by the exceedingly large ash-content of 7.8 gm. per 1,000 gm. of milk as against 2 gm. in 1,000 gm. of mother's milk. Not only does cow's milk contain more ash, but in vastly different proportion of mineral constituents than mother's milk, as will be seen by the following table when compared with the preceding table showing mineral contents of the ash of mother's milk. In 1,000 gm. of cow's milk there is:

13. Camerer and Soldner: Cited by Albu-Neuberg, Mineralstoffwechsel, p. 51.
14. Blauberg: Cited by Langstein and Meyer Säuglingsernährung und Säuglingsstoffwechsel, Wiesbaden, 1910, page 15.
15. Bunge: Cited by Albu-Neuberg, Mineralstoffwechsel, p. 51.
16. Soldner: Cited by Freund, in Pfaundler and Schlossman, p. 377.

	Bunge[16] Gm.	Soldner[13] Gm.	Hoobler Gm.	Soldner[17] Gm.
K_2O	1.766	1.720	.....	1.885
Na_2O	1.110	0.51	.....	0.465
CaO	1.599	1.980	1.600	1.72
MgO	0.210	0.20	0.167	0.205
Fe_2O_3	0.004	.....	.....	0.021
P_2O_5	1.974	1.82	2.140	2.437
Cl	1.697	0.98	1.86 (NaCl)	0.820
S	....	.....	0.33638	....

It will be seen that in the same quantities of milk, that of the cow contains over twice as much potassium, five times as much sodium, phosphorus and calcium, four times as much magnesium and chlorin and six times as much sulphur. And, further, these salts are not in the same organic combination in one as in the other, as shown by Keller,[18] and also by Schlossman,[19] as relates to phosphorus, and when we consider that it is the organically bound salts only, as shown by Lunin,[4] which are available, this factor is a very important one.

Not only are the salts organically bound, but there is a peculiar specificity about the whey containing the salts of mother's milk. Meyer[20] has shown that not only the protein and fat of mother's milk, but even the casein and fat of cow's milk, are well absorbed and retained when mixed with the whey of mother's milk. Children fed on the fat and protein of mother's milk mixed with the whey of cow's milk are not able to utilize these food products and do badly. It would seem that some constituent in mother's milk whey contains the essential dynamic force for making the casein and fat of both mother's and cow's milk available for nutritive purposes.

Having now considered separately the salts of the child's body and the salts of the two most common foods, let us study the processes which take place when these foods are ingested by the infant. It would contribute to a continuity of thought if we were to follow each individual salt through its various metabolic steps under perfectly normal conditions and discuss them under the heads of ingestion, absorption, retention and elimination, considering the results obtained by investigators in the use of mother's milk and cow's milk.

After having considered these steps in normal metabolism, I shall address myself briefly to abnormal conditions of metabolism, desiring rather to give most attention to the consideration of the normal. I shall take occasion to consider, along with the findings of literature, some results obtained by me in a series of metabolism studies which I have

17. Soldner: Cited by Langstein and Meyer, Säuglingsernährung und Säuglingsstoffwechsel, Wiesbaden, 1910, page 15.

18. Keller, A.: Arch. f. Kinderh., 1900, xxix.

19. Schlossman: Arch. f. Kinderh., 1905, xl.

20. Meyer, L. F.: Cited by Meara, Problems of Nutrition in Early Life, Arch. Pediat., xxvii, 401.

TOTAL ASH

Food	Intake	Elimination		Absorption			Retention		
		Feces	Urine	Gm.	Percent.	Per Kilo	Gm.	Percent. of Intake	Per Kilo
Mother's milk (Blauberg)	1.13	0.193	0.373	0.937	82.9	....	0.56	49.5	....
Mother's milk (Blauberg)	1.32	0.24	0.47	1.08	81.8	....	0.61	45.9	....
Cow's milk (Soldner)	6.841	2.686	3.1341	4.15	60.7	.....	1.013	14.8	....
Diluted cow's milk, 2.1% fat (Hoobler)	8.9691	4.2651	4.7966	4.7039	53.0	.565	....	....	....
Cow's milk, 4% fat (Hoobler)	9.4808	3.1390	3.0834	6.3418	66.8	.808	2.8917	43.5	.368
Cow's milk and cream, 5.4% fat (Hoobler)	8.7634	1.8675	4.1493	6.8059	78.6	.861	2.7465	37.8	.344
Cow's milk (Blauberg)	6.84	2.68	3.13	4.15	60.7	....	1.01	14.8	....

Figures given above are in grams in 24 hours.

176

carried out in the wards and laboratory of the Presbyterian Hospital on a perfectly healthy infant of 9 months who had been fed on cow's milk from the time of his birth, details of the experiment, as relates to nitrogen metabolism, having already been published.[22]

TOTAL ASH

I will first consider the figures covering the entire mineral metabolism as represented by total ash, and will then discuss its various phases.

INGESTION

First let us consider the intake. It should be remembered that mother's milk is relatively poor in ash-content while that of cow's milk is exceedingly rich, so that one is not surprised to note that the intake of total ash through breast feeding is very much less than with cow's milk feeding. From the figures of Blauberg, Soldner, and my own determinations, the ash intake in artificially fed children is from six to nine times greater than that of breast-fed children.

ABSORPTION OF TOTAL ASH

Various observers have recorded their findings of ash absorption in mother's milk, varying from 81.82 per cent. by Blauberg to 53 per cent. of intake by Schlossman; Biedert's determination was 77 per cent., and that of Rubner and Heubner 79.42 per cent., while the absorption of total ash of cow's milk by different authors is as follows (see also p. 115):

	Per cent.		Per cent.
Soldner	60.7	Biedert	65.1
Schlossman	70.	Hoobler	53.
Tangl	62.1	Hoobler	66.8
Blauberg	53.72	Hoobler	78.6

It will be seen that the absorption per cent. is 15 per cent. to 25 per cent. better on mother's milk, but because of the large intake the actual amount absorbed is very much larger in cow's milk feedings than in breast-fed. For example, 1.08 gm. was absorbed in twenty-four hours on mother's milk, while on cow's milk from 4 to 6 gm. were absorbed daily. Thus approximately four to six times more is absorbed in artificial feeding.

As we shall see later, this better absorption of mother's milk ash lies in the fact that calcium, magnesium and phosphorus are much better absorbed. As was demonstrated in my work on the various fat feedings, and now being published in the Presbyterian Hospital Report of this year, nitrogen, chlorin, sulphur and magnesium were absorbed in the same ratio as these elements existed in the food. The greatest variations from the ratio in the food occurred in calcium and phosphorus.

---

22. Hoobler: Arch. Pediat., 1910, xxvii, 853.

RETENTION

Without doubt the best criterion of availability and utilization of any given food-stuff is not its large per cent. of absorption, or even its large absolute amount of absorption; but rather the absolute amount retained. Literature does not yet contain reports which cover sufficient periods of investigation to feel quite sure that these so-called absolute retentions are permanent or simply transitory, since it takes weeks to utilize and eliminate the mineral salts. Therefore a prescribed diet should be carried out for weeks instead of days for most accurate results. However, the reports in literature show that the ash of mother's milk is well retained and this is but natural, for the salts come to the infant in much better form for utilization than in cow's milk.

In Blauberg's case on mother's milk (see total ash tabulation), the absolute retention was 0.61 gm., being 45.9 per cent. of the intake. In cow's milk feeding, the per cent. of retention is lower but the absolute amount is higher, owing to the much richer ash-content of the cow's milk. Blauberg's case on cow's milk feeding, having a retention of 14.8 per cent. of intake, represented an absolute amount of 1.013, being nearly twice the amount retained under mother's milk feeding. In my 9-month child there was retained 2.89 gm. or 43.5 per cent. intake. Blauberg found that with mother's milk feeding all the minerals were retained with the exception of sodium; in cow's milk there was a loss in Cl, S, and Na. It would seem that each child is a law unto itself so far as retention of mineral ash is concerned. It apparently takes it on just in accordance with the demands of physiologic growth.

In my determinations in connection with various strengths of fat in foods, I found that as compared with nitrogen retention, the retention of the mineral salts was relatively poorer. This poor retention was most marked on the lower fat food, better on the medium fat diet, and best as regards the absolute amount retained on the high (5.4 per cent.) fat diet. Retention of the salts in proportion to nitrogen was never in the same proportion as existed between the salts and nitrogen of the food.

ELIMINATION

The elimination through the feces and urine differs in amounts on mother's and cow's milk. In mother's milk feeding, one-third of the salts are eliminated through the feces and two-thirds through the urine, while in cow's milk feeding about half is eliminated by the urine and half by the feces, though the figures of different investigators vary. In my own figures the ash of the feces was three times as large on a 2.1 per cent. fat mixture as on a 5.4 per cent. mixture.

THE ANOMALIES IN THE METABOLISM OF TOTAL ASH

In the elaboration of Finkelstein's theory of food disturbances in infants and children, L. F. Meyer[23] has attributed to the mineral salts certain deleterious influences.

In each of Finkelstein's four stages of nutritional disturbance, Meyer finds that there is some anomaly in the salt metabolism. In the stage of *"Bilanzstörung,"* there is decreased retention of the alkaline earths. There is also a lessened retention of other salts.

In the stage of dyspepsia, the salt elimination by the feces is increased but the ash balance is not markedly changed. In the stage of decomposition the entire picture is determined by the loss of the mineral salts, particularly through the loss of the fixed alkalies. Through the fatty acids in the stools, the Ca and Mg are used up. The diarrheal stools of this period are due largely to alkali loss. The condition of relative acidosis of Steinits (and of alkalipenia of Pfaundler) takes place during this stage, due to the loss of alkali.

In the fourth stage, of intoxication, the salt metabolism is little known. There is a negative balance of chlorin and probably of the other mineral constituents. Whether the salt loss controls the water loss or vice versa is still a question, but since the urine is much decreased and the output of water by the feces is increased, it would seem that the salts were accountable for this diversion of the water elimination. It is evident that salts play an important part in every digestive disturbance of the infant and young child.

CALCIUM

The calcium need of the growing infant is well met through the abundance of its salts in the milk, either of mother's or of cow's. Calcium makes up one-fifth of the ash of mother's as well as of the ash of cow's milk. Calcium is taken into the body in organic and inorganic form. The organic combination is present in milk, yolk of eggs and vegetables, and the inorganic form in water used as a diluent and for drinking.

The importance of the calcium salts in the developing organism can hardly be overestimated. Physiologists[24] have shown that the calcium *ions* in the blood, though in small quantity, are yet absolutely necessary to the irritability of muscle. If calcium is present in too large quantities, as compared with Na and K *ions,* there is produced a tonic contraction known as calcium rigor.

Calcium has a definite specific action of its own and cannot be replaced by other earthy bases, as magnesium and strontium, as stated by Stewart.[25] The fact is well known that calcium is necessary to ferment action

23. Langstein and Meyer: Säuglingsernährung und Säuglingsstoffwechsel, Wiesbaden, 1910, pp. 111-166.

24. Howell: Physiology, Ed. 2, 1907.

25. Stewart: Physiology, Ed. 1910, p. 542.

as shown by the coagulation of blood and the precipitation of casein in milk. Calcium is much the largest mineral constituent of the body. Its most common salt is calcium phosphate, which makes up a large part of the bone salts.

Jacques Loeb[26] has shown the necessity of calcium salts for the development of the lower forms of life, and Blauberg has shown that children who cannot metabolize calcium cannot survive.

Mother's milk contains only about 20 per cent. as much calcium as cow's milk; therefore we would expect a considerable variation in its absorption and retention, as is shown by the following:

CALCIUM AS CaO

The calcium of mother's milk is 0.394 grams in 1,000 gm. I found calcium of cow's milk to be 1.6 grams in 1,000 gm., or nearly four times as much in cow's as in mother's milk. (See also tabulation page 120.)

It will be noted first that the calcium intake in cow's milk feeding is about eight times greater than in mother's milk; that the amount actually absorbed and retained is four times greater on cow's milk than on mother's milk. However, a much larger percentage of mother's milk calcium is retained. It is evident, therefore, that the calcium of mother's milk is much better metabolized than the calcium of cow's milk, and since a healthy nursing infant shows no signs of a deficiency of calcium, we may well consider the amount which it gets as being the true calcium need. The absorption of calcium depends in part on the presence of accompanying salts; for example, if much alkali bases are present in the intake the absorption is diminished, whereas NaCl assists in calcium absorption. Calcium is more readily absorbed on flesh than on a vegetable diet.

ELIMINATION

It should be noted that the elimination of calcium is almost entirely through the feces; only 5 to 10 per cent. of the intake appears in the urine. This does not mean that the calcium is not well absorbed, but that it is excreted into the large intestine, as is proved by the fact that larger quantities of calcium are found in the large intestine than in the small intestine. It was Voit[27] who showed that 0.15 gm. of calcium per day was excreted from the inner surface of the intestine.

The amount of calcium excreted in the urine of infants fed on breast and cow's milk does not vary greatly, but the amount which appears in the feces varies greatly, being in some instances twenty times greater. Calcium makes up a quarter or a third part of the dried feces of cow's-milk-fed children, as against a much smaller portion in breast-fed. The

26. Loeb, J.: Cited by Meyer, Jahrb. f. Kinderh., lxxi, 1.
27. Voit: Cited by Howell, Physiology, Ed. 2, p. 834.

CALCIUM AS CaO

Food	Intake	Elimination		Absorption			Retention		
		Feces	Urine	Gm.	Percent.	Per Kilo	Gm.	Percent.	Per Kilo
Mother's milk .... (Blauberg)	0.2884	0.0952	0.0127	......	....	....	0.176	62.4	....
Mother's milk .... (Blauberg 5 mos.)	0.2720	0.0660	0.0310	0.2060	75.8	....	0.175	64.5	.026
Cow's milk (R. & H. 7½)	2.0824	1.142	0.0166	0.9370	45.1	....	0.924	44.4	.122
Diluted cow's, 2.1% fat ... (Hoobler)	2.0536	2.2687	0.0301	Negative	....	....	Negative	....	....
Cow's whole milk, 4% fat..........	2.0500	1.6962	0.305	0.3538	17.2	.045	0.3233	15.7	.041
Cow's milk and cream, 5.4% fat	2.0923	0.9515	0.0085	1.1408	54.5	.142	1.1322	54.1	.142

Figures given above are in grams in 24 hours.

form in which the calcium usually appears in the feces is that of the insoluble soaps, or in the form of calcium phosphate.

In my series of studies the elimination of calcium in the feces was greater on milk of lower fat content. As fat was increased in the food, the calcium was diminished in the feces. The calcium eliminated in the urine appears along with magnesium, bound with phosphoric, carbonic and uric acids. Iron is another mineral constituent which is excreted very poorly through the urine, and this leads one to group these two constituents together and to inquire if there are other characteristics. It should be noted that their presence in many organs, for example the thyroid gland, the liver, the spleen and the ovaries, suggests physiologic and chemical affinities as pointed out by Albu and Neuberg.[28] The internal secretions which play such a part in intermediary metabolism of the mineral salts, may be largely affected by the relationship of these two minerals. Calcium and phosphorus are closely allied in the bones, in the ovaries, and in the thyroid gland.

THE ANOMALIES OF CALCIUM METABOLISM

As a rule there is a great individual difference in the amount of calcium absorbed, and a further difference in the ability to retain the calcium absorbed. Rarely is such a condition due to the lack of calcium in the food, although many artificial foods are very poor in calcium. A diet containing less than 1 to 1.5 gm. CaO daily should be considered calcium-poor, except when on mother's milk feeding.

It has been shown that when calcium is purposely withheld from the diet of young puppies, rachitis develops, and the bones of young pigeons fed on calcium-poor diet are very fragile (Forster[3]). In the bones, in rachitis the mineral constituents are depleted, particularly calcium and phosphorus. The total ash of bones which normally is 65 per cent. falls to as low as 25 per cent. and the main loss falls on the calcium phosphate. The calcium loss in rachitis is largely through the intestine, with but little change in urinary calcium. In feces of rachitis, there is an increased elimination over that of healthy children, as shown by J. A. Schabad.[29] In rachitis particularly the weak point in the metabolism cycle may be the inability of the bones themselves to take up and build into bony tissue the calcium and phosphorus brought to them by the fluids, as has been pointed out by Albu and Neuberg.[28] The fact that calcium has much to do with the function of the nervous system has been shown by the calcium disturbances in tetany, as demonstrated by Schabad.[30] Further, the large proportional content of the brain tissue of the new-born in calcium

28. Albu-Neuberg: Mineralstoffwechsel, Berlin, 1906, p. 70.

29. Schabad, J. A.: Arch. f. Kinderh., liii, 241.

30. Schabad, J. A.: Monatschr. f. Kinderh., ix, No. 1; Jahrb. f. Kinderh., l, No. 1.

(0.168 per cent. CaO), as compared with an 8-year-old child's brain (0.05 per cent.) speaks further confirmation of this. There is a very appreciable loss of calcium from the nerve structures during the first year of life. Quest[31] found less calcium in the brains of children who died of tetany than of children of the same age without tetany.

Schloss[32] has more recently shown that subnormal body temperature in some cases depends on the presence of calcium *ions*. In the symptom-complex which Finkelstein calls *Ernährungstörung*, during the stage of *Bilanzstörung*, Meyer[23] has shown that there is a decreased retention of calcium due in part to the fact that the fats of the stools are increased, and these demand the alkaline earth to neutralize the fatty acids. There may be such a demand that not only will no calcium and magnesium be retained, but there may be an actual withdrawal of these salts from the body. This may account for a portion of the loss of weight in this stage of food disturbance.

IRON

Cow's milk and mother's milk contain about the same amounts of iron. Each is very poor in iron, and were it not for the relatively large amount stored in the liver and blood of the new-born there would be a deficiency in the early months of feeding. The following table shows that the form in which the iron is present has a large bearing on its availability. The iron of goat's milk is poorly absorbed and poorly retained, while the iron of mother's milk is well absorbed and well retained. Iron is eliminated almost entirely through the feces but a very small quantity through the urine.

Iron plays an important part in metabolism. It is specially important in the formation of the hemoglobin molecule. It acts as a catalyst in oxidation processes, especially in the group of nucleoproteins, as has been shown by Spitzer[44] and by Manchot.[45] Iron is presented for consumption in both the organic and inorganic form. The organic forms occur in the nucleoalbumins, in milk, yolk of eggs and in many vegetables.

IRON AS Fe_2O_3

In 1,000 gm. mother's milk, .02 gm. to .04 gm.
In 1,000 gm. cow's milk, .021 gm. (Abderhalden).

Food	Intake	Elimination Feces	Urine	Absorption Gm.	%	Retention Gm.	%
Mother's milk	.00705	.00084	.00055	.00621	88.09	.00566	82.28
Goats' milk	.00344	.00259	.00009	.00085	24.71	.00076	22.09

Figures given above are in grams in 24 hours.

31. Quest: Cited by Freund, in Pfaundler and Schlossman, i, p. 285.

32. Schloss: Cited by Langstein and Meyer, Säuglingsernährung und Säuglingsstoffwechsel, Wiesbaden, 1910, p. 21.

44. Spitzer: Cited by Albu and Neuberg, Mineralstoffwechsel, Berlin, 1906, p. 151.

45. Manchot: Cited by Albu and Neuberg, Mineralstoffwechsel, p. 151.

MAGNESIUM AS MgO

In 1,000 gm. mothers' milk there is 0.068 gm. MgO.
In 1,000 gm. cows' milk there is .205 gm. MgO.

Food	Intake	Elimination			Absorption			Retention		
		Fœces	Urine	Gm.	Gm.	Percent.	Per Kilo	Gm.	Percent.	Per Kilo
Mother's milk (Blauberg)	0.047	0.0157	0.014	....	....	.....	.....	0.0175	37.2	.....
Cow's milk (Soldner)	0.15017	0.0944	0.03718	....	....	.....	.....	0.017	11.5	.....
Diluted cow's milk, 2.1% fat (Hoobler)	0.10843	0.0058	0.0134	.10258	94.6	.123		0.0891	82.1	.011
Whole cow's milk, 4% fat (Hoobler)	0.07755	0.0300	0.04861	.04746	61.3	.045		Negative	.....	.....
Cow's milk and cream, 5.4% fat (Hoobler)	0.14999	0.0828	0.01909	.06719	44.7	.008		0.04809	32.0	.006

Figures given above are in grams in 24 hours.

184

MAGNESIUM

Magnesium and calcium are very closely connected in the metabolic function. They occur in the organism in much the same places and as salts of the same acids. Their proportion is CaO:MgO::40:1. Magnesium has a little wider distribution in the body tissues than does calcium. The latter occurs almost entirely—at least 99 per cent.—in the bones, while magnesium is found in muscle-tissue as high as 0.04 per cent. The part which magnesium plays in bone structure is important. Magnesium makes up about 10 to 15 per cent. of the total ash of bone. The relation of magnesium in these structures is about 1:9. The magnesium table on page 123 indicates that the Mg need of the growing infant on mother's milk is 0.047. Bunge, as cited by Albu and Neuberg, gives the magnesium need as 0.6. This seems rather high, for, since there is about 0.06 gm. Mg in a litre of mother's milk, it would require 10 litres to satisfy this need. Blauberg's breast-fed infant got but 0.047 gm. daily. The intake when fed on cow's milk varied; according to Soldner the daily intake was 0.15 gm., while my determinations showed intake varying from 0.07 to 0.15.

ABSORPTION

The absorption of magnesium which takes place through the small intestine is relatively very good. My determinations gave 94.6 as the per cent. of intake which was absorbed when feedings were low in fat. As the fat content of the food was increased, there was relatively poorer absorption, the percentages being 61.3 on a 4 per cent., and 44.7 on 5.4 per cent. fat mixture.

RETENTION

The retention of magnesium in my series was better on 2.1 per cent. fat mixture than on the 5.4 per cent. mixture. This retention varied inversely with the calcium retention so far as the amount of the fat in the food is concerned. In my findings for calcium, retention was poorest on lower fat mixtures and improved on the higher fat mixtures.

ELIMINATION

Excretion occurs both through urine and feces. On mother's milk in Blauberg's case, the excretion through either channel was about the same, while in cow's milk in some instances it was higher in urine and in others it was higher in the feces. In any event, the excretion is very small and that through the urine occurs as triple phosphates.

ANOMALIES OF RETENTION

There is more or less relation between Ca and Mg in the formation of oxalic acid concretions. It has been found that if the ratio of CaO to MgO be as 1 to 0.8 the concretion may be kept in solution. The smaller

PHOSPHORUS AS P_2O_5

				Total Gm.	Organically Bound, Gm.
In 1,000 gm. mother's milk				.294	42.3
In 1,000 gm. cow's milk				2.437	46.
In 1,000 gm. cow's milk (Hoobler)				2.140	....

Food	Intake	Elimination		Absorption			Retention		
		Feces	Urine	Gm.	Percent.	Per Kilo	Gm.	Percent.	Per Kilo
Mother's milk	0.2768	0.0363	0.0481	......	...	...	.192	69.13	.....
Mother's milk, 5 mos.	0.2030	0.0220	0.088	0.1810	89.1	...	.093	45.9	.0138
Cow's milk	1.4429	0.5352	0.5003	......	...	...	.4074	30.7	.....
Cow's milk (Keller's 2¾ mo)	0.8248	0.1073	0.4106	0.7174	87.1	...	.3068	37.2	.0626
Cow's milk (Blauberg's 7½ mos.)	2.0605	0.9627	0.5899	1.098	53.28	...	.5079	24.2	.0671
Diluted cow's milk, 2.1% fat (Hoobler)	2.2155	0.7648	1.152	1.4507	67.0	.174	.3320	14.5	.040
Cow's milk, whole, 4% fat (Hoobler)	2.7418	0.59914	2.009	2.1426	78.1	.274	.1336	4.8	.0171
Cow's milk and cream, 5.4% fat (Hoobler)	2.2346	0.3789	1.336	1.8556	83.0	.235	.6196	27.7	.0657

Figures given above are in grams in 24 hours.

the calcium and the larger the Mg content the easier becomes the solution of calcium oxalate.

PHOSPHORUS

Of all the mineral elements, perhaps none has been studied more assiduously than phosphorus. Phosphorus is brought into the body in two very different forms, viz., that which is organically bound, occurring in milk, eggs and legumes, and a small part as phosphoric acid. When in organic combination it is found as nucleoalbumin, nuclein, vitellin, casein and lecithin.

The source in which we are most interested is that of mother's and cow's milk, and these two foods differ considerably in the amount of organically bound phosphorus. Mother's milk contains 0.31 to 0.45 gm. per liter of P_2O_5, while cow's milk contains 1.81 gm. P_2O_5 per liter. Keller[33] has shown that of the phosphorus of mother's milk 77 per cent. is organically bound, while in cow's milk only 27.9 per cent. is so bound. Of this organically bound phosphorus 54 per cent. occurs as nucleophosphorus in mother's milk, and but 13.4 per cent. in cow's milk, so that it is very evident that the phosphorus of cow's milk, though larger in actual quantity, is not in such form as to be available, as is the case of mother's milk. The nucleins of milk make up 41.5 per cent. of the total phosphorus of mother's milk, while of cow's milk only 6 per cent. is in that form. In mother's milk 35 per cent. of total phosphorus is in the form of lecithin, while the lecithin of cow's milk is but 5 per cent. according to Stocklasa.[34]

The form in which the phosphorus reaches the organism is important for Salkowski has shown that the organism has not the power to build from phosphorus-free albumin, or from inorganic phosphates, cells which require as an integral part organically bound phosphorus.

Indeed, it has been shown that the phosphorus absorption is not in the least affected by the presence or absence of inorganic phosphates, but, on the other hand, the phosphorus absorption may be greatly increased when a child is fed on yolk of egg as shown by Cronheim and Muller.[35]

Phosphorus is in demand in the body, particularly in glandular structures and bones, and for the central nervous system, and we should expect to find a considerable daily need on the part of the growing organism. This need seems satisfied in the healthy breast-fed infant on an intake varying from 0.7 to 0.8 gm. as a minimum and 1 to 2 gm. as a maximum. This is a wide variation, but we should consider that phosphorus is one of the minerals which becomes a definite part of the tissue structures throughout the body, and by virtue of its close connection

---

33. Kellar, A.: Arch. f. Kinderh., xxix, Stuttgart, 1900, p. 1.
34. Stocklasa: Ebenda, 1897, xxiii.
35. Cronheim and Muller: Ztschr. f. diät. u. physik. Therap., 1903, vi.

with the albumin molecule must likewise suffer destruction along with the albumin, therefore it varies with the protein need.

The investigators who have determined phosphorus balances on infants are Blauberg, Michel, Keller, Cronheim and Muller and Schlossman. Let us consider some of their findings in comparison with the determinations which I have made.

ABSORPTION

It will first be noted that the intake of phosphorus is nearly ten times as great for cow's milk as for mother's milk and that in both forms of milk feeding the per cent. of intake absorbed indicates a very good absorption ability. In mother's milk, the absorption per cent. is 89.2 and that of cow's milk 53.2 in Blauberg's case. My determinations were 67.0 per cent., 78.1 per cent. and 83.0 per cent. on low, medium and high fat feeding. From this it would seem that phosphorus is more readily absorbed in the presence of increasing quantities of fat. The amount of the absorption depends more on the kind of phosphorus than on the quantity. The absorption of phosphorus is hindered when there is a relatively high ratio of accompanying alkaline earths and alkalies in the food; for example, when vegetables are fed a large calcium intake is present. This forms insoluble salts of phosphorus in the intestine and thus absorption is prevented. However, when these two elements meet within the body, they are joined in exceedingly close metabolic activity.

From my own determinations it appears that the phosphorus and nitrogen absorption varied considerably from the ratio in which these elements occurred in the food. Phosphorus absorption was relatively less than nitrogen absorption, during the low (2.1 per cent.) fat feeding, and was best in the medium fat feeding (4 per cent.), where it approximated the ratio which existed between nitrogen and phosphorus in the food.

RETENTION

The retention of phosphorus is one of great importance to the existence of life, for in conditions of starvation the organism clings tenaciously to its phosphorus—perhaps more so than to any other mineral constituent, except NaCl. This is probably due to its close connection with the central nervous system, for at the end of long periods of starvation the phosphorus content of nervous tissue is very little impoverished. This retention is, no doubt, in proportion to the need, and not only the present need, but it is stored up for an emergency; for the animal organism when fed on phosphorus-rich diet not only brings itself into phosphorus equilibrium, but retains a part of this excess phosphorus. The retention keeps step with the need and gradually diminishes when the skeleton is well formed.

As in the case of absorption, the phosphorus is retained not so much in proportion to its amount as according to the kind present. Its retention runs parallel with that of nitrogen in cases studied by Keller,[33] but L. F. Meyer[36] has been unable to confirm this finding, and in my determinations phosphorus and nitrogen were not retained in proportional amounts, i. e., 29.5 per cent. food-nitrogen was retained while only 4.8 per cent. of food-phosphorus was retained.

ELIMINATION

The elimination of phosphorus takes place both through the feces and through the urine. In most instances it is about equally divided between these two channels of excretion. However, great variations occur, for example, in children on a vegetable diet which contains much calcium, the phosphorus is largely excreted through the feces, since the calcium forms insoluble salts with the phosphorus and thus absorption is inhibited, while children on a generous flesh diet will excrete most of the phosphorus through the kidneys. The amount excreted through the urine on mother's milk varied from 0.04 to 0.08 gm., while on cow's milk it was much higher, being 0.589 gm. in Blauberg's case and as high as 2.009 gm. in one of my determinations. (See phosphorus tabulations.)

In the feces from mother's milk feedings, the elimination varied from 0.02 gm. to 0.036 gm., while on cow's milk it was 0.962 in Blauberg's case. My own determinations were 0.7648, 0.5991 and 0.3789 gm., the larger quantity appearing with the lower fat-content of feeding and diminishing as the fat was increased.

A number of investigators have tried to show that the elimination of phosphorus and nitrogen was parallel, arguing from the fact that with cell destruction both N and P were released; and, indeed, this is true for certain groups of tissues, and could we estimate their catabolism separately, this would be our result. However, since N is only influenced in the protein wear and tear of the body, and since phosphorus has many influences other than is brought about by its connection with nitrogen in the albuminous molecule, as a number of observers have shown—Ehrstrom, and more recently L. F. Meyer[36]—there may be nitrogen retention with a phosphorus loss, and vice versa. The fact, too, that phosphorus is retained so tenaciously, while nitrogen is more readily given up, is another reason why the ratio of $N:P_2O_5$ in the urine is of little value as an index to cellular metabolism. The phosphorus balance obtained by considering the intake and elimination through feces and urine can only be depended on for correct interpretation of metabolic activity of phosphorus, and, indeed, the same may be held for any of the food constituents.

36. Meyer, L. F.: Ztschr. f. physiol. Chem.. 1904. xliii.

ANOMALIES IN PHOSPHORUS RETENTION

The anomalies related under the head of calcium retention are all shared in by phosphorus. Indeed, the pathologic conditions which affect one nearly always affect the other. As has been stated, in rachitis and osteomalacia there is a disturbance of retention of the phosphorus, particularly that part bound with calcium and magnesium. In these diseases the giving of calcium increases the retention of phosphorus and the giving of phosphorus increases the retention of calcium, proving undoubtedly their chemical and physiologic affinity.

Phosphorus has a close connection with intermediary metabolism, as shown by its large content in the thyroid gland, the ovaries and the testes. So great is the necessity for phosphorus in the functioning of the testes and ovaries that castration is sometimes employed in order to divert the phosphorus to the use of the bones, as has been done occasionally in osteomalacia.

In that anomaly known as phosphaturia, in which the ratio of P_2O_5 to CaO changes from 12:1 to 4:1, if a calcium-poor diet is given, the phosphates quickly disappear. Phosphorus may be retained in abnormally large quantities as pointed out by L. F. Meyer.[37]

SODIUM AND POTASSIUM

The relationship of potassium and sodium to the maintenance of the alkalinity is a very interesting and important one. The study of the influence of their *ions* on muscle-contractility and nervous irritability is yielding valuable data. The power of their *ions* to influence body weight, body temperature, pulse and even leukocyte count is a most important contribution made by L. F. Meyer[37] and S. Cohn.[23]

We will first discuss the problems of alkalinity into which Na and K enter, since these elements form the fixed alkalies. Under the anomalies of alkalinity we will discuss the problems which relate to variations of this alkalinity.

It should be remembered that both alkaline and acid solutions exist within the same body; that the blood, various secretions, as well as each body cell has a definite amount of alkali, and can vary only within very narrow limits in order that they may perform their proper functions. This automatic regulation of alkalinity of the tissues and fluids is one of the marvels of the human mechanism, and it is remarkable how rarely it varies sufficiently to produce a pathologic condition. It is for the maintenance of this stupendously important work that the fixed alkalies, sodium and potassium, are used. Albu and Neuberg[28] have explained this self-regulation thus: Through the tearing down of the albumin of the body and the albumin taken in in the food, sulphuric and phosphoric

37. Meyer, L. F.: Deutsch. med. Wchnschr., 1905, No. 37.

acids are set free and must be neutralized by the alkalies of the blood. These acids would draw out the fixed alkalies were it not for the supply of carbonate derived from the carbonic acid and from the vegetable salts taken in the food. At certain times when the breaking down of albumin is excessive, ammonia is also set free and this is used along with the carbonates for the fixing of the acids. By means of this sort of neutralization, the acids become a constituent of the body, the fixed alkalies remain untouched, and the alkalinity of the tissues is unchanged. Should this reaction suffer the least change, either through a lessening of the bases or an increase of the autogenous acids, the organism becomes at once in danger.

The constant chemical reaction is also necessary for the ferment action which takes place throughout the body. The alkalies act also as carriers of the carbonic acid in the blood-stream.

The *ions* of potassium and sodium have an important bearing on the heart action, as shown by Overton.[38] K *ions* do not seem an absolutely necessary accompaniment of rhythmical action, but if present in too large numbers they cause a depression, even to complete inhibition. On the other hand, Na *ions* are necessary to contractility and irritability of heart-muscle. If present alone they produce muscular relaxation.

Jacques Loeb[26] has shown how closely developing life is dependent on exact proportions of NaCl in solution as shown by his experiments in sea-water, physiologic salt solution and in water with no NaCl in it.

Let us, therefore, study the sources of supply of these important elements, and see if we can determine the daily need for the growing infant. (See tabulation on page 131.)

In mother's milk there is much less sodium and potassium than in cow's milk. There is more potassium than sodium in each of these milks. The daily need of the nursing infant as represented by the intake is for sodium 0.5877 gm., and for potassium 1.1032 gm. In cow's milk feeding the sodium intake was below the intake on mother's milk and the potassium intake was considerably above that on mother's milk.

ABSORPTION

The absorption is relatively good on both milks. On absorption the Na salt takes its place in the blood and tissue fluids, while the potassium, displaying its selective action, takes its place in the various body-cells and in the blood-cells. Its most common salts are potassium phosphate, which is the chief mineral constituent of red blood corpuscles, and potassium chlorid, which is found in the body-cells. The potassium salts make up 0.4 per cent. of the total blood and 0.65 to 0.8 per cent. of fresh muscle tissue. It is evident therefore that for the production of

---

38. Overton: Arch. f, d. ges. Physiol. Bonn (Pflüger), 1902, xcii, 346.

Potassium as K_2O

In 1,000 gm. mother's milk 0.69 gm. K_2O.
In 1,000 gm. cow's milk 1.885 gm. K_2O.

Food	Intake	Elimination		Absorption		Retention	
		Feces	Urine	Gm.	Per cent.	Gm.	Per cent.
Mother's milk (Klotz)	1.1032	0.2842	0.1591	....	....	0.6598	74.2
Cow's milk (Meyer)	1.9605	0.2033	1.4411	....	....	0.8161	16.12
Cow's milk (Blauberg)	1.57	0.271	1.12	1.30	82.8	0.180	11.5

Figures given above are in grams in 24 hours.

Sodium as Na_2O

In 1,000 gm. mother's milk there is .049 gm. Na_2O.
In 1,000 gm. cow's milk there is .465 gm. Na_2O.

Food	Intake	Elimination		Absorption		Retention	
		Feces	Urine	Gm.	Per cent.	Gm.	Per cent.
Mother's milk	0.5877	0.1924	0.1481	....	....	0.2471	67.2
Cow's milk	0.478	0.075	0.3305	....	....	0.0725	15.27
Cow's milk (Soldner)	0.409	0.098	0.343	.311	75.9	Negative	....

Figures given above are in grams in 24 hours.

the muscle of the growing child an adequate supply of potassium salts must be given.

RETENTION

The retention in per cent. of intake in mother's milk is very good, being 67.0 per cent. for sodium and 74 per cent. for potassium, while the retention on cow's milk is relatively poor, being 15.27 per cent. for sodium and 16.12 per cent. for potassium.

ELIMINATION

K and Na are eliminated through the urine and feces. The potassium in the urine is bound with Cl and with phosphorus and the sodium chiefly as NaCl. The sodium of the urine largely depends on the sodium intake in the food, while the potassium in the urine depends on the destruction of tissue; hence K metabolism is parallel with tissue destruction. This is explained by the fact that K is in the cells and is more closely bound, while Na is held in solution in the blood and tissue fluids and, therefore, more readily excreted. The normal ratio of Na to K in the urine is 3:1, 2:1 and some authors place it as 5:3.

ELIMINATION THROUGH THE FECES

About 15 to 25 per cent. of the intake of K and N are eliminated through the feces. These amounts vary considerably with the kind of diet, whether it is rich in alkali or not, or whether it is vegetable or made up of a considerable part of meat.

ANOMALIES OF RETENTION OF FIXED ALKALI

There is at times an over-retention of potassium salts to the point of potassium intoxication, and some authors[28] have attempted to build a theory for uremia on this fact. In such cases the potassium salts are retained in the blood-stream rather than taking their places in the tissue structure. But the most common anomaly is not that of over-retention but of marked withdrawal of the fixed alkalies. Against such a contingency the organism of the carnivora has builded up a strong resistance. First in the use of the carbonate of the tissue fluids and blood, and, as a last resort, in the production of ammonia. As has been previously stated, under normal conditions the carbonates with the help of a small amount of ammonia, are sufficient to care for the normal production of acids in the body. Under abnormal production of acids, as occurs in diabetes and in conditions of acidosis in certain infants fed on high fat mixtures, and in some older children fed on a mixed diet containing a quart or more of rich milk, there is a demand for a large quantity of ammonia to protect the fixed alkali.

A vast number of researches have been carried on covering the field of conditions of acidosis. It was Salkowski in his experiments on dogs

CHLORIN AS NaCl

In 1,000 gm. mother's milk, 0.294 gm. Cl.
In 1,000 gm. cow's milk, 0.82 gm. Cl.
In 1,000 gm. cow's milk (Hoobler), 1.8678 gm. NaCl.

Food	Intake	Elimination		Absorption			Retention		
		Feces	Urine	Gm.	Percent.	Per Kilo	Gm.	Percent.	Per Kilo
Mother's milk	0.3297	0.0135	0.1776	0.3162	95.4	....	0.1386	58.0	....
Diluted cow's milk, 2.1% fat (Hoobler)	2.3178	0.042	2.2421	2.2758	98.1	.274	0.0337	1.4	.004
Whole cow's milk, 4% fat (Hoobler)	2.3926	0.1567	2.3328	2.2359	93.4	.286	Negative	....	....
Cow's milk and cream, 5.4% fat (Hoobler)	2.3428	0.06031	2.1340	2.2824	97.3	.288	0.14849	6.3	.018

Figures given above are in grams in 24 hours.

194

who first pointed out that the self-produced body acids were bound by the withdrawal of the fixed bases of the body, and thus there would be impoverishment of these indispensable mineral constituents were it not for the fact that the carnivora are protected by this increased ammonia excretion; but this protection is only within narrow limits.

Not only is the withdrawal of alkali accomplished through the overproduction of acids, but it has been shown that a diet rich in fats will cause a withdrawal of alkali for the purpose of combining with the fatty acids of the stools. The fatty acids will first utilize such alkaline earths (Ca and Mg) as are available, and then for further neutralization will call on the fixed alkali of the body. This in turn demands the production of ammonia for the protection of the fixed alkali. This often occurs in healthy infants when on a high fat mixture, but it takes place preeminently, as shown by L. F. Meyer,[23] in the stage of decomposition of Finkelstein's *Ernährungstörung*. In this condition not only does the fat cause loss of alkali, but even sugar produces the same result.

SODIUM CHLORID

Of all the mineral constituents, sodium chlorid has the most varied and important functions to perform. The function of maintaining osmotic pressure has been the one most studied, and its relation to the retention and excretion of water is well known. In recent years to the Na *ions* and the Cl *ions,* acting either separately or in conjunction, have been assigned various results. L. F. Meyer[23] has shown that the intake of Na *ions,* especially when bound with the halogen group, particularly with chlorin, when in certain concentration, viz., 3 gm. NaCl to 100 c.c. water, always produced an increase of temperature in a young infant. There is a marked decrease in the body weight when fed on milk freed of salts; also the pulse and leukocyte count are affected. Just what the daily need of this salt is depends largely on the kind of food ingested. There is a certain demand for this salt and when the intake is cut off the body retains with great tenacity what it has until further intake occurs.

The chlorin intake in mother's milk is 0.3297 gm., while on cow's milk the chlorin intake in terms of NaCl was 2.3926. The tabulation on page 133 shows the chlorin metabolism in terms of NaCl.

The demand for NaCl is greater in herbivora than in carnivora, because of the greater consumption of K carbonates, as was pointed out in the classic observation by Bunge.[39] His concise explanation of this phenomenon is that with a large intake of K carbonate there is formed in the blood the salts of sodium phosphate and potassium chlorid. Both being foreign, they are eliminated, leaving a loss of NaCl which must be replenished.

---

39. Bunge: Cited by Albu and Neuberg, Mineralstoffwechsel, p. 164.

NaCl is ingested in large quantities. It being well absorbed, there is an increased quantity in the blood, hence its isotonicity is disturbed and either there must be a holding back of water until the solution is isotonic, or an increased elimination of the NaCl. Both of these processes may take place.

ABSORPTION

The absorption of salt is found to be excellent—usually above 90 per cent. of the intake is absorbed. The retention of NaCl is only sufficient to cause a balance to be maintained under normal conditions. In my determinations I found that there was utilized but 1.4 per cent. to 6.3 per cent. of the intake.

ELIMINATION

The elimination takes place almost entirely through the kidneys. But a very small quantity appears in the feces, so well is it absorbed. In my determinations there was a little over 2 gm. excreted through the urine daily, while less than 0.1 gm. appeared in the feces.

It has been observed that salt solution when injected subcutaneously is more quickly eliminated than when taken by mouth. With the excretion of NaCl there must accompany it a certain amount of water, and, therefore, the intensity of diuresis depends on the molecular concentration within the body. Not only does salt affect the retention and withdrawal of water, but it holds a very close relation to nitrogen.

Voit's original work seemed to show that with increasing retention of NaCl there was an increased retention of nitrogen; later investigations have not agreed with this. Belli[40] sums up his findings with the statement that in small amounts, as in the food normally, it hastens and increases protein retention, but in greater quantities it tends to lessen the nitrogen retention.

THE ANOMALIES OF NaCl RETENTION

There are a number of conditions which seem markedly affected by sodium chlorid. The most important is that of nephritis. Von Noorden[41] was the first to work on this important condition. He noted a variation in different cases. Some retained and others did not retain NaCl. Halpern[42] has shown that both in acute and chronic nephritis the salt content of the urine is dependent on the salt content of the food. In cases in which there is edema there is marked lessening of the edema when the patient is put on a salt-free diet, and there appears in the urine an increase in the NaCl elimination. The use of salt-free diet, whether

40. Belli: Cited by Albu and Neuberg, Mineralstoffwechsel, Berlin, 1906, p. 170.

41. Von Noorden: Lehrbuch d. Pathologie d. Stoffwechsels, Berlin, 1893.

42. Halpern: Cited by Albu and Neuberg, Mineralstoffwechsel, Berlin, 1906, p. 174.

with or without edema, brings about more or less of a dechloruration of the body. It would seem that in these cases the NaCl retention always precedes the water retention and that the edema consequent on water retention is due to the NaCl retained. However, no hard and fast rules can be laid down in regard to use of salt-free diet, as in some cases it will not reduce edema, and in some cases a salt-rich diet will not always produce NaCl retention.

L. F. Meyer[23] believes that many of the symptoms present in food disturbances of infants may be traced to the deleterious influence of sodium chlorid, acting not only as salt, but also in the capacity of the respective *ions*. He believes particularly that the rises of temperature during the stage of intoxication of Finkelstein's *Ernährungstörung* is due to the action of these *ions*. In children with food disturbances smaller quantities of NaCl solution will raise temperature more quickly than in healthy children.

Fisher[43] has shown that the injection of salt solution of one-sixth molecular strength may produce glycosuria, and that this glycosuria may be stopped by injecting a calcium chlorid solution.

Abderhalden[6] believes that every cell has particular salts in specific apportionment and that a disturbance of this relation, as would take place in Fisher's experiment just quoted, would cause considerable trouble in the life processes of the cell.

SULPHUR

Of all the mineral salts, sulphur has been the last to receive due attention at the hands of investigators. What we know of sulphur metabolism is largely due to Freund[46] and his pupils. Sulphur presents itself for ingestion in the food in two different forms, viz., in the inorganic salts, and organically bound with albumin. The inorganic salts have little or no effect on metabolism and need not be considered. It is that sulphur which is organically bound which is the important part and which supplies the daily need of the growing infant.

Whether or not sulphur is necessary for the maintenance of life is still a question, but any substance so closely associated with nitrogen may be assumed to have a distinct function, though as yet this function is obscure.

The total sulphur intake of infants fed on mother's milk is .04 gm., while on cow's milk the daily intake is about 0.44 gm., according to my recent researches. The sulphur of mother's milk is very well absorbed, as is also that of cow's milk. My determinations show that it is absorbed in from 88.2 to 95.7 per cent. of intake. This absorption is quite in

43. Fisher: Cited by Abderhalden, Lehrbuch d. physiolog. Chemie, Berlin, 1909, p. 358.
46. Freund: Zeit. f. phys. Chem., Strassburg, 1900, xxix, 24-46.

SULPHUR IN TERMS OF S

In 1,000 gm. mother's milk, total sulphur .0572 gm.
In 1,000 gm. cow's milk (Hoobler), total sulphur .33538 gm.

Food	Intake	Elimination		Absorption			Retention		
		Feces	Urine	Gm.	Percent.	Per Kilo	Gm.	Percent.	Per Kilo
Mother's milk	.0396	.0096	.026	.0298	75.5	....	.0039	9.8	....
Cow's milk	.5832	.01484	.2019	.0436	74.5	....	Negative	....	....
Diluted cow's milk, 2.1% fat (Hoobler)	.46308	.0542	.3777	.4089	88.2	.491	Negative	....	....
Whole cow's milk, 4% fat (Hoobler)	.4411	.02430	.26589	.4168	94.2	.531	.15091	34.2	.019
Cow's milk and cream, 5.4% fat (Hoobler)	.4444	.01901	.30585	.42546	95.7	.533	.11961	26.9	.015

Figures given above are in grams in 24 hours.

keeping with the facility with which nitrogen is absorbed, and this is probably due to the fact that its connection with the albumin molecule is so close. (See tabulation, page 137.)

The absorption takes place through the small intestine, and some of it is again eliminated into the large intestine, making up the sulphur found in the feces.

Schwarz[47] found in a 5-year-old child on a mixed diet that the absorption was very good, being 92.2 per cent. of the intake. My normal child on a milk diet had an absorption of 92.4 per cent. of the intake. Identical methods of determination were used by both of us.

RETENTION

The retention of sulphur in mother's milk feeding is very good, while with cow's milk the retention is relatively poor. In one of my determinations there was a negative balance and in two others 34.2 and 26.9 per cent. of the intake was retained. Schwarz,[47] in a normal 5-year-old child on a mixed diet found that sulphur retention was relatively poor, being 31.1 per cent. of the intake.

ELIMINATION

The elimination of sulphur occurs mostly through the urine. In cow's milk feeding ten times as much appeared excreted through the urine as through the feces.

The sulphur in the feces appears as iron sulphate and alkali sulphate, while in the urine there are recognized four different forms, viz., the inorganic sulphate sulphur, the ethereal sulphate sulphur, neutral sulphur and basic sulphur. The first named is by far the most abundant in the urine, making up about 80 per cent. of the total sulphur. Ethereal sulphate sulphur makes up about 8 per cent. of the total sulphur and the neutral and basic sulphurs the balance.

Just what significance should be assigned to total sulphur and to each of the various sulphurs making up the total, has been the subject of much speculation.

Because of the connection between sulphur and albumin in tissues, the sulphur metabolism has been taken as the index to protein metabolism. The normal ratio is $N : H_2SO_4 : : 5 : 1$.

The relative amount of ethereal sulphate sulphur has been taken as an index of the degree of albuminous putrefaction going on in the intestine, and also for the breaking down of albuminous cells in the body.

The neutral sulphur appears to be increased on a vegetable diet and decreased on a meat diet. Investigators have shown that in periods of starvation, as well as in other conditions of protein break-down, there is an increase in the per cent. which neutral sulphur holds to total sulphur.

---

47. Schwarz: Jahrb. f. Kinderh., 1910, lxxii, p. 549.

Lepine[48] is the authority for believing that neutral sulphur has its origin partly from the taurin of the bile. This is first excreted into the intestine, reabsorbed, and again eliminated through the urine. In those conditions of disturbed oxidation, if below normal, neutral sulphur is low; if above normal, then the neutral sulphur is increased. In my determinations of neutral sulphur it appears that on cow's milk containing 2.1 per cent. fat the neutral sulphur averaged 7.2 per cent. of the total sulphur, but that on feeding 4 per cent. and 5.4 per cent. fat mixtures the neutral sulphur was increased to as high as 15 per cent., more than doubled. This might be explained by the fact that during these higher fat feedings small amounts of acetone, diacetic acid and beta-oxybutyric acid were found in the urine, forecasting an impending acidosis, in which already tissue albumin had begun to disintegrate.

ANOMALIES OF SULPHUR RETENTION

Schwarz has shown that in rachitis the total sulphur absorption in two cases was 76.9 and 83 per cent., which was somewhat lower than in his normal case, which showed 92.2 per cent. absorption. The retention in one case was 30.9 per cent. and in the other 26.1 per cent. of the intake. This was about the same as in his normal case, viz., 31.1 per cent.

There was eliminated through the urine 55 per cent. of the total sulphur in one case and 54.1 in the other, while in the urine of his normal case 61.1 per cent. was thus eliminated. The elimination by the feces in two of his cases of rachitis showed a marked change from his normal case—23.1 per cent. and 17 per cent. in rachitis and but 7.8 per cent. in the normal.

Of the various forms of sulphur in the urine, the only one which showed much variation from the normal was that of the neutral sulphur, which in two of his cases was considerably increased, being 18.5 per cent. and 18.6 per cent., while his normal showed 7.8 per cent. of the total sulphur. In one of his rachitic cases no variation from the normal occurred.

A further anomaly of sulphur metabolism is that of cystinuria. Bunge has shown that in the catabolism of cystin, albumin, which has sulphur in it, sets sulphur free, which usually unites with bases and is eliminated as sulphates; but if the bases are lacking, then alkali is drawn from the cells of the body.

SUMMARY

1. Salts are necessary to maintain life.
2. Salts are best absorbed and utilized when in organic combination with food stuffs.

48. Lepine: Cited by Albu and Neuberg, Mineralstoffwechsel, Berlin, 1906, p. 148.

3. There are marked differences in the salt content of mother's and cow's milk which should be considered in artificial feeding.

4. Certain pathologic conditions arise in which certain of the salts are not absorbed, even though in abundance in the food.

5. In certain other pathologic conditions salts are actually withdrawn from the body to such an extent as to impoverish the organism and produce grave disturbances of nutrition.

6. The various salts, with the exception of iron, are present in sufficient quantities and proper proportions in mother's milk. In most of the dilutions of cow's milk there is an excess of salts which may be neglected in feeding normal infants, but which plays an important rôle in the feeding of children already suffering from nutritional disturbances. The conditions under which the salt content of feedings should be altered and in just what degree each or all should be varied, are still unsolved problems.

131 East Sixty-Seventh Street.

18

Reprinted from Am. J. Dis. Child., 28, 574–581 (1924)

THE RELATION OF CALCIUM AND PHOSPHORUS IN THE DIET TO THE ABSORPTION OF THESE ELEMENTS FROM THE INTESTINE *

W. J. ORR, M.D.; L. E. HOLT, JR., M.D.; L. WILKINS, M.D.

AND

F. H. BOONE, M.D.

BALTIMORE

The problem of absorption from the intestine has taken on a new significance since it has been appreciated that the failure of calcification in rickets is coincident with and apparently dependent on the absorption of minerals. The experiments of Schabad,[1] Schloss [2] and others, including us,[3] have shown that active rickets is associated with defective absorption of calcium and phosphorus, and that as the disease heals, large quantities of these elements are retained. Moreover, it seems clear that the absorption of these elements can be increased in at least two ways: (1) by the administration of a factor contained in certain animal fats, of which cod liver oil is the best example; and (2) by the use of ultra-violet rays. Both of these measures are effective, even though the quantity of calcium and phosphorus supplied varies greatly. It has been supposed that these substances act by altering in some way the permeability of the intestinal wall toward these particular elements.

Although cod liver oil and ultraviolet rays are the methods by which the absorption of these elements has been effected experimentally, still there are other factors which may presumably influence the process, such as the concentration of calcium and phosphorus supplied in the diet, the reaction of the intestinal contents, variations in the concentration of other salts, changes in temperature, etc. It would seem that considerable light

---

* Received for publication, July 29, 1924.

* From the Department of Pediatrics, Johns Hopkins University, and the Harriet Lane Home, Johns Hopkins Hospital.

1. Schabad, J. A.: Ztschr. f. klin. Med. 66:454, 1908-1909; ibid. 68:94, 1909; ibid. 69:435, 1910; Berl. klin. Wchnschr. 46:823, 1909; ibid. 46:923, 1909; Jahrb. f. Kinderh. 72:1, 1910; ibid. 74:511, 1911; Arch. f. Kinderh. 52:47-68, 1909; ibid. 53:380, 1910; ibid. 54:83, 1910; Ztschr. f. Kinderh. 2:117, 1911; Monatschr. f. Kinderh. 11:63, 1912. Schabad and Soroschowitch: Monatschr. f. Kinderh. 9:659, 1911; ibid. 10:12, 1912; Arch. f. Kinderh. 57:276, 1912.

2. Schloss, E.: Deutsch. med. Wchnschr. 39:1505, 1913; Arch. f. Kinderh. 63:359, 1914; Jahrb. f. Kinderh. 78:694, 1913; ibid. 79:40, 194, 1914; ibid. 82:435, 1915; ibid. 83:46, 1916. Frank and Schloss: Jahrb. f. Kinderh. 79:539, 1914; Biochem. Ztschr. 60:378, 1914; Monatschr. f. Kinderh. 13:271, 1914.

3. Orr, W. J.; Holt, L. E.; Wilkins, L., and Boone, F. H.: The Calcium and Phosphorus Metabolism in Rickets, with Special Reference to Ultraviolet Therapy, Am. J. Dis. Child. 26:362 (July) 1923.

might be thrown on the process of absorption in general by an investigation of these various factors separately. In this instance we have studied only the effect of varying the concentrations of calcium and phosphorus in the diet on the absorption of these elements.

Considerable work has already been done on this subject but much of it is open to criticism, either because the variation of the elements in the diet was so small that little significance could be attached to the results, or because the effect of other factors, such as cod liver oil and light rays, were not excluded.

Largely as a result of the earlier work [4] on the subject, the conclusion has been accepted that feeding an excess of one element impairs the absorption of the other, although an increased amount of the element fed in excess may be retained. There is, however, contradictory evidence [5] on this point. Metabolism experiments have been the means employed to study the question. In more recent years studies of the blood have furnished additional information in regard to the absorption of these particular elements, a rise of concentration in the serum being taken as an indication of increased absorption, and a fall, of impaired absorption.

Data are available in regard to the alterations in the concentrations of calcium and phosphorus in the blood, produced by varying the intake of these elements. Boggs [6] reports an increase in blood calcium in dogs after feeding calcium lactate. Meigs, Blatherwick and Cary [7] report experiments with cattle, in which calcium chlorid or disodium phosphate was added to the diet. Excessive calcium in the diet caused an increase in the plasma calcium but a diminution of the plasma phosphorus; while, on the other hand, excessive phosphate in the diet raised the phosphorus concentration of the plasma.

The production of experimental rickets in rats by McCollum, Simmonds, Shipley and Park [8] on a diet high in calcium but low in phosphorus has furnished more evidence that calcium absorption is thus improved and phosphorus absorption impaired, for Howland and Kramer [9] have shown that in these animals the calcium concentration of the blood serum is raised and that of the inorganic phosphorus

4. Bertram, J.: Ztschr. f. Biol. **14**:335, 1878. Hammarsten: Text Book of Physiologic Chemistry, Ed. 7, 1915, 762. Forbes, E. B., et al.: Ohio Agric. Exp. Sta., Tech. Bull. **6**:66, 1915. Meyer and Cohn: Quoted by Blühdorn, Footnote 15.

5. Quoted by Blühdorn, Footnote 15.

6. Boggs, T. R.: Bull. Johns Hopkins Hosp. **19**:201, 1908.

7. Meigs, E. B.; Blatherwick, N. R., and Cary, C. A.: J. Biol. Chem. **37**:63, 1919.

8. McCollum, E. V.; Simmonds, N.; Shipley, P. G., and Park, E. A.: J. Biol. Chem. **47**:507 (Aug.) 1921.

9. Howland, J., and Kramer, B.: Bull. Johns Hopkins Hosp. **33**:313 (Sept.) 1922.

lowered. Furthermore, when rickets is produced by a diet low in calcium and relatively high in phosphorus,[10] the concentration of serum phosphorus is increased and that of the calcium diminished.[9]

Thus all of the reported experiments [11] on animals confirm the original suggestion that an excess either of calcium or phosphorus in the diet exercises an unfavorable influence on the absorption of the other element from the intestine. The natural assumption that has been made to explain this is, that an excess of one element in the diet causes precipitation of the other element in the intestine in the form of insoluble calcium phosphate, which is eliminated in the feces.

We have been able to find records of very few experiments in man which are free from error or at least criticism. Schabad [12] reported observations on a child to whom he gave an excess of sodium phosphate, with resulting improvement in the phosphorus retention, but with definite impairment of the calcium balance. He also tried the effect of feeding calcium acetate, with the result that an excessive loss of phosphorus occurred in the feces. Bosworth and Bowditch [13] performed a somewhat similar experiment. They gave a child an excess of calcium chlorid and found an increased retention of calcium, but a marked loss of phosphorus in the feces.[14]

The work of Blühdorn,[15] however, would suggest an entirely different conclusion. He studied the metabolism of two children who received a normal diet, diets with an excess of calcium and those with an excess of phosphorus. He concluded from his experiments that calcium and phosphorus absorption run parallel. An excess of either element in the diet caused an increase in the quantity of both retained. He found no evidence for an unfavorable effect of excessive calcium on the phosphorus metabolism, or of excessive phosphorus on the calcium metabolism.

10. McCollum, E. V.; Simmonds, N., and Kinney, E. M.: Am. J. Hygiene **2**:97 (March) 1922.

11. Since this was written, the experiments of Salvesen, Hastings and McIntosh on dogs have been published (J. Biol. Chem. **60**:311-327 [June] 1922). They, too, find that oral administration of phosphates cause a rise of inorganic phosphorus in the serum, and a drop in the serum calcium. Their experiments with oral administration of calcium salts, however, did not give such striking results.

12. Schabad, J. A.: Arch. f. Kinderh. **54**:83, 1910.

13. Bosworth, A. W., and Bowditch, H. I.: Boston M. & S. J. **177**:864 (Dec. 20) 1917.

14. In this connection the studies of Howland and Kramer on tetany are of interest (Tr. Am. Ped. Soc., 1922, p. 204). These observers found that feeding calcium raised the concentration of the calcium in the blood serum, but caused a coincident fall in the phosphorus content of the serum. The mineral metabolism of their patients was not studied, but the results were nevertheless highly suggestive.

15. Blühdorn, K.: Ztschr. f. Kinderh. **29**:43 (April) 1921.

These results of Blühdorn seemed so surprising and so much in conflict with animal experiments and the few other uncomplicated experiments with children, that we undertook to investigate this point further,

TABLE 1.—*Experiments on Child with Rickets*

B. G., colored child, aged 18 months, clinical signs of rickets. Admitted March 26, 1923.

Serum determinations, 3/26/23: Ca = 10.2 mg./100 c.c.; P = 2.8 mg./100 c.c.

First Metabolism Period: Four days (4/4/23—4/8/23) normal milk diet.

Ca intake	3.98 gm.	P intake	2.84 gm.
Ca urine output	0.03 gm.	P urine output	1.46 gm.
Ca stool output	2.86 gm.	P stool output	0.72 gm.
Total Ca output	2.89 gm.	Total P output	2.18 gm.
Ca retention	1.09 gm.	P retention	0.66 gm.
Per cent. retained	27.1	Per cent. retained	23.4
Per cent. output in urine	1.3	Per cent. output in urine	66.9

Ratio Ca/P retained 1.65

Serum determinations, 4/8/23: Ca = 8.4 mg./100 c.c.; P = 4.0 mg./100 c.c.

Second Metabolism Period: Four days (4/16/23—4/20/23) Diet: milk + CaCl₂.

Ca intake	9.20 gm.	P intake	2.80 gm.
Ca urine output	0.30 gm.	P urine output	1.22 gm.
Ca stool output	7.12 gm.	P stool output	1.16 gm.
Total Ca output	7.42 gm.	Total P output	2.38 gm.
Ca retention	1.78 gm.	P retention	0.42 gm.
Per cent. retained	19.4	Per cent. P retained	15.1
Per cent. output in urine	4.0	Per cent. P output in urine	51.

Ratio Ca/P retained 4.2

Serum determinations, 4/19/23: Ca = 10.2 mg./100 c.c.; P = 3.1 mg./100 c.c.

Third Metabolism Period: Four days* (4/30/23—5/3/23) Diet: milk + Na₂HPO₄.

Ca intake	3.41 gm.	P intake	5.42 gm.
Ca urine output	0.04 gm.	P uterine output	1.49 gm.
Ca stool output	3.26 gm.	P stool output	3.47 gm.
Total retention	3.30 gm.	Total P output	4.96 gm.
Ca retention	0.11 gm.	P retention	0.46 gm.
Per cent. retained	3.2	Per cent. P retained	8.4
Per cent. output in urine	1.2	Per cent. P output in urine	30.0

Ratio Ca/P retained 0.24

Serum determinations, 5/4/23: Ca = 7.55 mg./100 c.c.; P = 4.1 mg./100 c.c.

Subsequent Course: Antirachitic treatment was started immediately after third metabolism period, with resulting cure of the rickets.

Serum determinations, 5/14/23: Ca = 10.0 mg./100 c.c.; P. = 4.0.

Serum determinations, 5/23/23: Ca = 10.8 mg./100 c.c.; P = 5.0.
Child discharged in good condition 5/24/23.

---

* Child developed diarrhea on the third day and the experiment was stopped. Results calculated to four-day period (multiplied by ⁴⁄₃) for the sake of comparison.

in order to determine if the conditions found in the lower animals are applicable to man.

Two subjects were selected for this study: one a child with incipient rickets, the other a normal child who had previously suffered from a

mild nutritional disturbance. The calcium and phosphorus intake and
output of these children was determined on three different diets: a
normal diet, a high calcium diet, and a high phosphorus diet. Suitable
intervals were allowed to elapse between these periods of study.
Determinations of the calcium and phosphorus of the serum were made

TABLE 2.—*Experiment on Undernourished Child*

C. S., colored child, aged 14 months, somewhat undernourished. Admitted
April 1, 1923.

Serum determinations, 4/4/23: Ca = 10.0 mg./100 c.c.; P = 4.9 mg./100 c.c.

First Metabolism Period: Four days (4/4/23—4/8/23) on normal milk diet.

Ca intake	3.98 gm.	P intake	2.84 gm.
Ca urine output	0.09 gm.	P urine output	1.37 gm.
Ca stool output	2.86 gm.	P stool output	0.68 gm.
Total Ca output	2.95 gm.	Total P output	2.05 gm.
Ca retention	1.03 gm.	P retention	0.79 gm.
Per cent. retained	26.0	Per cent. retained	27.6
Per cent. output in urine	3.1	Per cent. output in urine	66.6

Ratio Ca/P retained 1.30

Serum determinations, 4/16/23: Ca = 9.0 mg./100 c.c.; P = 5.4 mg./100 c.c.

Second Metabolism Period: Four days (4/16/23—4/20/23) Diet: milk +
$CaCl_2$.

Ca intake	7.29 gm.	P intake	2.13 gm.
Ca urine output	0.41 gm.	P urine output	1.02 gm.
Ca stool output	4.84 gm.	P stool output	0.94 gm.
Total Ca output	5.25 gm.	Total P output	1.96 gm.
Ca retention	2.04 gm.	P retention	0.17 gm.
Per cent. Ca retained	27.9	Per cent. retained	8.0
Per cent. output in urine	7.7	Per cent. output in urine	52.0

Ratio Ca/P retained 12.0

Serum determinations, 4/21/23: Ca = 10.0 mg. 100 c.c.; P = 3.3 mg./100 c.c.

Third Metabolism Period: Four days (4/30/23—5/4/23) Diet: Milk +
Na_2HPO_4.

Ca intake	3.95 gm.	P intake	6.36 gm.
Ca urine output	0.05 gm.	P urine output	2.96 gm.
Ca stool output	3.50 gm.	P stool output	2.82 gm.
Total Ca output	3.55 gm.	Total P output	5.78 gm.
Ca retention	0.40 gm.	P retained	0.58 gm.
Per cent. retained	10.3	Per cent. retained	9.2 gm.
Per cent. output in urine	1.3	Per cent. output in urine	51.0

Ratio Ca/P 0.69

Serum determinations, 5/4/23: Ca = 10.4; P = 5.0
5/7/23: Ca = 10.5; P = 4.3

Discharged 5/8/23 in good condition.

---

in connection with each period of study. The details of our procedure
and the methods used were as reported in a previous publication.[3]
Protocols of these experiments are given in Tables 1 and 2.

COMMENT

It is quite evident from these experiments that increasing the intake
of calcium causes more calcium to be retained; the serum calcium rises
if it is low, and more calcium is lost in the urine. At the same time the

phosphorus retention is definitely diminished, considerable amounts of phosphorus are diverted from the urine to the stools, and there is a diminution of the concentration of phosphorus in the serum.

The effect of high phosphorus intake is almost equally striking. Although the actual amount of phosphorus retained is not increased and may even be somewhat diminished, the concentration of phosphorus in the serum is definitely increased. There is a very marked decrease in the amount of calcium retained, a great increase in the calcium of the stools, a marked diminution of the calcium in the urine, and in one case a definite fall in the concentration of calcium in the serum.

The fact that absorption of calcium and phosphorus does not run parallel is perhaps most clearly demonstrated by examination of the ratio of the retained calcium to the retained phosphorus. It will be seen that on a normal milk diet this ratio is about 1.3, that is, a little more calcium is retained than phosphorus. On the high calcium diet, in one case four times as much calcium as phosphorus is retained, and, in the other case, twelve times as much. On the high phosphorus diet considerably more phosphorus is retained than calcium.

Our results, therefore, seem to contradict the findings of Blühdorn and confirm those of Schabad, of Bowditch and of Bosworth, and the numerous investigators who have worked with lower animals. It would appear that an excess of either calcium or phosphorus in the diet tends to increase the output of the other element in the intestine, and the natural assumption that has been made is that this is due to the precipitation of insoluble phosphates of calcium in the intestine. Apparently only calcium ions, the various types of phosphate ions and molecular phosphates of calcium in solution can pass through the intestinal mucosa, but insoluble phosphates of the calcium cannot be absorbed. If this is true, it should follow that any factor which favors solution of calcium phosphate should promote the absorption of both calcium and phosphorus from the intestine (when they are present in any fixed concentrations). Such factors are: (1) increased acidity of the intestinal contents, with resulting production of the more soluble primary phosphate from the insoluble secondary and tertiary forms; (2) reduction of temperature; (3) increase in the total salt concentration [16] and (4) specific ion effects.

It is, of course, not possible to measure directly the changes in the hydrogen-ion concentration of the intestinal contents, but indirect evi-

---

16. It has been shown by Brønsted and others that the solubility of sparingly soluble salts is often increased by the presence of foreign salts, and sometimes even by the addition of salts containing a common ion. That this is true of at least one form of insoluble calcium phosphate, the tricalcium phosphate, $Ca_3(PO_4)_2$, has been shown by the unpublished experiments of one of us (L. E. H.).

dence on this point is not wanting. For instánce, it has been shown [17] that foods which are acid forming improve calcium retention, while base forming foods have the opposite effect. Moreover Sato [18] noted an unfavorable effect on calcium metabolism when alkali was added to the dietary of an infant. Unfortunately, the phosphorus metabolism was not followed in either of these studies. The experiments of Orr,[19] however, furnish evidence that both phosphorus and calcium absorption are unfavorably influenced by diets that increase the alkalinity of the stools.

The effect of changes in temperature on the absorption of calcium and phosphorus has not been studied, but it would seem that they might exert both a direct and an indirect influence on the process. The solubility of tertiary calcium phosphate is diminished by heat, and one would therefore expect that a rise in temperature would impair absorption. The work of Yllpö [20] suggests that temperature changes may also exert an indirect effect, namely, by altering the reaction of the gastro-intestinal contents. Yllpö has recently shown that fever is often accompanied by decreased acidity in the stomach, and it seems possible that the reaction of the intestinal contents might also be altered.

So far, there have been no investigations of calcium and phosphorus metabolism in which the variable factor has been the total salt concentration.

There is, however, evidence which might be interpreted as indicating that specific ion effects play a part in absorption from the intestine. Goldschmidt and Dayton [21] and Goldschmidt and Binger [22] have shown great differences in the ease with which sodium chlorid is absorbed by the intestine, depending on the presence and concentration of sodium sulphate or calcium lactate. Although these observers interpreted their results as indicating an alteration of the intestinal wall by these latter salts, it seems equally possible, in the light of recent chemical work,[23] that specific interaction of ions might play a part in such phenomena.

We have, then, considerable evidence that absorption of calcium and phosphorus from the intestine depends on the concentration of calcium and phosphate ions, and the presence of soluble undissociated phosphates of calcium. Such physicochemical factors as alter these concentrations of salts or ions or their activities may greatly influence the absorption

17. Bogert, L. J., and Kirkpatrick, E. E.: J. Biol. Chem. **54**:375 (Oct.) 1922.
18. Sato, A.: The Effect of Alkali and Malt Preparations on the Retention of Calcium in Infancy, Am. J. Dis. Child. **16**:293 (Nov.) 1918.
19. Orr, W. J.: Am. J. Dis Child. To be published.
20. Yllpö, A.: Acta Pediat. **3**:213 (Feb.) 1924.
21. Goldschmidt, S., and Dayton, A. B.: Am. J. Physiol. **48**:459 (May) 1919.
22. Goldschmidt, S., and Binger, C. A. L.: Am. J. Physiol. **48**:473 (May) 1919.
23. Brønsted, J. N.: J. Am. Chem. Soc. **42**:761, 1448, 1920; ibid. **43**:2265, 1921; ibid. **44**:877, 938, 1922; ibid. **45**:2898, 1923.

of these elements. The question still remains: how do cod liver oil and ultraviolet light effect the absorption of these elements so profoundly?

SUMMARY

1. It is shown by metabolism studies that excessive amounts of calcium in the diet tend to increase the total absorption and retention of calcium, but tend to impair phosphorus retention.

2. Excessive amounts of phosphorus in the diet exercise an unfavorable influence on the calcium metabolism, and are accompanied by an increase in the calcium lost in the feces.

3. The retention of one element in the intestine by an excessive amount of the other in the diet is best explained by the formation of insoluble phosphates of calcium which cannot be absorbed.

19

Reprinted from *Am. J. Dis. Child.*, **86**(5), 553–567 (1953)

USE OF FERRIC AND FERROUS IRON IN THE PREVENTION OF HYPOCHROMIC ANEMIA IN INFANTS

W. L. NICCUM, M.D.

R. L. JACKSON, M.D.

AND

GENEVIEVE STEARNS, Ph.D.

IOWA CITY, IOWA

THE INCIDENCE of deficiency disease in infants has decreased concurrently with increase and dissemination of nutritional knowledge. However, hypochromic anemia continues to occur commonly in the latter half of the first year of life. It is desirable, therefore, to prevent rather than treat hypochromic anemia. This study was undertaken to determine the amount and form of iron needed for this purpose.

Since the studies of Elvehjem and co-workers,[1] Stearns and co-workers,[2] Heath and Patek,[3] and McClean,[4] iron preparations have been employed more frequently during the early months of postnatal life to prevent depletion of iron stores and to insure the availability of sufficient iron to maintain optimum hemoglobin values during infancy. Various amounts and types of iron have been advised as a daily dose. McClean[4] recommends 50 to 60 mg. of iron daily as ferrous sulfate; Elvehjem, 25 mg. of iron daily as ferric pyrophosphate and 1 mg. of copper daily as copper sulfate, and Stearns,[5] 5 to 10 mg. of iron daily as ferric ammonium citrate. In recent months excellent reports[6] of iron metabolism in normal, premature, and ill infants and children have been published which adequately review the literature and discuss the diagnosis and treatment of hypochromic anemia.

This study was supported by a grant from Mead Johnson & Company.

From the Department of Pediatrics, State University of Iowa College of Medicine.

1. (*a*) Elvehjem, C. A.; Peterson, W. H., and Mendenhall, D. R.: Hemoglobin Content of the Blood of Infants, Am. J. Dis. Child. **46**:105, 1933. (*b*) Elvehjem, C. A.; Siemers, A., and Mendenhall, D. R.: Effect of Iron and Copper Therapy on Hemoglobin Content of Blood of Infants, ibid. **50**:28, 1935.

2. (*a*) Stearns, G., and McKinley, J. B.: The Conservation of Blood Iron During the Period of Physiological Hemoglobin Destruction in Early Infancy, J. Nutrition **13**:143, 1937. (*b*) Stearns, G., and Stinger, D.: Iron Retention in Infancy, ibid. **13**:127, 1937.

3. Heath, C. W., and Patek, A. J., Jr.: The Anemia of Iron Deficiency, Medicine **16**:267, 1937.

4. McClean, E. B. Iron Therapy in Hypochromic Anemia, Pediatrics **7**:136, 1951.

5. Stearns, G.: College of Medicine Symposium on Infant Feeding: Nutritional Requirements During Infancy, J. Iowa M. Soc. **40**:154, 1950.

6. (*a*) Smith, C. H.; Schulman, I., and Morgenthau, J. E.: Iron Metabolism in Infants and Children, in Advances in Pediatrics, edited by S. Z. Levine and others, Chicago, Year Book Publishers, Inc., 1952, Vol. 5, p. 195. (*b*) Moore, C. V.: Iron Metabolism and Hypochromic Anemia, Currents in Infant Care, Nutrition, and Medicine, 1950, Vol. 2, p. 78.

The amount of iron available for the production of hemoglobin during early infancy is derived primarily from two sources. Iron is stored in the liver of the fetus during the latter half of the third trimester, and the amount is influenced considerably by the nutritional status of the mother.[7] Under optimum conditions, approximately 50 mg. of iron is stored in the fetal liver. Inasmuch as the amount of iron stored is related directly to the length of gestation, infants born prematurely or immaturely have less iron storage. Iron is made available after birth from the hemolysis of excess red blood cells. If it is assumed that the blood volume of a full-term infant at birth is approximately 450 ml., then an additional 150 to 180 mg. of iron would be made available for storage in this manner. There is very little loss of this iron, and it should be sufficient to aid in the production of another 300 to 450 ml. of whole blood.

It has been shown[8] that if the umbilical cord is not clamped until all pulsations cease approximately 100 ml. of blood will enter the infant's body which, during its breakdown, will make available approximately 45 mg. more iron for storage. This amount of iron may seem insignificant, but it approximates the amount of iron in the diet of many an infant during the first six months of extrauterine life. C. A. Smith and co-workers[9] have concluded, from their study of transplacentally acquired radioactive iron from maternal erythrocytes of healthy mothers, that the full-term infants whose cords were clamped late would have sufficient iron stored to prevent anemia for the first six months.

Guest[10] has observed that there is little likelihood of an iron-deficiency anemia developing in the first year of life in normal full-term infants without infection if an adequate amount of iron was provided during the intrauterine life. He believes an iron-deficiency anemia will not occur, even though the infant is fed a diet devoid of iron supplements. McCance and Widdowson,[11] basing their opinion on animal studies primarily and with the aid of mathematical determinations, have come to the conclusion that full-term infants have sufficient storage of iron to meet only 60% of their needs for the first six months after birth and that the other 40% might be obtained from human milk. This possibility seems doubtful, as mature human milk contains 0.07 to 0.36 mg. of iron per 100 ml.

Differences of opinion exist as to the relative efficiency of ferrous and ferric iron preparations in the prevention or treatment of iron-deficiency anemia. The investigations of Darby and Hahn,[12] in which they used radioactive ferrous chloride

7. Strauss, M. B.: Anemia of Infancy from Maternal Iron Deficiency in Pregnancy, J. Clin. Invest. 12:345, 1933.

8. Wilson, E. E.; Windle, W. F., and Alt, H. L.: Deprivation of Placental Blood as a Cause of Iron Deficiency in Infants, Am. J. Dis. Child. 62:320, 1941.

9. Smith, C. A.; Caton, W. L.; Roby, C. C.; Reid, D. E.; Caswell, R. S., and Gibson, J. G., II: Transplacental Iron: Its Persistence During Infancy as Studied Isotopically, Am. J. Dis. Child. 80:856, 1950.

10. Guest, G. M.: Hypoferric Anemia in Infancy, in Symposium on Nutrition: Nutritional Anemia, Cincinnati, Robert Gould Research Foundation, Inc., 1947, p. 161.

11. McCance, R. A., and Widdowson, E. M.: The Metabolism of Iron During Suckling. J. Physiol. 112:450, 1951.

12. (a) Darby, W. J.; Hahn, P. F.; Kaser, M. M.; Steincamp, R. C.; Densen, P. M., and Conk, M. B.: The Absorption of Radioactive Iron by Children 7 to 10 Years of Age, J. Nutrition 33:107, 1947. (b) Hahn, P. F.; Carothers, E. L.; Cannon, R. O.; Sheppard, C. W.; Darby, W. J.; Kaser, M. M.; McClellan, G. S., and Densen, P. M.: Iron Uptake in 750 Cases of Human Pregnancy Using the Radioactive Isotope Fe^{59}, Fed. Proc. 6:392, 1947.

(2 to 3 mg. of $FeCl_2$ containing Fe^{59}, 47-day half-life, reduced with a slight excess of ascorbic acid and given orally) indicated that ferrous iron is utilized more efficiently by the intestinal mucosal cells. This work corroborates the clinical observations of Moore [13] in earlier experiments. Stearns and Stinger,[2b] in earlier studies, had observed that ferric iron, when given in small amounts in the form of ferric ammonium citrate, was retained and utilized well by healthy infants. Small amounts of ferric iron apparently are reduced to ferrous iron in the gastrointestinal tract. The utilization of iron from such foods as egg yolk and fortified cereals (the iron in egg yolk is 1.0 to 1.5 mg. ferrous iron in an organic form and in the fortified cereal, 8.5 mg. of ferrous iron per ounce) was also studied by the latter group of investigators. The total intake required to insure retention of iron was found to be 0.5 mg. per kilogram of body weight, and intakes up to 1.0 to 1.5 mg. per kilogram allowed ample retention for hemoglobin formation.

The gradient of absorption of iron is thought to be greater in the duodenum and upper ileum,[14] and excretion of iron by the gastrointestinal tract is probably a function of the colon.[15]

Granick has reviewed [16] the literature on absorption of iron which supports the conclusion that ferrous is more readily absorbed than ferric iron. He attempts, from his experimental data, to explain the exact role of ferritin in the regulation of absorption and excretion of iron. It is his opinion that the amount of iron in the ferrous state that is absorbed by the mucosal cell is regulated by a factor called the mucosal block, which in turn is related to the relative or absolute amount of ferrous iron contained in the cell and indirectly to the amount of ferritin contained therein. He further reports that the quantity of ferric iron being released from the cell to the blood stream is dependent on the relative "redox" level of that cell and observed this to be a function of the reduced oxygen tension in the blood stream. The fraction of the blood plasma protein transporting the iron is designated as siderophilin. Schade and Caroline [17] have isolated chemically a globulin fraction of plasma, which they believe aids in the transport of iron in the ferric state and is presumably the siderophilin described by Granick.

Human or cow's milk contains small and varying amounts of iron, with mean values reported respectively as 0.07 and 0.18 mg. per 100 ml.,[18] 0.010 and 0.50 mg.

13. Moore, C. V.; Dubach, R.; Minnich, V., and Roberts, H. K.: Absorption of Ferrous and Ferric Radioactive Iron by Human Subjects and by Dogs, J. Clin. Invest. **23**:755, 1944.

14. Footnote 13. McCance, R. A., and Widdowson, E. M.: Absorption and Excretion of Iron Following Oral and Intravenous Administration, J. Physiol. **94**:148, 1938. Hahn, P. F.; Jones, E.; Lowe, R. C.; Meneely, C. R., and Peacock, W.: The Relative Absorption and Utilization of Ferrous and Ferric Iron in Anemia as Determined by Radioactive Isotope, Am. J. Physiol. **143**:191, 1945.

15. Hahn, P. F.; Bale, W. F.; Hettig, R. A.; Kamen, M. D., and Whipple, G. H.: Radioactive Iron and Its Excretion in Urine, Bile, and Feces, J. Exper. Med. **70**:443, 1939. Footnote 4.

16. (a) Granick, S.: Ferritin: Increase of Protein Apoferritin in the Gastrointestinal Mucosa as a Direct Response to Iron Feeding; The Function of Ferritin in the Regulation of Iron Absorption, J. Biol. Chem. **164**:737, 1946; (b) Structure and Physiological Functions of Ferritin, Physiol. Rev. **31**:489, 1951.

17. Schade, A. L., and Caroline, L.: An Iron-Binding Component in Human Blood Plasma, Science **104**:340, 1946.

18. Marriott, quoted by Brennemann, J.: Artificial Feeding of Infants, Brennemann's Practice of Pediatrics, Hagerstown, Md., W. F. Prior Company, Inc., 1948, Vol. 1, Chap. 26.

per 100 ml.[19] and 0.36 and 0.13 mg. per 100 ml.[20] Supplemental foods commonly given during the first year of extrauterine life that contain appreciable amounts of iron are the following: egg yolk, 1 to 2 mg. per yolk as ferrous iron; pureed meats, 1 to 4 mg. per ounce as ferrous iron and fortified cereals, averaging 8.5 mg. as ferrous iron per ounce of dried cereals. Fruits and vegetables which contain appreciable amounts of iron [4] are the following: peaches, prunes, green beans, peas, sweet potatoes, and carrots. The form of iron in these foods is difficult to ascertain.

The average daily requirements of iron for the first year of life, recommended by the Food and Nutrition Board of the National Research Council, is 6 mg. per day.[21] The form of iron advised is not specified.

This study was undertaken to determine both the desirability of using iron prophylactically and the relative effectiveness of ferric and ferrous salts, by observing the hemoglobin response of full-term, immaturely born, and prematurely born infants receiving nutritionally adequate diets of known content, supplemented by small prophylactic doses of ferric or ferrous salts.

MATERIALS AND METHODS

Eighteen full-term infants were observed in the metabolism ward for 6- to 12-month periods, from June, 1949, until June, 1952. Two premature infants were observed in the metabolism ward during this period whose birth weights were 5 lb. 1 oz. (2,300 gm.) and 4 lb. 8 oz. (2,040 gm.). The records of 115 full-term infants who were in the metabolism ward for 6- to 12-month periods during the years 1939 to 1949 were reviewed. The records of a set of twins, whose birth weights were 6 lb. (2,720 gm.) each, and of a set of triplets, whose birth weights were 3 lb. 14 oz. (1,760 gm.), 3 lb. 10 oz. (1,640 gm.), and 3 lb. 11 oz. (1,670 gm.), were reviewed.

Nineteen full-term infants also were observed in the well-baby clinic. Two premature infants also were observed in the well-baby clinic whose birth weights were 3 lb. 15 oz. (1,790 gm.) and 4 lb. 6½ oz. (2,000 gm.).

Ferric ammonium citrate was fed to all infants in the metabolism ward during the first 10 years of the study. The dose given was 5 mg. of iron daily at 3 months of age, increased to 10 mg. of iron daily after 6 months of age. All of the other infants observed in the metabolism ward and outclinic received a concentrated ferrous sulfate preparation [22] fed in exactly the same manner. All iron was given to the infants in their formulas.

The diets of all infants in the metabolism ward were weighed and measured, and aliquot specimens were examined chemically for other metabolic studies. Modified whole-milk feedings were given. During several of the periods, such feedings as protein hydrolysates, soybean formulas, and varying amounts of vitamin D were given these children. The infants observed in the well-baby clinic were from intelligent families of the higher socioeconomic groups. The diet schedule and other supplements given these infants are reported by one of us elsewhere.[23] All infants made satisfactory growth in height and weight, and all progressed normally in their neuromotor development.

19. Jeans, P. C., and Marriott, W. Mc.: Infant Nutrition: A Textbook of Infant Feeding for Students and Practitioners of Medicine, Ed. 4, St. Louis, C. V. Mosby Company, 1947, p. 158.

20. Macy, I. G.; Kelley, H., and Sloan, R.: The Composition of Milks: A Compilation of the Comparative Composition and Properties of Human, Cow, and Goat Milk, Colostrum, and Transitional Milk, Bulletin of the National Research Council, No. 119, 1950, p. 23.

21. Food and Nutrition Board, National Research Council: Recommended Dietary Allowances, Revised 1948, Reprint and Circular Series No. 129, 1948, p. 16.

22. Solution containing 125 mg. ferrous sulfate or 25 mg. of ferrous iron per cubic centimeter labeled Fer-In-Sol, supplied by Mead Johnson & Company.

23. Jackson, R. L.: College of Medicine Symposium on Infant Feeding: Feeding of Healthy Infants, J. Iowa M. Soc. **40**:159, 1950.

Some of the infants observed in the metabolism ward acquired upper respiratory infections of varying degrees of severity and duration. Prior to the availability of antibacterial agents, more severe and prolonged infections occurred. Mild upper respiratory infections also occurred in some of the infants observed in the well-baby clinic.

The hemoglobin values of infants with respiratory infections are tabulated separately. The infections were classed as severe if a complication such as otitis media or pneumonitis developed or a prolonged low-grade infection was recorded. These severe or chronic infections usually began between the 20th and 25th weeks of life. All of these infants were in the group fed ferric ammonium citrate. Infections other than those noted above were slight; no infant had more than three mild infections with or without fever, often consisting only of a slight rhinitis.

TABLE 1.—*Data on Infants Fed Ferric Ammonium Citrate Who Were Observed in the Metabolism Ward with No Infection*

Age, Wk.	No. Determinations	Hemoglobin, Gm./100 Ml. (Mean)	Age, Wk.	No. Determinations	Hemoglobin, Gm./100 Ml. (Mean)
1	2	19.5	27	27	11.6
2	9	17.2	28	24	11.8
3	22	15.6	29	23	11.9
4	20	13.7	30	23	11.6
5	24	13.3	31	24	11.5
6	25	12.3	32	23	11.4
7	27	10.8	33	22	11.4
8	27	11.4	34	21	11.7
9	31	11.0	35	19	11.4
10	32	10.2	36	17	11.5
11	34	10.9	37	14	11.6
12	27	10.9	38	16	11.7
13	31	10.9	39	15	11.7
14	33	11.8	40	15	11.2
15	34	11.3	41	12	11.3
16	35	11.3	42	11	11.5
17	33	11.6	43	11	11.2
18	36	11.4	44	10	11.2
19	36	11.8	45	7	10.8
20	34	11.6	46	6	11.5
21	36	11.9	47	6	11.5
22	34	11.7	48	5	11.1
23	32	11.9	49	5	11.3
24	30	11.8	50	5	11.2
25	28	11.4	51	1	11.3
26	29	11.7	52	1	11.8

All infants in the metabolism ward were subjects of other metabolic studies and because of this were having repeated venipunctures. During the early part of the study, when vitamin D requirement was studied, approximately 10 to 15 ml. of blood was drawn every four to six weeks. After 1949, only 5 to 10 ml. of blood was withdrawn from each infant every four to six weeks. It was calculated that the total amount of serum iron withdrawn from these infants during the period of this study amounted to approximately 15 to 16 mg., which would not result in significant difference in the hemoglobin values of the two groups of infants.

Hemoglobin determinations were made by the Newcomer method,[24] with a visual colorimeter up to 1945, and a Klett-Summerson photoelectric colorimeter after that time. The instruments are standardized with oxyhemoglobin and carbon monoxide hemoglobin. Hemoglobin values were determined, for the most part, at weekly intervals on all infants in the metabolism ward, and at monthly intervals in the outpatient group.

The mean hemoglobin values with number of determinations and age in weeks of all infants are tabulated in Tables 1 to 5, inclusive. The mean hemoglobin values have been plotted and a

---

24. Newcomer, H. S.: Absorption Spectra of Acid Hematin, Oxyhemoglobin, and Carbon Monoxide Hemoglobin: A New Hemoglobinometer, J. Biol. Chem. **37**:465, 1919.

TABLE 2.—*Data on Infants Fed Ferric Ammonium Citrate Who Were Observed in the Metabolism Ward with Mild Infections*

Age, Wk.	No. Determinations	Hemoglobin, Gm./100 Ml. (Mean)	Age, Wk.	No. Determinations	Hemoglobin, Gm./100 Ml. (Mean)
1	2	19.5	26	31	11.7
2	11	17.3	27	30	11.5
3	23	16.2	28	31	11.7
4	23	14.5	29	29	11.8
5	24	13.5	30	30	11.6
6	27	12.4	31	25	11.9
7	24	11.2	32	23	11.9
8	24	11.5	33	25	11.5
9	28	11.0	34	24	11.8
10	30	11.0	35	21	11.9
11	28	10.9	36	17	11.7
12	34	11.1	37	17	11.2
13	33	11.3	38	16	11.8
14	36	11.1	39	13	12.2
15	40	11.3	40	13	12.3
16	38	11.3	41	12	12.5
17	35	11.3	42	11	11.8
18	37	11.4	43	10	11.7
19	32	11.4	44	9	11.8
20	36	11.4	45	8	11.6
21	38	11.9	46	7	12.0
22	35	11.5	47	7	11.2
23	34	11.4	48	4	11.7
24	33	11.5	49	3	12.4
25	36	11.8	50	3	12.3
			51	2	11.6

TABLE 3.—*Data on Infants Fed Ferric Ammonium Citrate Who Were Observed in the Metabolism Ward with Severe Infections*

Age, Wk.	No. Determinations	Hemoglobin, Gm./100 Ml. (Mean)	Age, Wk.	No. Determinations	Hemoglobin, Gm./100 Ml. (Mean)
1	..	....	25	13	11.5
2	3	17.5	26	15	11.3
3	7	17.4	27	14	11.3
4	9	15.4	28	14	11.9
5	12	13.0	29	17	11.7
6	12	11.6	30	11	11.3
7	12	11.1	31	12	11.5
8	12	10.8	32	11	11.9
9	12	10.9	33	9	11.3
10	14	10.7	34	9	11.0
11	14	10.3	35	9	10.8
12	13	10.8	36	8	10.9
13	14	11.5	37	9	10.5
14	13	11.3	38	9	10.6
15	12	10.8	39	8	10.7
16	12	11.2	40	7	11.3
17	12	11.0	41	7	11.2
18	12	11.0	42	7	10.8
19	12	11.6	43	7	11.3
20	13	11.4	44	7	10.8
21	14	12.1	45	6	11.0
22	13	11.6	46	3	10.8
23	13	11.7	47	2	11.6
24	14	11.3	48	3	11.2

smoothed mean curve drawn to demonstrate the values obtained (Charts 1 and 2). The two groups of published data [25] to which our data are compared are so labeled where they appear. A scatter pattern of the values obtained for the metabolism-ward infants who received ferrous salts is shown in-Chart 3.

TABLE 4.—*Data on Infants Fed Ferrous Sulfate Who Were Observed in the Metabolism Ward*

Age, Wk.	No. Determinations	Hemoglobin, Gm./100 Ml. (Mean)	Age, Wk.	No. Determinations	Hemoglobin, Gm./100 Ml. (Mean)
1	7	16.2	28	6	12.5
2	7	15.4	29	5	12.7
3	7	13.4	30	5	12.5
4	7	12.6	31	6	12.5
5	8	11.2	32	5	13.1
6	6	11.7	33	5	13.2
7	8	11.1	34	4	12.1
8	8	10.2	35	4	13.5
9	10	11.2	36	5	13.2
10	8	10.6	37	5	13.2
11	9	11.0	38	7	13.0
12	8	11.4	39	4	13.0
13	7	11.4	40	3	13.2
14	9	11.4	41	3	12.6
15	7	11.6	42	3	12.5
16	7	11.7	43	4	12.8
17	9	11.2	44	3	12.7
18	9	12.2	45	4	11.8
19	5	12.0	46	4	13.0
20	5	12.2	47	3	12.7
21	11	12.7	48	2	12.4
22	6	12.3	49	2	12.8
23	8	12.6	50	1	11.2
24	8	12.6	51	3	12.4
25	9	12.5	52	1	12.6
26	8	12.1	53	1	11.2
27	7	13.0	54	1	12.4

TABLE 5.—*Data on Infants Fed Ferrous Sulfate Who Were Observed in the Well-Baby Clinic*

Age, Mo.	No. Determinations	Hemoglobin, Gm. 100 Ml. (Mean)
2	9	12.0
3	3	10.3
4	15	11.6
5	7	12.1
6	7	12.0
7	3	11.9
8	3	11.9

Representative standard deviations have been calculated on our data at 29 weeks and 38 weeks for all the infants in the metabolism ward in order to make comparisons between our data and those reported by other investigators. The group of infants seen in the well-baby clinic was small, and the number of values did not lend itself to statistical analysis.

In late infancy, the number of hemoglobin values for each week was too small to give reliable means for certain of the groups studied. As mean hemoglobin values for adjacent weeks were nearly identical, the data for two to three weeks have been combined (Table 6).

25. Footnotes 1 and 16*b*.

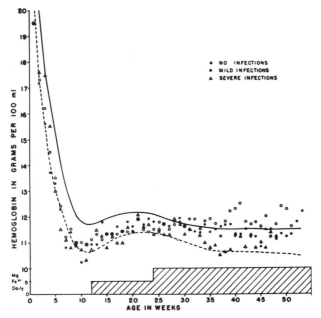

Chart 1.—Mean hemoglobin determinations of all infants receiving ferric ammonium citrate in the dosage shown. The solid line represents the mean values reported by Elvehjem and the broken line the mean values reported by Kato. Comparison is made between patients with and without infection and the severity of infection.

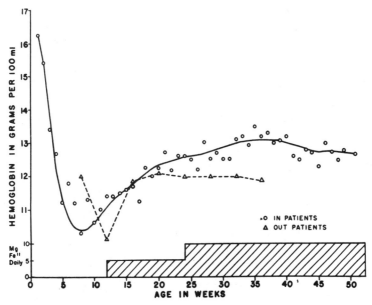

Chart 2.—Mean hemoglobin values of all infants fed ferrous sulfate in the dosage shown. Refer to Chart 1 for mean values reported by others.

217

The formulas used for determining standard deviation, standard error of the mean, and "significant ratio t" are those in common usage.[26]

RESULTS

A total of 2,804 hemoglobin determinations were made on the blood of 115 infants who were fed ferric ammonium citrate from the 12th to the 52d weeks of life or longer. This group was subdivided into 54 infants with 1,105 hemoglobin determinations who had no infections, 45 infants with 1,213 hemoglobin determina-

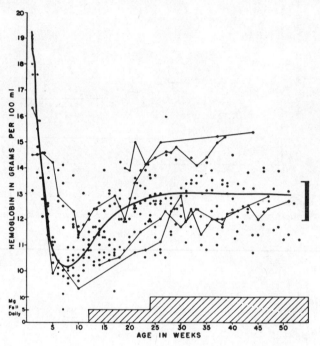

Chart 3.—A scatter pattern of the 305 hemoglobin values for patients receiving ferrous sulfate in the dosage shown. The heavy line represents the mean hemoglobin value of the group and the light lines are values for individual infants. Vertical bar at the right shows the range of values reported by Elvehjem after 26 to 30 weeks of age.

TABLE 6.—*Means, Standard Deviations, and Standard Errors of Means for Groups of Infants as Designated in Tabulation*

Wk.	Group	Classification	Mean	S. D.	S. E. of Mean	No. Determinations
			Hemoglobin, Gm./100 Ml.			
28-29-30	FeSO₄	No severe infection	12.7	1.06	0.26	16
37-38-39	FeSO₄	No severe infection	13.1	1.24	0.31	16
29	F. A. C.*	No severe infection	11.8	1.37	0.19	52
38	F. A. C.	No severe infection	11.7	1.15	0.20	32
29	F. A. C.	Severe infection	11.7	1.34	0.39	12
37-38	F. A. C.	Severe infection	10.5	1.32	0.31	18

* Ferric ammonium citrate.

26. Hill, A. B.: Principles of Medical Statistics, Ed. 4, London, The Lancet, Ltd., 1948.

tions who had mild infections, and 16 infants with 486 hemoglobin determinations who had severe infections (see above for classification of types of infections). A total of 304 hemoglobin determinations were made on the blood of 18 infants who were fed ferrous sulfate and were observed in the metabolism ward for a similar number of weeks. None of the infants in this group had severe infections. In addition, 53 hemoglobin determinations were made on the 19 infants fed ferrous sulfate who were observed in the well-baby clinic. The hemoglobin values of four infants born prematurely, two followed in the metabolism ward, and two observed in the well-baby clinic, are reported separately. The immature infants in our series consisted of a set of twins and a set of triplets, all of whom were observed in the metabolism ward. Their hemoglobin values are graphed separately. The premature infants were fed ferrous sulfate and the immature infants were fed ferric ammonium citrate.

Chart 1 demonstrates that no difference, graphically or statistically, exists between the hemoglobin value of the two groups of infants fed ferric ammonium citrate, in one of which there were no infections and in the other, mild infections. Therefore, these two groups are combined in the remainder of the discussion. Furthermore, since there were no severe infections in the ferrous sulfate group, all of the values for this group are dealt with in a similar manner.

At 29 weeks of age the mean hemoglobin value of the group of infants given the ferric salts who had no infection was identical to that of those who had severe infection, 11.8 and 11.7 gm. per 100 ml. (Chart 1), respectively. The mean hemoglobin value was significantly higher, 12.7 per 100 ml. (Chart 2) in the group of infants fed ferrous iron. At 38 weeks of age the mean hemoglobin values of the infants given ferrous and ferric iron who had no severe infection were 13.1 (Chart 2) and 11.8 gm. per 100 ml. (Chart 1) respectively, and the difference at both age periods was significant at the 1 per cent level of confidence. These values tend to support the experimental data of Darby and Hahn,[12a] Hahn and Carothers,[12b] and Moore [27] that ferrous iron is utilized more efficiently than ferric iron.

It is well recognized that infection tends to lower the hemoglobin value of infants [6a] and, indeed, at times is the only clinical factor that can be found as the cause of an iron-deficiency anemia. By 30 weeks of age the mean hemoglobin value of the infants with severe infections given ferric iron had decreased to 10.6 gm. per 100 ml. The most severe infections occurred at this period. In the latter weeks of the study the mean hemoglobin value of this group of infants approached 11.5 gm. per 100 ml.

The scatter graph (Chart 3) is informative in that the spread of hemoglobin values of the infants fed ferrous iron is shown. The range of values is indicative of the variation in hemoglobin levels among the group of infants, rather than degree of fluctuation in one infant, as is shown by the light lines indicating values for each of four infants. There is no adequate explanation why hemoglobin values of infants fed similar amounts of iron, living in a controlled environment and receiving carefully constructed diets, might level off at 11.5 gm. or at 13 gm. per 100 ml. after the fourth month of life unless it could be differences in storage of iron during

27. Footnotes 6b and 13.

pregnancy, which is dependent on the maternal diet and the maturity of the infant. A definite trend toward increasing hemoglobin values occurred from the fourth to the sixth month of life, whether the highest level at four months was 11.5 or 13.0 gm. After 6 months of age, very little change was noted in the hemoglobin values obtained from a given infant.

The hemoglobin values of four infants born somewhat prematurely are shown in Chart 4. The smallest infant had a birth weight of 4 lb. 6 oz. (1,980 gm.), so that these infants did not differ markedly from full-term infants. None required transfusions, and with the small amounts of supplemental ferrous iron given, each

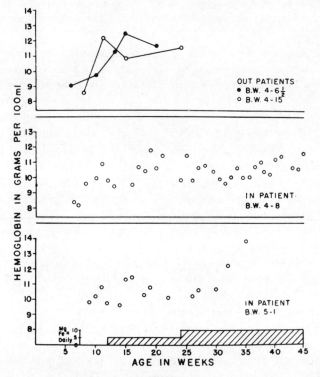

Chart 4.—Hemoglobin values of the four premature infants studied. All received ferrous sulfate in the dosage shown. There is a progressive rise in hemoglobin values. No small premature infants were studied. *B. W.* indicates birth weight in pounds and ounces.

was able to maintain hemoglobin values greater than 10 gm. per 100 ml. There is no agreement as to how soon premature infants are able to utilize supplemental iron in their diets, but evidence is accumulating to the effect that prematurely born infants are able to utilize iron when given in the form of pureed meats as early as the sixth week of extrauterine life.[28]

28. Levine, S. Z.: Protein and Amino Acid Nutrition in Pediatrics and in Pregnancy, in Proteins and Amino Acids in Nutrition, edited by M. Sahyun, New York, Reinhold Publishing Corporation, 1948, Chap. 10. Sisson, T. R. C.; Emmel, A. F., and Filer, L. J., Jr.: Meat in the Diets of Premature Infants, Pediatrics **7**:89, 1951.

All three of the triplets studied (Chart 5) required small whole-blood transfusions at 20 to 25 weeks of age, after which 10 mg. of ferric iron daily sufficed to maintain hemoglobin values above the 10 gm. level. The whole-blood transfusion given the girl twin at 18 weeks of age caused an immediate rise of hemoglobin to 16.2 gm. per 100 ml. The hemoglobin values then decreased in a manner parallel to that of the first eight weeks of postnatal life, thus increasing the amount of stored iron. In retrospect, it might have been the procedure of choice to have given transfusions to the boy twin also. However, he was making a satisfactory weight gain and was suffering apparently no ill effects from the low hemoglobin levels found, and he showed a progressive rise of hemoglobin value in the latter weeks of the study.

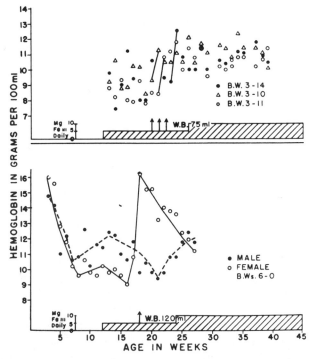

Chart 5.—Hemoglobin values of a set of triplets and a set of twins. Whole blood transfusions were given as shown by the arrows. They all received ferric ammonium citrate supplements to their diets. Note the rapid fall of hemoglobin in the female twin after transfusion and the similarity of slope to the curve plotted at the time of physiological hemolysis of red blood cells shortly after birth.

COMMENT

The published data with which we compare our results are those of Elvehjem [1] of Wisconsin, and Kato [29] of Chicago.

Elvehjem and his group had obtained approximately 2,000 hemoglobin values on 750 children from birth to 5 years of age. The diets of these children were supervised. These infants were seen in the child health centers of Madison, Wis.

29. Kato, K., and Emery, O. J.: Hemoglobin Content of Blood in Infancy: Study of 780 Cases from Birth to 2 Years, with 1,065 Determinations, Folia haemat. **49**:106, 1933.

The mean hemoglobin value for infants at 52 weeks was 11.5 gm. per 100 ml. At the end of the study, 18 children were fed iron supplements consisting of egg yolk at 3 months of age and fortified cereals at 4 months of age. In this group of infants an increase of hemoglobin from an average of 11.5 to an average of 12.4 gm. per 100 ml. was noted. The authors subsequently added 25 mg. of iron as ferric pyrophosphate and 1 mg. of copper as copper sulfate to the diets of a third group of infants of comparable ages and found an elevation of hemoglobin content of the blood from 12.0 to 13.5 gm. per 100 ml. at 52 weeks of age.[1b] The former curve is used in comparison with our data (Chart 1) because weekly results were not listed in the latter article. The range of hemoglobin values reported for the infants given iron and copper will be compared grossly to our ferrous sulfate group (Chart 3).

Kato and Emery [29] studied 180 infants in the age period of birth to 2 years and obtained 1,065 hemoglobin determinations. These infants were not given additional iron, and the diets were not described. The patients were from the lower socioeconomic group of Chicago and were seen in the child-welfare clinics of the University of Chicago or in the newborn service of Cook County Hospitals (Chart 1).

Our standard deviations of the hemoglobin values at 29 and 38 weeks, presented in Table 6, compare favorably with those reported by the above investigators, namely, 1.4 gm. per 100 ml. (Kato at 7 to 8 months and 9 to 12 months); 1.24 (Elvehjem at 24 to 28 weeks), and 1.51 (at 52 to 56 weeks).

No statistical difference exists between the mean hemoglobin values of the group of well infants fed ferric ammonium citrate when compared to those of Elvehjem's series at either 29 or 38 weeks. There is, however, a statistical difference between Kato's values and those of the infants reported herein at these two age periods. This difference is significant at the 1% level of confidence.

Elvehjem's later publication discussed the addition of both 12.5 mg. of iron and 0.5 mg. of copper and also 25 mg. of iron and 1 mg. of copper daily in the form of ferric pyrophosphate and copper sulfate, beginning at 3 weeks of postnatal life. Fifty-five patients were the subjects of this report and were studied in the Dungreen school clinic. He observed a consistent increase of hemoglobin from the previously reported 9 to 11 gm., to 12 to 13.5 gm. per 100 ml. of whole blood with the larger doses given. With the smaller dosage not as consistent or uniform an increase occurred. No tables of data were published in this paper, so a statistical analysis cannot be made. However, it can be seen that with only 10 mg. of iron as ferrous sulfate without added copper we obtained exactly the same hemoglobin values. These results indicate that if copper is needed in addition to that supplied by the diet, the amount required is minute and is provided by the copper-contaminating U. S. P. iron salts. Evidence exists [30] that the absorption of iron is decreased in the presence of excessive phosphate. The choice by Elvehjem's group of a ferric instead of a ferrous salt, and a salt containing phosphate ion may have contributed to the poorer utilization of iron by their subjects. Also much has been written

30. Hegsted, D. M.; Finch, C. A., and Kinney, T. D.: The Influence of Diet on Iron Absorption: The Interrelation of Iron and Phosphorus, J. Exper. Med. **90**:147, 1949. Darby, W. J.: Iron and Copper, Council on Foods and Nutrition, J. A. M. A. **142**:1288, 1950.

lately,[31] in regard to the major role of protein in the manufacture of red blood cells and hemoglobin synthesis. The protein content of the diets fed in Elvehjem's study is not reported. All the infants reported in the present study were artificially fed, and it is the practice in this clinic to offer a high-protein intake of 3 to 4 gm. per kilogram.[2a] The high-protein feeding might well be an important factor to explain the satisfactory results obtained with smaller amounts of iron.

Hemoglobin values of infants have shown the customary initial fall from high values (18 to 22 gm. per 100 ml.) to a minimum value at 10 to 12 weeks of age (10.5 to 11.5 gm. per 100 ml.). During the next 10 weeks the usual progressive secondary rise of hemoglobin values is observed. However, after about the 20th week of life a slow secondary fall of hemoglobin occurs, and the values continue to fall slowly throughout the remainder of infancy unless iron-containing foods or medicinal iron is given. If one had only the data of these representative curves of hemoglobin values it would seem likely that the secondary rise indicates utilization of stored iron, and that the secondary fall indicates the need for additional dietary iron, in the form of either iron-containing foods or supplementary elemental iron. The full-term infants in this study receiving small amounts (5 to 10 mg.) of ferric or ferrous iron did not demonstrate the secondary fall of hemoglobin values. The infants with more severe infections showed a progressive slow rise of hemoglobin values during late infancy.

It is often stated [32] that iron is not absorbed when given in milk and with meals high in phytates or phosphates. The small amount of ferrous or ferric iron used in the study was added to the milk, and satisfactory hemoglobin responses were obtained. The iron did not cause changes in the milk and there were no symptoms of gastrointestinal tract intolerance to the preparation used. One major exception should be pointed out, however. At one time the ferric ammonium citrate preparation used in this study was found to be contaminated by mildly pathogenic organisms and was thought to be responsible for a mild epidemic of diarrhea in the metabolism ward. More concentrated ferrous iron solutions have been prepared, such as the one used in this study,[22] which do not support bacterial growth.

CONCLUSIONS AND SUMMARY

One hundred fifteen full-term infants were given ferric iron as ferric ammonium citrate, and 37 full-term infants were given ferrous iron as ferrous sulfate. Seven immature or prematurely born infants were studied. No instance of gastrointestinal irritation due to the iron was observed.

Ferrous iron in the same dosage permitted significantly higher hemoglobin values in well infants than did ferric iron.

The small amounts of iron given daily were sufficient to maintain hemoglobin values at a constant level throughout the latter half of infancy in all full-term

31. Lynch, H. D., and Snively, W. D., Jr.: Hypoproteinosis of Childhood. J. A. M. A. **147**:115, 1951. Stare, F. J., and Thorn, G. W.: Protein Nutrition in Problems of Medical Interest, ibid. **127**:1120, 1945. Jacobs, H. M., and George, G. S.: Evaluation of Meat in the Infant Diet, Pediatrics **10**:463, 1952.

32. McCance, R. A.; Edgecombe, C. N., and Widdowson, E. M.: Phytic Acid and Iron Absorption, Lancet **2**:126, 1943. Footnote 30.

infants. Even in those infants who had severe infections, marked anemia did not develop, but hemoglobin values were maintained above 10 mg. per 100 ml.

Prematurely born infants and infants of multiple birth may need more assistance in the prevention of anemia than is provided by these small daily quantities of iron. A small transfusion at 15 to 20 weeks of age was efficacious in bringing the hemoglobin value to near normal, after which 10 mg. of iron daily maintained hemoglobin at normal levels.

This study corroborated the findings of others that severe infectious illness in infancy is accompanied by significant decrease in the hemoglobin level. Mild infections, on the other hand, caused no significant decrease in the hemoglobin level.

The amount of iron storage at birth depends on the adequacy of the mother's diet, the length of gestation, and the watchfulness of the obstetrician that the umbilical cord not be clamped until all pulsations cease, so that the baby receives the maximum amount of blood possible. The infant born at term of a healthy well-fed mother will maintain a good hemoglobin level at least up to 6 months of age. If he receives some iron-containing foods daily after the fourth month of life, probably no other iron supplements are necessary. An infant receiving only the iron of milk generally shows a slow decrease in hemoglobin level during the latter half of infancy and, if his original iron store is poor, an iron-deficiency anemia will occur in late infancy. However, in view of the many variables involved in determining the iron available to the infant and the difficulty in evaluating each variable it seemed wise to study the effect of a daily dosage of iron maintained at a level sufficiently low to be given in the formula. Five milligrams of iron was given daily to infants 3 to 6 months of age and 10 mg. daily to the older infants, which prevented the development of hypochromic anemia.

RESPIRATORY METABOLISM IN INFANCY AND IN CHILDHOOD

XXI. DAILY WATER EXCHANGE OF NORMAL INFANTS

S. Z. LEVINE, M.D.

M. A. WHEATLEY, M.D.

T. H. McEACHERN, M.D.

H. H. GORDON, M.D.
AND
E. MARPLES, B.A.

NEW YORK

The importance of water in the preservation of health and in the treatment of disease in infancy and in childhood has been recognized for many years. The infantile organism is especially hydrolabile, probably because of its high content of body water; this content comprises over 70 per cent in the newly born infant, as against less than 60 per cent in the adult. This hydrolabile tendency is exemplified by the wide fluctuations in daily body weight of healthy infants while on constant diets, by the ready development of dehydration fever in newly born and in older infants temporarily deprived of water and by the occurrence of anhydremia as a frequent accompaniment of infantile diarrhea.

Despite the importance of water to infants, knowledge of their fluid requirements has in large measure been deduced from measurements of the average amounts of milk voluntarily withdrawn from the breast by nursing infants. These observations were later supplemented by studies of water balance, which for the most part were incomplete, since all sources of incoming and outgoing water were not directly determined. The validity of the assumption that the value for fluid intake obtained in these incomplete studies represents the optimal fluid intake for all normal infants can be assessed more accurately through continuous and complete studies of the water exchange throughout the twenty-four hours under varying conditions of diet and environment.

This paper presents the results of 28 such measurements of the water exchange of 16 healthy infants. Seven observations on 3 of the infants were made in conjunction with previously reported twenty-

The early observations were made in collaboration with Dr. J. R. Wilson and Dr. T. C. Wyatt.

From the New York Hospital and the Department of Pediatrics, Cornell University Medical College.

four hour measurements of their energy and organic (protein, fat and carbohydrate) exchanges.[1]

APPARATUS AND METHODS

A detailed description of the methods employed for analysis of the diet and excreta (urine and feces), for measurement of the twenty-four hour insensible loss from skin and lungs, for determination of the daily respiratory exchange and for calculation of the composition of the metabolic mixture was given in previous papers.[2]

In a study of the exchange of water between the body and the environment, all sources of incoming and outgoing water must be known.[3] The incoming water comprises (1) the water ingested as such, (2) the preformed water of the so-called solid foods and (3) the water of combustion derived from the oxidation of organic foodstuffs within the body.[4] A fourth item, tissue water, sometimes included in the available sources, is the fraction held in physical combination with body protein, fat and glycogen. Since this moiety is already present in the body as water, shifts in it will be reflected solely in alterations of extracellular and intracellular fluid and will not affect the net water exchange between the body and the environment.

Outgoing water comprises the quotas eliminated through (1) urine, (2) feces and (3) skin and lungs.[5] The difference between incoming

1. Levine, S. Z.; McEachern, T. H.; Wheatley, M. A.; Marples, E., and Kelly, M. D.: Respiratory Metabolism in Infancy and in Childhood: XV. Daily Energy Requirements of Normal Infants, Am. J. Dis. Child. **50**:596 (Sept.) 1935.

2. Levine, S. Z., and Wheatley, M. A.: Respiratory Metabolism in Infancy and in Childhood: XVII. Daily Heat Production of Infants; Predictions Based on the Insensible Loss of Weight Compared with Direct Measurements, Am. J. Dis. Child. **51**:1300 (June) 1936. Levine and others.[1]

3. Newburgh, L. H.; Johnston, M. W., and Falcon-Lesses, M.: Measurement of Total Water Exchange, J. Clin. Investigation **8**:161 (Feb.) 1930. Wiley, F. H., and Newburgh, L. H.: Improved Method for the Determination of Water Balance, ibid. **10**:723 (Oct.) 1931.

4. The constants of Newburgh [3] were used to calculate the water of oxidation. One gram of protein, of fat and of carbohydrate when oxidized in the body releases as end products 0.41, 1.07 and 0.60 Gm. of water, respectively. The composition of the metabolic mixture of 3 infants (H. S., J. F. and J. C.) was determined directly in the respiration chamber on the final day of each of 7 observations (17 through 23). In the remaining observations, the daily metabolic mixture was calculated from the energy exchange measured for periods of from two to four hours, the dietary carbohydrate, the urinary nitrogen and the daily behavior records of the infants.[1]

5. The water loss through skin and lungs was determined from the total insensible perspiration by deducting the difference between exhaled carbon dioxide and inhaled oxygen. $CO_2 - O_2$ was considered to equal $0.41\ C + 0.08\ P - 0.08\ F$, when C, P and F represent the grams of carbohydrate, protein and fat, respectively, in the metabolic mixture.[3]

and outgoing water provides a direct measure of the water balance during the period of observation (table 1).

The technic of measurements was essentially as follows:

At the start of the observation and at the same time on succeeding days until the end of the period, the infant, the daily intake and the daily output in urine and feces were weighed on a specially constructed balance with a capacity of 10 Kg. and an accuracy of 50 milligrams.[6] Between daily weighings, the infants reclined on a metabolism bed, which, with competent nursing, insured quantitative collections of urine and feces over prolonged periods. The bed and the collecting apparatus, both of which were designed by Dr. Hoag, were fully described by him in a previous communication.[7] The difference between the initial weight of the baby plus the weight of the intake on the one hand and the final body weight plus the weight of the urine and feces on the other afforded an accurate measure of the daily loss through skin and lungs, provided other losses, such as loss through vomiting, did not occur during the period.

TABLE 1.—*Items in a Water Balance Sheet*

Direct Measurement (Modified after Newburgh[5])

Sources of available water	Outgoing water
1. Intake as such	1. In urine
2. In solid foods	2. In feces
3. Of oxidation:	3. In insensible perspiration:
Protein $\times$ 0.41	Insensible perspiration $-$ ($CO_2 - O_2$)
Fat $\times$ 1.07	($CO_2 - O_2$) = (P $\times$ 0.08) $-$ (F $\times$ 0.08) $+$
Carbohydrate $\times$ 0.60	(C $\times$ 0.41)

Indirect Measurement

Total change in body weight minus change in weight due to:
1. Protein intake $-$ (feces $+$ metabolized)
2. Fat intake $-$ (feces $+$ metabolized)   } = water balance
3. Carbohydrate intake $-$ (metabolized)

This method of weighing afforded quantitative data on the total intake, on the total outgo and on changes in body weight during the observation. The individual increments of outgo through urine, feces and skin and lungs were also available, and a complete weight balance of the infant could be tabulated. By analysis of the intake and the excreta (urine and feces) for their water content and by determination of the composition of the metabolic mixture either through direct measurement of the respiratory exchange or through calculation,[8] a water balance was concurrently obtained.[9]

---

6. Levine, S. Z.; Wilson, J. R., and Kelly, M. D.: Insensible Perspiration in Infancy and in Childhood: I. Its Constancy in Infants Under Standard Conditions and the Effect of Various Physiologic Factors, Am. J. Dis. Child. **37**:791 (April) 1929.

7. Hoag, L. A.: Apparatus for the Quantitative Collection of Urine and of Stools in Male Infants, Am. J. Dis. Child. **44**:770 (Oct.) 1932.

8. Footnotes 4 and 5.

9. The following methods were employed in triplicate for analysis of the diet and, when indicated, of the urine and feces: the macro-Kjeldahl method for

(Footnote continued on next page)

Concurrent measurements of the total change in body weight with the balance and of the water balance, obtained by chemical analysis of the diet and the excreta (urine and feces) in conjunction with measurements of the twenty-four hour energy metabolism in the respiration chamber on the final days of 7 observations (17 through 23), afforded a means of checking the reliability of the direct method of measurement of the daily water exchange (table 1). The comparative results are shown in table 2.

The similarity of the average figures for the twenty-four hour change in body weight secured in toto with the balance (64 Gm.) and by algebraic summation (50 Gm.) of the individual components (protein, fat, carbohydrate and water) attests to the reliability of the water balances reported in this paper.[10] When one recalls the magnitude of

TABLE 2.—*Comparison of the Organic Balance plus the Water Balance with the Actual Change in Body Weight (in Grams per Twenty-Four Hours)*

			Balance*					Actual Change in Weight[‡] (6)	Differ-ence (6 — 5) (7)
Subject	Obser-vation No.	Date	Organic			Water (4)	Total[†] (1+2+3+4) (5)		
			P (1)	F (2)	C (3)				
H. S.	17a	11/16/31	5.8	17.0	—0.9	82	104	117	13
J. F.	18a	1/ 8/32	4.6	14.5	—4.5	40	55	80	25
J. C.	19a	2/19/32	5.4	17.4	—2.1	14	35	46	11
J. C.	20a	2/26/32	—1.9	—9.1	0.2	—3	—14	—5	9
J. C.	21a	3/ 4/32	4.3	25.9	—1.1	39	68	83	15
J. C.	22a	4/15/32	4.6	9.0	1.4	2	17	25	8
J. C.	23a	4/21/32	0.3	10.2	—1.7	79	88	103	15
Average							50	64	14

* Balance is positive except where indicated.
† Balances of organic materials and of water were determined by measurement of the respiratory exchange for from twenty and one-half to twenty-three hours and chemical analysis of urine, feces and diet.[1]
‡ Actual change in body weight was determined by weighing the infant just before and after observation in the respiration chamber.

the items involved in the balances (approximating 1,000 Gm. each in the intake and output for these observations) and the diverse technics employed in obtaining the two series of measurements, one is impressed

nitrogen; the Roese-Gottlieb method (Association of Official Agricultural Chemists: Official and Tentative Methods of Analysis Compiled by the Committee on Editing Methods of Analysis, Washington, D. C., Association of Official Agricultural Chemists, 1930, p. 217) for fat; the official gravimetric method of the Association of Agricultural Chemists (id., p. 216) for lactose, and prolonged drying to constant weight for water. The dietary calories were determined by multiplying the grams of protein (N × 6.25), fat and carbohydrate, as analyzed, by the customary constants, 4.1, 9.3 and 4.1, respectively.

10. Balance studies of a number of inorganic substances (sodium, potassium, chlorine, calcium and phosphorus) were made concurrently on a number of infants, but the amounts of these substances are so trivial on the basis of weight that they may for practical purposes be disregarded in estimating the materials involved in total changes of body weight.

by the narrow range of deviations shown in the table. Differences between actual and calculated values for change in body weight ranged between 8 and 25 Gm. daily in individual observations and averaged 14 Gm. for the entire series. Unless one assumes that the various sources of error fortuitously arranged themselves to compensate for each other, the results may be accepted as a check on the accuracy of the chemical and metabolic operations and the methods of calculation.

EXPERIMENTAL PROCEDURE

Studies of the water exchange of 16 male infants ranging in age from 3 to 11½ months were made in 28 observations of from one to seven days' duration for a total of eighty-five days. The age and nutritional status of the infants are shown in table 3. They were all in good health during the periods of study.

Observations were begun after foreperiods of constant diet of at least two and usually more days. The diets consisted of mixtures of cow's milk, cane sugar or dextrimaltose and water; thoroughly mixed, pooled samples of dried milk preparations were almost invariably used. The composition of the diets is shown in table 3.

Fourteen infants resided in a metabolism ward, described in previous papers.[11] The environmental conditions were maintained as constant as possible without the aid of an air-conditioned room, and the water balances of the infants while on adequate diets and under varying conditions of diet (both fluid and caloric intake) were studied. The effect of environmental temperature and humidity on water exchange was determined in 2 infants (I. R. and F. L.), who were studied in an air-conditioned room which permitted rigid control of external conditions. In the series of observations on the effect of diet and environmental conditions on water balance, the same infant was used throughout successive periods and all variables except the one under investigation were maintained constant.

RESULTS

Detailed data of the observations are presented in table 4.

The Water Exchange of Healthy Infants on Adequate Diets.—In order to establish the magnitude and range of the water balances of normal infants receiving formulas customarily employed in infant feeding, 14 healthy infants were studied in 17 observations of from two

11. Levine, S. Z., and Wilson, J. R.: Respiratory Metabolism in Infancy and in Childhood: I. Basal Metabolism of Children, Am. J. Dis. Child. **31**:323 (March) 1926. Wilson, J. R.; Levine, S. Z., and Rivkin, H.: Respiratory Metabolism in Infancy and in Childhood: II. Ketosis and the Respiratory Exchange in Children, ibid. **31**:335 (March) 1926.

TABLE 3.—*Nutritional Status, Daily Diet and Rectal Temperature of Subjects*

Subject	Date	Observation No.	Period, Days	Nutritional Status — Age, Mo.	Weight, Kg.	Height, Cm.	Daily Diet — Calories	Protein, Gm.	Fat, Gm.	Carbohydrate, Gm.	Fluid,* Gm.	Average Rectal Temperature, F.	Environmental Conditions — Average Temperature, C.	Average Humidity, Percentage
W. B.	2/ 6/28	1	5	8½	6,748	70.5	844	27	33	104	956	99.0	25	30
	2/11/28	2	6	8½	6,895	71.0	844	27	33	104	1,316	98.5	24	35
J. N.	2/23/28	3	7	11½	6,281	…	861	40	48	61	1,215	98.5	25	22
K. F.	4/25/28	4	3	5½	6,119	…	834	34	39	81	976	98.4	24	25
E. B.	5/18/28	5	4	10	7,725	…	825	35	42	71	1,018	99.0	25	50
J. H.	12/14/28	6	3	7	6,520	…	861	40	48	61	1,029	98.8	25	39
W. A.	11/18/29	7	2	5½	7,545	70.0	810	30	35	88	1,042	98.5	25	41
K. B.	12/15/29	8	2	8½	7,742	…	810	30	35	73	1,079	99.0	25	40
K. M.	1/ 2/30	9	2	8	7,256	71.0	700	30	30	73	962	98.7	25	
J. S.	1/ 8/30	10	2	8	7,475	…	700	30	30	73	994	98.0	26	
W. D.	3/24/30	11	2	9	5,223	69.0	376	26	18	25	1,037	98.9		
	3/26/30	12	2	9	5,173	69.0	311	22	14	22	1,597	98.4		28
W. L.	5/ 5/30	13	3	5	4,427	64.0	275	18	16	13	1,381	98.0		
	5/ 6/30	14	1	5	4,453	64.0	272	18	16	13	1,683	98.1	29	
	5/ 7/30	15	1	5	4,508	64.0	397	26	23	19	1,701	98.0		
	5/ 8/30	16	1	5	4,533	64.0	414	27	24	20	2,035	97.8		
H. S.	10/12/31	17	4	6½	6,978	67.0	907	34	40	72	1,173	99.8	26	40
J. F.	1/ 5/32	18	3	9	7,166	71.0	863	37	42	78	1,132	99.9	24	43
J. C.	2/16/32	19	3	4½	6,283	65.0	682	30	34	59	1,093	99.7	24	28
	2/23/32	20	3	4½	6,100	65.0	341	15	17	30	1,032	98.8	24	25
	3/ 1/32	21	3	5	6,602	65.0	863	37	42	78	1,027	98.3	23	35
	4/12/32	22	3	6½	7,320	68.0	678	30	34	58	1,081	98.9	24	30
	4/19/32	23	2	6½	7,243	68.0	678	30	34	58		98.6	24	35
I. R.	4/22/32	24	1	6½	7,407	68.0	503	22	25	44	619	101.3	24	35
	2/13/33	25	5	3	3,741	58.5	562	22	23	63	1,275	99.6	22	60
F. L.	2/20/33	26	5	3	4,048	58.5	555	22	23	61	845	98.7	22	60
	10/ 4/33	27	3	7	6,394	61.5	792	31	34	85	896	98.6	29	40
	10/ 9/33	28	5	7	6,656	62.5	792	31	34	85	1,041	98.8	22	80

* The figures recorded in this column represent the total weights of the intake.

TABLE 4.—*Detailed Data on Water Exchange in Terms of Twenty-Four Hours*

Subject	Observation No.	Metabolic Mixture* Calories	Protein, Gm.	Fat, Gm.	Carbohydrate, Gm.	Available Water Intake, Gm.	Oxidation,† Gm.	Total, Gm.	Outgoing Water Total, Gm.	Urine, Gm.	Feces, Gm.	Skin and Lungs,‡ Gm.	Total Insensible Loss, Gm.	Water Balance, Gm.	Change in Body Weight, Gm.
W. B.	1	566	25	4	104	822	77	899	876	228	125	523	567	+ 23	+ 20
	2	566	25	4	104	1,232	77	1,309	1,277	513	186	578	622	+ 32	+ 32
J. N.	3	508	22	18	61	1,091	65	1,156	1,138	548	50	540	565	+ 18	+ 21
K. F.	4	511	30	6	81	863	67	930	847	317	48	482	517	+ 83	+ 84
E. B.	5	637	30	24	71	916	81	997	924	182	190	552	582	+ 73	+ 89
J. H.	6	516	24	18	61	925	66	991	955	486	92	377	402	+ 36	+ 45
W. A.	7	630	25	16	92	896	83	979	924	519	42	363	401	+ 55	+ 56
K. B.	8	628	30	16	92	961	85	1,046	982	398	12	572	611	+ 64	+ 48
K. M.	9	637	30	19	80	833	81	934	862	299	37	526	560	+ 72	+ 44
J. S.	10	420	30	20	80	888	82	970	929	333	71	525	559	+ 41	+ 40
W. D.	11	420	23	24	25	959	50	1,009	1,061	571	78	412	422	+ 52	+ 47
	12	332	23	24	25	1,527	50	1,577	1,606	1,135	66	405	415	− 29	− 26
W. L.	13	348	9	28	13	1,328	41	1,369	1,367	909	68	390	394	+ 2	+ 7
	14	411	9	28	13	1,630	41	1,671	1,637	1,220	31	386	390	+ 34	+ 38
	15	400	16	29	19	1,630	49	1,679	1,611	1,108	50	453	460	+ 68	+ 73
	16	570	14	28	20	1,975	48	2,023	2,041	1,543	57	441	448	+ 18	+ 24
H. S.	17	585	26	18	72	1,003	73	1,076	1,088	424	117	547	577	− 12	+ 34
J. F.	18	483	28	16	78	960	75	1,035	1,014	455	90	469	502	+ 21	+ 63
J. C.	19	409	22	16	59	957	62	1,019	1,021	590	67	364	389	− 2	+ 36
	20	536	15	24	30	964	50	1,014	1,033	756	21	256	288	− 19	+ 20
	21	521	30	10	78	851	70	921	916	401	108	407	441	+ 5	+ 53
	22	548	23	20	39	945	66	1,011	1,007	591	32	364	388	+ 4	+ 34
	23	566	27	21	59	483	69	552	582	−197	45	340	365	− 30	+ 5
	24	364	26	30	44	1,172	69	1,241	1,000	319	39	642	660	+241	+240
I. R.	25	360	13	6	62	735	49	774	752	417	69	266	292	+ 22	+ 39
	26	522	13	6	61	767	48	755	744	216	58	470	496	+ 11	+ 41
F. I.	27	536	22	9	85	881	70	951	930	498	61	371	407	+ 21	+ 52
	28		23	10	85	881	71	952	941	449	67	425	461	+ 11	+ 47

* The metabolic mixture was determined directly in the respiration chamber throughout the twenty-four hours of the final day of observation 17 through 23. In the remaining observations it was estimated from the dietary carbohydrate, the urinary nitrogen (× 6.25), the respiratory quotient obtained in periods of from two to four hours and the daily activity records of the infants.

† The water of oxidation was determined from the metabolic mixture by use of the constants of Newburgh:[3] $(P \times 0.41) + (F \times 1.07) + (C \times 0.60)$.

‡ The water loss through skin and lungs was determined from the total insensible loss by deducting the fraction contributed by exhaled carbon dioxide less inhaled oxygen:[3] $(CO_2 - O_2 = (C \times 0.41) + (P \times 0.08) - (F \times 0.08))$.

to seven days each for a total of sixty days. The ages of the infants ranged from 3 to 11½ months and the weights from 3.7 to 7.7 Kg. The protein, the caloric and the fluid content of the milk mixtures employed averaged 4.8 Gm., 118 calories and 160 Gm. per kilogram of body weight per twenty-four hours (2.1 Gm., 53 calories and 2.4 ounces per pound) and ranged from 3.9 to 6.4 Gm. of protein, from 94 to 150 calories and from 132 to 225 Gm. per kilogram, respectively. Such diets are generally accepted as adequate to cover the physiologic requirements of infants. The results are summarized in table 5.

Of the average total of 150 Gm. of water available in the intake of these 14 infants, 65, 13 and 68 Gm. per kilogram of body weight were eliminated by way of urine, feces and skin and lungs, respectively, leaving a balance of 4 Gm. per kilogram for retention. In terms of percentages of available water, the partition of outgoing water averaged 43 per cent through the urine, 9 per cent through the feces and 45 per cent through the skin and lungs; 3 per cent of the incoming water was retained within the body. The notable fraction contributed by the skin and lungs to outgoing water emphasizes the importance of this avenue of elimination and the inaccuracy of clinical estimates of water balance based only on intake of fluid and volume of urine.

It should be noted that the cited figures represent averages for total periods and that the distribution of water elimination through the different channels varied not only in individual infants on comparable diets (tables 3 and 4) but even in the same infant on successive days (not shown in tables). These fluctuations in water elimination from day to day are in accord with the clinically recognized hydrolability of infants, and they reaffirm the importance of prolonged observations for valid interpretation of results of studies of water exchange in these subjects. The greater elasticity of the compartment of urinary water (range, from 24 to 111 Gm. per kilogram; coefficient of variability, $\frac{\sigma}{mean} = 32$ per cent) as compared with the excretion through skin and lungs (range, from 48 to 86 Gm.; coefficient of variability, 19 per cent) will be more fully discussed in a later section.

Although individual infants varied in their elimination of water through the different avenues, an equilibrium or positive water balance was obtained in all except 2 observations (observations 17 and 19). Of particular significance is the correlation of water balance to total change in body weight with these diets. The total gain in body weight of the 14 infants averaged 46.5 Gm. daily, of which water constituted 32.7 Gm., or 70 per cent. The demonstration that the average proportion of retained water to total accretion of body weight coincides with the water content of the infantile body provides, in conjunction with previously reported data,[1] experimental evidence that the relative and the absolute amounts of organic materials and of water deposited in

TABLE 5.—*Water Balance and Partition of Excretion of Healthy Infants on Adequate Diets per Kilogram of Body Weight per Twenty-Four Hours*

Subject	Observation No.	Period, Days	Average Weight, Kg.	Daily Diet Protein, Gm.	Daily Diet Calories	Daily Diet Fluid,* Gm.	Available Water,† Gm.	Partition of Outgoing Water Urinary Gm.	Urinary %‡	Fecal Gm.	Fecal %‡	Skin and Lungs Gm.	Skin and Lungs %‡	Total, Gm.	Water Balance Gm.	Water Balance %‡
E. B.	5	4	7,725	4.5	107	132	129	24	18	25	19	71	55	120	9	7
K. M.	9	2	7,236	4.1	96	133	129	41	32	5	4	72	56	118	11	8
J. S.	10	2	7,475	4.0	94	133	130	45	34	9	7	70	54	124	6	4
W. A.	7	2	7,545	4.0	107	138	130	69	53	6	4	48	37	123	7	6
K. B.	8	2	7,742	3.9	105	139	135	51	38	2	1	74	55	127	8	6
W. B.	1	5	6,748	4.0	125	142	133	34	25	19	14	78	58	131	2	3
J. C.	22	3	7,320	4.1	93	148	138	81	58	7	5	50	36	138	0	0
	21	3	6,602	5.6	131	156	140	61	44	16	12	62	44	139	1	1
J. F.	18	3	7,166	5.2	120	158	144	63	44	13	9	65	45	141	3	2
J. H.	6	3	6,520	6.1	132	158	152	75	49	14	9	58	38	147	5	4
K. F.	4	3	6,119	5.6	136	160	152	52	34	8	5	79	52	139	13	9
F. L.	27	3	6,394	4.8	124	163	149	78	52	10	6	58	39	146	3	2
H. S.	17	4	6,978	4.9	116	168	154	61	39	17	11	78	51	156	−2	−1
J. C.	19	3	6,283	4.8	109	174	162	94	58	11	7	58	36	163	−1	0
J. N.	3	7	6,281	6.4	137	193	184	87	47	8	4	86	47	181	3	2
W. B.	2	6	6,895	3.9	122	200	190	74	39	27	14	84	44	185	5	2
I. R.	25	5	3,741	5.9	150	225	207	111	54	18	9	71	34	200	7	3
Average			6,752	4.8	118	160	150	65	43	13	9	68	45	146	4	3

* Total weight of intake.
† Includes ingested water and water of oxidation.
‡ The figures in these columns represent percentages of available water.

233

the body by means of the diets customarily employed in infant feeding are both qualitatively and quantitatively compatible with adequate growth.

Effect of Variations of Fluid Intake on the Water Exchange of Infants.—The effect of augmentation of the fluid intake on the water balance is graphically presented in charts 1 and 2. In chart 1 the observations of table 5 have been arranged in three groups, in which the daily fluid intake averaged 136, 157 and 192 Gm. per kilogram of body weight (range: 130 to 145, 146 to 165 and 166 to 225 Gm. per kilogram). No augmentation is noted in the water balance with increasing fluid intake, the water available for retention averaging 7, 4 and 3 Gm. per kilogram, respectively, for the low, moderate, and high normal levels of intake. The fecal and the insensible quota likewise remained relatively constant, but the urinary quota rose from 44 to 68 to 85 Gm. per kilogram of body weight.

The response of the different compartments of outgoing water to enhanced fluid intake was even more strikingly demonstrated in 4 infants (J. C., observations 22 and 23; W. B., observations 1 and 2; W. D., observations 11 and 12; W. L., observations 13 and 14 and observations 15 and 16) whose caloric intake remained constant in each pair of observations (table 3) but whose fluid intake was raised in successive periods from a daily minimum of 85 Gm. (J. C., observation 23) to a daily maximum of 449 Gm. per kilogram of body weight (W. L., observation 16). Here again, enhancement of the fluid intake resulted in notable increases in the urinary output of each infant, with relatively small or negligible alterations in water balance or in the fecal and insensible compartments of water elimination. Practically all of the excess water of the intake in each pair of observations was eliminated in the urine.

The evidence suggests that the compartment of urinary water is the most labile of all avenues of water elimination and that in a state of health and with ordinary conditions of diet and environment, alterations of fluid intake are reflected primarily in this fraction. That additional fluid in the diet did not augment the retention of water within the body lends further experimental support to the practice of feeding healthy infants approximately 150 cc. of fluid per kilogram of body weight (2 to 3 ounces per pound). Routine administration of fluid beyond this level serves merely to dilute the urine.

The water elimination through skin and respiratory passages, on the other hand, was essentially independent of the fluid intake in these observations, suggesting that this avenue of elimination was under the control of a more stable, physiologic mechanism than that of water regulation. Data demonstrating that this mechanism is concerned with the

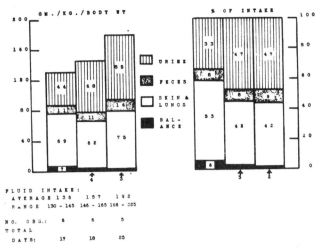

Chart 1.—Water balance of normal infants on adequate diets (arranged according to fluid intake). The total height of the columns indicates the total available water; the vertically lined compartments, the output of water in the urine; the dotted areas, fecal water; the blank areas, loss of water through the skin and the lungs. The difference between incoming and outgoing water is designated by the shaded areas and represents shifts in body water. The same designation is used in the following figures.

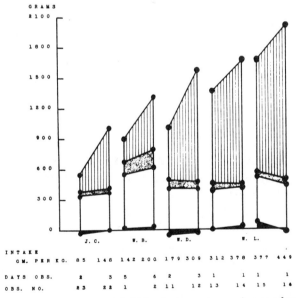

Chart 2.—Effect of increasing fluid intake on water exchange of normal infants. Each vertical line is a single observation.

regulation of body temperature will be presented in the following sections.

The present studies on water exchange with increasing fluid intakes were made with one exception (observation 23) at levels well above the accepted minimal fluid requirements of infants. In one observation, infant J. C., with a daily fluid intake of 85 Gm. per kilogram of body weight, had typical dehydration fever, his rectal temperature reaching 39.3 C. (102.8 F.) on the third day of reduced fluid intake. The pathogenesis of dehydration fever in infants and its relation to water and electrolyte exchange are at present under investigation.

Effect of Variations of Caloric Intake on the Water Exchange of Infants.—A series of 4 observations (19 through 22, table 3), each of

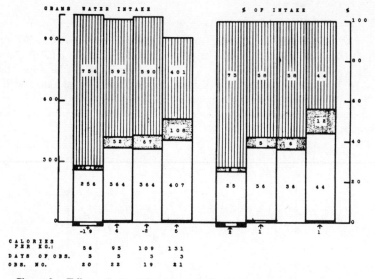

Chart 3.—Effect of alterations in caloric intake on water exchange of a healthy infant (J. C.).

three days, was made on 1 infant (J. C.) to determine the effect on his water exchange of changes in caloric intake when the amount of fluid in the diet was constant. This infant received milk mixtures of the usual qualitative composition and containing constant and adequate amounts of fluid (approximately 150 Gm. per kilogram), but the caloric intake was progressively raised from the low level of 56 to 93, 109 and finally 131 calories per kilogram of body weight. The results are graphically shown in chart 3.

When the diet was adequate both in calories and in fluid (observations 19 and 22), 58 per cent of the water intake was eliminated in the urine, 6 per cent in the feces and 36 per cent in the insensible perspiration. A reduction in the intake from the maintenance levels of 93 and

109 calories to the submaintenance level of 56 calories per kilogram (observation 20) was accompanied by a sharp decline in the fecal and the insensible loss of water and by a striking augmentation of the urinary loss. Conversely, with the hypermaintenance level of 131 calories per kilogram (observation 21), the fecal and the insensible loss increased notably and the urinary water fell to a distinctly lower level.

The parallelism between fecal output and food intake is in accord with expectation. It is generally recognized that the total bulk of the stool and presumably of the fecal water depends on the amount of ingested food. The correlation between insensible loss of water and caloric intake is also readily explained if one recalls the relationship which exists between insensible perspiration and energy metabolism. The low, normal and high caloric diets stimulated the metabolism to different degrees, so that the daily heat production, as actually measured throughout the final day of each experimental period, totaled 395,460,510 and 530 calories, respectively. These increases in energy exchange in turn augmented the insensible perspiration,[13] the insensible water rising from 256 to 364 to 407 Gm. daily. With a constant fluid intake and with no marked change in the water balance in the different periods, this increase in insensible and in fecal loss was necessarily reflected in a corresponding reduction of urinary water (from 756 to 590 to 401 Gm. in twenty-four hours).

These results are consistent with the conception that at levels of fluid intake well above the minimum for adequate urinary secretion, the output of urinary water represents a claim on available water which is subordinated to the need for regulating body temperature by vaporization through the skin and lungs. The clinical counterpart of these observations is seen in the diminution of urinary secretion accompanying the high metabolism of fever, and they point to the necessity for administering extra fluids to febrile infants in order to maintain urinary secretion and flow at a level adequate to remove the end products of the heightened metabolism.

Effects of Variations in Environment on Water Exchange.—The effect of variations in environmental temperature and relative humidity is shown in chart 4.

Elevation of the environmental temperature in 1 infant (I. R., observations 25 and 26) from 22 to 29 C. (from 72 to 84 F.), with the relative humidity constant at 60 per cent, markedly increased the water loss through skin and lungs (from 266 to 470 Gm., or from 34 to 62 per

---

13. It was shown in a previous paper [2] that under environmental conditions which could not be rigidly controlled this relationship was not sufficiently consistent except under strictly basal conditions to permit prediction of the total daily metabolism of infants from their measured water of vaporization.

cent of the intake), with a corresponding decrease in the urinary water
(from 417 to 216 Gm., or from 54 to 29 per cent of the intake).
Increase of the relative humidity from 40 to 80 per cent with the
temperature maintained constant at 22 C. (72 F.; infant F. L.) resulted
in a similar but less striking increase in the water lost through the skin
and lungs (from 371 to 425 Gm., or from 39 to 45 per cent of the intake),
while the urinary water fell from 498 to 449 Gm., or from 52 to 47 per
cent of the total intake. The fecal water remained relatively constant,
and in each five day period the daily water balance remained positive
(from 11 to 22 Gm. per day).

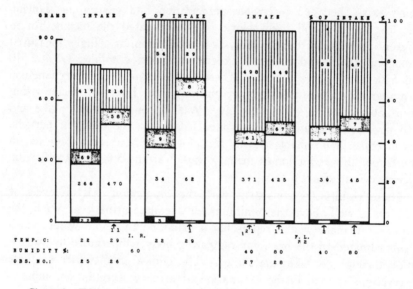

Chart 4.—Effect of alterations in environment (temperature and humidity) on
water exchange of normal infants.

These observations supplement the dietary studies in calling attention to the auxiliary role of the kidneys in the excretion of water in
health and under usual conditions of diet. The necessity for regulating
body temperature by extra vaporization of water from skin and lungs
at the high levels of external temperature and humidity represented a
prior claim on the supply of available water, with the result that water
was shunted from renal to extrarenal channels, leaving adequate sur-
pluses for retention in all periods. Under conditions of more limited
fluid intake or more extreme environment, sufficient water might not
be available for adequate vaporization from skin and lungs, for urinary
flow and for deposition of body water, with resultant development of
fever, retention of waste products and dehydration, singly or in combination.

COMMENT

This paper presents a comprehensive system for the metabolic measurement of water exchange in infants modified after the methods elaborated by Newburgh.[3] Direct measurement for from twenty and one-half to twenty-three hours in 7 observations in the respiration chamber of the oxygen consumption, the carbon dioxide production and the water elimination through skin and lungs, combined with chemical analyses of the diet for water, nitrogen, fat and carbohydrate, of the urine for water and nitrogen, and of the feces for water, nitrogen and fat, afforded a means of checking the reliability of the revised methods for calculating water exchange.[14] The close agreement between the daily change in weight measured in toto with the balance and the sum of the organic and the water balance (table 2) substantiates the validity of the technical procedures.

The difficulties inherent in measuring the respiratory exchange of infants have prompted a number of investigators to employ total weight balances as a means of measuring the water exchange. These workers have assumed that the total weight of the intake, including solid constituents, may be substituted for the water intake as such plus the water of oxidation and that, on the outgoing side, the total insensible loss plus the total weight of the excreta may be estimated as water, the fractions ascribable to carbon dioxide less oxygen in the former and to solids in the latter being omitted from consideration.

Justification for the use of this simple method of weighings in the study of the water exchange of infants resides in the fact that water naturally forms a considerable fraction of both the intake and the excreta of infants (87 per cent of milk, 98 per cent of urine, 80 per cent of feces, from 85 to 95 per cent of the insensible loss) and of the total change in body weight (70 per cent of tissues).

In the 17 observations on normal diets reported in this paper, the water balance obtained by direct measurement averaged 33 Gm. daily and the total gain in body weight 47 Gm. (table 5). Although the absolute difference of 14 Gm. is small, the figure for total gain in weight represents a deviation of 43 per cent from the figure for the directly determined water balance. In addition, inconsistencies of the correlation between the two series of measurements were demonstrable in individual infants. These inconsistencies, jointly with the probably greater disparity which would prevail in abnormal states of body hydration, impair the clinical usefulness of the method of simple weighings for determining the water exchange of infants. The conclusion is justified that more precise knowledge than can be derived by use of this method is needed in

---

14. Lavietes, P. H.: Metabolic Measurement of Water Exchange, J. Clin. Investigation **14**:57 (Jan.) 1935. Peters, J. P.: Body Water: The Exchange of Fluids in Man, Springfield, Ill., Charles C. Thomas, Publisher, 1935.

careful studies of the fate of water in the body not only in health but especially in the hydrolabile states accompanying disease. Studies designed to correlate shifts in body water with electrolyte change will be presented in a future publication, which will serve as further substantiation of the reliability of the methods used in the metabolic measurement of water exchange.

SUMMARY

Metabolic measurements of the water exchange were made in 28 observations of from one to seven days each on 16 healthy, full term male infants from 3 to 11½ months of age.

Twenty-four hourly determinations of the energy exchange in the respiration chamber, chemical analyses of the diet and excreta (urine and feces) and concurrent measurements of body weight served to control the validity of the methods employed for calculation of the water exchange. The magnitude of the disparity between the water balance and the weight balance was briefly discussed.

With normal diets (118 calories, 4.8 Gm. of protein, 160 Gm. of fluid per kilogram in twenty-four hours) and ordinary conditions of environment, 65, 13 and 68 Gm. of water per kilogram of body weight were eliminated through urine, feces and skin and lungs, respectively. Urinary water averaged 43 per cent, fecal water 9 per cent and extrarenal water (skin and lungs) 45 per cent of the total available water, leaving a surplus of 3 per cent for retention within the body.

The water retained within the body by subjects receiving the normal diets averaged 33 Gm., which is compatible with the building up of 47 Gm. of new tissue daily. (Water content of infantile tissue equals 70 per cent.)

Augmentation of fluid intake resulted in a notable increase in urinary water without appreciably enhancing the water balance or the water elimination through other channels.

Augmentation of food intake increased the elimination of water through the skin and lungs and the feces at the expense of urinary water.

Elevation of the environmental temperature from 22 to 29 C. (72 to 84 F.) in one observation strikingly increased the water eliminated through the skin at the expense of urinary water. Increasing the relative humidity from 40 to 80 per cent in another observation caused similar but less striking changes. In neither instance was fecal or retained water markedly affected.

CONCLUSIONS

A comprehensive system for studying the water exchange of infants and the results when average conditions of diet and environment prevail are presented. The results in conjunction with data previously reported [1] indicate that the customary diets employed in infant feeding, containing approximately 120 calories, from 4 to 5 Gm. of protein and 160 Gm. of fluid per kilogram of body weight, are adequate to ensure the deposition within the body of organic materials and water which qualitatively approximate the chemical composition of infantile tissue and which quantitatively fulfil the requirements for satisfactory growth. The effects on the water exchange of variations in caloric and fluid intake and of environmental temperature and relative humidity were also studied. Such studies are a prerequisite for investigations of the water exchange of premature and of sick infants.

525 East Sixty-Eighth Street.

Part VI

VITAMINS

Editor's Comments
on Papers 21 Through 27

Rickets and scurvy, the most commonly described vitamin-deficiency states, were well known for their physical characteristics by the end of the nineteenth century. The chemical delineation of the vitamins and their precise role in nutrition, together with the minimum daily requirements, had to await new techniques of analytical biochemistry and the combined studies of many researchers. Space does not permit inclusion of all the key articles that detail the unraveling of the vitamin story. At least one third of this volume could be subtitled "From Rice to Rats," and profitably be devoted to the decade of original work reported by McCollum et al. (1915,

1922). The practical application of the results of their studies on vitamins A and D in cod liver oil probably still leaves an oily taste in the mouth of anyone over fifty reading this section.

Jeans' meticulously researched review of the literature in this field (Paper 25) is of exemplary merit. The reason for selecting the other articles presented here is self-evident from the titles.

21

Reprinted from *Lancet*, 685–687 (Nov. 16, 1878)

THREE CASES OF SCURVY SUPERVENING ON RICKETS IN YOUNG CHILDREN

W. B. Cheadle, M.D., F.R.C.P.

PHYSICIAN TO THE HOSPITAL FOR SICK CHILDREN, GREAT ORMOND-STREET; SENIOR ASSISTANT-PHYSICIAN AND LECTURER ON PATHOLOGY AT ST. MARY'S HOSPITAL.

THE outbreak of scurvy during the late Polar Expedition, on which it had so disastrous an influence, has specially associated the disease in the public mind with an arctic climate. The amateur pathology of naval officers has, moreover, been directed to show that scurvy is not dependent upon any defect of diet, but essentially connected with extreme cold, prolonged absence of sunlight, and severe physical exertion. Yet scurvy in its most severe and typical form breaks out in tropical climates as well as within the Arctic Circle, and under the full glare of a summer sun as well as in the protracted gloom of a six months' night. Cold and darkness and fatigue may favour its development, but that is all. They are not invariable factors in the production of the scorbutic condition. There *is*, however, an invariable factor, without the presence of which all other casual and irregular factors are powerless to set up the disease. This essential factor, it has been proved over and over again, is the absence of certain elements in food. If the body is deprived of these elements, the scorbutic condition is produced. What these elements are has not yet been absolutely settled with scientific precision, but we know positively that they exist in fresh vegetables, in lime-juice, in milk, and in less considerable degree, perhaps, in some other fresh animal foods. Dr. Baly suggested that the essential elements consisted of the organic acids, such as the citric, malic, and tartaric acids, which exist plentifully in fruits and vegetables of the most powerful antiscorbutic virtue. Later Dr. Garrod found that these acids pure and alone, separated from the fresh fruits and vegetables which yield them, and the alkaline bases with which they are combined, possess no antiscorbutic properties, and he essayed to show that potash was probably the essential ingredient. This hypothesis fails, however, for many substances rich in potash, such as beef-tea, for instance, possess little or no antiscorbutic power. Dr. Buzzard upon this put forward another hypothesis founded upon the facts that both the organic acids and potash are found largely in all the best antiscorbutics — viz., that neither alone, but a combination of the two together, constituted the essential element. This theory has been further developed by Dr. Ralfe, physician to the Seamen's Hospital at Greenwich, who has recently investigated the subject clinically and experimentally. The results of these observations have been published in THE LANCET, and throw much fresh light upon the physiologico-chemical effects of a scorbutic diet upon the condition of the urine, and presumably therefore upon the blood also. The primary change in scurvy Dr. Ralfe believes to be "a general alteration between the various acids, inorganic as well as organic, and the bases found in the blood, by which (*a*) the neutral salts, such as the chlorides, are either increased relatively at the expense of the alkaline salts, or (*b*) that these alkaline salts are absolutely decreased. The primary change, therefore," he concludes, "is a chemical alteration in the blood, consisting essentially in a diminution of its alkalinity." This condition produces dissolution of the blood-corpuscles, and fatty degeneration of the muscles and the secreting cells of the liver and kidney, just as in experiments on animals a similar condition is produced by injecting acids into the blood or feeding them with acid salts. The change must affect other tissues also, such as those of the bloodvessels, which become fragile and easily rupture, and the mucous membrane of the gums, which swells and softens. With regard to this hypothesis, I may remark that, whether ultimately confirmed or not, it seems to explain not only why fresh vegetables are antiscorbutic by virtue of the alkaline salts which they contain, but also why salted provisions, although not essential to the production of scurvy, by the neutral salts which they contain, favour so powerfully the development of the scorbutic state.

This relation between the nature of the food ingested and the production of scurvy, and the absolute power of prevention exercised by the presence of certain elements of food in the diet, have lately been in some danger of being overlooked, or at any rate greatly underestimated. Three cases of scurvy which I have lately met with appear to me especially significant and instructive at this juncture, since they exhibit the development of the disease under the simplest conditions. Most of the surrounding influences which exist in the ordinary circumstances under which scurvy is developed, and which complicate the question of its genesis, were absent. The subjects were all children, from sixteen months to three years old. There was no protracted exposure to great cold or prolonged darkness; no severe and exhausting physical exertion. All the conditions of existence were fairly normal and healthy, with the single exception of diet. In the most extreme case of the series, indeed, the general conditions of life, apart from this, were unusually good; the others were fully up to the average amongst the poor. The one defect present in each instance, the common factor of disease, was a deficiency in certain essential elements of food.

CASE 1.—For the first case I am indebted to my friend, Mr. W. A. Sumner, with whom I saw it on the 12th of January last, and who has kindly supplied me with the chief particulars of its history and subsequent course. The patient, G. S——, aged sixteen months, was the first child of well-to-do parents of the middle class, living in a healthy part of St. John's-wood. At the time I saw the child he presented a very striking and extraordinary aspect. Dark-red, soft, and gelatinous masses protruded from the mouth between the lips, and gave the child the appearance of being engaged in sucking pieces of raw flesh. On examination these projections were seen to be the gums swollen to this extreme degree, soft, spongy, and bleeding. The mucous membrane of the mouth was spongy and swollen also to such an extent that it was almost in contact with the tongue as it lay on the floor of the cavity. The breath was extremely offensive, the legs œdematous, the skin harsh and unhealthy-looking, the complexion sallow and anæmic. The limbs were tender on being handled, the muscles flabby, but no muscular or periosteal swellings could be detected. The child was muscularly so feeble that it could not sit up, but fell over immediately when placed in an upright position. It was exceedingly rickety, the fontanelle widely open, the ends of the long bones enlarged, the ribs beaded, and the walls of the thorax falling in deeply with each inspiration, which was laboured and stridulous.

I learnt that the child was apparently healthy when born, the parents being also healthy, with the exception that the mother had suffered from some uterine affection before marriage. The baby had been fretful for the first few months, but, on the whole, kept very well until it was about ten months old—i. e., about six months previously, when it began to be weakly. For the first three months of life it had the breast, with some Swiss milk in addition after the first five weeks. At the end of three months oatmeal gruel made with water was substituted for the condensed milk, which the mother thought did not agree with the child; but she continued to suckle it as before. The breast-milk and the oatmeal and water were thus continued together until the sixth month, when the child was completely weaned. From this date it had no more milk of any kind for the next four months —i. e., from the time it was six months old until it was ten months, it was kept entirely on oatmeal and rusks. At ten months old a little mutton-broth was given in addition, because the child appeared to be growing weakly, and this diet was maintained without any change until the fourteenth month, at which period the child was first seen by Mr. Sumner. From the sixth month then, when the child was weaned, until it was fourteen months old, or for a period of eight months, it had no milk, no meat, no potatoes—nothing but oatmeal, rusks, and water, with a little mutton-broth. Its chief food was the oatmeal, which the mother considered the most strengthening. I think there need be no wonder that the child grew rickety and more and more feeble, until Mr. Sumner was called in at fourteen months, when he found the gums had begun to swell, and a state of scurvy had fairly set in. Chlorate of potash and bark were prescribed, and subsequently the syrup of iodide of iron. The swelling, however, increased, with occasional hæmorrhage from the mouth, and alum and glycerine were applied to the gums locally. This failed to have any effect. The swelling of the gums still got more and more excessive, until the whole of the soft parts of the upper and lower jaws seemed to be involved, and the bleeding became more profuse. The treatment was then changed to the perchloride of iron and cod-liver oil internally, and glycerine of tannin was applied to the spongy excrescences. The local application speedily reduced the swelling to some extent, but the child grew weaker in spite of the iron and cod-liver oil, and was unable to sit upright. The feet and legs began to swell, and there was much dyspnœa, stridulous respiration, especially during sleep, occasionally developing into the paroxysms of laryngismus.

Such was the history of the case up to the time of my visit, and it threw abundant light upon the nature of the affection from which the child was suffering. It had been enfeebled by no exhausting disease or wasting fever. All the conditions of life under which it was placed were healthy, except that of diet. It was well nursed, well clothed, lived in airy well-ventilated rooms in an open healthy situation. It had also had food in ample quantity; but the quality was clearly defective. For eight months, with the exception of some broth occasionally, it had been limited to one kind of food only—viz., farinaceous food. That it would become rickety on such a diet might have been foretold with absolute certainty. The diet was, however, more than a rickety diet—it was a scurvy diet. It comprised neither milk nor fresh vegetables nor fresh meat; milk is an excellent antiscorbutic, fresh vegetables are an absolute specific against scurvy. The disease, moreover, rarely breaks out on an abundant fresh meat diet. Most children get a certain amount of milk, at any rate, until they become old enough to take more solid food, and then they usually have a little meat or gravy, and almost invariably potatoes, in addition to the staple farinaceous food, and their diet is thus rendered antiscorbutic. But in this case the child was deprived of all these usual antiscorbutic elements, both the milk of earlier life and the potatoes of the later period, and scurvy followed accordingly. The treatment consisted in substituting new milk with rusks for the oatmeal and water, the milk being given in small quantities at first on account of its being stated not to have agreed previously, and gradually increased to the full allowance of two pints in the twenty-four hours. In addition to this a tablespoonful of raw meat very finely minced and sweetened with a little sugar was ordered to be given every day. The cod-liver oil was continued, with steel wine and glycerine, and, in addition, five grains of bromide of potassium with a view of relieving the laryngismus. The child was also directed to be sponged every morning with tepid—almost cold—water.

The result of these measures has proved highly satisfactory. Mr. Sumner writes to me under the date of the 7th of March :—" The child is decidedly improving. Sponginess of the gums has completely disappeared, and he can sit up now without any inconvenience;" and later, " Since you saw him the child has greatly improved. The fontanelle is all but closed ; the swelling &c. of the gums have entirely disappeared, so that I have for a long time discontinued the tannic acid. The spine is straighter and firmer, and he can sit upright, and even move about the floor, though not as yet able to stand. I have had partially to discontinue the bromide, as the skin became irritated. He has more or less continued the diet you recommended, and I have now allowed his parents to take him to Margate to try the effect of salt-water bathing." I have since learnt that the child is running about thoroughly strong and well.

CASE 2.—A. S——, aged sixteen months, was admitted into the Children's Hospital, Great Ormond-street, on March 9th, 1877. His legs were swollen and œdematous, the gums were swollen and projected as dark-red, spongy excrescences between the lips. They were stained with submucous hæmorrhages, and bled on the least touch. Some hard swellings could be felt deeply seated in the flesh of each thigh, and the shafts of the long bones felt enlarged and swollen. One of his swellings was attributed to a blow four months before. The skin looked muddy and unhealthy, but there were no ecchymoses there. There were however, two unhealthy-looking superficial sores, one on the right wrist and another on the forefinger. The legs were highly œdematous and swollen. The child was fretful and irritable, and disliked being handled, there being evidently general tenderness. The temperature was below the normal—viz., 97·2°. The urine contained a small quantity of albumen. The history obtained from the mother was as follows :—The child was the youngest of seven, two of whom had died, one while teething, and another from wasting and diarrhœa. The other surviving children were said to be " weak at the chest," but none affected in the same way as this. The parents lived in fair comfort, in healthy quarters at Hampstead. The child was born healthy, but had always suffered from cold feet and hands. He was brought up entirely by hand, the mother stating that until the time he was ten months old he had a quart of milk to himself. Then he began to take bread and Dr. Ridge's food, with a share of a pint of milk, which served the whole family of seven. The child has had no meat, would not eat potatoes and gravy, and thus he had lived solely on bread, with a little butter, and this small quantity of milk for the last six months. Ever since birth he had had double otorrhœa. When four months old there was an attack of diarrhœa, and about this time he brought up about a teaspoonful of blood five or six times. About three months ago —i. e., when the child was thirteen months old and had been three months upon the bread and water diet—red lumps appeared on the gums, about the double teeth, some of which he was cutting, and a little later the legs began to swell. The spongy excrescences of the gums increased, and about four weeks ago they began to bleed freely, so as to saturate three or four handkerchiefs a day.

The case was clearly, like the preceding, one of scurvy supervening upon rickets, both conditions being due to deficiency in certain important elements of food. As before, diet had not only been a rickety diet, but a scorbutic one also.

The treatment consisted in a full allowance of milk, with mashed potatoes beaten up in milk, raw meat, and the juice of two oranges. A mixture, containing one grain of citrate of iron and quinine, with a drachm each of syrup and lemon-juice, was given every four hours. The gums were ordered to be freely painted over, three times a day, with a solution containing fifteen minims of glycerine of tannin to the ounce.

The food was taken very well with the exception of the orange-juice, and in three days' time the gums began to look more healthy ; the hæmorrhage ceased ; the gums were less swollen. Two days later, or on the fifth since admission, the urine became free from albumen, which never returned. On the eighth day the swelling of the gums had quite gone down, there having been no hæmorrhage since admission, but there was still slight œdema of the feet. The temperature remained always below the normal, varying from 97° to 98°F., except on the day after admission, when it reached 99·5° F. in the evening.

The general health and condition of the child improved in a most remarkable degree ; its skin became more natural, its lips gained colour, and it increased in weight rapidly, gaining 3 lb. in less than three weeks—a very large increase considering its small original weight for a child of that age. When weighed a week after admission it was 16½ lb. ; in seventeen days it weighed 19½ lb.; in the next seventeen days it gained only one pound more. The recovery continued without any drawback. The skin of the swollen legs peeled off in large flakes, but there was no general desquamation. On April 19th, six weeks after admission, the child was sent to Highgate, having for some time shown all the signs of perfect health and vigour. The deep-seated swellings in the thighs and the thickening round the bones had entirely disappeared.

In the third case the symptoms were somewhat less extreme, but the scorbutic condition was unmistakable, and the diet corresponded most closely with that in the preceding cases.

CASE 3.—Emma W——, aged three years, the child of parents living in Deptford, was admitted into the Children's Hospital on April 30th, 1877, suffering from great debility, and bleeding at the mouth. On examination, the gums were found to be fungous, bleeding, and swollen to such a degree that they formed a wall on each side of the teeth, almost hiding them. This was especially prominent and fleshy at the inner part of the upper incisors, where it was about a quarter of an inch thick. The breath was offensive. There was slight but clearly-marked œdema of the ankles. There were no ecchymoses under the skin, which was muddy and unhealthy-looking, nor was there hæmorrhage from any mucous surface, except from the fungous gums. A pinch on the leg produced no bruise. The signs of rickets were well marked, but not extreme. The ends of the long bones were enlarged, the ribs beaded, the fontanelle was not quite closed, and the teeth were decaying and many broken off short. The muscles were flabby, but there were no deep-seated swellings to be detected. The urine was free from albumen. The temperature was normal. The history obtained from the mother was that this was the second of three children, one of whom had just died from bronchitis. The father and mother were healthy. This child was suckled up to two years old, and fed on bread-and-butter in addition, with a little beef-tea. From the time of its being weaned, at two years old, its diet had consisted of bread-and-butter and tea, with occasionally German sausage, of which it was very fond, and a little brandy-and-water. It never took potatoes; never had vegetables of any kind or fruit. Never had any fresh meat or gravy; never any milk, except a very small quantity in the tea. Three months ago the child had scarlet fever, not very severely. Was only ill a fortnight, but remained weaker after the attack, and unable to use her legs properly. The gums soon commenced to swell and bleed, and for the last six weeks this has increased, having reached its height during the last three days. For the last few weeks also the left arm and right leg have been noticed to be tender to the touch, and the child has refused to have its boots on. It sweats profusely about the head at night, screams and jumps during sleep. The bowels have been rather confined, but the motions natural.

The case was one of scurvy supervening on rickets, the food on which the child had been kept being a sufficient cause for the development of the scorbutic state.

The treatment consisted in a diet of two pints of milk, potatoes mashed and broken up with milk, and raw meat. Three grains of citrate of iron and quinine and a drachm each of syrup and of lemon-juice were given every six hours. The gums were ordered to be well brushed over three times a day with a solution of glycerine of tannin and glycerine of carbolic acid, fifteen minims of each to the ounce.

On the 5th of May, the sixth day since admission, the gums were already decidedly less swollen, and bled only when touched; but the child was feverish, and suffering from bronchial catarrh. By the 9th the gums had contracted to their normal size, although still a little spongy and red. The œdema had disappeared, the child improved in spirits and appearance, had gained weight, and, in fact, had quite returned to the healthy state by the first week in June, when symptoms of measles appeared, and it had to be removed from the hospital owing to the quarantine wards being not yet open.

These three cases show a remarkable agreement in their symptoms and in the conditions under which the morbid state was developed. All these children were rickety, and in all the most prominent symptoms of scurvy had been superadded to those of rachitis. In all the diet had been such as is known to produce the rachitic condition with the greatest regularity and certainty—viz., one consisting almost entirely of farinaceous food without a sufficient quantity of milk, or other food containing an adequate amount of animal oil. This I believe to be the chief essential ingredient the want of which in the food gives rise to rickets, rather than the want of mineral matter. It is known that in the diet of all these children the mineral element would be deficient also. In the first case the earthy salts in the food would be chiefly contained in the bran of the oatmeal, which would pass through undigested. In the two remaining instances the bread used would be probably of the finer kind most affected by the poor. All white bread is poor in earthy salts, and in the finest and whitest known these are at the lowest.

One of the most interesting points with regard to this series is the supervention of scurvy on this pre-existing state of rickets. Rachitis is the most common of all the morbid conditions we meet with amongst the patients of the Children's Hospital; yet cases of scurvy are extremely rare. Why did these particular rickety children out of all the number alone become scorbutic? I believe the explanation lies in the fact that, curiously enough, in each of these cases one factor usually present in the diet of children was omitted in addition to those ordinarily wanting in a simple rachitic diet—viz., potatoes. The common antiscorbutic element in the food of infants is milk; but after they are weaned, or if brought up by hand at an early age, the children of the poor get very little milk; it is too expensive. They soon begin to feed with their parents, and potatoes and gravy are almost invariably given them. This does not prevent them becoming rickety, but it seems to keep off scurvy; potatoes,

as the late Dr. Baly proved, being an excellent antiscorbutic. The children in the present cases had no antiscorbutic. Milk was not given at all in the first case, no fresh meat, no fresh vegetable of any kind. In the other two cases a very minute quantity of milk, and that probably watered, was alone given; but no fresh meat, no fresh vegetables of any kind.

I have said that cases of scurvy are rare amongst children in large towns, and instances of the fully-developed disease undoubtedly are so. It seems to me possible, however, that the cases of ulcerative stomatitis, which are not infrequent amongst ill-nourished, neglected children, may be due to the scorbutic condition — i.e., imperfectly-developed scurvy. The foul ulceration of the gums closely resembles the condition of these parts presented by cases of scurvy where the swelling of the severest stage has subsided, and the general cachectic condition is analogous to that which exists in scorbutic disease.

22

INFANTILE SCURVY: THE BLOOD, THE BLOOD-VESSELS AND THE DIET

ALFRED F. HESS, M.D., AND MILDRED FISH

NEW YORK

[*Editor's Note:* In the original, material precedes this excerpt.]

DIET

The infants in the group which we are particularly considering were being fed on various preparations of milk, and their diet was in no wise changed, excepting, as has been stated, that an attempt was made to do without orange-juice. Most of them were receiving mixtures of milk and barley water, the milk being "Grade A Pasteurized," that is, heated for thirty minutes to 145 F. Some were receiving malt soup, others Schloss milk and a few Eiweissmilch. It is interesting to note that all four children who were being fed on malt soup developed scurvy; this may have been mere chance, as these infants all had exudative diathesis, but can also be accounted for by the fact that in the preparation of this food the milk had been heated twice, the pasteurized milk having been brought to the boiling-point. As Neumann pointed out, this two-fold heating probably plays an important rôle in the production of scurvy. It is also possible that the malt should not be disregarded in this connection. Whether cereal, which was used in the form of barley-water, tends to the production of scurvy has never been definitely determined. This point must be borne in mind, how-

249

ever, in view of the classical paper of Holst and Froelich[5] on experimental scurvy produced by the giving of cereals, and on reflecting how large a part proprietary foods played in the statistics of the American Pediatric Society. As regards the cases which developed on an Eiweiss-milch diet, little need be added. This is not a criterion of the efficacy or usefulness of this food, which was devised not as a permanent diet, but as a therapeutic agent.

During the past three years we have had a considerable number of cases of scurvy develop in infants being fed on pasteurized milk. In 1912, when the first cases were noted, we were pasteurizing the milk in our own diet kitchen, heating it to a temperature of 165 F. for twenty minutes. At this time several cases of scurvy developed, owing to the fact that through an oversight orange-juice was not given. During the past year we have been supplied by one of the large dealers with a pasteurized milk that has been heated only to 145 F. for thirty minutes. Nevertheless, we had several cases of scurvy develop on this diet. In most of the cases the infant was receiving two-thirds milk and one-third barley-water, with the addition of sugar. In two instances, whole milk was being given without the addition of barley water. There were other patients in the same ward on the identical diet who did not develop scurvy. In other words, the pasteurized milk was not the sole factor in the production of the disease. That the pasteurization did play an important rôle, however, was shown by substituting raw, unheated milk for the pasteurized milk, the formula and the amount of food remaining unchanged. In this case the scorbutic symptoms began to disappear within a week of giving raw milk and had altogether vanished in two weeks. Whatever the predisposing factor of scurvy (this infant had exudative diathesis), a case with this clinical course can be interpreted only as being, in a large measure, the result of pasteurized milk.

Raw cow's milk must not, on the other hand, be considered as having potent antiscorbutic properties. Its effect cannot be compared to the miraculous change which is brought about by giving orange-juice. This is especially striking when we take into consideration the small amount of orange-juice necessary to bring about a cure and compare it with the large amount of raw milk which is given. Raw milk, however, contains sufficient of the essential substances to prevent the development of scurvy.

It is possible that in addition to the pasteurization there are other factors in connection with the milk which enter into the causation of scurvy. Plantegna has laid emphasis on the freshness of the milk

---

5. Holst, A., and Froelich, T.: Ztschr. f. Hyg. u. Infektionskrank., 1912, lxxii, 1.

both before and after pasteurization. This factor may be found to resolve itself into a question of reaction, of greater or less acidity, which experiments on animals have shown to be of importance. Against the justification of attributing scurvy to the heating of milk, the favorable statistics given by Variot and other French authors, including thousands of cases of infants fed on boiled milk, have always seemed conflicting evidence. Whatever may be the explanation of their results, it must be remembered that these statistics refer to patients treated in the dispensaries, and that they were not observed under ideal conditions. There can be no doubt that milk loses some of its antiscorbutic qualities as the result of heating; pasteurized to the degree which we are considering, 145 for thirty minutes, it seems to lose only a portion of its essential properties. The cases that developed in our wards on this diet were for the most part very mild. They showed petechial hemorrhages, some tenderness of the bones, a very slight degree of peridental hemorrhage, but they did not evince a tendency to progress. There seems to have been almost, but not quite, a balance between the demands of the body and the supply in the diet of the essential substances on which scurvy depends. They were not all, however, of this mild or immature type of case; two of the severest cases developed in infants receiving two-thirds pasteurized milk.

DIETETIC THERAPY

We have come to a consideration of dietetic treatment, which at once suggests the efficacy of orange-juice. Last year we gave, as routine, orange-juice that had been boiled for five or ten minutes and found that we were able to obtain satisfactory results. One ounce was given daily and, as far as we could judge, boiling did not lessen its therapeutic value. This year, for orange-juice we substituted the juice of orange-peel, which was prepared as follows:

The orange-peel was finely grated and 1 ounce of it was added to 2 ounces of water, a small amount of sugar being added to overcome the slightly bitter flavor. The juice of orange-peel seems to serve the same purpose as the juice of the orange itself. It is being used at the asylum at the present time, and after a trial of several months, we have come to the conclusion that it has marked antiscorbutic power. At first we made use of the peel to test its value, but have continued its use because it allows us to serve the oranges to the older children in the institution, and in this way is somewhat economical.

According to our experience, the efficacy of vegetables cannot be compared to that of orange-juice. Two cases of scurvy developed among the infants over one year whose diet included vegetables, mainly carrots. It is impossible to state how much vegetable the nurses gave these two children; there is no reason to believe, however, that they received less than the twenty-eight other children in the ward. It is probable that they had a peculiar susceptibility to scurvy; one had exudative diathesis. When we reflect that sporadic cases of beriberi have been reported in which vegetables had been given that had been cooked for a long time, we must consider whether it is not possible that vegetables may also lose their antiscorbutic properties if cooked to a high degree. The experiments of Holst and Froelich[5] would also seem to caution us in this regard; they found that the juice of white cabbage lost its antiscorbutic value when heated even to 60 C. for ten minutes.

One of the patients, an infant receiving malt soup, developed scurvy in spite of the fact that it was given a teaspoonful of cod-liver oil three times a day for one month before the disease manifested itself. It will also be noted that in the case of recurrent scurvy which we cited, the patient had been receiving cod-liver oil for some weeks previous to the onset of the second attack. Evidently this valuable therapeutic agent cannot be relied on as an antiscorbutic. This is of interest in view of the experiments of Osborne and Mendel[6] showing the ability of cod-liver oil to promote growth in rats which had been stunted by means of a standard diet. Olive-oil certainly does not possess any antiscorbutic power. In the severest case of our group the patient had obtained a teaspoonful of olive-oil three times a day for a month before the development of scurvy.

The potency of potato was tried in some cases. It will be remembered that, in the scurvy of adults, the value of potato has been greatly lauded, and that epidemics of this disease have been reported to have followed a failure of the potato crop. First we made some trials with potato flour which is sold in the market; this was prepared with water and added to the milk in the same proportion as barley-water. It was soon evident, however, that potato flour cannot cure scurvy. We next employed mashed potato; a tablespoonful of boiled potato was added to a pint of water, using for this purpose the water in which the potato was boiled. In other words, instead of using a tablespoonful of barley to a pint of water, mashed potato was substituted. This was found very efficacious. The scorbutic symptoms quickly disappeared, although it did not seem to bring about the sudden change that is sometimes seen when orange-juice is given. It is probable that baked potato is just as valuable as an antiscorbutic.

In view of what has been outlined, at what age should we begin to give infants an antiscorbutic? There is no doubt that if an infant is fed solely on heated cow's milk the tissues begin to lose antiscorbutic substances — there is a negative balance of this material — from the

6. Osborne, T., and Mendel, L. B.: Jour. Biol. Chem., 1914, xvii, 401.

very first days of life. Such being the case, it would seem that these essential substances should be supplied to the infant as soon as it is possible. As far as is known, there is no physiologic reason why orange-juice or potato should not be given in small quantities to an infant a few weeks of age. Two years ago, it was clearly shown[7] by means of an examination of the duodenal contents, that starch-splitting ferments are present in the intestine of infants at birth, and are secreted in large measure after the first few weeks of life. It would also seem worthy of trial to substitute potato water for barley-water in the mixtures of pasteurized milk which are being distributed with such great benefit by the various diet kitchens in the larger cities. This will obviate the necessity of constantly admonishing the mothers not to omit orange-juice from the daily diet of their infants.

COMMENT

The chemical processes involved in scurvy are as yet unknown. There have been a few metabolism experiments connected with this disease, but they do not agree in their results. Lust and Klocman[8] found a positive balance of mineral salts in the course of scurvy and a negative balance during convalescence. They describe a disturbance of elimination of the salts of the body, which is quite the opposite to what is found in rickets.

A more recent study of metabolism is that of Bahrt and Edelstein[9] which is based, not on examinations during life, but on chemical analysis of the organs after death. These authors found a decrease of ash in the bones, especially of calcium and phosphorus very much as in rickets. A test of this nature, of the organs of the body, ought to afford reliable information. It should be noted, however, that in the case in question the patient had been under treatment for six weeks prior to death and that the tissues may therefore not have been in the active stage of the disease at the time of death. Further tests must decide which of these views is correct; from a clinical point of view, it is difficult to associate a marked deficiency of calcium salts with a disease in which fracture of the bones is a classical symptom, followed by a normal formation of callus. It should be emphasized that metabolic studies of this kind at present are necessarily incomplete, that after the various salts and organic substances are quantitatively analyzed, there is no doubt that more substances have been omitted than included in the chemical tests. This disease, furthermore, sharply emphasizes the fact that although an estimation of the caloric value

---

7. Hess, A. F.: The Pancreatic Ferments in Infants, AM. JOUR. DIS. CHILD., October, 1912, p. 205.

8. Lust, F. and Klocman. L.: Jahrb. f. Kinderh., 1912, lxxv, 663.

9. Bahrdt, H., and Edelstein, F.: Ztschr. f. Kinderh., 1913, ix, 415.

of food is important, it may omit the very substances which are essential to health and life. In some of our cases the caloric value of the food was as high as 120 calories per kilo, body weight, but nevertheless there was a development of scurvy, accompanied by loss of weight and failure of nutrition.

In this connection we must mention the very interesting and suggestive studies of Funk.[10] This author has coined the word "vitamines" for substances which are essential to the health and life of the body, and the lack of which produces a group of diseases which he has termed the "avitaminosen," including beriberi, scurvy, pellagra and rickets. The vitamines, Funk asserts, are crystallized nitrogen containing bodies of very complicated structure which are chemically defined, but concerning the exact structure of which we as yet know little. They are essential to life, although present in very small amounts. Such is the definition which Funk gives of the substances which he considers play an important and even vital part in nutrition.

Similar studies have been made by others, notably Stepp,[11] who terms these substances "lipoids," by which he means substances soluble in alcohol and in ether. He also found that animals could not live when deprived of these substances. Although these "vitamines" have not been satisfactorily isolated from a chemical point of view, and exception has therefore been taken to the term, there is no doubt from experiments on animals that these substances play an important rôle in the nutrition of the body. When they are removed from the diet the animals develop various nutritional disturbances, and regain their normal condition only when they are again added to the diet. These vitamines are thermolabile and are supposed to constitute a group of which there are various members. It is probable that one of this group is the vitamine which prevents the development of scurvy. It would also seem that this material is supplied in the mother's milk, and that this accounts for the fact that nursing infants do not develop scurvy.

SUMMARY

Infantile scurvy is a disorder characterized clinically by hemorrhage, for example, the classical bleeding into the gums and the subperiosteal hemorrhages of the long bones. A study of the cause of this bleeding, which must include a consideration of the clotting-power of the blood, forms the nucleus of this investigation.

For the coagulation tests blood was aspirated directly from the blood-vessels and oxalated. This plasma showed a slight diminution in clotting-power. This defect did not seem, however, to be the result of an insufficiency of calcium. The antithrombin was not increased.

10. Funk, C.: Die Vitamine, 1914, J. F. Bergmann, Wiesbaden.
11. Stepp, W.: Deutsch. med. Wchnschr., 1914, No. 18, p. 892.

Small amounts of blood were also obtained by puncture of the finger. Examinations of this blood revealed a normal number of blood platelets. In other respects the picture was that of a simple secondary anemia, except that the hemoglobin was diminished out of proportion to the red blood-cells. A marked regeneration of these cells during convalescence, leading to a polycythemia, was also noticed.

These various departures from the norm are insufficient to account for the hemorrhages associated with the disease. The integrity of the blood-vessels was therefore investigated by means of a device which may be termed the *"capillary resistance test."* This test consists in subjecting the capillaries and vessels of the arm to increased intra-vascular pressure, by means of an ordinary blood-pressure band, and of observing whether this strain results in the escape of blood through the vessels — the appearance of petechial hemorrhages into the skin. The vessels of normal infants were found to withstand, without apparent disturbance, 90 degrees of pressure for three minutes, whereas the vessels of infants suffering from scurvy gave way under this pressure. The test is not specific for scurvy, but is a method of demonstrating a weakness of the vessel walls, whatsoever may be its cause.

In the course of an exceptional opportunity to observe scurvy in its incipiency, numerous petechial hemorrhages of the skin or mucous membranes were frequently noted as one of the earliest signs of the disease; no sign, however, should be regarded as preeminently the primary symptom of scurvy.

It is generally recognized that scurvy has not only an exciting cause, but a predisposing cause. *The well-known "exudative diathesis" of Czerny was found definitely to predispose to the development of scurvy.* Whether there are other predisposing factors remains to be determined.

Several cases of scurvy developed in infants who were being fed on milk which was pasteurized to 145 F. for thirty minutes. They were cured by receiving fruit-juices or raw milk.

Orange-juice was found not to lose its efficacy as the result of being boiled for ten minutes. The juice of the peel was successfully substituted as an antiscorbutic for the juice of the orange.

Potato proved to be an excellent antiscorbutic. It is suggested that it be added to pasteurized milk as potato-water instead of the barley-water which is now commonly used as a diluent. In this way the necessity will be obviated of giving orange-juice.

Cod-liver oil or olive-oil, although given for weeks, did not prevent the development of scurvy.

23

Reprinted from *J. Biol. Chem.*, **34**(3), 537–551 (1918)

MILK AS A SOURCE OF WATER-SOLUBLE VITAMINE.*

By THOMAS B. OSBORNE and LAFAYETTE B. MENDEL.

WITH THE COOPERATION OF EDNA L. FERRY AND ALFRED J. WAKEMAN.

(*From the Laboratory of the Connecticut Agricultural Experiment Station and the Sheffield Laboratory of Physiological Chemistry in Yale University, New Haven.*)

(Received for publication, April 13, 1918.)

In our early feeding experiments with isolated food substances the failure either to induce substantial growth in young rats or to satisfy completely the maintenance requirement of older animals during long periods on the mixtures then tested led us to study the value of milk in the diet.[1] Having secured very favorable results with a food paste consisting of dried milk powder, starch, and lard, we proceeded to prepare what was termed "protein-free milk"[2] which enabled us to undertake a large number of trials of different proteins for their nutritive significance. The use of about 28 per cent of protein-free milk as the sole source of inorganic salts and what may now be termed water-soluble vitamine in the food mixtures—a procedure which was successful in many hundreds of experiments on rats—was based on the favorable results previously obtained with the food pastes containing the equivalent proportion of milk, in the form of 60 per cent of the dried milk powder. We continued to use this quantity because experience had shown that "addition of not inconsiderable portions (5 to

---

* The expenses of this investigation were shared by the Connecticut Agricultural Experiment Station and the Carnegie Institution of Washington, D. C.

[1] Osborne, T. B., and Mendel, L. B., Feeding Experiments with Isolated Food-Substances, *Carnegie Institution of Washington, Publication 156*, pts. i and ii, 1911.

[2] Osborne and Mendel, *Carnegie Institution of Washington, Publication 156*, pt. ii, 1911, 80. Attention is here called to an error in the description of the preparation of protein-free milk on p. 81, line 1, in which 1.64 cc. should read 164 cc.

256

30 per cent) of the actual milk food to the earlier inefficient protein mixtures is incapable of bringing about growth in any degree equal to that at once initiated when the protein-free milk is added in relative abundance."[3]

In attempting to study the rôle of lipoids in nutrition Stepp[4] had found that milk restored the nutritive efficiency of diets which, by thorough extraction with alcohol and ether, had been rendered inadequate for the nutrition of mice. A little later Hopkins[5] published his noteworthy observations on the effect of additions of fresh milk in securing growth in rats which otherwise failed to grow upon so called "synthetic" dietaries consisting of mixtures of purified proteins, fats, carbohydrates, and salts. From present day standards it is assumed that the addenda of milk used by the different investigators promoted nutrition and growth by furnishing accessory factors or vitamines rather than any of the long familiar nutritive dietary units. Hopkins' experiments differ from our own particularly in respect to the astonishingly small amount of milk that sufficed to render adequate an otherwise ineffective food mixture. This is even more striking in view of the fact that most of the milk solids consist of substances which fall into the categories of the common foodstuffs. Thus Hopkins says:

"In my experiments, while the artificial diet consisted of casein, fat, starch, sugar and inorganic salts, the addendum consisted of milk itself; but this was given in such small quantity that the total solids contained in it amounted to no more than from 1 to 3 or 4 per cent of the whole food eaten. This small addition induced normal growth upon dietaries which without it were incapable even of maintenance. A special feature of my experiments was the rigorous use of controls. In each and every experiment two sets of rats, chosen carefully so as to show correspondence in the weight, sex, and origin of the individuals contained in them, were fed side by side. The sole difference in treatment consisted in the administration of the minute ration of milk to one of the sets compared. In some experiments after the relative rates of growth had been compared for a week or two, the small milk ration was transferred to the set which had been previously fed without it. In all cases the influence of the milk upon growth

---

[3] Osborne and Mendel, *Carnegie Institution of Washington, Publication 156*, pt. ii, 1911, 83.

[4] Stepp, W., *Z. Biol.*, 1912, lvii, 135.

[5] Hopkins, F. G., *J. Physiol.*, 1912, xliv, 425.

was so large that it could not have been due to any alteration in the quality of the protein eaten or in its ratio, nor, in my own belief, to the presence of any known milk constituent."

The quantities of milk just referred to could yield at most an equivalent of 0.3 gm. of protein-free milk per day, thereby constituting no more than 5.2 per cent of the food mixture, in contrast with the 28 per cent which we have been accustomed to use when this product has served as the source of vitamine.

In a subsequent communication Hopkins and Neville[6] again describe the nutritive failure of rats on synthetic diets—a result which we can substantiate—and their improvement as the result of small additions of milk.   Thus they state:

"To six of the above set of rats, after the decline in their weight had begun, 2 cc. of milk *per diem* were given.   An immediate betterment of the general condition of the animals followed; growth was reestablished and the health then maintained.   In another experiment six rats were put upon Osborne and Mendel's diet, but were given milk from the first.   In each case the animal grew."

Hopkins and Neville further state, however:

"When the small ration of milk was given each day in advance of feeding with the Osborne and Mendel diet the food consumption remained of the same order, and did not rise to the amount consumed by the rats in Hopkins' earlier experiments.   The resulting growth though quite definite and steady was distinctly slower than in the experiments mentioned."

We were long ago impressed by the apparent discrepancies in the quantitative relations of the amounts of milk required to furnish the vitamine factor in our experiments in contrast with those of Hopkins.   This was especially true in view of our repeated failures to obtain equally satisfactory results when small proportions of protein-free milk were employed.   For example, even with 14 per cent in the diet the rats failed sooner or later; but, with very few exceptions, they responded promptly when 28 per cent was given.   With quantities varying from 0.28 per cent to 7 per cent the rats failed to complete their growth although some of them made very satisfactory gains during the first few weeks on such diets.   These experiments indicate that individual animals vary greatly in their requirements for this water-soluble

[6] Hopkins, F. G., and Neville, A., *Biochem. J.*, 1913, vii, 97.

vitamine. We have noted the same variability with respect to the quantities of yeast which must be fed to different animals to induce similar amounts of growth.

28 per cent of protein-free milk in the food mixture supplies the equivalent of 30 to 50 cc. of whole milk per day for rats eating from 6 to 10 gm. of food per day when the composition and calorific value of the food approximate that employed by both Hopkins and us. Hopkins himself has commented upon the apparent discrepancies between our earlier results and his. A careful study of his charts will show that the animals which received 5 cc. of milk made better gains than those receiving smaller quantities, and particularly so when the less purified "protene"—a commercial casein product from milk—was employed in his food mixtures. Furthermore the growth of Hopkins' rats even with the larger milk additions was, as a rule, less rapid than is true of rats on our successful food mixtures. Without some information regarding the rate of normal growth of the animals in Hopkins' colony it would be unfair to assume that his experimental animals were far behind the average. In any event the contrast between his experiments with and without milk is sufficiently striking to overshadow the secondary consideration as to whether the quantities of milk employed by him permitted the *maximum* growth which we have taken as our standard.

Newer experiments in which dried *whole* milk was used by us as the source of water-soluble vitamines have indicated that less than 24 per cent is unsatisfactory for inducing rapid growth in food mixtures of the following general type:

	per cent
Casein	18
Milk powder	24
Salt mixture	3
Starch	28
Butter fat	9
Lard	18

This mixture contains the equivalent of 10 per cent of protein-free milk. McCollum and Davis[7] have reported experiments in which smaller proportions of *skimmed milk* powder added to diets containing polished rice induced growth in animals. From a

[7] McCollum, E. V., and Davis, M., *J. Biol. Chem.*, 1915, xxiii, 181.

quantitative standpoint the results are somewhat conflicting; and the records are not directly comparable with those of Hopkins or ourselves owing to the absence of data regarding food intakes. Presumably, however, even under the most favorable conditions in McCollum and Davis' experiments the milk equivalent of the *skimmed milk* powder fed by them was of decidedly larger magnitude than in the case of Hopkins' experiments.

In searching for a tenable explanation of the (quantitatively) inferior results obtained by us we have thought of the possibility that the manipulations, and particularly the heating, incident to the preparation of the dried protein-free milk, as well as the milk powder, might produce a deterioration or loss of the vitamine factor. This seemed somewhat plausible in view of the alleged destruction of the antiscorbutic properties of milk through pasteurization. Accordingly we attempted to duplicate the experience of Hopkins by feeding diets consisting of casein or edestin, starch, a salt mixture, lard, and butter fat, along with which fresh milk was offered in varying quantities to the animal. When 2 cc. of milk per day were given the animals were rarely able to make more than very slight gains in weight, and many of them were barely maintained. Inasmuch as most of the market milk locally available is pasteurized prior to delivery we took the added precaution of securing unpasteurized milk from a high class dairy farm. This did not alter the outcome of our experiments; indeed we have no reason to believe that the nutrition-promoting properties of milk are lost by brief periods of heating.

Comparative trials made with approximately equivalent amounts of protein-free milk as such, and of fresh milk not incorporated with the food mixture, have shown substantially similar outcomes (see Charts I and II). Not until at least 16 cc. of fresh milk per day were supplied along with the food mixture, was anything approaching a normal rate of growth secured. Even this amount sometimes failed. We were at first inclined to attribute such failure to the considerable volume of fluid intake which this addendum entailed, so that the additional quantities of the basal ration sufficient to permit rapid growth were not consumed by the animals. This hypothesis was soon negatived, however, by the demonstration that the further addition of a small amount of brewer's yeast (about 25 mg.) per day served to facilitate growth by markedly raising the food intake in addition to the continued ingestion of the fluid milk.   16 cc. of milk per day had not therefore limited the rats' ability to *eat* sufficient food for growth.

That the deficiency of diets containing the lesser amounts of milk involves the vitamine factor is rendered more than probable by the fact that these comparatively small additions of yeast, the highly efficient growth-promoting power of which we have discussed elsewhere,[8] sufficed to render the previously inadequate ration satisfactory for growth.   As a rule the most significant outcome of the yeast additions (which were fed apart from the rest of the food and therefore could not have altered its flavor) was a larger food intake.   We are not prepared to assert, however, that an augmented food intake is the sole effect of the incorporation of these vitamine-containing products in the dietary.

We are at a loss to explain the apparent differences, in respect to the efficiency of milk as an accessory or vitamine factor in the diet, in the experiments of Hopkins and ourselves.   It scarcely seems plausible that milk from different sources, even though produced by cows on unlike feeds, should account for the wide variations noted; in fact we have used samples from several local sources, always with the same result.   However, it may be recalled that according to McCollum, Simmonds, and Pitz,[9] the efficiency of milk to promote the growth of the young of the same species is believed to be dependent upon a suitable intake of vitamines with the diet, thus suggesting that they are not produced *de novo* in the body of the lactating animal.

It is stated that the vitamines "pass into the milk only as they are present in the diet of the mother, and that milks may vary in their growth-promoting power when the diets of the lactating animals differ widely in their satisfactoriness for the growth of young."[9]

Protein factors cannot be involved here, inasmuch as we have shown that even on a diet inadequate with respect to its protein, the milk of the mother may be suitable for the growth of her young.[10]

[8] Osborne and Mendel, *J. Biol. Chem.*, 1917, xxxi, 149.
[9] McCollum, E. V., Simmonds, N., and Pitz, W., *J. Biol. Chem.*, 1916, xxvii, 33.
[10] Osborne and Mendel, *J. Biol. Chem.*, 1912, xii, 473.

The evidence of various investigators regarding the antineuritic value of milk, however, is not at variance with our experience in the study of growth.   Cooper[11] found milk far inferior to various animal tissues in curing or preventing avian polyneuritis.   According to Gibson and Concepción[12] in feeding experiments with fowls, pigs, and dogs, in the Philippines, the results obtained showed the antineuritic vitamines to be present in milk in slight amounts only, and that the continued feeding of either fresh or autoclaved milk without suitable additions to the diet induced symptoms of beri-beri.   The authors conclude that the antineuritic powers of milk are so slight that in infant feeding the diet should be extended as soon as possible; and that the young of healthy mothers are probably born with a reserve supply of the so called vitamine substances sufficient to maintain them in good nutritive condition until the time when they begin to eat other foodstuffs.

From a practical standpoint a more precise understanding of the quantitative relations of the vitamines is highly desirable.   The fact that such diverse cellular structures as yeast, wheat embryo, corn germs, and glandular tissues[13] show a surprising richness in growth-promoting properties aside from their protein and mineral content, is of immediate significance at a time when milk is still so uniquely valued for its nutrient virtues.   Of course, the problem of the fat-soluble vitamine in milk is not here considered.   It is not unlikely, however, that the need of children and other growing animals for the water-soluble vitamine, beyond the earlier stages of development when milk admittedly satisfies the nutritive requirements, may not be adequately filled by some of the current or enforced dietary practices.   Thus with a too scanty allowance of milk, a liberal inclusion of products from cereals rendered poor in vitamine by milling, of sugar, fats, and few additional animal products other than meat (which has been shown to contain relatively little of the water-soluble vitamine[14]), it is not surprising if disasters sometimes manifest themselves.

In view of the results of Hopkins' experiments it has become

[11] Cooper, E. A., *J. Hyg.*, 1912, xii, 436; 1914, xiv, 12.
[12] Gibson, R. B., and Concepción, I., *Philippine J. Sc.*, *B*, 1916, xi, 119.
[13] Osborne and Mendel, *J. Biol. Chem.*, 1917, xxxii, 309; 1918, xxxiv, 17.
[14] Osborne and Mendel, *J. Biol. Chem.*, 1917, xxxii, 209.

generally believed that milk is one of the richest sources of the water-soluble vitamines among our food products. Whatever explanation may ultimately be found for the much larger amounts of milk needed to promote normal growth in our rats compared with Hopkins' rats, it seems advisable for the present in practice to use a liberal amount of milk when this is depended on to supply any considerable proportion of this most necessary food factor.

A particular case of this kind is that of infant feeding where it is customary to reinforce the supply of calories by diluting top milk and adding milk sugar. Under these circumstances the child is supplied with a food that contains a relatively smaller proportion of the water-soluble vitamine than does the original cow's milk. While milk thus modified may contain sufficient vitamine as long as the food intake is normal, if for any reason the child's appetite fails the vitamine supply is reduced and endless dietary troubles may easily result. It is not improbable that a large part of the difficulties of artificially feeding babies is due to this cause, and that these can be obviated as successfully by securing an adequate supply of this indispensable constituent of a suitable diet as has been the case in feeding animals on artificial diets since we have learned how properly to provide this food factor.

This is a practical question which deserves prompt investigation, for the best way to reinforce the vitamine content of the diluted milk is not yet evident, chiefly owing to our still limited knowledge of the distribution of this vitamine in nature. Such investigations as have been made demonstrate that the proportion of water-soluble vitamine in the various vegetable and animal tissues differs greatly, and it is probable that sooner or later some way will be found to a solution of the problem of successful infant feeding.

[Editor's Note: Page 545 is a blank page.]

CHART I. The records in Series A show the comparative effect of additions of varying quantities—2 to 16 cc.—of fresh cow's milk to a diet otherwise devoid of water-soluble vitamine and consisting of

		per cent
Casein		18.0
Salt mixture*		4.5
Starch		50.5
Butter fat		9.0
Lard		18.0

It will be noted that continued vigorous growth was not attained until the larger quantities of milk were supplied. When addition of 16 cc. of milk failed to promote growth on the above diet a small amount of yeast (25 mg. of brewer's yeast, dried) often sufficed to improve nutrition, and the effect of its removal was promptly manifested (see Rats 4438, 4443). That the milk furnished some vitamine is shown by the speedy decline after its removal from the diet, in Rat 4434, despite the presence of the yeast. Without milk at least 100 mg. of yeast per day were required to promote growth in the rats on this diet, as shown in the final periods for Series A, Rats 4434, 4438, 4443.

Series B likewise shows the slight promoting effect of 2 cc. of milk in the first periods, in contrast with the experience of Hopkins. When fresh milk was replaced by protein-free milk (in the periods indicated by the dotted lines) no better results were obtained until larger quantities, i. e. more than 5.6 per cent, of the food were furnished. Small supplements of yeast, as well as increments in the quantity of protein-free milk sufficed to facilitate growth.

In Series B the food consisted of

		per cent
Edestin		18.0
Salt mixture*		0.0– 4.5
Protein-free milk		28.0– 0.0
Starch		25.0–48.5
Butter fat		9.0
Lard		20.0

* The composition of the salt mixture is given in *J. Biol. Chem.*, 1917, xxxii, 317.

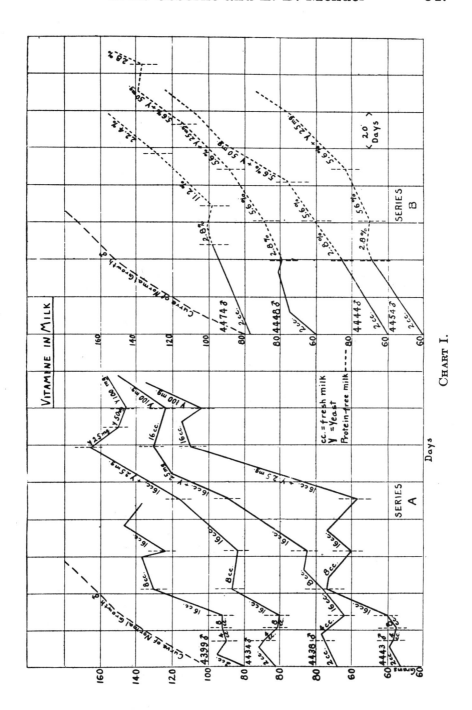

CHART I.

Chart II. Showing the comparative effect of supplements of fresh milk (unbroken lines) or protein-free milk (dotted lines) as sources of water-soluble vitamine added to diets consisting of

	per cent
Casein or edestin......................................	18.0
Protein-free milk.....................................	0.0–22.4
Salt mixture*..	4.5– 1.0
Starch...	47.7–31.6
Butter fat...	9.0
Lard...	18.0–20.0

It will be noted that growth was not vigorous until considerable quantities of fresh milk or protein-free milk were used. Small quantities comparable to the amounts of fresh milk used in Hopkins' experiments were of little avail. The use of yeast (Y) even in small quantities always promoted the nutritive result.

Rat 4484 which grew unusually well on a diet containing only 5.6 per cent of the protein-free milk illustrates the occasional variations which are observed whenever large numbers of nutrition experiments are made to ascertain the minimum of some essential dietary factor. Generalizations should, therefore, only be drawn from a considerable number of individual trials.

* The composition of the salt mixture is given in *J. Biol. Chem.*, 1917, xxxii. 317.

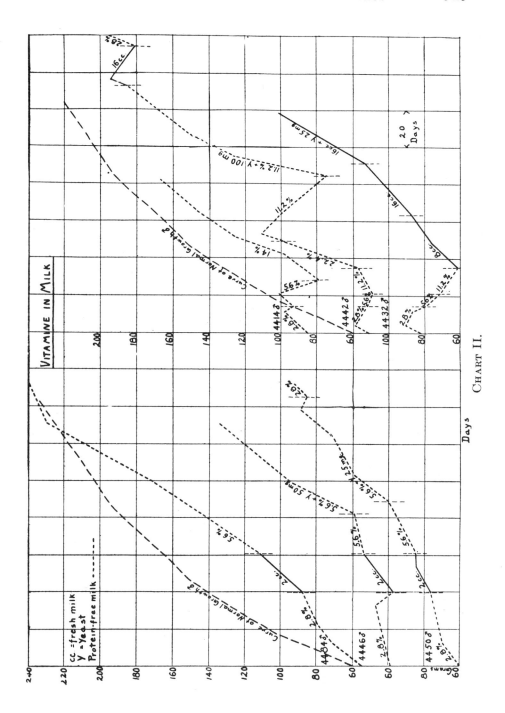

CHART II.

CHART III. Showing the effect of additions of varying amounts of milk (recorded in cc.), milk powder (per cent), or yeast (Y), as sources of water-soluble vitamine in a diet consisting of

	per cent
Casein	18.0
Milk powder	0.0–48.0
Salt mixture*	4.5– 1.0
Starch	50.0–18.0
Butter fat	9.0
Lard	18.0

As in Charts I and II, growth was far from satisfactory until the milk additions were considerable in amount. Yeast invariably augmented the effect of the milk.

* The composition of the salt mixture is given in *J. Biol. Chem.*,1917. xxxii, 317.

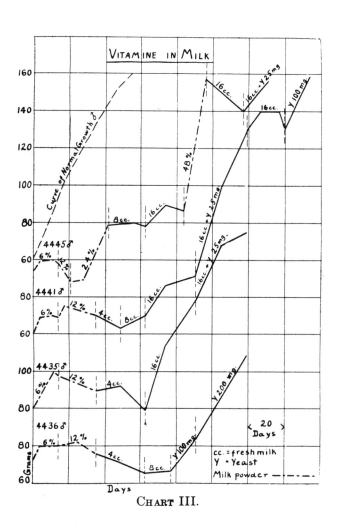

CHART III.

24

Reprinted from *Lancet*, 407–412 (Mar. 15, 1919)

AN EXPERIMENTAL INVESTIGATION ON RICKETS

Edward Mellanby, *The Brown Institute, London University*

LECTURE I.

HAVING described in the first two lectures of this course the experimental results obtained in a Research on Alcohol for the Central Control Board (Liquor Traffic), I propose in the next lectures to deal with another social evil—rickets—and to give an account of an experimental investigation made for the Medical Research Committee with the object of finding the essential cause of this disease.

THE SERIOUS RESULTS OF RICKETS.

It is but little realised how great and how widespread is the part played by rickets in civilised communities. If the matter ended with bony deformities obvious to the eye it would be bad enough, but investigations have demonstrated that such deformities only represent a small part of the cases affected. Schmorl's histological investigations on children dying before the age of 4 years showed that 90 per cent. had had rickets. Again, Lawson Dick's examination of the children in London County Council schools, and more particularly the examination of their teeth, led him to state that 80 per cent. of such children had had rickets. The relation between rickets and defective teeth has been placed on an experimental basis recently by the work of my wife,[1] and there can be little doubt that any remedy which would exclude the one would almost certainly improve and might eradicate the other. The rachitic child, in fact, carries the stigma of the disease throughout life in the form of defective teeth.

Nor is this the most serious part of the evil, for the reduced resistance to other diseases of the rachitic child and animal is so marked that the causative factor of rickets may be the secret of immunity and non-immunity to many of the children's diseases which result in the high death-rate associated with urban conditions. It is a striking fact to remember that in the West of Ireland, where the death-rate is only 30 per 1000, rickets is an unknown disease, whereas in poor urban districts of this country where rickets is rife the death-rate in children varies from 100 to 300 per 1000. It is at least suggestive that there may be some relation between rickets and the enormous death-rate of towns, even although the disease in itself does not kill.

The experimental work I wish to describe in these lectures has shown that the rachitic condition need not be at all advanced before the animal's whole behaviour is transformed. It becomes lethargic and is far more liable to be affected by distemper and broncho-pneumonia and is very susceptible to mange. The low resistance of animals which develops as the result of conditions which ultimately lead, under favourable circumstances, to rickets is impressive.

So many of the conclusions regarding the ætiology of rickets have been based on a small number of experiments that it may not be out of place to record that this investigation, undertaken for the Medical Research Committee, has already involved the use of 200 puppies and is still incomplete.

On referring to the literature at the beginning of the research it was soon obvious that the number of hypotheses put forward to explain the ætiology of rickets was legion, while discussion on the subject with those having clinical knowledge only emphasised the completely speculative nature of the ideas held by those whose business it is to deal with the disease.

A considerable number of experiments were first made in an attempt to see whether the ætiology of rickets was to be sought along non-dietetic lines and it was only after failure that the dietetic solution was resorted to. This type of work has continued and has clearly shown that, however important other factors may be, and that there are other factors is not denied, the dietetic problem is the primary key to the situation. In the next lecture some of the more commonly held hypotheses of rickets will be mentioned and discussed in relation to the results obtained in this work.

EXPERIMENTAL METHODS.

Although it is well recognised that different breeds of

[1] THE LANCET, 1918, ii., 767.

dogs vary considerably in their susceptibility to rickets, no special type has been used in this work. In some ways this may be disadvantageous; but, on the other hand, to be driven to associate rickets with a particular breed is in itself unsatisfactory and obviously leads the investigator into a blind alley if the ultimate object is to extend the results to children.

The experimental methods used to detect rickets have depended on (1) X ray examination of the bones; (2) calcium estimation of the bones after death; (3) histological preparations of the bones.

The calcium estimation of the bones has been made by Cahen and Hurtley's modification of the oxalate method. In comparative estimations it is useful; but, since it is well recognised that the calcium content of bones varies considerably and independently of the rachitic condition, this method can never be used alone and must always be controlled by histological examination. [In the lecture further details of the methods were described and X ray photographs and histological specimens were demonstrated by means of the epidiascope].

In these lectures I propose to illustrate the normality and degree of rickets obtained by means of the calcium oxide content of the bones. Histological preparations can be seen if desired and also the X ray photographs of many of the dogs. In all cases histological preparations of the bones were made and corresponded, in comparative experiments, with the CaO results given.

[A series of puppies with and without rickets was then shown]. In the puppies exhibited it will be observed that the differences between normal and rachitic puppies are similar to the differences between normal and rachitic children. Like the rachitic child, the puppy shows abnormally large swellings at the epiphyseal ends of the bones; it has a marked rickety rosary, its tendons and ligaments are loose, the bones tend to bend, and thereby help to exaggerate the leg deformity. The amount of deformity often depends on the weight of the animal. Again, the rachitic puppy is lethargic and does not jump about; its power to run, apart from the leg deformity and before this develops, is comparatively limited; there is, in fact, a general loss of tone of the musculature. Similarly, just as the rachitic baby is a good baby and does not cry much, so also the dog in this condition seldom barks or makes the superfluous efforts practised by the normal healthy puppy.

The puppies were started on their diets after leaving the mother, the ages varying between 5 and 8 weeks, the latter being the more usual. They were kept for varying periods according to the type of experiments. In the earlier periods they were usually killed after five to six months, but as the work progressed and the diets became more rachitic this time was considerably shortened.

DETERMINATION OF RACHITIC DIET.

Having determined to see what part diet played as a causative factor in rickets, it was necessary to get a standard diet which would always produce this condition in the experimental animals. The first diet used consisted of whole milk (175 c.cm. per diem) and porridge made up of equal parts oatmeal and rice, together with 1–2 g. NaCl. The oatmeal and rice was later replaced by bread and found to be as effective and easier to use. This second diet was afterwards modified as the experimental results were obtained. The following four diets (Table I.) have therefore been used

TABLE I.—*Rachitic Diets.*

Diet I.	Diet II.	Diet III	Diet IV.
Whole milk, 175 c.cm.	Whole milk, 175 c.cm.	Separated milk, 175 c.cm.	Separated milk, 250–350 c.cm.
Oatmeal, rice. 1–2 g. NaCl.	Bread ad lib.	Bread (70 per cent. wheaten) ad lib.	Bread (70 per cent. wheaten) ad lib.
		Linseed oil, 10 c.cm.	Linseed oil, 5–15 c.cm.
		Yeast, 10 g.	Yeast, 5–10 g.
		NaCl, 1–2 g.	Orange juice, 3 c.cm.
			NaCl, 1–2 g.

during the course of the work, each one of which is a rachitic diet under laboratory conditions.

The modifications of the diets were carried out in order to : (1) ensure a more rapid development of rickets ; (2) to be compatible with better health and better rate of growth. As will be seen later, the better the animal grows on a rachitic diet the more easily is rickets produced or rather the more difficult it is to stop. In the close examination of foodstuffs from this point of view, this is eminently desirable. It is undesirable in such work to have animals in a semi-starved condition involving a high mortality due to broncho-pneumonia and marasmus. Puppies, like all young animals, tend to develop these diseases unless the diet is well chosen.

RESULTS OF ADDITION OF VARIOUS SUBSTANCES TO RACHITIC DIET.

Having obtained diets which normally produce rickets, various substances were added and the effect on the development of the disease noted. In the following tables the quantity of calcium estimated as CaO present in the shaft of the femurs of the animals fed on these diets is given. In the last column the histological findings of the bones examined are added.

TABLE II.—*Diet I. plus more Whole Milk.*

No. of experiment	Diet.	Duration. Months.	Initial weight.	Final weight.	Gain.	CaO in femur shaft. Dry.	CaO in femur shaft. Fresh.	Histology results.
			g.	g.	g.	%	%	
43	Diet I.	4	905	2187	1282	23·5	—	Rickets.
52	,,	8	1745	5200	3455	23·5	—	,,
53	,,	7½	1765	4245	2480	22·5	—	,,
56	+ 325 c.cm. milk.	5	1810	5280	3470	31·8	—	Normal.
57	+ 325 ,,	5	1330	4980	3650	29·2	—	,,

TABLE III.—*Diet II. plus Meat and Meat Extracts.*

No. of experiment	Diet.	Duration. Months.	Initial weight.	Final weight.	Gain.	CaO in femur shaft. Dry.	CaO in femur shaft. Fresh.	Histology results.
73	Diet II.	4	3950	6110	2160	20·7	—	Rickets.
96	+ dog biscuit.	5½	1905	4200	2295	22·1	9·38	,,
97	,,	5½	1375	3295	1920	16·03	5·90	,,
68	+ Wat. ext. of meat.	4	4000	6540	2540	32·8	—	Normal.
69	+ Meat protein.	5	4840	7630	2790	21·7	—	Rickets.
70	+ 80 % alc. ext. of meat.	5	4577	6695	2118	30·2	—	Normal.
93	+ 10 g. meat.	5½	1220	7450	6230	29·53	15·43	,,

TABLE IV.—*Diet II. plus Yeast and Malt Extract.*

No. of experiment	Diet.	Duration. Months.	Initial weight.	Final weight.	Gain.	CaO in femur shaft. Dry.	CaO in femur shaft. Fresh.	Histology results.
96	Diet II.	5½	1905	4200	2295	16·03	5·90	Rickets.
94	+ 10-20 g. yeast.	5½	1590	5000	3410	23·05	11·33	,,
95	,,	6	2410	6000	3590	18·02	9·75	,,
75	+ Malt ext.	4	3350	5240	1890	31·2	—	Normal.
86	,,	7	1810	4500	2690	18·68	12·64	Slight rickets.

TABLE V.—*Diet II. plus Different Fats.*

No. of experiment	Diet.	Duration. Months.	Initial weight.	Final weight.	Gain.	CaO in femur shaft. Dry.	CaO in femur shaft. Fresh.	Histology results.
73	Diet II.	4	3950	6110	2160	20·7	—	Rickets.
71	+ 10-20 g. butter.	6	2150	6930	4780	29·04	15·5	Normal.
76	+ 10 c.cm. cod-liver oil.	3	2715	8000	5285	27·41	16·82	,,
80	+ 10 c.cm. linseed oil.	5	2535	6115	3580	16·22	8·08	Rickets.
81	,, ,,	5	2875	5320	2445	13·33	6·08	,,
109	+ 10 c.cm. peanut.	5½				26·35	15·60	Normal.
102	+ Wat. ext. of butter.	6				16·64	6·95	Rickets.

TABLE VI.—*Diet III. with Various Fats instead of Linseed Oil.*

No. of experiment	Diet.	Duration.	Initial weight.	Final weight.	Gain.	CaO in femur shaft. Dry.	CaO in femur shaft. Fresh.	Histology results.
		Weeks.						
138	Diet III.	3	1755	2685	930	16·58	7·14	Rickets.
140	,,	3	1060	2100	940	20·46	7·36	,,
148	With cod-liver oil.	17	1735	3890	2155	27·78	16·51	Normal.
146	With butter.	17	1920	3765	1845	26·95	15·89	,,
147	With olive oil.	17	1445	2625	1180	23·79	13·22	Slight rickets.
163	With peanut.	17	2350	4020	1670	18·88	13·81	,,
145	Diet III.	17	1830	3605	1775	21·60	12·35	Rickets.

TABLE VII. *Diet III. Plus Meat and Meat Extracts.*

No. of experiment	Diet.	Duration.	Initial weight.	Final weight.	Gain.	CaO in femur shaft. Dry.	CaO in femur shaft. Fresh.	Histology results.
141	Diet III. + 5 g. meat.	17	2490	5820	3330	17·48	7·19	Rickets.
143	+ 20 g. meat.	17	2890	4400	1510	17·83	9·48	,,
144	+ 50 g. meat.	17	3690	8825	5135	15·74	10·72	,,
160	+ Watery ext. of 50 g. meat.	12	2005	3825	1820	13·88	7·20	,,

Using Diet I., we see in Table II. that increasing the whole milk from 175 to 500 c.cm. per diem prevents the development of rickets. In other tables are experimental results obtained by means of Diet II.

On Diet II. not only does meat but both the watery and alcoholic (80 per cent.) extracts have an inhibitory effect. (Table III.) On the other hand, the protein residue after loss of extractives allows rickets to develop.

Table IV. shows the effect of adding malt extract and yeast to Diet II. Yeast therefore has no protective influence. Malt extract has some inhibitory action and delays the onset of rickets when added to Diet II.

A large number of experiments were now made in which the effect of different fats were analysed. A few of the results are given in Table V. Many other fats and margarines, animal and vegetable, were tested, but almost uniformly they prevented rickets, the only undoubted exception being linseed oil. The results allowed the evolution of Diet III., in which separated milk was used in order to eliminate the milk fat, whose place was taken by linseed oil. Yeast was also added to the diet. Using this diet, a closer analysis of the effect of different fats was possible. (Table VI.) Now we see from the calcium results, which are an accurate indication in this case of the rachitic picture, that the value of the oils is graded, cod-liver oil being the best and linseed oil the worst ; the vegetable oils, olive and arachis, are not so good as butter.

It was found that adding orange juice (¼ orange per diem) did not prevent rickets. Further, that the addition of 5 g. calcium phosphate, or doubling the separated milk and so increasing the calcium intake in this form was without preventive action on the development of the disease. In Diet IV., therefore, the separated milk was doubled and 3 c.cm. orange juice per diem also given. On Diet IV. the growth and general health of the puppies seemed better, and both these factors are of importance in such an investigation. Another improvement was to substitute 5 g. of yeast by a small quantity of a commercial yeast extract (3–4 g. per diem).

On Diets III. and IV. it was found that small quantities of meat and meat extract did not prevent rickets developing, as they have previously been observed to do when used in addition to Diet II. Table VII. illustrates some of these results. Although meat did not prevent rickets, a closer analysis of these and other results showed that it did have some inhibitory effect. It will be noticed, for instance, that the CaO present in the fresh femur shaft of Exp. 144, where 50 g. of meat was eaten, is higher than in Exp. 141. where only 5 g. of meat was added to Diet III. The action of small quantities of meat (10 g. per diem) is best seen when given with quantities or types of fat otherwise ineffective in preventing rickets. It will often be seen to keep the growth normal, whereas in its absence rickets would develop. This, no doubt, explains the experimental results obtained when meat was added to Diet II. The small amount of butter—i.e., about 5 to 7 g.—in the milk of this diet had its anti-rachitic effect enhanced by the small amount of meat.

On Diet III. it was seen that the action of the fats as regards rickets was graded, the animal fats being more anti-rachitic than the vegetable fats and the latter differing from each other greatly. The best of the vegetable fats in preventing rickets are arachis (peanut) and olive oils. The worst of those examined include linseed, cottonseed, babassu oils, a hydrogenated fat, and cocoanut oil. These oils were all refined.

IMPORTANCE OF DIETETIC FACTOR.

The above dietetic results indicate that diet plays an important part in the etiology of rickets. An examination of the results obtained suggests that rickets is a deficiency disease which develops in consequence of the absence of some accessory food factor or factors.

Of the three factors known, fat-soluble A, water-soluble B, and antiscorbutic, two of these can be at once excluded. Yeast has no preventive influence on the development of the disease, and in consequence water-soluble B cannot be considered as of importance. Again, orange juice, sufficient to exclude any possibility of scurvy when considered with the rest of the diet, did not inhibit the disease, and this therefore allows the exclusion of the antiscorbutic factor. On the other hand, the anti-rachitic substances for the most part have been found, so far as the rickets experiments have gone, to be similar to those in which, according to the experiments on growth, of McCollum, Osborne, Mendel, and others, fat-soluble A is present. It therefore seems probable that the cause of rickets is a diminished intake of an anti-rachitic factor which is either fat-soluble A, or has a somewhat similar distribution to fat-soluble A. The facts are not all in favour of this hypothesis as it stands, and these will be discussed in the next lecture.

Another point which has been definitely established in the course of this work is that rickets develops much more readily in the fast-growing puppies than in those growing slowly. As might be expected, therefore, the prevention of rickets in a rapidly growing dog requires more anti-rachitic factor to keep the growth straight. This point is brought out in the case of two puppies of the same litter (Exps. 173 and 174) fed on the same diets (Diet IV. + 10 g. meat). The larger puppy grew much more rapidly than the other. Puppy (K) 173 increased from 1130 to 2240 g.—i.e., a gain of 1110 g. in 10 weeks, whilst L (Exp. 174) increased in weight from 1800 to 3970 g.—i.e., a gain of 2170 g. in the same period. It will be seen in the X ray photographs that rickets is more strongly developed in the faster growing dog, although both are rachitic, the diets being deficient in the anti-rachitic factor. Puppies of the same litter which received 10 g. of butter in addition to the diets received by Nos. 173 and 174 were normal.

LECTURE II.

We saw in the last lecture the manner in which the experiments were carried out, together with some of the main results. Substances which had no preventive action on the development of rickets included separated milk, bread, the protein of meat, yeast, linseed and babassu oils, and hydrogenated fat. Substances with well-marked preventive action included cod-liver oil, butter, and suet. Then there were other substances whose preventive action was definite but not so great as that possessed by the above animal fats. In this group were meat, meat extract, malt extract, lard, arachis and olive oils.

THE PART PLAYED BY FAT-SOLUBLE A.

The results seemed to favour the hypothesis that experimental rickets can be prevented by diets containing an abundance of anti-rachitic factor and that the anti-rachitic factor and fat-soluble A have somewhat similar distributions. There are, however, several points which are not in harmony with the ordinarily accepted views about fat-soluble A. Three of these will be discussed.

Relation of Rapidity of Growth to Development of Rickets.

Rickets develops best in rapidly growing animals, this fact being in harmony with the clinical observation that large and rapidly growing children most often suffer from rickets, whereas marasmic children generally escape. It is, therefore, difficult at first sight to associate a disease of rapid growth with a deficiency of fat-soluble A which is, according to accepted teaching, necessary for growth. For it has been shown, in the case of rats by McCollum, that both fat-soluble A and water-soluble B are essential for growth. Before fat-soluble A and the anti-rachitic factor can be held to be the same thing, further consideration is necessary.

The first point to emphasise is that some of the fastest growing dogs in these experiments have had very little fat-soluble A in their diet. Here are two examples :—

	Exp. 144.	Exp. 175.
Diet III. + 50 g. of meat per diem ...	....	–
Initial weight	3690 g.	–
Increase in weight in 13 weeks...	5135 g.	4585 g.
Rickets	Marked	Very slight.

If the milk were completely separated, Diet III. ought to have contained no fat-soluble A. Meat is reputed to contain little or no fat-soluble A when devoid of fat. The fat was dissected off as completely as possible, but there was undoubtedly a little not removed.

The following experiments show that when only 10 or 5 g. of meat were added, or even without any meat, good growth was obtained.

In experiments 186 and 185 no meat was present in the diet and yet the puppies grew considerably, though, it is true, not to quite the extent of Exp. 190 where the fat eaten was cod-liver oil, which is known to contain fat-soluble A.

—	Exp. 176.	Exp. 141.	Exp. 186.	Exp. 185.	Exp. 190.
Diet	D. III. + 10 g. meat.	D. III. + 5 g. meat.	D. IV. (Linseed oil).	D. IV. (Olive for linseed).	D. IV. (Cod-liver for linseed).
Increase in weight ...	2930 g. in 10 weeks.	2720 g. in 10 weeks.	1200 g. in 5 weeks.	1100 g. in 5 weeks.	1525 g. in 5 weeks.
Condition ...	Rickets.	Rickets.	Rickets.	?	Normal.

These results cannot fail to raise the question as to the necessity of fat-soluble A being present in the diet before growth is possible. As the experiments were not carried out from the point of view under discussion I do not naturally deny that fat-soluble A is necessary for growth, more especially as the separation of the milk in the diets was not always perfect. I think, however, that it can be definitely stated that the amount of growth a puppy experiences has no relation to the amount of fat-soluble A in the diet, although a small minimum amount may be necessary. It is, of course, possible that puppies can make use of considerable stores of fat-soluble A in their own tissues, which will allow growth for some months even in the circumstances of deficient fat-soluble A in the diet.

It has, however, been already pointed out in this work that large and rapidly growing puppies require more anti-rachitic factor to prevent the development of rickets. If, therefore, fat-soluble A and the anti-rachitic factor are identical the presumption is that the function of fat-soluble A in the diet of puppies is not so much to ensure growth as to promote correct growth ; in other words, to keep the growth straight : and the greater the amount of growth in any period the greater is the amount of fat-soluble A necessary to keep it along normal lines. If this view is correct, then it can hardly be claimed that fat-soluble A is in any different category from the point of view of growth than the antiscorbutic factor, for, even in the absence of this latter, the rate of growth diminishes and there is often rapid loss of weight.

The Action of Meat and Meat Extracts.

The second difficulty involved in considering the anti-rachitic factor and fat-soluble A as identical is the part which meat and meat extracts play in the development of rickets. It has been seen that, although when added to Diet II. these substances prevent rickets, in the case of Diet III. rickets develop. Yet even in the Diet III. and IV. experiments, the action of meat is undoubtedly inhibitory in nature and, when 50 g. of meat are given, will almost prevent rickets in a small puppy. Just as in the last section it was seen that meat has a stimulating action on the growth of puppies far beyond its fat-soluble A content, so also it appears now that the anti-rachitic action of meat is in a greater measure than any fat-soluble A it is reputed to contain. Either we must recognise that meat contains more fat-soluble A than the rat-feeding experiments have led us to believe or we must endeavour to find another explanation of the action of meat in rickets. It seems to me that another explanation is possible.

It is known that meat has one action on metabolism, which is more strongly developed than in any other food-stuff. This is its specific dynamic action or power to stimulate the total chemical exchanges taking place in the body. In having this stimulating action it will increase the effectiveness of any fat-soluble A in the diet and will tend to prevent the storing up and deposition of this substance in the subcutaneous and other tissues. Again, any fat-soluble A in the tissues will be more readily mobilised under the stimulating influence of the metabolising meat. It is probable that the anti-rachitic action of meat may therefore be due more to its making the fires burn more brightly, and thereby increasing the effectiveness of any fat-soluble A present in the body, rather than to the fat-soluble A it possesses in itself. If this explanation of the action of meat be true, then it is still possible to regard fat-soluble A and the anti-rachitic factor as identical.

The Different Effects of Vegetable Oils.

The third difficulty, which is probably of less importance than the two foregoing, is the widely different action of the vegetable fats as regards the development of rickets. In the growth experiments of previous workers all the vegetable fats are described as deficient in fat-soluble A, and the impression is received that there is but little difference between them. On the other hand, their anti-rachitic influence varies considerably, being obviously present in arachis and olive oils and absent in linseed and babassu oils. Other vegetable oils like cocoanut and cottonseed occupy an intermediate position. If the anti-rachitic factor is fat-soluble A, then it must be accepted that the type of experiment described in this work is a more delicate test for fat-soluble A than previous work involving the growth of rats.

The difficulties have now been stated and briefly discussed. On the whole, it will probably be agreed that they are not formidable, and not more than might be expected under the circumstances.

Since this is probably the first research on growth factors carried out on dogs, it might be expected that the facts would not be identical with those met with in rats. Again, a superficial survey of the question suggests that particular difficulties would be met with. For we know something of the part played by accessory food factors in such deficiency diseases as beri-beri and scurvy, and we know something of the part played by these substances in growth, but in the case of rickets we are apparently up against a combination of both a deficiency disease and growth, rickets, in fact, being a disease accompanying growth. Whether the anti-rachitic factor is fat-soluble A as previously understood is therefore undecided, but, on the whole, these substances appear to be identical. It is at least certain that the distribution of the two substances is remarkably similar.

REVIEW OF SOME EARLIER HYPOTHESES AS TO ÆTIOLOGY.

It is interesting to see how the facts brought out in this work fit in with some of the most commonly held hypotheses of the ætiology of rickets. I think it will be agreed that the accessory factor hypothesis allows many of these older hypotheses to be so focussed that a common and simple image is visible.

Dietetic Hypothesis.

Rickets as a disease due to deficiency of fat.—The work of Bland-Sutton on the lion cubs at the Zoological Gardens has left its impress on English thought as regards rickets and, together with the acknowledged efficacious results that follow the treatment of rachitic children with cod-liver oil and other fats, has brought about a general acceptance of the view that rickets is due to deficient fat in the diet. The results recorded here make it clear why this view is so commonly held, but demonstrate that the efficacy of the treatment—curative or preventive (as regards the latter the work of Hess and Unger is of particular interest)—does not depend on fat *per se*, but rather on the type of fat, and whether it contains an abundance of the anti-rachitic factor, animal fats being superior to vegetable fats.

Excess of carbohydrate in the diet.—When a diet contains excess of carbohydrate it means that it is made up largely of cereals. Now cereals, and more particularly cereals like wheat, rice, and oats, which have undergone transformation in the course of manufacturing processes, are most deficient in anti-rachitic factor. A diet, therefore, of such substances is quite unbalanced and most effective in producing rickets.

Deficiency of fat and excess of carbohydrate.—This condition comprises the first two hypotheses, and what is said about them can be extended with further emphasis to this suggestion. Such a combination would most certainly involve a deficiency of anti-rachitic factor.

Deficiency of calcium salts in the diet.—It has been seen previously that abundance of calcium in the diet, either in the form found in separated milk or in calcium phosphate, will not prevent rickets when the diet is deficient in anti-rachitic factor. Similarly, it has been found by some workers that a diet deficient only in calcium salts, but otherwise adequate, will not produce rickets. It is, however, more than probable that a deficient calcium intake associated with deficient anti-rachitic factor will bring about a more acute production of rickets, and must always be an adjuvant factor to be considered in the ætiology of rickets.

The "Domestication" Theory of Rickets.

Von Hansemann's "theory of domestication" includes in a comprehensive way all the unhygienic conditions associated with life in civilised and more particularly in crowded communities. The difficulty is that we have not yet complete knowledge as to what is unhygienic in the environment of civilisation. There is something subtle about the problem, and many of the factors about which we hear so much may be of little or no importance when compared with factors about which nothing is at present known. Modern mode of life, and particularly of urban life, has involved two main changes in environment: (1) diet; (2) greater confinement and lack of fresh air. My experimental results have indicated that the dietetic changes are of prime importance in bringing about the widespread development of rickets, although, according to the researches here described, diet must be considered from an entirely new point of view.

Effects of Confinement.

At this point I wish to consider the part played by confinement in the ætiology of rickets, more particularly because in recent years the experimental work of Findlay has indicated that it may be of importance. Findlay's work involved the use of 12 dogs fed on a diet of oatmeal porridge and milk (amount not stated). It will be seen that this diet is similar to Diet I. used in my experiments, a diet which normally produced rickets in experimental puppies. (Diet I. was composed of whole milk 175 c.cm., oatmeal and rice, and 1-2 g. NaCl.) On this diet, then, the confined dogs were rachitic, the dogs obtaining exercise normal.

It seems to me that, working with such a diet, which approaches a rachitic diet, experimental results can only show that want of exercise is a factor in the production of rickets, but cannot be regarded as proof that it is the primary factor. Before the acceptance of this hypothesis is possible it must be shown that confinement on an adequate diet—that is to say, one compatible with the best health, always brings about rickets. Certainly the porridge and milk diet, unless the milk is large, cannot be considered healthy (in three months two of Findlay's confined puppies died of broncho-pneumonia and one of marasmus).

The beneficial effect of freedom in the case of dogs on an inadequate diet is what might be expected and is not, in my opinion, discordant with a dietetic hypothesis. The constant movement must raise the whole metabolic changes in the body and, in the first place, prevent or delay the deposition of fat with its accessory food factor in the subcutaneous and other depôts and, secondly, bring into activity any anti-rachitic factor normally stored away and ineffective. Exercise, in other words, must give a greater opportunity to any anti-rachitic factor in the food or tissues of the animal to play its part in the animal economy. In addition to this, exercise or the possibility of exercise undoubtedly improves the animal's health, and it is almost certain that a rachitic diet is more effective in producing rickets when the animal's health is subnormal as it may be following continuous confinement.

A strongly rachitic diet after a few weeks has a decided effect on the animal's activity, and it is difficult to give any real exercise to a puppy that is rachitic even though the bony and ligamentous changes may not be the disability which limits the movement. On the other hand, confinement generally fails to prevent a well-fed puppy from taking abundant exercise. The analogy can probably be applied with greater force to children; a well-fed child between 9 months and 2 years can get exercise whatever its environment, whilst a child with active rickets will show the same lethargy in a slum or the middle of Hyde Park. The activity of an infant is not to be measured by the amount of running it performs, but by its small movements. My own experience is that confinement will not produce any symptoms of rickets in adequately fed puppies.

Results of Investigation in Glasgow.

It may not be out of place to refer to the recent statistical account of an investigation made by Miss Ferguson on rickets, more particularly in Glasgow. The results of this work are against the hypothesis that rickets is a dietetic deficiency disease and the general conclusion, although undetermined in a definite sense, is that the factors favouring the development of rickets are: (1) Insufficient space in houses; (2) confinement in such houses; (3) imperfect parental care. No support is given to the dietetic hypothesis. It is interesting, however, to examine some of the results relating to family budgets in this paper.

Below are given the tables relating to the "average consumption of food" (p. 68) in rachitic and non-rachitic families.

Now let us consider the tables, obtained by Miss Ferguson, in the light of the accessory factor hypothesis. First, what are the substances in the diets which allow rickets—i.e., are

Average Consumption per "Man" per Day of the Chief Articles of Diet in Grammes.

(1) Rachitic families.   (2) Non-rachitic families.

—	(1)	(2)	—	(1)	(2)
Flour	387·9	376·2	Other cereals	15·6	26·9
Potatoes	291·0	236·8	Margarine or butter	33·6	38·5
Milk	256·0	309·0	Fish	15·7	35·9
Meat	89·1	92·6	Eggs	15·1	30·4
Sugar	91·4	84·0	Cheese	6·7	8·2
Oatmeal	40·4	36·0			

deficient in anti-rachitic factor? The answer is flour, potatoes, sugar, oatmeal, and other cereals. On the other hand, what are the anti-rachitic substances? Milk, meat, margarine or butter, fish, eggs, and cheese. The following table shows how the diets of rachitic and non-rachitic families differ as regards these articles. The rachitic families received :—

Substances allowing rickets.	Substances delaying or preventing rickets.
11·7 g. more flour.	53·0 g. less milk.
54·2 g. „ potatoes.	3·5 g. „ meat.
7·4 g. „ sugar.	5·9 g. „ margarine or butter.
4·4 g. „ oatmeal.	20·2 g. „ fish.
11·3 g. less other cereals.	15·3 g. „ eggs.
	1·5 g. „ cheese.

Is it a coincidence that except as regards "other cereals" there is an increase in the diet of the rachitic families of the substances allowing rickets and, what is of greater importance, a decreased amount of substances having an anti-rachitic influence? It will, of course, be answered that the differences are too small in amount to be regarded as of importance. As a matter of fact, a moment's consideration will show that the real state of affairs is probably more emphatic than the figures represent. The outstanding fact brought out in Miss Ferguson's paper is that rickets is often associated with the more careless parents. It is clear that the infants below 2 years old will not get from such parents their proper share of the "good things" of the articles of the above budgets. The good things happen to be those substances containing the anti-rachitic factor. The children will undoubtedly be put off with an undue proportion of bread and the commoner foodstuffs which produce rickets.

It is improbable, however, that family budgets will ever decide the course of rickets in individual cases, but sufficient has been said to make it clear that in the appraisement and criticism of this statistical work too little attention has been given to this side of the problem and too much to the exercise and confinement factors.

GENERAL CONSIDERATION OF RICKETS AS A DEFICIENCY DISEASE.

It will be noticed that, although rickets has been interpreted on the basis of my experimental results as primarily a deficiency disease of a dietetic nature, this has not prevented other conditions from receiving attention and being considered as of some importance. A knowledge of general metabolism would not allow the exclusion of other factors ; for dietetic problems must always be regarded as a whole, and the idea that accessory food factors can be considered separate and apart from other elements of the diet and from the general metabolism is unsound.

An adequate diet is itself a unit, and its soundness, to a large extent, consists of the mutual assistance and interplay in the metabolic changes the elements experience in the body. The absence of, or deficiency in, one element means the ineffectiveness of another. For instance, the absence of carbohydrate involves a defective oxidation of fat, and probably an inefficient protein metabolism. Similarly, it is possible to imagine an abundance of accessory food factors in the diet which may, however, be ineffective because of some wrong balance in the energy-bearing materials. The same argument applies where the metabolism varies for reasons other than diet.

These few words are all the more necessary because recent work on accessory food factors has appeared too self-contained and, if persisted in, may be responsible for a period of disbelief in their existence with subsequent lack of progress in the study of a subject which is obviously of prime importance both from the academic and practical points of view.

The Dietetic Problem.

There is some danger in applying laboratory results to a clinical condition, more especially when the results are new and for the most part uncontrolled by clinical observation. But some remarks are necessary in this connexion, for, if experimental research can point to the real cause of a disease. then not only is the curative treatment controlled, but, what is of much greater importance in the case of rickets, it ought to be possible to indicate why rickets is widespread and to direct knowledge along preventive lines.

It appears, then, from this work that the foodstuffs of an infant ought to contain a maximum amount of anti-rachitic factor. Since, further, the dietetic problem is one of balance, foodstuffs which contain no anti-rachitic factor cannot be considered as neutral, but as positively rickets-producing, for the more of them that is eaten the greater is the necessity for foods containing the factor. Since there is a limit to what a child can eat, the inference is obvious. It is probable that bread is the worst offender, and to allow bread to form too large a part of an infant's dietary seems to me to be courting disaster. The same statement may apply to other cereals, but this has not been worked out to any extent.

Another point of importance is the type and amount of fat eaten by children. Since the above remark as to the limited amount of food a child can eat applies with even greater force to fat, it is necessary to give children the best fat from the point of view under consideration. They should therefore not be given vegetable margarines or any other vegetable fat. The natural fat for a child is the fat of milk, and to give it a vegetable fat not only limits the amount of butter it can eat, even if procurable, but also weighs down the diet in the rachitic direction. If additional fat is given to that normally eaten, then cod-liver oil is the best.

Milk as an Anti-rachitic Factor.

Undoubtedly milk ought to remain the staple article of diet not only until weaning, but for some years after this time. Milk is undoubtedly better than the corresponding amount of butter. Under normal circumstances the child would then be assured of a good supply of anti-rachitic factor. Not, however, under all circumstances is this certain, for the work of McCollum, Simmonds, and Pitz has shown that before an abundance of fat-soluble A appears in the milk the mother must have a good supply of this substance in her food. This means that the animal's power of synthesising these accessory food factors is small or absent. Grass is a good source of fat-soluble A for the cow, and a well-fed cow, from this point of view, will give good milk. The mother drinks this milk, and the accessory food factors are passed on to her mammary glands, thereby allowing the breast-fed child to get an adequate supply.

The problem therefore reverts largely to the feeding of the cow, and it is probable that the cow fed in the stall largely on vegetable oil-cakes will give a milk deficient in accessory food factors. If, therefore, a nursing mother's diet is deficient in the anti-rachitic factor, it is easy to understand how the breast-fed child develops rickets, for it is probable that the same argument applies even if it should subsequently prove that the anti-rachitic factor and fat-soluble A are not identical. Recently Hess and Unger have shown that the diet of the negro women in New York, whose breast-fed children are nearly always rachitic, is very often deficient in fat, the amount of milk they drink being small. These suggestions may also explain why rickets develops more commonly in the winter months, when the cow's diet is more artificial.

Other Foodstuffs.

As for the action of other foodstuffs, it has been pointed out that meat has an anti-rachitic effect to some extent and even in small quantities (10 g. a day to a puppy) will render a slightly rachitic diet safe, probably by making the anti-rachitic factor in the diet more effective. Vegetable juices seemed also to have some inhibitory action on the development of rickets.

In these days, when proprietary articles are so commonly used as foods for children, it is of vital importance that these substances should be judged by their accessory food-factor content in addition to the ordinary analysis as to any protein, fat, carbohydrate, and salts they may contain.

Synthetic milks, especially such as contain linseed and other vegetable oils, ought to be discountenanced as foodstuffs unless it can be satisfactorily shown that their accessory food factors are abundant. Similarly, the dispensing of vegetable oils instead of cod-liver oil to children, often rachitic when the oil is given, may do much more harm than good. This is most certainly the case, as I pointed out at the Physiological Society's meeting in January, 1918, when the type of Marylebone cream containing linseed oil is given. If children are to have the best chance for a healthy existence, until further work extends or modifies my experimental results, it would be safer to exclude all vegetable oils from their dietary.

Finally, it is necessary to point out that this experimental work is far from complete, and no doubt in the near future much further knowledge will be forthcoming. The subject is of great importance and will not end with rickets. For instance, the researches of my wife on the action of accessory food factors on the development of teeth show how 'necessary it is that throughout the whole period of calcification of the teeth—i.e., up to the eighteenth year—there should be abundance of anti-rachitic factor in the diet, and a deficiency at any period will be reflected in the calcification and probable uneven arrangement of the teeth. Still further points of practical interest will come to light soon.

REFERENCES.

Schmorl: Verhandlungen der deutsch. path. Gesellsch., 1909, 58.
Dick: Proc. of Roy. Soc. Med., 1915.
Cahen and Hurtley: Biochem. J., 1916, x., 308.
Osborne and Mendel: Various papers in J. Biol. Chem., 1912-19.
McCollum and co-workers: Various papers in J. Biol. Chem. and Amer. J. Physiol., 1912-19.
Hess and Unger: J. Amer. Med. Assoc., 1917, lxix., 1583; and 1918, lxx., 900.
Von Hansemann: Berliner klin. Woch., 1906, 20 and 21.
Findlay: Brit. Med. J., 1918, July 4th.
Ferguson: Pub. of Med. Research Comm., Spec. Report Series, 20.
McCollum, Simmonds, and Pitz: J. Biol. Chem., xxvii., 33.

25

Reprinted from *JAMA*, **106**(25), 2150–2159 (1936)

THE RELATIVE VALUE OF DIFFERENT VARIETIES OF VITAMIN D MILK FOR INFANTS: A CRITICAL INTERPRETATIVE REVIEW

Philip C. Jeans, M.D.

Iowa City

CLINICAL OBSERVATIONS

In the abstracts that follow, the quantities of vitamin D are stated in terms of U. S. P. or International units. In most instances conversion from other unitage statements has been necessary. It is to be recognized that conversion factors are to some extent arbitrary and that the results by the older methods of assay vary in different laboratories. The variations are presumably due to factors beyond the control of the most careful experimenters and may be so great as to lead to the conclusion that the older methods are inaccurate. No doubt some of the confusion that now exists concerning the relative values of vitamin D from different sources is dependent on the inaccuracies of assay of this vitamin by the older methods.

Daniels, Stearns and Hutton,[22] 1929: This was an inpatient balance study in which slightly better retentions of calcium and slightly poorer retentions of phosphorus were obtained with irradiated milk than with 5 cc. of cod liver oil. The authors conclude that cod liver oil in the amount used was less effective than irradiated milk. It is the reviewer's interpretation that the retention values represent a low vitamin D intake for both the cod liver oil and the irradiated milk groups. Calcium retentions of from 35 to 39 mg. per kilogram are about what may be expected from approximately

---

22. Daniels, Amy L.; Stearns, Genevieve, and Hutton, Mary K.: Calcium and Phosphorus Metabolism in Artificially Fed Infants, Am. J. Dis. Child. **37**: 296 (Feb.) 1929.

276

135 units of vitamin D and the milk intake stated,[16] and considerably less than approximately 50 mg. per kilogram to be expected when from 340 to 350 units (one teaspoonful of cod liver oil) is given.[23] In the study under consideration the potency of none of the vitamin D preparations was determined. The milk was irradiated under a quartz lamp for a period sufficient to have a strong flavor develop, and the cod liver oil was an unrefined product purchased especially because of crudeness.[24] No conclusions can be drawn from this study for the purpose of this review.

Barnes, Brady and James,[25] 1930: In an outpatient study, rickets was cured or prevented in 95 per cent of sixty-four babies receiving 840 units of vitamin D daily as cod liver oil. At the end of the study, 98 per cent of the babies were either well or benefited. Rickets was cured or prevented in only 44 per cent of fifty-seven babies receiving 750 units of vitamin D as irradiated ergosterol. The results in the latter group "were not significantly better than those for the control group of untreated subjects." The cod liver oil and viosterol used were assayed for vitamin D content. Roentgenograms and serum calcium and phosphorus were the criteria. Lack of cooperation is stated for the mother of one of the two babies who developed rickets on the cod liver oil regimen.

De Sanctis and Craig,[26] 1930: This study is difficult to interpret because the potency of the cod liver oil was only estimated and rickets was diagnosed entirely by means of clinical signs. With viosterol at a daily level of 810 units of vitamin D, rickets developed in 23 per cent of the babies. With cod liver oil at an estimated vitamin D level of from 380 to 460 units of vitamin D daily, rickets developed in 3 per cent of the babies. Subsequent reports by the same authors give essentially the same type of results.

Hess, Lewis and Rivkin,[27] 1930: In this preventive study sixty infants from 4 to 12 months of age and housed in an institution were given 10 or 20 drops daily of viosterol in oil, beginning in the autumn and ending in March. It is estimated from data given by Bills[28] that 10 drops of viosterol in oil contained 2,860 units. The babies were outdoors almost daily. The proportion of infants receiving either dosage is not stated. The criteria were physical examinations from time to time and roentgenograms and calcium and phosphorus levels in the blood at the end of the study. The authors state that the type of disorder generally recognized as rickets was almost completely prevented but that as judged by the more refined methods the protection was not absolute. Of the entire group, ten developed mild rickets; two of these received 10 drops of viosterol in oil and eight received 20 drops. When the cases of clinical rickets are excluded and only those with roentgenographic rickets are considered, there remained three infants with slight rickets and one with slight to moderate rickets, all having received 20 drops

of viosterol in oil. The authors conclude that the dosage employed in this study (5,700 units) was inadequate.

The baby with slight to moderate rickets after the ingestion of 20 drops daily of viosterol in oil for two and one-half months was given six teaspoonfuls of cod liver oil daily. Slight healing was noted in ten days and complete healing in three weeks. The authors state that the 20 drops of viosterol in oil were equivalent to ten teaspoonfuls of cod liver oil on a rat unit basis. In this instance rapid healing was produced by approximately 2,100 units as cod liver oil in an infant whose rickets developed while he was receiving approximately 5,700 units as viosterol.

Hess, Poncher, Dale and Klein,[29] 1930: Viosterol in oil (286 units to the drop[28]) was administered in an outpatient preventive experiment to fifty-one infants in doses of 1, 2, 3, 5, 10, 15 and 20 drops daily. Cod liver oil was given to forty-one infants in doses of 1, 2 and 3 teaspoonfuls and 2 tablespoonfuls daily. The prematurely born infants of the study are excluded from this discussion. The only infant of the entire group who developed roentgenographic rickets was one of seventeen receiving two teaspoonfuls of cod liver oil daily. A distaste for cod liver oil was noted in this case. It is stated that ten drops of viosterol in oil (2,860 units) was the smallest dose that prevented a fall in both the calcium and the phosphorus of the blood from the first to the later months of the first year of life. This amount is stated as the minimum dose for prophylaxis.

Apparently the lowering of the blood values for calcium and phosphorus represented variations within the normal range, in some instances the later values being slightly less than earlier ones, but still good values. Roentgenographic rickets did not develop in any of six infants receiving one drop of viosterol in oil (286 units) or in any of seven infants receiving one teaspoonful of cod liver oil (approximately 350 units[28]), while rickets was evident in nine of thirty-four control infants.

Hess, Lewis, McLeod and Thomas,[30] 1931: This was an outpatient preventive and curative study of milk from cows fed irradiated yeast and from cows fed irradiated ergosterol. Roentgenograms were used as the criterion. Each variety of milk was produced at levels of 215 and 430 units of vitamin D to the quart and was fed to four groups of infants at a constant level of approximately 24 ounces daily. The vitamin D intake was approximately 160 and 320 units daily. The study group consisted of infants from 1½ to 6 months of age and the observations were made from January to March inclusive. "Thirty-three of the infants had previously been getting cod liver oil, twenty-three of the preventive group and ten of the rachitic group, but this was discontinued, although the amounts were so small as to be inconsequential." The data for the preventive study are not given, but it is stated that rickets was prevented in all infants except two of an unstated number receiving 160 units daily as "yeast milk." Prevention was successful with 160 units as "viosterol milk" in an unstated number of infants, in sixteen infants receiving 320 units as "yeast milk" and in seventeen receiving 320 units as "viosterol milk." The curative study group included thirteen infants; three

23. Jeans, P. C., and Stearns, Genevieve: Growth and Retentions of Calcium, Phosphorus and Nitrogen of Infants Fed Evaporated Milk, Am. J. Dis. Child. **46:** 69 (July) 1933. Nelson, Martha, V. K.: Calcium and Phosphorus Metabolism of Infants Receiving Undiluted Milk, ibid. **42:** 1090 (Nov.) 1931.
24. Personal communication from one of the authors.
25. Barnes, D. J.; Brady, M. J., and James, E. M.: The Comparative Value of Irradiated Ergosterol and Cod Liver Oil as a Prophylactic Antirachitic Agent When Given in Equivalent Dosage According to Rat Units of Vitamin D, Am. J. Dis. Child. **39:** 45 (Jan.) 1930.
26. De Sanctis, A. G., and Craig, J. D.: Comparative Value of Viosterol and Cod Liver Oil as Prophylactic Antirachitic Agents, J. A. M. A. **94:** 1285 (April 26) 1930.
27. Hess, A. F.; Lewis, J. M., and Rivkin, Helen: Newer Aspects of the Therapeutics of Viosterol (Irradiated Ergosterol), J. A. M. A. **94:** 1885 (June 14) 1930.
28. Bills, C. E.: Physiol. Rev. **15:** 1 (Jan.) 1935.

29. Hess, J. H.; Poncher, H. G.; Dale, M. L., and Klein, R. I.: Viosterol (Irradiated Ergosterol). J. A. M. A. **95:** 316 (Aug. 2) 1930.
30. Hess, A. F.; Lewis, J. M.; MacLeod, Florence L., and Thomas, B. H.: Antirachitic Potency of the Milk of Cows Fed Irradiated Yeast or Ergosterol, J. A. M. A. **97:** 370 (Aug. 8) 1931.

in each of the two groups receiving "yeast milk" and two and five infants respectively in the groups receiving 160 and 320 units as "viosterol milk." In two of the three infants receiving 160 units as "yeast milk" the rickets became worse for a period of from one to two months before signs of healing were noted. In all other infants healing was marked or complete at the close of the experiment. No difference is noted between the 160 and the 320 unit "viosterol milk" groups or between either of these groups and the 320 unit "yeast milk" group. Accurate comparison of the relative values of these two varieties of milk does not seem possible. Inferiority of 160 units as "yeast milk" is indicated.

Wyman and Butler,[31] 1932: This was an inpatient curative study of two infants and two children with advanced active rickets. They were kept for a control period of from ten to twenty-three days without antirachitic agents. Serum calcium and phosphorus and roentgenograms were used to determine the amount of healing. During the experimental period the only antirachitic agent used was from 32 to 40 ounces of "yeast milk." The unitage of the milk is not stated, but a succeeding article[32] reports the potency at 430 units to the quart. One of the four subjects showed some small degree of healing in the control period. This child was given pasteurized "yeast milk" and later "yeast milk" boiled for five minutes. The rate of healing was increased over that of the preliminary period. The remaining three children showed evidence of deposition of bone demonstrable by roentgenograms within two weeks of beginning treatment. The authors conclude that "yeast milk" is an effective source of antirachitic substance.

Hess and Lewis,[33] 1932: The study group consisted of ninety-eight infants from 1½ to 6 months of age, mostly Negroes. A few of the babies were in an orphanage, but the majority were outpatients. The study was both preventive and curative and was carried on from January to April. The criterion was roentgenograms. The babies received from 24 to 32 ounces of irradiated milk daily, containing 135 units of vitamin D to the quart. The preventive study concerned thirty-six infants, including one prematurely born, without roentgenographic evidence of rickets at the beginning of the study. Of the remaining sixty-two infants, fourteen had roentgenologic evidence of rickets and forty-eight had clinical signs of rickets without roentgenologic changes. All the infants with roentgenologic evidence of rickets showed signs of healing within from four to six weeks; four of these had not healed completely at the end of the experiment. In the ten cases in which the rickets healed, the average time for healing was fifty-five days. In the discussion of the preventive experiment the authors mention the occurrence of rickets in only the prematurely born baby. The authors conclude that irradiated milk is highly satisfactory both from a prophylactic and from a curative point of view. An examination of the tabular data reveals that in addition to the prematurely born baby, two others (E. H. and P. U.) developed rickets six weeks and two months after the start of the experiment. Because of these two cases the conclusion would seem warranted that irradiated milk was not completely protective against rickets even for full term infants.

Gerstenberger and Horesh,[34] 1932: Two hospitalized rachitic infants were fed 500 cc. daily of vitamin D milk produced by feeding Holstein cows 540,000 units of vitamin D daily as irradiated ergosterol. The unitage of the milk was not stated, but the fat of the milk contained 6.75 units per gram. Assuming that the milk had a fat content of 4 per cent, it may be estimated that the infants received 135 units daily. The vitamin D milk was supplemented with ordinary skimmed milk. These two infants had slight evidences of healing as shown by roentgenograms in three and four weeks respectively, but the process had not healed when the experiment was forced to close after ten and eleven weeks. The blood phosphorus had not reached a normal value in either child by ten weeks. It seems fair to conclude that the level of vitamin D fed approached closely or was below the minimum curative dose.

Mitchell, Eiman, Whipple and Stokes,[35] 1932: This was a study of irradiated milk and milk from irradiated cows, conducted from February to October. The babies were admitted to the study from February to April and each baby was studied from six to eight months. The infants were kept indoors except for three months in the summer, when they were outdoors for two hours daily in a low-roofed, screened pavilion so placed with reference to surrounding buildings that no direct sun touched it and skyshine was also excluded. All antirachitic agents were excluded for six weeks before the experiment. The irradiated milk used contained 175 units to the quart as determined by assay of the separated fat. The irradiated milk group consisted of thirteen infants with no roentgenologic evidence of rickets. Roentgenograms were made at regular intervals, but only the final results (October) are recorded. The tabulated data show two children with mild and one child with moderate rickets, all healed. It is stated also that "a small group of markedly rachitic infants have been treated in the ward of the University and Children's Hospitals with irradiated milk as the only antirachitic agent. Prompt healing has occurred in each instance."

The milk from irradiated cows contained 60 units of vitamin D to the quart as determined by assay of the separated fat. The experimental group included twenty infants with no roentgenologic evidence of rickets and one with moderate rickets. The tabulated results of the preventive experiment show three infants with mild and three with moderate rickets, all healed. In the curative experiment the rickets healed, though slowly. The amount of vitamin D received by this group is not stated, but the statement is made that the 95 to 110 units which the youngest babies in the 1932 study of Hess and Lewis must have received is not far in excess of the number of units administered to this group of twenty-one infants. The authors state that the twenty infants of this preventive study were protected.

The authors say: "It is customary in the institution to give from one-half to one teaspoonful of cod liver oil daily and among the older infants and young children the presence of moderate rickets is seen frequently, and severe rickets occasionally." It would be most interesting if this observation were confirmed by a controlled experiment.

On the basis of the data given, the conclusion seems justifiable that neither of the milks studied was completely protective. Evidently rickets developed in both

31. Wyman, E. T., and Butler, A. M.: Antirachitic Value of Milk from Cows Fed Irradiated Yeast, Am. J. Dis. Child. **43**: 1509 (June) 1932.
32. Wyman, E. T.: New England J. Med. **209**: 889 (Nov. 2) 1933.
33. Hess, A. F., and Lewis, J. M.: Milk Irradiated by the Carbon Arc Lamp, J. A. M. A. **99**: 647 (Aug. 20) 1932.

34. Gerstenberger, H. J., and Horesh, A. J.: J. Nutrition **5**: 479 (Sept.) 1932.
35. Mitchell, J. M.; Eiman, John; Whipple, Dorothy V., and Stokes, Joseph, Jr.: Am. J. Pub. Health **22**: 1220 (Dec.) 1932.

groups and was healed by October. The reviewer is leaving out of consideration any possible influence indirect summer sunshine may have had, and the unusually high vitamin D unitage of the irradiated milk.

Barnes,[36] 1933: This was an outpatient curative study, roentgenograms being used as the criterion, in which milk fortified with 400 units of a vitamin D concentrate (Vitex) to the quart was given as the sole antirachitic agent in treating fifteen rachitic infants. The amounts of vitamin D ingested were from 300 to 400 units daily. All the infants recovered promptly. No individual data are given. From this study it may be concluded that cod liver oil concentrate milk with 400 units to the quart will bring about complete healing of rickets under the unrecorded conditions of this experiment.

Hess and Lewis,[37] 1933: This was an outpatient, winter, curative study of irradiated milk, "yeast milk," viosterol in oil and cod liver oil. A large proportion of the infants were Negroes, mostly Puerto Ricans. The babies were from 2 to 17 months of age. Irradiated milk with from 135 to 160 units of vitamin D to the quart was fed at levels of 115 and 75 units (24 and 16 ounces of milk). The criterion was roentgenograms. The 115 unit group included four infants of 17, 13, 9 and 4 months of age. The three older infants had severe rickets, and after four weeks of feeding with irradiated milk the healing was recorded as 3 plus and 2 plus. The youngest infant had slight rickets and the healing was recorded as 1 plus. The 75 unit group included six infants of 9, 9, 6, 4, 3 and 2½ months of age. The 6 months old infants had marked rickets and the healing was questionable. One 9 months old infant had moderate rickets and the healing was 1½ plus. The remaining infants had slight rickets and the healing after four weeks was 2, 1½, 1 and 1 plus.

In the study of "yeast milk" two groups of five infants each were given 24 ounces daily of milk containing 325 and 215 units of vitamin D to the quart respectively. The two groups received 245 and 160 units daily respectively. The five infants of the 245 unit group were 8, 6, 5, 6 and 4 months of age. At the start the rickets was moderate in three and slight to moderate in two infants. After four weeks the healing was 2½, 2, 1½, 1 and 1 plus. The infants of the 160 unit group were 11, 5, 6, 5 and 6 months of age. At the start the rickets was moderate in two, slight to moderate in one and slight in two. After four weeks the healing was 2, 2, 1, 1½ plus and 0. Healing was present in six weeks in the baby who showed no healing at four weeks.

In the study of viosterol preparations eight babies from 2 to 12 months of age were given 865 units daily (as viosterol in oil). The amount of milk is not stated. On the assumption that the amount of milk was the same as for most of the associated observations, viosterol showed a distinct inferiority as compared with irradiated milk and "yeast milk." The 865 units as viosterol permitted one-third as much healing as did 115 units as irradiated milk and one-half as much as 160 units as "yeast milk."

The results with cod liver oil were discarded by the authors because they were irregular and unsatisfactory. The authors concluded that irradiated milk has about twice the effectiveness of "yeast milk" and fifteen times the effectiveness of viosterol on the basis of equal unitage. Their conclusions otherwise, as based on the data presented, cannot be determined for the reason

that the discussion of the vitamin D situation is based on all the previous experience of these authors.

From the data presented it is obvious that irradiated milk with from 135 to 160 units to the quart produces improvement in rickets. A valid comparison between the 75 unit irradiated milk group and the other groups is difficult for the reason that the milk intake of the 75 unit group was reduced in proportion to the vitamin D reduction. When the healing results are averaged, only a slight advantage is evident in favor of the larger over the smaller unitage of "yeast milk," the difference between 1.3 and 1.6 plus. When the 115 unit irradiated milk group is compared with the 160 unit "yeast milk" group, there appears to be two-thirds as much healing in the "yeast milk" group with four-thirds the amount of vitamin D. Thus it may be considered that for these two groups of babies irradiated milk seems approximately twice as effective as "yeast milk." It may be concluded also that 24 ounces of "yeast milk" containing either 215 or 325 units of vitamin D to the quart produces improvement in rachitic infants, the latter being somewhat more effective.

In this and other publications by these authors, comparisons are made between the various antirachitic agents as regards relative effectiveness for man. Among the agents compared is cod liver oil. These comparisons, especially of irradiated milk with cod liver oil, have been quoted extensively. For comparison it would seem desirable that the values to be compared be determined with some degree of accuracy. So far as the reviewer can ascertain, these authors have determined neither the minimum protective nor the minimum curative dose of cod liver oil, but a value has been assigned to this substance and the assumed value has been used for comparison. If actual data available from other sources indicate conclusions at variance with those of these authors as regards cod liver oil, it seems appropriate to give preference to the conclusions based on data.

Wyman,[32] 1933: This was a metabolic study of a 16½ months old rachitic infant who was given "yeast milk" containing 430 units of vitamin D to the quart in amounts of from 940 to 1,180 cc. (430 to 540 units) daily. The control period was in April and the experimental period from April 23 to June 9. The serum calcium and phosphorus at the end of the control period were 9.7 and 2.4 mg. per hundred cubic centimeters respectively; after twelve days of the experimental period the values became 11.8 and 5.5 mg. respectively. The retentions of calcium and phosphorus in the control period were 0.078 and 0.020 Gm. daily, and during the experimental period 0.855 and 0.592 Gm. These results indicate that "yeast milk" with 430 units of vitamin D to the quart allows ample for good healing of rickets when the infant receives a quart or more of milk. The increase in serum calcium and phosphorus is very satisfactory for the time allowed. The retention indicates rapid deposition of calcium.

Kramer and Gittleman,[38] 1933: This was an inpatient curative study comparing irradiated milk and milk from cows fed irradiated yeast. The criteria consisted of roentgenograms and determinations of the calcium and phosphorus of the serum. The study was carried into early summer. Most of the infants were Negroes; all were housed in such a manner as to minimize the effect of sunshine, and the results with control patients indicated a negligible effect from extraneous vitamin D

36. Barnes, D. J.: J. Michigan State M. Soc. **32**: 242 (April) 1933.
37. Hess, A. F., and Lewis, J. M.: An Appraisal of Antirachitics in Terms of Rat and Clinical Units, J. A. M. A. **101**: 181 (July 15) 1933.

38. Kramer, Benjamin, and Gittleman, I. F.: New England J. Med. **209**: 906 (Nov. 2) 1933.

factors. Thirteen infants from 3 to 22 months of age were chosen as subjects and were kept without antirachitic treatment for a period to preclude spontaneous healing. Three infants showed evidence of healing in the preliminary period. The remaining ten infants were used for the experiment. Each infant ingested 1 quart of milk daily. Two infants received "yeast milk" containing 150 units; three received "yeast milk" containing 110; three received irradiated milk at the 150 unit and two at the 110 unit level. At the levels fed, the authors observed no significant difference in effectiveness between "yeast milk" and irradiated milk.

This was a well controlled experiment. Whether significant or not, it is of interest to note the ratios of effectiveness as determined by the time required to produce the first signs of healing by roentgen rays. At each level the irradiated milk showed a slight superiority over the "yeast milk." For the 150 unit groups the ratio was 1 : 1.4 and for the 110 unit groups 1 : 1.45. At the same time the expected differences appear between 110 and 150 units of each group. The 110 unit irradiated milk produced approximately the same initial healing results as the 150 unit "yeast milk." The experiment was not continued to complete healing, though the healing was far advanced in those cases in which it was not complete. The blood calcium and phosphorus values were not yet normal in some of the infants at the close of the experiment. Failure to produce normal values after from one to one and one-half months of treatment indicates a relatively low degree of effectiveness.

Jeans and Stearns,[39] 1934: This was an inpatient, metabolic, preventive study. The study group included seven infants from 3 weeks to 15 months of age. Irradiated evaporated milk, evaporated milk with cod liver oil concentrate (Vitex or Zucker concentrate) and evaporated milk together with cod liver oil given separately were the three diets used for the observations. Food intakes were known accurately. Each of the three experimental diets was given to a group of infants of the same age and milk intake; in the course of the observations, each infant received each diet in turn. The criteria used were calcium retention, rates of growth, roentgenograms and serum calcium and phosphorus. The study included forty metabolic periods. The youngest infants received only 60 units of vitamin D daily at the beginning of the study; by 16 weeks of age all the infants were receiving 135 units daily. During the study, no infant developed rickets. The calcium retentions on the three diets showed the same range. No source of vitamin D proved superior in any way to either of the other two as regards retentions. The average calcium retention of the group was lower by 10 mg. per kilogram than the retention observed with infants given the same milk intakes per kilogram but 340 units of vitamin D as cod liver oil. The growth and development of the study group was definitely slower than in control groups given 340 units of vitamin D. The authors conclude that the three sources of vitamin D studied are apparently equivalent, unit for unit. It is implied also that 135 units of vitamin D to the quart of reconstituted evaporated milk does not allow sufficient intake of vitamin D to permit the best development of infants, even though it is indicated that this amount of vitamin D will prevent rickets.

Wilson,[40] 1934: This was a clinical outpatient study of cod liver oil concentrate (Vitex) milk containing 400 units to the quart. The study group consisted of thirty-three infants from 6 to 13 weeks of age at the start, including two pairs of twins, three prematurely born and one infant probably born prematurely. With one exception, none had had antirachitic treatment before the test period. The feeding was undiluted milk with from 8 to 10 per cent added sugar. The milk ingestion varied from 17 to 32 ounces daily (215 to 400 units). The criteria consisted of monthly roentgenograms and body weights and lengths. The progress and general development of the infants were generally normal and satisfactory. All had attained at least the average length and weight for their ages before the end of the study. Musculature and appearance were excellent. Some of the infants developed what is termed mild or doubtful rickets; for the purpose of this review and for reasons stated in the preceding discussion, these cases are classed as normal. Two infants developed rickets of moderate and significant severity. One of these two infants was "probably premature." Prematurity might be a partial explanation of the result even though the regimen prevented rickets in three other babies prematurely born and in two pairs of twins. The other rachitic infant developed rickets in a home with such poor conditions that removal from the home became desirable; it recovered from rickets very promptly after removal while receiving vitamin D milk as the only antirachitic agent. The rapid recovery suggests strongly that the previous intake of vitamin D milk may have been different from that which was assumed. Accepting these two cases of rickets at their face value, the study shows that cod liver oil concentrate milk containing 400 units of vitamin D to the quart prevented rickets in twenty-eight of twenty-nine full term infants and in three of four infants prematurely born. The rapid recovery of the one full term infant from rickets after it was brought under better control favors holding in abeyance the full acceptance of this case.

Drake, Tisdall and Brown,[41] 1934: This was an outpatient preventive study carried on from October to May. It concerned the effects of cod liver oil, viosterol and irradiated milk. Roentgenograms were the criterion. Growth in weight was reported as normal, and above or below normal. A group of 137 infants received cod liver oil; one infant receiving two teaspoonfuls (700 units) and two receiving three teaspoonfuls (1,050 units) developed moderate or marked rickets; none receiving one teaspoonful (350 units) developed this degree of rickets. A group of 186 infants received from 270 to 2,160 units of vitamin D as viosterol in oil. Of these no infant developed moderate or marked rickets at any level fed. A group of 141 infants received irradiated milk. None developed moderate or marked rickets. Thirty-eight of these infants under 4 months of age at the beginning of the experiment received 20 ounces of milk (95 units). The absence of moderate rickets in this group is contrasted with observations on thirty-one untreated infants, four of whom developed moderate or marked rickets. The authors do not draw any comparative conclusions concerning the relative values of the various sources of vitamin D, nor do such comparisons seem possible because the three types employed were not given in similar unitage. No distinction is made between babies breast fed and those artificially fed except in the irradiated milk group. Some of the infants received egg yolk. This study is illustrative of the weaknesses

39. Jeans, P. C., and Stearns, Genevieve: Proc. Soc. Exper. Biol. & Med. **31**: 1159 (June) 1934.
40. Wilson, W. R.: Prevention of Rickets by Milk Fortified with Vitamin D from Cod Liver Oil, J. A. M. A. **102**: 1824 (June 2) 1934.

41. Drake, T. G. H.; Tisdall, F. F., and Brown, A. G.: Canad. M. A. J. **31**: 368 (Oct.) 1934.

inherent in outpatient studies in general. One might infer that 95 units as irradiated milk is superior to 1,050 units as cod liver oil, though such an inference is invalidated by the results with 350 units as cod liver oil. A reasonable conclusion is that irradiated milk was apparently effective in preventing rickets, as was also cod liver oil in the amount of one teaspoonful daily (350 units) and viosterol in oil at the level of 270 units daily.

Barnes,[42] 1934: This was an outpatient preventive and curative study conducted from November to April. The study groups included twenty-two white and ten Negro infants without rickets and four white and two Negro infants with mild rickets. The infants varied in age from 1½ to 12 months; the average age at the start being about 6 months. No infant had had any antirachitic therapy except casual exposure to the sun during the preceding summer. During the experiment each infant, regardless of the total milk intake, received 135 units of vitamin D as cod liver oil concentrate (Vitex) in milk. Biweekly weights and roentgenograms were the criteria. A group of twenty-five infants, twelve white and thirteen Negroes, served as controls; these had had no antirachitic therapy through the winter and had a roentgenologic examination in April. The average age of the controls in April was 6.2 months. Fourteen (56 per cent) of the control group were rachitic as determined by the x-rays. Of the experimental groups the thirty-two normal infants were completely protected; the weight gains were satisfactory. The six infants who showed slight signs of rickets at the beginning of the experiment showed progressive improvement. In no case did the patient grow worse during the study. Healing occurred in from eight to sixteen weeks. On the basis of these observations it may be concluded that cod liver oil concentrate milk will prevent and cure rickets when the amounts of milk are adequate and the vitamin D intake is maintained at a constant level of 135 units daily. The slow healing of rickets suggests that this level approaches the minimal effective amount.

Wyman, Eley, Bunker and Harris,[43] 1935: This was an inpatient, curative study conducted from January to March, comparing irradiated milk and milk from cows fed irradiated yeast. The irradiated milk averaged barely 135 units and the "yeast milk" varied from 160 to 175 units to the quart. Roentgenograms and determinations of serum calcium and phosphorus were made at weekly intervals. The six infants observed were kept without vitamin D for a preliminary period to preclude spontaneous healing. Three infants, 6, 7 and 26 months of age, were given irradiated milk and three infants, 8, 9 and 22 months of age, were given "yeast milk," both milks in daily amounts of from 26 to 32 ounces. Each infant showed some healing within four weeks; they were not studied to complete healing. From examination of the roentgenograms and the rate of increase of the calcium × phosphorus product the authors conclude that the two milks are equivalent, unit for unit.

In this experiment the "yeast milk" contained from 20 to 30 per cent more vitamin D to the quart than did the irradiated milk, and the babies of the "yeast milk" group received approximately 20 per cent more vitamin D than did the babies of the irradiated milk group. Despite this disparity in the amounts of vitamin D the blood phosphorus curves, when plotted against time, showed a much steeper rise for the irradiated milk

group. The comparison obviously indicates a superiority for irradiated milk. The superiority is something more than 20 per cent.

Gerstenberger, Horesh, Van Horn, Krauss and Bethke,[44] 1935: This was an inpatient, curative study of irradiated milk and milk from cows fed irradiated yeast. The criteria used were roentgenograms, the time required for complete healing, and the serum calcium, inorganic phosphorus and phosphatase. It was originally intended to have the two milks at the same unitage level of vitamin D; viz., 148 units to the quart. The preliminary assays indicated an equal unitage, but later check assays showed a content of 216 units to the quart for the irradiated milk and 148 units for the "yeast milk," a ratio of approximately 1.5:1. In the clinical trial thirteen rachitic infants (twelve Negro, one white) were kept for from two to four weeks without antirachitic treatment to preclude spontaneous healing. Irradiated and "yeast" milks were then fed at levels of 720 and 480 cc., the total milk intake being kept approximately the same by the addition of skimmed milk to the diet. Both levels of feeding produced healing of rickets, the lower level much more slowly than the higher. From a comparison, in infants of the same age and severity of rickets, of the times required for healing as judged by roentgenograms and the production of normal blood values, the authors estimate that the irradiated milk was one and one-half times as potent as the "yeast milk." This ratio is the same as that found by assay of the milks. The authors conclude that the two types of milk seem of equal efficacy, unit for unit, for healing rickets in infants. They express the opinion that, if some difference does exist, it is the irradiated milk that is slightly superior. The belief is stated that 75 units of vitamin D daily is very close to the minimal amount required for ultimate healing of active rickets. In this experiment, vitamin D in the amount of 110 units daily was sufficient to heal rickets in from nine to twelve weeks and to produce normal serum calcium and phosphorus values in from seven to nine weeks.

This study is a good example of a well controlled curative experiment. The authors present a critical discussion of criteria for this type of study and offer an explanation of the lack of agreement between the results presented and some of those previously published by others. Some data are given as the basis of a discussion of the minimum preventive and curative dose of cod liver oil. In comparing irradiated milk to cod liver oil, the authors state that their data would probably establish the ratio at 1:1.

The data presented in this publication permit interpretations in addition to those presented. When the time for bone healing is used as the criterion, no difference is established between the 108 unit irradiated milk and the 108 unit "yeast milk" groups or between the 108 unit irradiated milk and the 162 unit irradiated milk groups. When the time required to establish normal blood values is used as the criterion, definite differences are observed. Irradiated milk supplying 108 units seems superior to "yeast milk" supplying 108 units, and the irradiated milk supplying 162 units seems superior to irradiated milk supplying 108 units. When the time required to establish normal blood calcium and phosphorus values is used as the criterion, the ratio of effectiveness of irradiated milk as compared to "yeast milk" is 1:1.3; when phosphatase values are used the ratio is 1:1.4. From the point of view here presented,

42. Barnes, D. J.: Rickets, Am. J. Dis. Child. **48**: 1258 (Dec.) 1934.
43. Wyman, E. T.; Eley, R. C.; Bunker, J. W. M., and Harris, R. S.: New England J. Med. **212**: 257 (Feb. 7) 1935.

44. Gerstenberger, H. J.; Horesh, A. J.; Van Horn, A. L.; Krauss, W. E., and Bethke, R. M.: Antirachitic Cow's Milk, J. A. M. A. **104**: 816 (March 9) 1935.

the author's opinion as to the possible superiority of irradiated milk seems confirmed.

Lewis,[45] 1935: Observations are reported which compare irradiated ergosterol in corn oil with irradiated ergosterol in milk. The preparation used was "crystalline vitamin D (calciferol)." This was an outpatient curative study. The study group included thirty-six infants, divided into four groups. Nine infants received 243 units of this vitamin D in oil, ten received 2,430 units in oil, nine received 243 units in milk and eight received 121 units in milk. Each baby received 24 ounces of milk daily. The criterion was the amount of healing at four, six and eight weeks as shown by roentgenograms. The author concluded that better results were obtained with 121 units in milk than with 243 units in oil and that 243 units in milk gave better results than 2,430 units in oil. He believes that the results obtained offer an explanation for the greater effectiveness of antirachitic milks as compared with viosterol in oil. Irradiated ergosterol in the amount of 121 units in milk was below the minimum curative level, as was also 243 units in oil. However, 243 units in milk was an adequate curative dose; this amount approximates three times the amount the author believes effective when administered as irradiated milk.

Tisdall, Drake and Brown,[46] 1935: Two infants with acute rickets were treated with irradiated cholesterol in corn oil. This substance in the amount of 750 units daily produced rapid healing. Good deposition of new bone was observed in two weeks and complete cure by seven weeks.

Rapoport, Stokes and Whipple,[47] 1935: This was an inpatient preventive and curative study of irradiated evaporated milk containing 125 units of vitamin D to the 14½ ounce can. The study group consisted of twenty-three infants under 5 months of age at the beginning of the experiment. The study was conducted from January 2 to May 15. Five infants had mild rickets at the beginning of the study. All the infants were fed nonirradiated evaporated milk for about one month. They were then divided into two groups according to the presence or absence of rickets by roentgenographic examination. The preventive group comprised nine infants and the curative group thirteen. One infant is considered separately because he failed to develop rickets after twelve weeks of feeding with nonirradiated milk that contained 30 units of vitamin D to the 14½ ounce can.

The nine infants of the preventive group received amounts of milk which permitted the ingestion of from 88 to 127 units of vitamin D daily. One developed mild rickets after eight weeks of irradiated milk feeding; the rickets healed in another four weeks. One infant developed moderate rickets, which later began to heal under the same regimen. The latter infant was one of twins and weighed 6 pounds 13 ounces (3,091 Gm.) at 5 weeks of age when the experiment started. He was then given nonirradiated milk for eight weeks without the development of rickets. With the irradiated milk he received 92 units of vitamin D daily. For the entire group the duration of irradiated milk feeding varied from four and one-half to thirteen weeks.

Of the thirteen infants in the curative experiment, two had complete healing, three slight healing, two an

advance of the rachitic process followed by slight healing, four no healing and two an advance of the process without healing.

The authors conclude that irradiated evaporated milk containing 125 units of vitamin D to the 14½ ounce can appeared to be adequate for the prevention of rickets in infants. They conclude also that the same milk appears to be unreliable for the cure of rickets in infants.

The results with two of the babies in the preventive group raise a question as to the adequacy of the protection provided by the product used. At least it is indicated that the amount of vitamin D given approaches the lowest level of a preventive dose. The curative results are in distinct contrast to those of other studies of this review. The fact that rickets increased in severity in 30 per cent of the infants of the curative study indicates a low preventive effectiveness.

Jeans and Stearns,[48] 1935: This was an inpatient, winter, metabolic study. The study group consisted of five white infants. When the experiment was started, one infant was 11 weeks, one was 6 weeks and the remaining three were from 10 to 20 days old. They were given evaporated milk containing cod liver oil concentrate (Vitex) with 400 units to the reconstituted quart. The daily intake of vitamin D varied from 245 to 400 units. The rate of growth of each infant both in weight and in length was above the Kornfeld averages and equal to the rate of growth of infants kept under similar conditions but given 340 units of vitamin D as cod liver oil. The infants were precocious in dentition and muscular achievement. The roentgenograms showed no rickets. The per kilogram retentions of calcium for thirty-four metabolism periods were reported. The retention for each intake was within the range and averaged approximately the same as the retention of a larger group of infants (200 periods of study) given 340 units of vitamin D as cod liver oil, and about 10 mg. per kilogram higher than the retentions observed in a similar group of infants given 135 unit milk. From this study it was concluded that evaporated milk containing cod liver oil concentrate sufficient to allow 400 units of vitamin D to the reconstituted quart prevents the development of rickets and permits high retentions of calcium and excellent growth and development of infants.

Strong, Naef and Harper,[49] 1935: This was an outpatient, preventive study carried on in New Orleans from December 1933 to November 1934. The study group consisted of twenty-two infants who were fed irradiated evaporated milk in such quantities that from 70 to 160 units of vitamin D was ingested daily, the amount being proportionate to the age of the infant. The infants were mostly in the first six months of life. The results were determined by roentgenograms, a single examination being made for each baby after a period of observation of from four to seven months. Roentgenograms were not made of two of the twenty-two infants. Of the remaining twenty infants the roentgenograms were made as follows: one in April, three in May, twelve in June, one in July, two in August and one in October. One baby examined in August was reexamined in November. Slight evidence of rickets was present in two infants, one examined in April and one in June. A control group given from 10 to 15 drops of viosterol daily (from 865 to 1,300 units) had no evidence of rickets. The authors con-

45. Lewis, J. M.: J. Pediat. **6**: 362 (March) 1935.
46. Tisdall, F. F.; Drake. T. G. H., and Brown, A. G.: Canad. M. A. J. **32**: 490 (May) 1935.
47. Rapoport, Milton; Stokes, J., Jr., and Whipple, Dorothy V.: J. Pediat. **6**: 799 (June) 1935.
48. Jeans, P. C., and Stearns, Genevieve: Proc. Soc. Exper. Biol. & Med. **32**: 1464 (June) 1935.
49. Strong, R. A.; Naef, E. F., and Harper, I. M.: J. Pediat. **7**: 21 (July) 1935.

clude that irradiated evaporated milk should be supplemented with additional vitamin D. Presumably they held the slight amount of rickets found as of significance. A preventive study in the summer can be of no significance if rickets is not found. The finding of definite rickets would be important. The question arises as to how definite the rickets was in these two cases.

Compere, Porter and Roberts,[50] 1935: This was an inpatient curative study of irradiated yeast in comparison with cod liver oil. It was conducted from January 1 to April 1. The study group consisted of twenty-one infants from 5 months to 2½ years of age. The infants were divided into five groups. Group 1 served as the control and group 2 received 2,061 units of vitamin D as cod liver oil. The remaining groups received irradiated yeast in amounts which supplied 2,252, 6.755 and 13,511 units of vitamin D. Roentgenograms were taken and determinations of calcium and phosphorus in the serum were made. The authors conclude that from 1.1 to 3.3 times as much of the vitamin D of irradiated yeast as of the vitamin D of cod liver oil is needed to produce the same curative results as determined by roentgenograms.

The reviewer is unable to evaluate this study on any basis employed in this review. More than half of the babies apparently had rickets of the mild and doubtful variety, which has been excluded from consideration in this review. Even by the exacting criteria employed, one baby had "little evidence of rickets." Further difficulties in evaluation are encountered in that the dosages employed are far above what are generally considered to be minimum effective levels.

Peterman and Epstein,[51] 1935: This was an orphanage study of evaporated milk containing 400 units of vitamin D to the 14½ ounce can (13 fluidounces). The observations began in January 1934 and continued to February 1935. As infants were discharged from the study group, replacements were made. The babies ranged in age from 2½ to 18 months at the beginning of the study. The criteria were roentgenograms and calcium and phosphorus values of the serum. The lowest average daily intake of vitamin D for any baby for any tabulated period was 308 units and the highest was 620 units. The authors found that no infant had any clinical, chemical or roentgenographic sign of rickets during the period of the study, and they concluded that the milk was amply protective.

From the tabulated data it may be calculated that the twelve babies with which the experiment started in January had at the beginning an average of 9.10 mg. of calcium and 6.08 mg. of phosphorus per hundred cubic centimeters of serum. In April, approximately three months after the experiment started, the average values for the same babies were calcium 10.12 mg. and phosphorus 3.54 mg. per hundred cubic centimeters. In February 1935 the average values for all the babies remaining in the group (ten infants) were calcium 10.35 mg. and phosphorus 4.74 mg. per hundred cubic centimeters. Such results can scarcely be considered satisfactory. The April values are such as might be expected with little or no vitamin D and are distinctly at variance with those of other studies of this review in which an equivalent or smaller quantity of vitamin D was used as cod liver oil or cod liver oil concentrate.

Drake, Tisdall and Brown,[52] 1936: This was an outpatient winter study of 103 infants from 1 to 6 months of age who received irradiated evaporated milk. The milk contained 9.8 units of vitamin D to the ounce. The amount of milk received by the babies varied from 6 to 20 ounces. Few babies received more than 16 ounces. Moderate or marked rickets was not observed; 17 per cent developed mild rickets. Of fifty-two babies receiving evaporated milk without vitamin D, 10 per cent developed moderate or marked rickets and 29 per cent developed mild rickets. Of fifty-two babies receiving pasteurized fresh milk without vitamin D, 23 per cent developed moderate or marked rickets and 25 per cent developed mild rickets. Concerning the slight and mild rickets, the authors state: "In the interpretation of the x-ray from the clinical standpoint it must be kept in mind that the 'extremely slight rickets' are so slight that most physicians would classify these x-ray plates as normal. Those grouped as 'mild rickets' also do not show changes which would cause any great concern from the clinical standpoint." For the purpose of this review the cases of mild rickets are excluded from consideration. The authors state that the babies gained weight faster than the usual rate. Growth data are not given.

Rapoport and Stokes,[53] 1936: This was an inpatient winter study of ten infants receiving irradiated evaporated milk and of nine infants receiving irradiated fresh milk. For eighteen of the infants the experiment was preventive and for one curative. At the beginning of the experiment the infants were from 2 weeks to 5½ months of age, with an average age of 2 months. The evaporated milk contained 125 units of vitamin D to the 14½ ounce can and the fresh milk 140 units to the quart. For both groups of infants the vitamin D intake varied from 100 to 145 units daily. The observations were made over a period of four and one-half months. No infant developed rickets. The one infant who had mild rickets at the beginning of the study had slow healing; healing was first noted at thirteen weeks and was complete at eighteen weeks. The authors call attention to the lack of agreement between the clinical and the x-ray signs of rickets. It is stated that excellent growth and development of the infants were observed.

The results of this experiment indicate that irradiated fresh milk and irradiated evaporated milk are of equal value. The slow healing of rickets indicates a close approach to a minimum effective level of vitamin D. As nearly as can be determined from the data given, the rates of growth correspond closely to Kornfeld's averages with the exception of two babies who made greater growth progress.

Lewis,[54] 1936: This report concerns the effect of crystalline vitamin D administered in milk, in oil and in propylene glycol, in an outpatient preventive study conducted from December to the end of April. The 255 infants were distributed into eight groups. Between 50 and 60 per cent of the babies of each group were Negroes. Nearly 50 per cent of the babies were either partially or wholly breast fed, but none of these were included in the groups receiving vitamin D in milk.

Rickets developed in three of fifty-eight babies (5.1 per cent) receiving 145 units of vitamin D in 28 ounces of milk, in six of forty-one infants (14.6 per cent) receiving 145 units of vitamin D in oil, and in six of forty-four infants (13.6 per cent) receiving the same

50. Compere, E. L.; Porter, Thelma E., and Roberts, Lydia J.: A Clinical Comparison of the Antirachitic Value of Irradiated Yeast and of Cod Liver Oil, Am. J. Dis. Child. **50**: 55 (July) 1935.
51. Peterman, M. G., and Epstein, Ely: Prevention of Rickets with a Cod Liver Oil Concentrate in Milk, Am. J. Dis. Child. **50**: 1152 (Nov.) 1935.

52. Drake, T. G. H.; Tisdall, F. F., and Brown, A. G.: J. Pediat. **8**: 161 (Feb.) 1936.
53. Rapoport, Milton, and Stokes, J., Jr.: J. Pediat. **8**: 154 (Feb.) 1936.
54. Lewis, J. M.: J. Pediat. **8**: 308 (March) 1936.

amount of vitamin D in propylene glycol. At the level of 290 units of vitamin D daily, rickets developed in one of fifty-one infants (1.9 per cent), in five of fifty-two infants (9.6 per cent) and in five of forty-five infants (11.1 per cent) who received the vitamin D respectively in milk, in oil and in propylene glycol. Of forty-two babies who received 1,450 units in oil, one (2.4 per cent) developed rickets. Of a control group of twenty-two babies receiving no vitamin D, eight (36.3 per cent) developed rickets. In a baby with rickets 290 units of crystalline vitamin D in 28 ounces of milk was effective, whereas previously in the same infant 290 units in a teaspoonful of milk produced no healing.

The author concluded that "crystalline vitamin D" is much more effective when dispersed in milk than when administered in a more concentrated state in oil or propylene glycol. He considers also that 1,450 units in oil is a satisfactory protective dose. Interpretation of this study is not aided by the fact that in a preventive experiment rickets developed at all levels of vitamin D administration and that an intake of vitamin D which permits rickets is considered satisfactory.

SUMMARY OF CLINICAL STUDIES

Cod Liver Oil.—DeSanctis and Craig found that cod liver oil at an estimated level of from 380 to 460 units prevented physical signs of rickets in 97 per cent of the babies studied. Barnes, Brady and James observed cure or prevention of rickets in all but two of sixty-four babies receiving 840 units of vitamin D as cod liver oil in an outpatient study; the mother of one of the rachitic infants was noncooperative. Also, in an outpatient study Drake, Tisdall and Brown obtained complete protection against moderate rickets with one teaspoonful of cod liver oil (350 units) daily, though complete protection was not attained with two and three times this amount. Julius Hess observed no rickets when one teaspoonful of cod liver oil (350 units) was fed daily. Jeans and Stearns[23] and Nelson[23] observed ample retentions of calcium and phosphorus and no rickets when one teaspoonful of cod liver oil was given. Jeans and Stearns found poorer retentions of calcium and phosphorus, though no rickets, with from 60 to 135 units of vitamin D as cod liver oil. The evidence presented can be interpreted to indicate that one standard teaspoonful of cod liver oil (350 units) is ample and that 135 units or less may prevent rickets, but it permits retentions of calcium and phosphorus definitely lower than the retentions obtained with a larger intake of vitamin D.

Irradiated Ergosterol.—The lowest level of irradiated ergosterol found successful in preventing rickets is 270 units, as reported by Drake, Tisdall and Brown, and 286 units as reported by Julius Hess. This is in contrast to the failure of Barnes to prevent rickets with 750 units and the failure of Alfred Hess to prevent rickets with 5,700 units: however, in the same experiment Hess observed rickets prevention with 2,860 units. Later, Alfred Hess obtained healing with 865 units. Lewis found 243 units as crystalline vitamin D in oil below the minimum curative level and later found 290 units in either propylene glycol or in oil to be below the minimum protective level. The data cited are too conflicting to allow satisfactory conclusions. If 270 units (Drake, Tisdall and Brown) daily is an adequate preventive dose, it may be considered that the minimum preventive dose has not yet been determined.

Cod Liver Oil Concentrate in Milk.—Using milk containing vitamin D as cod liver oil concentrate in the

amount of 400 units to the quart, Barnes found that from 300 to 400 units brought about prompt recovery from rickets. Later he found that 135 units daily in milk gave complete protection against rickets and produced slow but complete healing of rickets. Wilson obtained protection against moderate rickets with 400 unit milk in all full term infants studied except one not under good control. The experiments cited are with fresh milk. It may be concluded that fresh milk containing 400 units of cod liver oil concentrate to the quart when fed in customary amounts to full term infants will prevent rickets.

Evaporated milk with cod liver oil concentrate has produced results similar to those observed with fresh milk, with the exception of Peterman and Epstein's study. Jeans and Stearns observed not only prevention of rickets but high retentions of calcium and phosphorus when evaporated milk was fed with 400 units to the reconstituted quart. The retentions were of the same order as those observed when one teaspoonful of cod liver oil was given and considerably better than the retentions obtained with 135 unit milk. The retentions with 135 unit milk were believed to be suboptimal.

The results with fresh milk and with evaporated milk are sufficiently similar to permit their consideration as of one group. Though 135 unit milk prevents rickets, it may permit a suboptimal intake of vitamin D as judged by calcium retention. Milk containing 400 units to the quart seems entirely adequate.

Irradiated Milk.—Four preventive studies of irradiated fresh milk have been reported. In all four reports good results are claimed, but failure in complete prevention is recorded for two of the four studies.

The results with irradiated evaporated milk agree with those of irradiated fresh milk. In the study of Rapoport, Stokes and Whipple, rickets appeared in one or two of the nine subjects observed, and in the curative study rickets increased in severity in several cases. In the 1936 report of Rapoport and Stokes, better results are recorded. Drake, Tisdall and Brown report the prevention of moderate rickets. Two of twenty-two infants of Strong's study developed rickets. Jeans and Stearns report what are considered to be suboptimal retention of calcium with irradiated evaporated milk.

No reason has become evident for considering that irradiated fresh milk and irradiated evaporated milk have different antirachitic values. In the recent study of Rapoport and Stokes the two varieties were compared under the same conditions and appeared to be of similar value. In curative experiments with irradiated milk additional evidence is offered that vitamin D is present in amounts very close to the minimum effective level. The time required for healing is long and in some instances no healing occurred.

It may be concluded that irradiated milk will prevent rickets in most full term babies but that the amount of vitamin D present approaches closely the minimum preventive level and permits what is believed to be suboptimal retention of calcium.

"Yeast Milk."—Only one preventive study with "yeast milk" has been found (Hess, 1931). In this study rickets developed at a level of 160 units daily and was prevented at a level of 320 units. In this study two of the three babies observed on a curative basis had an increase in their rickets at the 160 unit level. In contrast to this curative observation, Kramer obtained healing at a level of 150 units and Gerstenberger at a level of 74 units. Wyman's studies show excellent antirachitic values for "yeast milk" with 430 units to the quart when a quart or more of milk is ingested.

Irradiated Ergosterol Milk.—Using milk from cows fed irradiated ergosterol preparations, Hess observed prevention of rickets with 160 and with 320 units daily. Gerstenberger observed slow and uncertain curative results with milk containing approximately 135 units to the quart. When crystalline vitamin D was added directly to milk, Lewis found 121 units daily to be below the minimum curative level and 243 units an adequate curative dose; later he found 290 units in milk to be a more or less adequate protective level. If 121 units daily is below the minimum curative level, an inferiority to irradiated milk and cod liver oil concentrate milk is indicated.

Animal Source Group.—Only three reports have been found in which two sources of vitamin D of animal origin are compared by use concomitantly in the same experiment. One of these (Daniels) may be disregarded because of unknown potency of the materials used. The study of Drake, Tisdall and Brown offers no basis for comparison. Cod liver oil at the lowest level fed, viz., one teaspoonful, protected against rickets. Irradiated milk fed at levels permitting 95 or more units daily gave protection. Jeans and Stearns compared cod liver oil, cod liver oil concentrate milk and irradiated milk with the conclusion that these are of equal value, unit for unit when the criterion is calcium retention.

Indirect comparisons also indicate equal values. Barnes prevented rickets with 135 units as cod liver oil concentrate in milk, and in several studies rickets was almost completely prevented with 135 unit irradiated milk.

Such evidence as is available may be interpreted to show that cod liver oil, cod liver oil concentrate milk and irradiated milk are of equal potency for the human being, unit for unit.

Vegetable Source Group.—Hess is the only one who has compared two sources of vitamin D of vegetable origin in the same experiment. He found 160 units as irradiated ergosterol milk to be protective whereas 160 units as "yeast milk" was not. He also found irradiated ergosterol in oil inferior to "yeast milk," the requirement for viosterol being ten times that for "yeast milk." Lewis reported the requirement of crystalline vitamin D in oil to be ten times that of crystalline vitamin D added to milk; the data of a later experiment indicate that the requirement for the crystalline vitamin D in oil is less than five times that for the crystalline vitamin D in milk; the minimum protective dose was not determined.

The comparisons cited between viosterol in oil and the vitamin D milks do not receive full support from studies of viosterol made by others. For example, the protection against rickets obtained by Drake, Tisdall and Brown with 270 units and by Julius Hess with 286 units as viosterol in oil is in striking contrast to the results reported by Alfred Hess and Lewis.

On the basis of Alfred Hess's report, an advantage might be interpreted in favor of irradiated ergosterol milk over "yeast milk." However, Kramer obtained curative results with 150 units as "yeast milk." The evidence available does not indicate any essential difference in relative human value between yeast milk and irradiated ergosterol milk.

Animal versus Vegetable Sources.—The reports of Barnes and DeSanctis indicate a superiority of cod liver oil over viosterol. The reports of Alfred Hess, of Kramer and of Gerstenberger and his associates may be interpreted to indicate that irradiated milk is from 1.3 to 2 times the value of "yeast milk." The report of Wyman indicates that irradiated milk is more than 20 per cent superior to "yeast milk" on a unit for unit basis.

On the basis that, unit for unit, yeast milk and irradiated ergosterol milk are of the same value, that irradiated milk and cod liver oil concentrate milk are of the same value, and that irradiated milk is superior to yeast milk, a group relationship has been established. Even granting these premises, the exact relationship between the two groups is not accurately determined. Whatever the difference, it seems to be small. On the basis of the evidence reviewed and its evaluation, the difference probably is not more than 1.5 : 1. This ratio of effectiveness is based entirely on curative experiments. Because of the possible inherent weaknesses already discussed for curative studies, corroboration by preventive experiments seems highly desirable.

Dispersion of Vitamin D in Milk.—The report of Lewis that crystalline vitamin D is of greater value in milk than in oil raises a new question for consideration. If the enhanced value is due to dispersion and consequent increased availability for utilization, all the vitamin D milks have this factor in common. Observations recorded in this review indicate that cod liver oil and cod liver oil concentrate in milk are of equal value. In Lewis's experiment 243 units of vitamin D in milk was amply effective in a curative experiment, while the same amount in oil was quite ineffective. In a later report 290 units in milk was relatively effective in a preventive experiment, whereas the same amount in propylene glycol or in oil seemed less effective. These observations may be contrasted with the observation of Drake, Tisdall and Brown that 270 units in oil seemed amply protective. As regards animal experiments, Haman and Steenbock[7] were unable to observe any difference in the chicken between irradiated ergosterol in oil and irradiated ergosterol in milk.

SUMMARY

Exclusive of purely laboratory products there may be only two varieties of vitamin D, one of animal origin and one of vegetable origin. All animal sources may have a vitamin D of the same value. The same is true for all vegetable sources. Vitamin D of animal source appears to be more potent for the human being than the vitamin D of vegetable source. The degree of superiority is not entirely established, but on the basis of evidence available it may be in the ratio of 1.5 : 1 when vitamin D milks are compared.

Animal source vitamin D milk with 135 rat units (U. S. P.) to the quart will prevent rickets, but this amount of vitamin D approaches closely the minimum effective level.

Prevention of rickets is not a criterion of adequacy of vitamin D intake. The amount of vitamin D that barely prevents rickets does not permit the best growth of infants, nor does it permit retentions of calcium and phosphorus as great as those considered desirable.

Animal source vitamin D in the amount present in one-standard teaspoonful of average high grade cod liver oil or in milk containing 400 units to the quart is adequate for the infant from the standpoint of calcium retentions and growth. The minimal amount that is adequate is not known.

Vegetable source vitamin D has not been used in a manner which would determine directly the minimum rickets-preventive dose or the amount that permits good growth and retentions.

Children's Hospital.

26

Reprinted from Acta Paediatr., Stockholm, 27, 209–218 (1939)

The prothrombin content in relation to early and late feedings of the newborn.

A preliminary report.

By

LEIF SALOMONSEN M. D. and **K. K. NYGAARD** M. D.

During recent years informations have been obtained forming a basis for the interpretation of the socalled hemorrhagic
disease of the newborn as originating in a quantitative hematologic disturbance. These informations further have precipitated
the application of vitamin K as a profylactic and curative
principle in this condition. This development may briefly be
summarized as follows:

1. The blood of the infants during the first year of life
is characterized by a lower prothrombin content as compared
to that of the adult. (Brinkhous et al. (1).)

2. There is a relative, transitory hypoprothrombinemia
between the second and the sixth day of life (Owen et al. (2),
Nygaard (3)). This explains satisfactorily the previous findings
of a transitory prolongation of the coagulation time of whole
blood during the identical period (Rodda (4), Maurizio (5),
Sandford et al. (6), Salomonsen (7)).

3. Clinical evidence of hemorrhagic disease of the newborn
is found to appear in the majority of cases during the same
period. (In Salomonsen's material 62 cases out of a total
of 66.)

4. Clinical evidence of hemorrhagic disease of the newborn
is found to occur in the presence of a prothrombin deficiency

markedly exceeding that characteristic for that particular stage of life (NYGAARD (3), DAM et al. (8)). This finding strongly suggests a pathogenetic relationship between the quantitative hematologic change and occurrence of hemorrhages. It further explains the previous findings of a prolongation of the cogulation time of whole blood in this group. (SCHLOSS and COMMISKY (9), LOVEGREN (10), SALOMONSEN (7)).

5. The relative, transitory hypoprothrombinemia during the first five days of life may be corrected by the administration of vitamin K to the infant right after delivery (WADDEL et al. (11), NYGAARD (3)). Unpublished data reveal that this may be accomplished also by administration of vitamin K to the mother before or during the first days after delivery. Vitamin K thus possibly constitutes a most promising principle in the prevention of hemorrhagic disease of the newborn.

6. The excessive hypoprothrombinemia in cases of hemorrhagic disease of the newborn can be corrected within 10—24 hours and the hemorrhages arrested by the administration of vitamin K to the infant (NYGAARD (3), DAM et al. (8)). On the basis of previously reported and further experience it may definitely be stated that vitamin K represents a most valuable therapeutic principle in this condition.

The recent rather abundant litterature on the subject of prothrombin content of the blood has presented evidence indicating that the prothrombin essentially may be formed by the liver in the presence of sufficient quantity of vitamin K. As far as is known at the present, a prothrombin content below the normal level may be caused by a marked impairment of liver function, by a reduction of absorbed vitamin K or by a combination of both factors. The quantity of vitamin K available for the metabolic processes of the liver may result from an inadequate intake of the vitamin, (dietary deficiency of the chicks) or by a faulty intestinal absorbtion (obstructive jaundice, sprue and mb. coeliacus, other intestinal disorders). It is only to be expected that future research may yield further essential informations regarding the physiology and pathology of the production of prothrombin and the mechanism governing the prothrombin level.

For a complete investigation into the prothrombin deficiency of the newborn the here mentioned possibilities necessarily will have to be particularly considered. This is not the intention of the present work. Our primary intention is to touch upon the endogenous production of a vitamin K-like principle as resulting from the metabolic processes of the intestinal flora.

ALMQUIST and coworkers (12, 13) have found that an anti-hemorrhagic factor similar to or identical with vitamin K is the metabolic product of certain species of bacteriae. This explains the necessity of preventing contamination of the food by the animal's own faeces in experiments of dietary vitamin K deficiency, as well as the difficulty of producing a low prothrombin level by dietary K-avitaminosis in animals with long intestinal tract and marked bacterial activity.

In recent publications (SALOMONSEN (7), DAM (8)) it is suggested that the prothrombin deficiency of the newborn may be related to a delay in the vitamin K production of the intestinal bacterial flora. It is known that no bacterial activity occurs immediately after delivery, further that its onset and later development is essentially governed by the intake of nourishment.

A complete and satisfactory investigation of the here presented problem would have to consider in detail, the development of the intestinal flora in relation to the prothrombin level of the blood. The present report may serve as a rough orientation as to the possibilities of the here outlined investigative approach which ultimately may prove to be a complex problem of no small magnitude.

Technic: For determination of the prothrombin of the blood the method of QUICK (14) has been employed. Instead of using his visual reading technic we have made use of an original apparatus (photelgraph (15, 16)) for photoelectric investigation of the process of coagulation. The photoelectric tracings obtained present the prothrombin time as the interval

from the addition of the calcium to the point of first formation of fibrin (point F of the tracing). The normal prothrombin
time as found to be 10—20 seconds with the non-essential
modifications as necessitated by the photoelectric investigation.

These investigations have been supplemented by daily
determinations of the coagulation time of whole blood according to the capillary method of Sabrazé.

Results: It is required to state the regular feeding regime
as followed in our institution. It has been customary to
depend solely on breast feedings except in cases where this is
impossible or may be contraindicated. The very first breast
feeding is given from 12—20 hours after delivery. Under
regular conditions no addition to the breast feedings is given
during the first week of life.

Table 1.

Account of prothrombin time at varying intervals post partum.

Group I: regular breast feeding from 12—20 hours post
partum. 12 observations in 12 cases.

Group II: extra feedings from two hours post partum. 10
observations in 13 cases.

	Prothrombin time in seconds			
	Days post partum			
	2nd.	3rd.	4th.	5th.
Group I.	28	30	17	27
	30	33	28	
		35	29	
		35	32	
			40	
Group II	17	15	16	17
	20	15		
	28	15		
		20		
		20		

Table 2.

Account of average, daily coagulation time (capillary method) at varying intervals post partum.

The two groups identical with those of table 1.

	Average coagulation time, in minutes							
	Days post partum							
	1	2	3	4	5	6	7	8
Group I. (12 cases) Average initial loss of weight 7.3 %	3.0	3.6	4.1	3.9	3.6	3.6	3.4	3.2
Group II. (13 cases) Average initial loss of weight 3.4 %	2.7	3.2	3.0	2.7	2.8	2.7	2.6	2.6

Table 3.

Account of coagulation time (capillary method) in three cases on restricted feedings post partum.

(The prothrombin time indicated in parenthesis.)

	Coagulation time, in minutes							
	Days post partum							
	1	2	3	4	5	6	7	8
Case 1.	4.5	5.5 (30)	5.0	5.5 (30)	—	4.5	4.0	3.5
Case 2	4.5	6.0 28)	6.5	6.5	5.5 (27)	4.5	3.5	—
Case 3. given vitamin K 80 hours p. p.	—	4.0 (25)	5.5	7.0 (65)	3.0	2.5	3.5	3.0

Investigations of the prothrombin time has been carried out in a group of 12 healthy, apparently normal infants, all maintained on this routine feeding regime (group I). As indicated in table 1, 11 of these present a prolongation of the prothrombin time as compared to the normal. These figures agree well with those of an identical series of 43 observations in a previously reported (3) group presenting evidence of the relative, transitory hypoprothrombinemia between the second half of first day and sixth day of life.

A second series comprised 13 infants who all were started on extra feedings of $^1/_2$ diluted cow's milk (boiled) two hours after delivery in addition to breast feedings. During the first day of life 10 cc. of diluted cow's milk was given six times daily, increasing with 10 cc. per feeding each day for four days after which time breast feedings only (group II). The results appear in table 1.

It appears that extra feeding of the infants from within two hours after delivery can prevent the development of the subsequent hypoprothrombinemia characteristic of the infants maintained on the regular breastfeedings as stated above.

Daily determinations of the coagulation time of whole blood by the capillary method seem to substantiate these findings in the group as a whole (table 2). As brought out by the same table the difference in the feeding regime of the two groups is evident also in the average initial loss of weight taking the groups as a whole, this loss being 3.4 per cent of the weight at time of birth in group II as compared to 7.3 per cent in group I.

For obvious reasons we have not deemed it justifiable to carry out investigations into a third group in which feeding was postponed beyond the 20 hour limit for onset of routine breast-feedings. We have however had occasion to investigate the coagulability in 3 infants who only received small quantities of sterile water during the first 30—34 hours of life, after which time regular breast feedings were given (table 3). In one of these cases, for some reason the fact was overlooked that the infant obtained practically nothing from the mother.

Due to a considerable initial drop in weight, our attention was called to this matter about 80 hours after delivery. The prothrombin time was then found to have increased from 25 to 65 seconds since 28 hours after delivery. The coagulation time of whole blood was found to be 7 minutes. It may be mentioned that this is the first case encountered in a total of a little better than 150 observations in which the prothrombin time exceeded 50 seconds without any clinical manifestation of hemorrhages. On this background vitamin K was immediately given and the infant started on extra feedings. No further sinus puncture was performed. The coagulation time was reduced rapidly. The further progress of the infant was fortunately satisfactory in every respect. Together with the mother it was dismissed in excellent general condition on the 11th day after delivery. We honestly admit that the here related experience has checked any desirability we may have harbored in investigating the prothrombin deficiency in relation to more pronounced delay of feedings in the newborn.

Comment: Although the present investigation admittedly has dealt with a limited number of cases, it still may have served the purpose of a rough orientation as explained at the outset. It appears that *extra feedings started within two hours after delivery can prevent the development of a subsequent hypoprothrombinemia.* It is further likely to assume that *normally at least a considerable period of absolut diet is required for the creation of a hypoprothrombinemia of the excessive degree found in cases of hemorrhagic disease of the newborn.*

In viewing these results on the background of present knowledge concerning vitamin K it appears that the variation of prothrombin here encountered can hardly be caused by a variation in the intake of vitamin K. Milk contains little vitamin K.

An understanding of the here presented findings may be obtained on the basis of the above quoted works by ALMQUIST. It seems suggestive *that early, extra feedings of the newborn may result in the hastening of the bacterial metabolism in the intestines, which thus creates a supply of vitamin K sufficient for*

the prevention of a relative, transitory hypoprothrombinemia other-
wise occurring.

It shall be stressed that the line of reasoning here presented can without serious reservations hardly be applied to
an interpretation of the excessive hypoprothrombinemia present
in cases with hemorrhagic disease of the newborn. For this
purpose a more extensive and varied investigative approach
is required. We are further fully aware of the lack of essential informations concerning prothrombin metabolism and vitamin K utilization in the infant.

We have however considered it opportunely in this connection to point out a few observations which, admittedly equivocal, may favor a certain relation to the here intimated
problem. Certain statistical data indicate that the onset of
the feedings may have occurred somewhat late in many of
the infants with hemorrhagic disease, as these infants exhibit
a more marked initial loss of weight as compared to the normals. In the 66 cases comprising the material of SALOMONSEN,
the initial loss of weight was 317 Gr. as compared to the
average loss of 279 Gr. in a control group of normals. Of
additional consequence may be the findings that hemorrhages
are relatively more frequent in infants whose mothers are
older primiparas, who have exhibited symptoms of intoxication
during the pregnancy or have undergone instrumental deliveries,
factors which *may* influence the requirements to a satisfactory
breast feeding. These points however can only be evaluated
by further investigations. Mention shall finally be made of
the statement made by SANFORD et al. (17) that no hemorrhagic disease of the newborn had been observed after the
institution of extra feedings with a formula of diluted cow's
milk from the fourth hour after delivery.

The no doubt complex problem of the interrelation of the
intestinal flora, endogenous production of the vitamin K-like
principle, the infant nourishment and the prothrombin deficiency
of moderate and marked degrees must be left open for further
investigation.

It is obvious that we are as yet not in the position to

state whether a similar early feeding regimen or vitamin K administration directly to the newborn or to the mother or both is the preferable procedure in the struggle for profylaxis of the hemorrhagic disease of the newborn. A consideration of this essential point is reserved for subsequent communications.

Summary and conclusions.

Judging from the results of prothrombin determinations in a series of newborns it appears that

1. The previously found transitory hypoprothrombinemia and prolongation of the coagulation time during the first 5 days of life can be corrected by early extra feedings of the infant from within two hours after delivery.

2. It is likely that a moderate period of absolute diet (up to 34 hours) is *normally* not followed by any *excessive* degree of hypoprothrombinemia, while this appears possible by a more prolonged period of absolut diet.

3. It is suggested that these quantitative hematologic variations may be an expression of the varied bacterial metabolism of the intestinal flora through the bacterial production of a vitamin K-like principle.

Litterature.

1. BRINKHOUS, K. M., SMITH, H. P. and WARNER, E. D.: Am. J. Med. Sc. 193, 475, 1937. — 2. OWEN, C. A., HOFFMANN, J. R., ZIFFRENS, S. E. and SMITH, H. P.: Proc. Soc. Exp. Biol. e. Med. 41, 181, 1939. — 3. NY-GAARD, K. K.: Acta obst. et gynec. Scand. 19, 361, 1939. — 4. RODDA, F. C.: Am. J. Dis. Child. 19, 269, 1920. — 5. MAURIZIO, E.: Z. bl. f. Gynäk. 54, 479, 1930. — 6. SANFORD, H. N., GASTEYER, T. H. and WYAT, L.: Am. J. Dis. Child. 43, 58, 1932. — 7. SALOMONSEN, L.: Acta pædiatrica. Vol. XXVII. Suppl. I 1939. — 8. DAM, H., TAGE-HANSEN, E. and PLUM, P.: Ugeskr. f. Læger. 11, 896, 1939. — 9. SCHLOSS and COMMISKEY: Am. J. Dis. Child. 1, 276, 1912. — 10. LÖVEGREN, E.: Jahrb. f. Kinderheilk. 78, 249, 1913. — 11. WADDELL, W. W. and GUERRY, DU PONT: J. Am.

Med. Ass. 112, 2259, 1939. — 12. ALMQUIST, H. J. and STOKSTAD, E. L. R.:
J. Biol. Chem. 111, 105, 1935. — 13. ALMQUIST, H. J., PENTLER, C. F. and
MECCHI, E.: Proc. Soc. Exp. Biol. a. Med. 38, 336, 1938. — 14. QUICK, A.,
STANLEY-BROWN, M. and BANCROFT, F. W.: Am. J. Med. Sc. 190, 501, 1935.
— 15. NYGAARD, K. K.: J. Lab. a. Clin. Med. 24, 517, 1939. — 16. NY-
GAARD, K. K.: The Lancet. In press. — 17. SANFORD, H. N., MORRISON,
H. J. and WYAT, L.: Am. J. Dis. Child. 43, 569, 1932.

27

Reprinted from *Fed. Proc.*, **9**, 371–372 (1950)

PYRIDOXINE DEFICIENCY IN THE HUMAN BEING

Selma E. Snyderman, Rosario Carretero, and L. Emmett Holt, Jr.

New York University College of Medicine

A pyridoxine-deficient diet, given for therapeutic reasons to two mentally defective infants for 76 and 130 days respectively, failed to produce clinical benefit but yielded information of nutritional interest. Both subjects developed evidences of pyridoxine deficiency, indicating that pyridoxine is a human dietary essential. The first change noted was the prompt disappearance of pyrdoxic acid from the urine and a reduction of the total urinary pyridoxine to low values ranging from 0.2 to 2 µg/day. Subsequently, both infants lost the ability to convert tryptophane to nicotinic acid, an effect which was desired in order to block a metabolic path for tryptophane that might be competing with normal tissue synthesis. A plateauing of the weight curve occurred 33 and 73 days after the institution of the regime. On the 76th day one subject developed a series of convulsions which were promptly relieved by the administration of pyridoxine. The other subject developed a hypochromic anemia at approximately the 130th day. This responded dramatically to pyridoxine; a rise in reticulocytes was noted after 72 hours reaching a peak in 4 days after which red cell count and hemoglobin rose to normal. Both subjects gained weight normally after supplementation. In marked contrast to the excellent and prompt clinical response to the administration of pyridoxine was a delay in the reappearance of the ability to convert tryptophane to nicotinic acid.

296

Part VII

ENERGY AND THE METABOLIC
BASIS FOR FEEDING

Editor's Comments
on Papers 28 Through 30

As the percentage method of feeding flourished in the United
States, the caloric calculation method of formula prescription,
based on the metabolic studies of Rubner and Heubner (1898) in
Germany, was acquiring its own disciples. Their recommendation
of approximately 100 calories per kilogram of body weight during
the first three months of normal infancy remains applicable to this
day. It was Heubner who coined the phrase "energy quotient,"
designating the relationship of the amount of food ingested in calories to the number of calories per kilogram of body weight expended per day. This energy quotient is often referred to in the
early literature and varies very little from study to study. The undisputed classic on the caloric basis of feeding is that of Powers (Paper 29).

The work of Talbot (Paper 28) has been selected for the precision and accuracy of his results, which were later expanded upon
by others only when refinements of instrumentation permitted,
and the team of Levine, McEachern, Wheatley, Marples, and Kelly
(1935) were able to fill in the details to complete the definition of
infant respiratory metabolism. Gordon and Levine are perhaps best
known for their exquisitely precise contributions to the metabolism of the premature infant. Their classic article, Paper 30, remains
unchallenged as the single most comprehensive, explicit guideline
for the metabolic basis of feeding the normal infant.

28

Reprinted from *Am. J. Dis. Child.*, **14**, 25–33 (1917)

TWENTY-FOUR-HOUR METABOLISM OF TWO NORMAL INFANTS WITH SPECIAL REFERENCE TO THE TOTAL ENERGY REQUIRE- MENTS OF INFANTS *

FRITZ B. TALBOT, M.D.

BOSTON

A series of investigations of the metabolism of normal infants were begun five years ago by Benedict and the writer at the Nutrition Laboratory of the Carnegie Institution of Washington with the object of obtaining a curve of the "basal" metabolism of normal infants. Some of these studies have already been published, and the rest are in the process of completion to be published later. Their primary object is to obtain the "basal" metabolism of infants (the metabolism at rest) for the purpose of comparing health with disease. The basal metabolism should mean that the subject is in complete muscular repose, and in the "postabsorptive" state, that is, when absorption of material from the alimentary tract has ceased. Since it is almost impossible to obtain a period of complete muscular repose in infants in the "postabsorptive" state and hungry, the term "basal" metabolism will be used in this communication in describing quiet periods shortly after food has been given. Since the results of these studies do not take into consideration the extra energy used up in muscular exercise, lost in the excreta or deposited in the body in the form of new tissue, they cannot be used as a definite measure of the food requirements of a normal growing infant. They contain information, however, which, with additional knowledge, helps in estimating the total caloric requirements of infants.

A careful review of the literature shows that there have been few instances in which an attempt has been made to obtain the twenty-four-hour metabolism of normal infants. The fundamental experiments of Rubner and Heubner[1] stand out as giving the only twenty-four-hour figures available for normal infants. They give records of three different normal infants weighing 5, 8 and 10 kg., the first and last being fed on human milk, and the second on a mixture of cow's milk. These infants were inside a respiratory chamber about twenty hours of the twenty-four-hour day. Unfortunately, complete records of the individual periods in these experiments showing the percentage increase in calories from rest to muscular activity are not available. Heubner, on

---

* Submitted for publication May 28, 1917.

* From the Nutrition Laboratory of the Carnegie Institution of Washington, Boston.

* Read at the meeting of the American Pediatric Society, White Sulphur Springs, W. Va., May 28, 1917.

1. Rubner and Heubner: Ztschr. f. biol., 1898, **36,** 1. Rubner and Heubner: Ztschr. f. biol., 1899, **38,** 315. Heubner: Berl. klin. Wchnschr., 1901, **38,** 449. Rubner and Heubner: Ztschr. f. exper. Path. u. Therap., 1905, **1,** 7.

the basis of these and other studies, maintains that an average normal infant requires per twenty-four hours, 100 calories per kilogram of body weight during the first three months of life, 90 calories during the second three months, and 80 or less calories during the last half of the first year of life. These figures are usually accepted as a basis from which to compute the energy requirements of normal infants.

The great difficulty of obtaining complete records of the respiratory metabolism for twenty-four hours accounts for the paucity of material reported above. The present investigation was carried on under Miss Alice Johnson and assistants, whose careful work and devotion day and night are responsible for the success of a very difficult piece of work, and without whose hearty cooperation it would have been impossible.

The purpose of the present investigation was to determine, if possible, how much extra energy was expended in the ordinary muscular activity of an infant during a twenty-four-hour day. It has been known for a long time that muscular activity increases the metabolism, but, on the other hand, there is no measure of how much of the day the infant is active. If the increase in metabolism due to muscular activity can be determined, if the factor of growth and the factor of energy lost in the excretions be established, this material could be used in conjunction with the average curve of the "basal" metabolism to estimate the number of calories in the food necessary for an infant in a twenty-four-hour day.*

The normal infants in the Directory for Wet-Nurses of the Boston Infants Hospital were selected for this purpose. The plan of the observation was to have the infant inside the respiratory chamber as many hours out of the twenty-four as possible so that an accurate measure of the total respiratory exchange could be obtained.

The periods were started at about 7 p. m., and run through the following twenty-four hours, stopping at the same time the next evening. Short periods were recorded so that it would be possible to select periods of absolute quiet as well as periods of activity. The cover was raised at regular intervals and the baby removed, nursed by his mother, and the diapers changed when soiled. It was due to the intelligent cooperation of the mothers that in one instance the infant was inside the respiratory chamber twenty-two hours and thirty-one minutes, and in the other, twenty-three hours and ten minutes. The flexibility of the apparatus made this possible without impairing the accuracy of the

---

* A tentative curve may be found in Morse and Talbot, Diseases of Nutrition and Infant Feeding, New York, 1915, p. 61. When such a curve is used the variations from the average should always be borne in mind, if it is applied to a single infant, because averages are made up from several subjects and the extremes may be as much as 10 per cent. one or the other side of the average figure.

results. The length of the actual observation compares very favorably with those of Rubner and Heubner, which were in all instances shorter.

E. L., girl, was born January 27, 1916, full term, the labor was normal and the baby weighed 3.71 kg. (8 pounds, 3 ounces) at birth. She was entirely breast fed up to date, receiving the breast every three hours. She had never been sick. Her weight April 20, 1916, was 5.03 kg. (about 11 pounds). The details of the twenty-four hours during which the respiratory exchange was measured are as follows:

```
                  6:48 p. m.—Nursed at breast
7:23 p. m. to  1:10 a. m.—In respiratory chamber. Quieted down. Slept
1:10 a. m. to  1:25 a. m.—Taken out, diapers changed.  Nursed nine minutes
                          Returned to chamber
1:25 a. m. to  2:02 a. m.—Restless
2:02 a. m. to  3:15 a. m.—Sleeping
3:15 a. m. to  3:51 a. m.—Moving about
3:51 a. m. to  4:30 a. m.—Quiet
4:46 a. m. to  6:40 a. m.—Moving and cried at intervals
6:40 a. m. to  6:54 a. m.—Taken out, given breast, diapers changed, wet with
                          urine.  Returned to chamber
6:54 a. m. to  7:54 a. m.—Played with hands and moved
7:54 a. m. to  8:39 a. m.—Asleep
8:39 a. m. to  9:26 a. m.—Moved hands and twisted body. Taken out, diapers
                          wet, changed. Nursed. Returned to chamber
9:46 a. m. to 10:40 a. m.—Moving and restless
10:40 a. m. to 11:14 a. m.—Quiet
11:14 a. m. to 12:31 p. m.—Grumbling, moving, waving hands, cooing
12:31 a. m. to 12:51 p. m.—Taken out, given breast.  Diaper soiled with small,
                          brownish yellow stool. Returned to chamber
12:51 p. m. to  1:45 p. m.—Gradually became quiet
1:45 p. m. to  3:00 p. m.—Twisted, grumbled or played with hands
3:00 p. m. to  3:29 p. m.—More restless
3:29 p. m. to  3:49 p. m.—Taken out, diapers changed, nursed.  Returned
                          to chamber
3:49 p. m. to  7:23 p. m.—Moderately active
                  7:23 p. m.—Taken out
```

She was weighed before and after each nursing and received amounts of breast milk as shown in Table 1.

TABLE 1.—AMOUNTS OF BREAST MILK RECEIVED BY INFANT E. L.
IN TWENTY-FOUR HOURS

Date	Time	Grams	Ounces
4/20/16	7:07 p. m.	90	3
4/21/16	1:21 a. m.	135	4½
4/21/16	6:50 a. m.	135	4½
4/21/16	9:42 a. m.	145	4¾
4/21/16	12:48 p. m.	90	3
4/21/16	3:45 p. m.	100	3¼
Total in 24 hr.		695	23¼

TABLE 2.—Results of the Measurements of Gaseous Metabolism of Infant E. L.

Period	Time	Length of Period, Min.	CO₂ Produced Measured, Gm.	CO₂ Produced Calculated to Hour Basis, Gm.	Average Pulse Rate	Respiratory Quotient
Preliminary	7:23 – 7:53 p. m.	30	2.88	5.76	126	
1st	7:53 – 8:28 p. m.	35	2.46	4.22	117	0.92
2d	8:28 – 9:03 p. m.	35	2.58	4.42	119	0.94
3d	9:03 – 9:39 p. m.	36	2.52	4.20	118	0.88
4th	9:39 –10:14 p. m.	35	2.46	4.22	116	0.86
5th	10:14 –10:51 p. m.	37	2.71	4.39	112	0.91
6th	10:51 11:27 p. m.	36	2.48	4.13	114	0.88
7th	11:27 p. m.–12:04 a. m.	37	2.31	3.75	115	0.80
8th	12:04 –12:38 a. m.	34	2.22	3.92	115	0.90
9th	12:38 – 1:10 a. m.	32	2.16	4.05	117	0.81
Preliminary	1:25 – 1:53 a. m.	28	2.80	6.00	132	
1st	1:53 – 2:32 a. m.	39	2.78	4.28	121	0.86
2d	2:32 – 3:09 a. m.	37	2.82	4.57	120	0.97
3d	3:09 – 3:58 a. m.	49	3.62	4.43	121	0.87
4th	3:58 – 4:49 a. m.	51	4.33	5.09	122	0.88
5th	4:49 – 5:39 a. m.	50	5.25	6.30	140	0.91
6th	5:39 – 6:15 a. m.	36	2.47	4.12	122	0.84
7th	6:15 – 6:40 a. m.	25	3.01	7.22	152	0.80
Preliminary	6:54 – 7:17 a. m.	23	2.50	6.52	145	
1st	7:17 – 7:56 a. m.	39	4.31	6.63	139	0.88
2d	7:56 – 8:31 a. m.	35	2.78	4.77	117	0.83
3d	8:31 – 9:26 a. m.	55	5.51	6.01	125	0.81
Preliminary	9:46 –10:04 a. m.	18	2.11	7.03	146	
1st	10:04 –10:32 a. m.	28	2.77	5.94	136	0.98
2d	10:32 –11:00 a. m.	28	1.92	4.11	115	0.86
3d	11:00 –11:33 a. m.	33	2.66	4.84	122	0.82
4th	11:33 a. m.–12:08 p. m.	35	3.87	6.63	143	0.90
5th	12:08 –12:31 p. m.	23	2.35	6.13	133	0.86
Preliminary	12:51 – 1:27 p. m.	36	2.87	4.78	119	
1st	1:27 – 2:16 p. m.	49	4.15	5.08	121	0.92
2d	2:16 – 3:29 p. m.	73	8.57	7.04	140	0.85
Preliminary	3:49 – 4:15 p. m.	26	2.84	6.55	128	
1st	4:15 – 4:47 p. m.	32	3.48	6.53	138	0.86
2d	4:47 – 5:14 p. m.	27	2.70	6.00	123	0.90
3d	5:14 – 6:19 p. m.	65	6.44	5.94	143	0.83
4th	6:19 – 6:52 p. m.	33	3.49	6.35	136	0.87
5th	6:52 – 7:23 p. m.	31	3.62	7.01	142	0.85
Total.		22 hr. 31 min.	120.80	....	...	0.87

302

The results of the measurements of the gaseous metabolism of E. L., aged 2 months, 3 weeks, weight 5.03 kg., for the twenty-four hours, April 20-21, 1916, are given in Table 2.

E. S., girl, was born at full term, Oct. 14, 1915. She weighed 6 pounds (2.72 kg.) at birth. She was always breast fed and did fairly well until February, 1916, when she had some indigestion and colic, and some facial eczema. These symptoms gradually straightened out, and on April 19, when 6 months and 1 week old, she weighed 5.76 kg. (the average weight for the age is 7.8). She finished nursing at 6:51 p. m., April 19, 1916. The program for the twenty-four-hour day was as follows:

```
              6:51 p. m.—Finished nursing
7:02 p. m. to 5:51 a. m.—Placed in chamber. Quickly went to sleep. Occa-
                         sional muscular movement recorded on
                         smoked drum
5:52 a. m. to 6:08 a. m.—Taken out, nursed, returned to chamber
6:08 a. m. to 8:13 a. m.—Asleep
8:13 a. m. to 8:51 a. m.—Moderate moves
8:56 a. m. to 9:08 a. m.—Taken out, nursed, returned to chamber
9:08 a. m. to 10:15 a. m.—Cooed, kicked, played, smiled, occasionally cried
10:15 a. m. to 12:14 p. m.—Quiet, very few moves
12:14 p. m. to 12:46 p. m.—More active
12:46 p. m. to 12:57 p. m.—Taken out, nursed, diapers changed, returned to
                         chamber.
12:57 p. m. to 2:08 p. m.—Kicking and waving hands
2:08 p. m. to 2:51 p. m.—Asleep
2:51 p. m. to 3:48 p. m.—Active, crying or laughing
3:48 p. m. to 4:00 p. m.—Taken out, nursed, diapers changed, returned to
                         chamber
4:00 p. m. to 5:19 p. m.—Played, moved and wiggled
5:19 p. m. to 7:03 p. m.—Asleep with the exception of a few minutes of play
```

She was weighed before and after each nursing and received amounts of breast milk as shown in Table 3.

TABLE 3.—Amounts of Breast Milk Received by E. S.
in Twenty-Four Hours

Date	Time	Grams	Ounces
4/19/16	6:51 p. m.	70	2¼
4/20/16	5:56 a. m.	135	4½
4/20/16	9:07 a. m.	125	4¼
4/20/16	12:54 p. m.	150	5
4/20/16	3:57 p. m.	135	4½
Total in 24 hr.		615	20½

The results of the measurements of the gaseous metabolism of E. S., aged 6 months, 1 week, weight 5.76 kg., for twenty-four hours, April 19-20, 1916, are given in Table 4.

TABLE 4.—Results of the Measurements of Gaseous Metabolism of Infant E. S.

Period	Time	Length of Period, Min.	CO₂ Produced		Average Pulse Rate	Respiratory Quotient
			Measured, Gm.	Calculated to Hour Basis, Gm.		
	April 19					
Preliminary	7:02 – 7:23 p. m.	21	1.99	5.69	135	
1st	7:23 – 7:59 p. m.	36	2.76	4.60	120	0.83
2d	7:59 – 8:34 p. m.	35	2.87	4.92	129	0.81
3d	8:34 – 9:04 p. m.	30	2.46	4.92	121	0.81
4th	9:04 – 9:36 p. m.	32	2.75	5.16	130	0.82
5th	9:36 – 9:44 p. m.	8	0.61	4.58	127	
2d Prelim.	9:44 –10:03 p. m.	19	1.59	5.02	129	
1st	10:03 –10:37 p. m.	34	2.73	4.82	128	0.81
2d	10:37 –11:07 p. m.	30	2.23	4.46	129	0.85
3d	11:07 –11:38 p. m.	31	2.33	4.51	130	0.80
4th	11:38 p. m. 12:15 a. m.	37	3.12	5.06	130	0.87
	April 20					
5th	12:15 –12:50 a. m.	35	2.83	4.85	130	0.88
6th	12:50 – 1:22 a. m.	32	2.79	5.23	136	0.86
7th	1:22 – 1:59 a. m.	37	2.87	4.65	126	0.84
8th	1:59 – 2:32 a. m.	33	2.77	5.04	139	0.85
9th	2:32 – 3:24 a. m.	52	5.07	5.85	136	0.79
10th	3:24 – 3:58 a. m.	34	2.62	4.62	141	0.88
11th	3:58 – 4:27 a. m.	29	2.68	5.54	143	0.85
12th	4:27 – 5:16 a. m.	49	4.74	5.80	146	0.84
13th	5:16 – 5:52 a. m.	36	3.67	6.12	154	0.79
Preliminary	6:08 – 6:28 a. m.	20	2.21	6.63	153	
1st	6:28 – 7:01 a. m.	33 '	2.88	5.24	137	0.84
2d	7:01 – 7:50 a. m.	49	4.49	5.50	131	0.85
3d	7:50 – 8:19 a. m.	29	2.53	5.23	118	0.84
4th	8:19 – 8:56 a. m.	37	3.64	5.90	124	0.80
Preliminary	9:08 –10:07 a. m.	59	7.64	7.77	151	
1st	10:07 –10:34 a. m.	27	1.87	4.16	120	0.79
2d	10:34 –11:05 a. m.	31	2.85	5.52	122	0.88
3d	11:05 –11:32 a. m.	27	2.05	4.56	119	0.79
4th	11:32 a. m. 12:02 p. m.	30	2.76	5.52	130	0.81
5th	12:02 –12:28 p. m.	26	2.05	4.73	118	0.78
6th	12:28 –12:46 p. m.	18	1.92	6.40	148	0.89
Preliminary	12:57 – 2:12 p. m.	75	8.90	7.12	142	
Preliminary	2:12 – 3:48 p. m.	96	10.19	6.37	137	
Preliminary	4:00 – 4:22 p. m.	22	2.80	7.64	135	
1st	4:22 – 4:54 p. m.	32	4.26	7.99	148	0.85
2d	4:54 – 5:25 p. m.	31	3.80	7.35	142	0.81
3d	5:25 – 5:56 p. m.	31	2.40	4.65	114	0.76
4th	5:56 – 6:36 p. m.	40	3.64	5.46	126	0.79
5th	6:36 – 7:03 p. m.	27	2.08	4.62	122	1.02
Total....................		23 hr. 10 min.	130.44	....	...	0.83

An average of the figures of the "basal" and of the maximum metabolism of E. L. are given in Table 5.

TABLE 5.—AVERAGE OF THE "BASAL" AND MAXIMUM METABOLISM
OF INFANT E. L.

	No. of Periods	Carbon Dioxid, Gm. per Hr., Average	Heat Computed (24 hr.) Calories			Average Pulse
			Total	Per Kg.	Per Sq. M. Lissauer	
"Basal" metabolism..............	12	4.15	285	57	944	117
Maximum metabolism............	20	6.24	428	85	1417	135

The "basal" metabolism of 285 calories was increased 143 calories by muscular activity. This corresponds to an increase of 67 per cent.

The average figures of the "basal" and of the maximum metabolism of E. S. are given in Table 6.

TABLE 6.—AVERAGE OF THE "BASAL" AND MAXIMUM METABOLISM
OF INFANT E. S.

	No. of Periods	Carbon Dioxid, Gm. per Hr., Average	Heat Computed (24 hr.) Calories			Average Pulse
			Total	Per Kg.	Per Sq. M. Lissauer	
"Basal" metabolism..............	18	4.75	338	59	1021	126
Maximum metabolism............	12	6.75	481	84	1453	143

The "basal" metabolism of E. S. was increased 143 calories by muscular activity which corresponds to an increase of 70 per cent. This is very close to the average increase of 65 per cent. found in the new-born infant.[2]

Since the infants were removed from the chamber at regular intervals during the twenty-four hours for their usual nursings, the metabolism obviously could not be measured during that time, but an estimate of what it would have been is justifiable. Considerable muscular work is performed in nursing, and if the average maximum metabolism for each infant is taken to represent the metabolism during that time, it cannot be far from the truth. Baby E. L. was out of the chamber one hour and twenty-nine minutes, and Baby E. S., fifty minutes. The estimated metabolism for fifty minutes for Baby E. S. would be found as follows:

2. Benedict and Talbot: Physiology of the New-Born Infant. Carnegie Institution of Washington, Publication 233, p. 112, Table 17.

The average maximum total metabolism is 481 calories; divide this by twenty-four hours and it will give 20 calories, the amount produced in one hour; 50/60 of 20 = 17 calories, or the amount theoretically excreted during the fifty minutes that E. S. was out of the chamber.

Tables 7 and 8 give the total number of calories used up by Infants E. L. and E. S.

TABLE 7.—Total Number of Calories Used by Infant E. L.

| Period | Carbon Dioxid, Gm. | Respiratory Quotient | Heat Computed (24 hr.) Calories | | | Pulse Rate |
			Total	Per Kg.	Per Sq. M. Lissauer	
Measured 22 hr., 31 min.	120.8	0.87	345	..	....	127
Estimated 1 hr., 29 min.	9.3	....	27			
Total....................	130	....	372	74	1232	

TABLE 8.—Total Number of Calories Used by Infant E. S.

| Period | Carbon Dioxid, Gm. | Respiratory Quotient | Heat Computed (24 hr.) Calories | | | Pulse Rate |
			Total	Per Kg.	Per Sq. M. Lissauer	
Measured 23 hr., 10 min.	130.4	0.83	387	..	....	127
Estimated 50 min.	5.6	....	17			
Total.....	136.0	....	404	70	1232	

What is measured is the actual heat produced by these infants. There are, however, other ways in which energy may be lost from the body, such as the potential energy of the urine and feces. This energy which is lost must be supplied in the food. An estimate of this loss is, of course, open to many objections, and the figure given here will be modified by future investigations. Presumably the greatest single factor to take into consideration is the fat lost in the feces, which with the urea in the urine should not exceed 15 per cent. of the total measured metabolism in a normal infant.

When the factor for the food lost in the excreta has been added to the total, and that amount of food given to the infant, it should neither gain nor loose weight, but should remain in an equilibrium. Extra food must, therefore, be added so that the baby may grow. This figure is also difficult to estimate. Clinically, when infants are receiving only slightly more food than is necessary to maintain an equilibrium, they gain very slowly in weight, whereas, if they are given more food they gain more rapidly. Rubner and Heubner's infants received a little less than 15 per cent. of the total measured calories for growth. If 20 per cent. is taken for the growth factor, it should give enough leeway for the infants to gain.

A rough estimate of the caloric requirements of a normal infant may be made by adding the calories used up by muscular activity to the basal metabolism. If the infant is very quiet, 15 per cent. should be added, if normally active 25 per cent., and if extremely active, about 40 per cent. To the result add 15 per cent. for energy lost in the excreta and 20 per cent. for growth. In the case of E. L. we know how many calories were actually used up in muscular exercise. Therefore, all that is necessary is to add the probable number of calories necessary to allow for growth and what is lost in the excreta. If 35 per cent. is added to the 74 calories per kilogram of body weight actually used by E. L., it is found that she needs about 100 calories per kilogram of body weight in her food. If the same thing is done for E. S., the food requirements are found to be about 94 calories per kilogram of body weight.

It is probable that infants fed on cow's milk, particularly on formulas containing large amounts of protein, will require even more food than infants fed on human milk, because the stimulating action of protein causes extra heat to be burned during digestion. The caloric requirements of normal infants obviously are not the same as those of the sick infant whose "basal" metabolism is higher per kilogram of body weight and who may use up additional energy because of increased restlessness from colic or discomfort, burn it up in fever, or may not absorb all the food given him, as happened in one infant who lost 20 per cent. of the food calories in the feces. Neither does it apply to the infant with a subnormal temperature, indicating depressed vital functions. These infants come under another category and require further study to answer many of the points now obscure.

29

Reprinted from Am. J. Dis. Child., **30**(4), 453–475 (1925)

COMPARISON AND INTERPRETATION ON A CALORIC BASIS OF THE MILK MIXTURES USED IN INFANT FEEDING *

GROVER F. POWERS, M.D.
NEW HAVEN, CONN.

Great progress in the study of nutrition has been brought about within the past two decades by new procedures in the feeding of experimental animals, particularly small animals. In earlier investigations, complex foods as they occur in nature were used, and important nutritive factors were often more or less unknowingly modified. In the more recent work, test rations of relatively simple foodstuffs, the proximate composition of which is known, are fed and the ensuing effect on the health and nutrition of the animals correlated with the variable or variables in the diet being studied. In this way, the rôle of certain nutrients in metabolic processes has been perceived. The method has reached its greatest refinement in the hands of Osborne and Mendel who, in their experiments on the rat, have employed "synthetic" diets of salts, vitamins and purified protein, carbohydrate and fat.

The adoption in infant feeding of the fundamental principles underlying the new method of approach in the study of nutritional problems would seem to promise fruitful developments; needless to say, application of the technic is more difficult with babies than with animals. However, some progress in this direction has been made in the Pediatric Clinic of Yale University. One of the necessary preliminary steps was to find out what the milk mixtures commonly used in infant feeding are when their constitution is expressed in terms of their actual nutrients independent of the medium, water, in which they are carried. Accordingly, the energy yielding food components were estimated in terms of their respective proportions of the total caloric value of the food mixtures as fed. This expression of the milk mixtures in terms of the unit of physiologic currency—the calory—has brought to light certain interesting and significant facts which will be described and discussed.

CURRENT DIETETIC METHODS OF EVALUATING FOODS

Foods are evaluated and compared in various ways according to the basic units used. The unit may be some other foodstuff or food component arbitrarily selected as a standard. More frequently, however, a

* Received for publication, May 22, 1925.
* From the Department of Pediatrics, Yale University, School of Medicine.

gravimetric standard, the ounce or gram, or the unit of energy, the calory, is employed.

The scientific use of food equivalents in dietetics has been largely limited to animal husbandry where the starch unit of food value is frequently used. Borrowing from the stockman's method, Pirquet developed a food unit system of dietetics for human beings and coined the term "nem" which he used as the unit of currency for food values. The expression of the nutritional value of all foods as multiples or fractions of the nutritive combustible value of 1 gm. of human milk of average composition (the "nem") may have great psychologic assets under certain circumstances, but the scientific value of the method is questionable. Physicians frequently illustrate to their patients the worth of various foods by comparing their nutritional value with that of an egg; the "nem" is helpful in just the same way.

The "formulas" of the food mixtures used in infant feeding are ordinarily expressed as the proportions by weight or volume, which the various food components are of the total mass of the food—the so-called "percentage system." So formulated, certain similarities and differences in foods may be suggested in a vague way but the essential fact inherent in "the percentage system," namely, that the values of the nutrients are ratios which express only degree of concentration, is often lost sight of. For comparative purposes, especially, it is difficult to perceive significant facts from small, often fractional, percentage values of protein, carbohydrate and fat which shift with changes in volume. More helpful data would be apparent if water were disregarded and the food constituents were expressed as proportions of the solids in the mixture. Protein, carbohydrate, fat and salts would then be shown as they are related to each other independent of their relation to the diluent. These points may be made clear by a simple example, as shown in the table.

Composition of Cow's Milk and Diluted Cow's Milk

	Percentage of Volume		Percentage of Solids	
	Cow's Milk	Cow's Milk and Water, Equal Parts	Cow's Milk	Cow's Milk and Water, Equal Parts
Protein	3.5	1.75	28	28
Carbohydrate	4.75	2.37	38	38
Fat	3.5	1.75	28	28
Salts	0.75	0.37	6	6
Solids	12.5	6.2	100	100
Water	87.5	93.73	700	1,500

If cow's milk, containing 3.5 per cent. protein, 3.75 per cent. carbohydrate, 3.5 per cent. fat, 0.75 per cent. salts, 12.5 per cent. total solids, and 87.5 per cent. water is diluted with an equal volume of water, the mixture contains 1.75 per cent. protein 2.37 per cent. carbohydrate, 1.75 per cent. fat, 0.37 per cent. salts, 6.2 per cent. total solids and 93.75 per cent. water. The emphasis is here not obviously on the essential difference in the two mixtures, namely, that the second contains about twice as much water as the first but rather on the apparent differences in the comparative amounts of protein, carbohydrate and fat. As a matter of fact, in both mixtures the protein, carbohydrate and fat are 28, 38 and 28 per cent. respectively, of the total solids, whereas the water in the second mixture (1,500 per cent. of the total solids) is approximately twice that in the first (700 per cent. of total solids). In this manner the actual comparative difference in the two mixtures is indicated to be exactly where it actually is, that is, in concentration. The energy yielding components do not appear to be affected relatively, as indeed they are not.

Although it is possible to establish a satisfactory means of comparative study of various foods on a quantitative basis, it is advisable to go further to a more fundamental unit for a common currency in infant feeding. The calory is the unit used everywhere by physiologists in the investigation of problems of nutrition. Itself a measure of energy, the calory is used constantly in metabolism studies and is also a physiologic unit. As such, it is greatly superior to the gram as the unit to which the protein, carbohydrate and fat food components may be reduced. The calory is a least common denominator of all energy-yielding food constituents and their derivatives. In this paper the caloric values of these derivatives have not been determined but it should not be thought that qualitative differences in the food constituents are considered unimportant, simply because interest is first directed to the relatively simple study of each of the three large groups of foodstuffs.

Briefly stated, in the analyses and comparisons of milk mixtures described in this paper, the total caloric value of a given amount of the food as fed is estimated, and the percentage relationships which exist between the total calories and the calories of protein, of carbohydrate and of fat are then determined. Thus, the energy yielding components are expressed and compared without confusing alliances with volumetric data.

Although a study of the protein, carbohydrate and fat components of food mixtures only is made in this paper, constituents which alone may be studied on a caloric basis, and emphasis has been placed on this method of approach, no undervaluation is implied of the importance in nutrition of water, vitamins and salts which are also food components.

EFFECT ON THE PROPORTION OF THE TOTAL CALORIES IN NUTRIENTS
WHEN WATER OR ENERGY YIELDING FOOD COMPONENTS
ARE ADDED TO MILK MIXTURES

The addition of water to any food mixture does not, of course, change the quantitative or calory relationships of the food components to each other. In whole cow's milk, for example, 22 per cent. of the total calories are in protein, 29 per cent. in lactose and 49 per cent. in fat (Chart 1). If water is added to whole cow's milk, the caloric value of each cubic centimeter of the mixture is thereby reduced but the proportions of the food components in the total energy valuation remain the same.

A very different result, however, is obtained when milk is "diluted" not with water, but with an energy yielding substance. The effect is to increase the value of the added component at the expense of those components which are unreinforced. The effect is shown in Chart 1. Carbohydrate, for example, when added in increasing amounts to a fixed volume of whole cow's milk, assumes an increasing percentage representation in the total energy value of the mixture at the expense of every other food component, protein, fat and lactose. These are "squeezed," as the chart suggests, by the added carbohydrate to smaller and smaller percentages of the total caloric valuation.

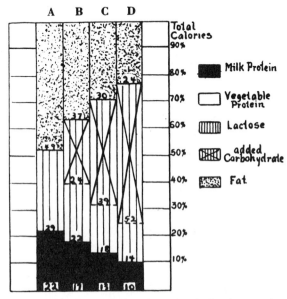

Chart 1.—Effect on the percentage of total calories in protein, carbohydrate and fat when various amounts of cane sugar are added to whole cow's milk: *A,* whole cow's milk, calories = 0.66 per c.c.; *B,* whole cow's milk, cane sugar, 5 per cent., calories = 0.86 per c.c.; *C,* whole cow's milk, cane sugar, 10 per cent., calories = 1.04 per c.c.; *D,* whole cow's milk, cane sugar, 17 per cent., calories = 1.32 per c.c. In each chart, the heavy black indicates milk protein; white, vegetable protein; straight lines, lactose; crossed lines, added carbohydrates, and dots, fat.

By subtraction, so to speak, of certain food components from mixtures, a reverse effect on the percentage representation of the other components in the total calories occurs. This is shown in Chart 2. If all the fat is removed from cow's milk (as in skimmed Cream-On), the percentages of the total calories in protein and lactose double their values in whole milk. If the milk has only part of its fat "subtracted" as in Dryco, then the percentage of the total calories in protein and lactose are also increased over their corresponding values in whole milk but not to the same degree as in fat-free milk.

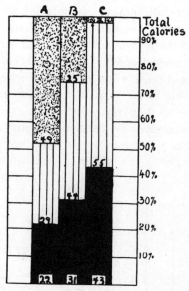

Chart 2.—Effect on the percentage of total calories in protein carbohydrate and fat when various amounts of fat are removed from cow's milk: *A*, whole cow's milk, calories = 0.66 per c.c.; *B*, Dryco, 1 part, water, 10 parts, calories = 0.42 per c.c.; *C*, skimmed Cream-on, 1 part, water, 10 parts, calories = 0.32 per c.c.

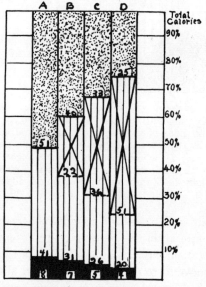

Chart 3.—Effect on the percentage of total calories in protein, carbohydrate and fat when various amounts of sugar are added to human milk: *A*, human milk, calories = 0.72 per c.c.; *B*, human milk, cane sugar, 5 per cent., calories = 0.92 per c.c.; *C*, human milk, cane sugar, 10 per cent., calories = 1.12 per c.c.; *D*, human milk cane sugar, 18 per cent., calories = 1.44 per c.c.

The effect of the addition of an energy yielding substance like sugar to breast milk is shown in Chart 3. · In breast milk, 8 per cent. of the total energy is in protein. As sugar is added, the protein, lactose and fat proportions of the total calories become smaller and smaller. When isodynamic amounts of sugar (18 per cent.) are added to human milk, protein constitutes only 4 per cent. of the total calories. The vitamins, salts and unknown factors are also proportionately reduced by the addition of sugar. Thus, this mixture, used particularly by Schick for premature and for feeble infants is probably not a safe food for use over any considerable period of time.

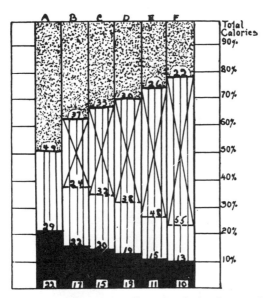

Chart 4.—Effect on the percentage of total calories in protein carbohydrate and fat when cane sugar in amount equivalent to 5 per cent. of the mixture is added to various dilutions of cow's milk with water: A, whole cow's milk, calories = 0.66 per c.c.; B, whole cow's milk, cane sugar, 5 per cent., calories = 0.86 per c.c.; C, whole cow's milk, 2 parts; water, 1 part; cane sugar, 5 per cent., calories = 0.62 per c.c.; D, whole cow's milk, 1 part; water, 1 part; cane sugar, 5 per cent.; calories = 0.53 per c.c.; E, whole cow's milk, 1 part; water, 2 parts; cane sugar, 5 per cent., calories = 0.42 per c.c.; F, whole cow's milk, 1 part; water, 3 parts; cane sugar, 5 per cent., calories = 0.36 per c.c.

When carbohydrate is added at a fixed percentage of the total volume to various water dilutions of cow's milk, the general effect on the distribution of calory percentages is identical with that demonstrated in the foregoing when carbohydrate is added in varying percentages of the total volume to undiluted cow's milk or to human milk (Chart 4). That is, as the mixtures in the series are made increasingly dilute while the volumes are kept the same, the percentage values in the total calories of protein, lactose and fat become progressively smaller, whereas that of the carbohydrate, always added in the same proportion of volume, becomes progressively larger. Thus, the addition of an energy yielding nutrient, such as sugar, at a fixed proportion of the total volume of mixtures identical in volume but containing diminishing amounts of energy yielding milk and increasing amounts of water, has the effect of actually adding to the mixtures relatively increasing amounts of sugar. On the other hand, if in the same water dilutions of milk, the ratio between the decreasing amount of milk and the added sugar is always the same, the percentage relationship of protein, fat, lactose,

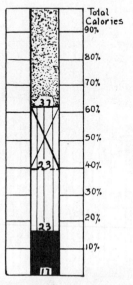

Chart 5.—Unaffected percentage of total calories in protein carbohydrate and fat when cane sugar in amount equivalent to 5 per cent. of the milk in mixture is added to dilutions of cow's milk: whole cow's milk, cane sugar, 5 per cent. of milk in mixture, calorie = 0.86 per c.c.; whole cow's milk, 2 parts; water 1 part, cane sugar 5 per cent. of milk in mixture, calories = 0.56 per c.c.; whole cow's milk, 1 part, water, 1 part, cane sugar, 5 per cent. of milk in mixture, calories = 0.43 per c.c.; whole cow's milk, 1 part, water, 2 parts, cane sugar, 5 per cent. of milk in mixture, calories = 0.28 per c.c.; whole cow's milk, 1 part, water, 3 parts, cane sugar, 5 per cent. of milk in mixture, calories = 0.21 per c.c.

and added carbohydrate in the total calories will be unaffected by water dilution. This is shown in Chart 5 where the added carbohydrate in the formulas is always 5 per cent., not of the volume of the mixture, but of the milk therein.

COMPOSITION AND COMPARISON OF MILK MIXTURES WHEN THE ENERGY YIELDING COMPONENTS ARE EXPRESSED IN PER-CENTAGES OF TOTAL CALORIES IN MIXTURES

With this preliminary discussion of some of the facts of general interest brought out by the method of food evaluation used in this study, a comparison and interpretation of the mixtures commonly used in infant feeding will now be made.[1]

Whey-Adapted Milk of Schloss ‡

Whole milk..	140.0 c.c.
Cream (20%)..	140.0 c.c.
Nahrzucker...	35.0 gm.
Flour...	15.0 gm.
Nutrose..	5.0 gm.
Water..	700.0 c.c.
Calories = 0.6 per c.c.	

Nine per cent. of total calories in protein, 49 per cent. in carbohydrate and 42 per cent. in fat. (Composition of cream:† protein, 3 per cent.; lactose, 3.9 per cent.; fat, 20 per cent.).

Artificial Mother-Milk of Friedenthal ‡

Water..	600.0 c.c.
Skimmed milk......................................	330.0 c.c.
Milk sugar...	58.0 gm.
Cream, q. s. to make a mixture containing 4.5 per cent. fat	
(If 16 per cent. cream is used, the required amount is 364.0 c.c.)	
Calories = 0.96 per c.c.	

Nine per cent. of total calories in protein, 37 per cent. in carbohydrate and 54 per cent. in fat. (Composition of skimmed milk:* protein, 3.2 per cent.; lactose, 4.5 per cent., and fat, 0 per cent. Composition of cream,* protein, 3.2 per cent.; lactose, 4.5 per cent., and fat, 16 per cent.).

Composition of Foods in Gravimetric Percentages

Food	Protein	Carbo-hydrate	Fat	Calories per 100 C.c. or Gm.	Per Cent. of Total Calories in: Pro-tein	Carbo-hydrate	Fat
Breast milk............................	1.5	7.3	4.0	72	8	41	51
Cows' milk.............................	3.5	4.7	3.5	66	22	29	49
Asses' milk *..........................	1.8	6.1	1.3	44	16	57	27
Ewes' milk *...........................	5.6	5.0	7.0	105	21	19	60
Reindeer milk *........................	10.9	2.8	17.1	207	21	5	74
Mares' milk *..........................	2.5	5.8	1.1	43	23	54	23
Goats' milk *..........................	4.6	4.3	4.0	71	25	25	50
Sows' milk *...........................	7.2	3.2	4.5	83	35	15	50
Eagle Brand condensed milk *..........	8.0	54.9	9.6	338	10	65	25
St. Charles evaporated milk *.........	8.8	10.9	8.7	157	22	28	50
Whey (König)†.........................	0.8	4.7	0.3	25	13	76	11
Dryco.................................	33.3	45.9	12.0	424	31	44	25
Klim (whole)..........................	27.0	38.0	28.0	512	21	30	49
Mammala..............................	24.0	54.0	12.0	420	23	51	26
Cream-On (skimmed)...................	39.0	49.6	0.5	359	44	55	1
Protein milk ‡........................	2.7	1.4	2.2	37	30	16	54
Mellins Food..........................	10.3	79.5	0.1	359	11	89	..
Malt soup extract (Borcherdt).........	6.4	69.2	....	302	8	92	..
Gaertner's milk §.....................	1.7	6.5	3.5	64	11	41	48
Backhaus milk §.......................	1.6	6.0	3.1	58	11	41	48
Ramogen..............................	7.0	34.6	16.5	314	9	44	47
Meigs mixture ⁵.......................	1.2	6.6	3.5	62	8	42	50
Rotch formula ⁵.......................	1.1	6.2	4.0	65	7	38	55
Lahmann's vegetable milk §............	10.0	38.5	25.0	419	9	37	54

* Morse, J. L., and Talbot, F. B.: Diseases of Nutrition and Infant Feeding, Ed. 2, New York, The Macmillan Company, 1920.
† Holt, L. E., and Howland, J.: The Diseases of Infancy and Childhood, Ed. 7, New York, D. Appleton & Co., 1916.
‡ Finkelstein, H.: Lehrbuch der Säuglingskrankheiten—Zweite Auflage, Berlin, J. Springer, 1921.
§ Fischer, L.: Infant Feeding in Health and Disease, Ed. 2, Philadelphia, F. A. Davis Company, 1901.

1. The data on which the study is based are summarized on the charts or in the tables which follow. The approximate physiologic fuel values of the food constituents were used, that is, protein, 4 calories per gram, carbohydrate, 4 calories per gram, and fat, 9 calories per gram. The fat content of butter was counted as 85 per cent. The protein content of wheat flour was counted as 10 per cent. (Sherman, H. C.: Chemistry of Food and Nutrition, Ed. 2, 1920, New York, The MacMillah Co.)

In Chart 6, the caloric evaluations of the milks of several species of animals are graphically shown, arranged in an ascending scale with reference to the protein percentage values in the total calories. The protein of human milk is markedly lower than that of any animals studied. The proportions of the total calories in protein of the milks of the sheep, reindeer, cow, horse and goat are strikingly similar, but the concentration of these milks varies greatly. It is noteworthy that the fat in the milk of the reindeer constitutes 74 per cent. of the total caloric value and the milk is highly concentrated; it has a caloric value of

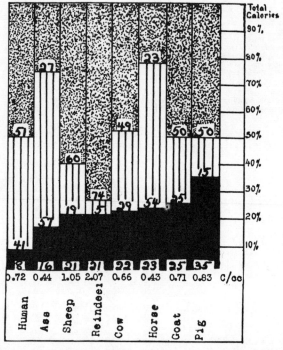

Chart 6.—Percentage of total calories in protein, carbohydrate and fat in the milk of animals of different species.

2 per cubic centimeter. No food used in infant feeding closely approaches reindeer's milk in this respect; the butter-flour mixtures of Moro represent the extreme point at present attained in concentration of milk mixtures fed to infants; in the foods described by Moro,[2] however, the caloric value is only about 75 per cent. of that of reindeer's milk. It is of interest to observe that of the milks of the various animals studied, no two, excepting those of the cow and of the goat, are similar in proportionate caloric configuration. As will be pointed out later, the

2. Moro, E.: Buttermehlbrei und Buttermehlvollmilch als Säuglingsnahrung. Monatschr. f. Kinderh. 18:97, 1920.

caloric percentage pattern of ass's milk is more nearly that of the milk mixtures commonly used in infant feeding than is that of any other natural milk.

In Chart 7 a series of infant foods and milk mixtures is shown, arranged also according to the ascending scale of the values of the protein percentages of the total calories. Breast milk is at one extreme and skimmed cow's milk at the other. It will be obvious from the analyses

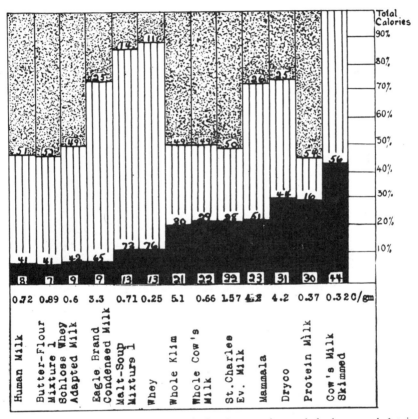

Chart 7.—Percentage of total calories in protein, carbohydrate and fat in several commonly used foods and feeding mixtures.

shown and graphically demonstrated in this paper that the mixtures studied fall rather readily into seven fairly well defined groups (Chart 8).

HUMAN MILK

Group 1.—Here the percentage representation in the total calories of protein, carbohydrate and fat are approximately 8, 41 and 51 per cent., respectively (Chart 3). Low protein combined with high fat is the outstanding characteristic of breast milk and no mixtures surpass it in respect to this combination.   In this group are the butter-flour mixtures,[3] most of the top milk mixtures with added sugar, most of the Winters,[4] Rotch and Meigs[5] mixtures, Ramogen and the avowed imitations of human milk—artificial mother's milk of Gaertner,[6] Backhaus,[6] Friedenthal,[7] whey-adapted milk of Schloss,[7] and synthetic milk adapted of Gerstenberger and Ruh.[8]   Excepting these modifications of cow's milk, which, after all, are either obsolete or restricted in their use. breast milk has no following among the mixtures used in infant feeding.   It stands alone among the vast majority of the successful mixtures, the caloric configuration of which is fashioned after a very different

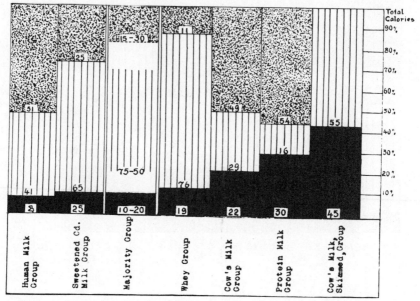

Chart 8.—Groups into which the milk mixtures commonly used in infant feeding may be assembled according to the similarity in their percentage distribution of protein, carbohydrate and fat in the total calories.

pattern from that of low protein, high fat and moderate carbohydrate. Quite the contrary result might have been anticipated and this method of analysis has revealed in a striking manner the uniqueness of breast

3. Czerny, A., and Kleinschmidt, H.:   Ueber eine Buttermehlnahrung für schwache Sauglinge, Jahrb. f. Kinderh. **87**:1, 1918.
4. Winters, J. E.:   Feeding in Early Infancy, Med. Rec. **63**:366, 1903.
5. Rotch, T. M.:   Infant Feeding — Weaning, Keating's Cyclopaedia of the Diseases of Children.   Vol. 1, Philadelphia, J. B. Lippincott Company, 1889.
6. Fisher, L.:   Infant Feeding in Health and Disease, Ed. 2, Philadelphia, F. A. Davis Co., 1901.
7. Finkelstein, H.:   Lehrbuch der Säuglingskrankheiten Zweite Auflage, Berlin, J. Springer, 1921.
8. Gerstenberger, H., and Ruh, H. O.:   Studies in the Adaption of an Artificial Food to Human Milk, Am. J. Dis. Child. **17**:1 (Jan.) 1919.

milk.   Human milk stands apart from the commonly used infant feedings, indeed, more conspicuously so than does cow's milk itself, in spite of the endeavor of most pediatricians to approach as near as possible to the one and to flee as far as possible from the other.   A study of Chart 9 shows that all [9] of the so-called butter-flour mixtures of Czerny and Kleinschmidt [3] and Moro [2] are essentially foods having the percentage caloric apportionments to protein, carbohydrate and fat of human milk; regardless of variations suggested by their diverse

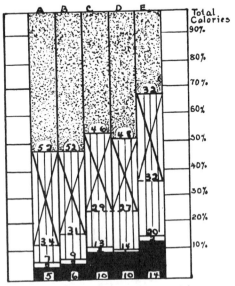

Chart 9.—Various butter-flour mixtures expressed in terms of the percentage of total calories in milk protein, vegetable protein, carbohydrate and fat: *A*, butter-flour food I (Czerny-Kleinschmidt), butter, 4.6 gm., wheat flour 4.6 gm., cane sugar 3.3 gm.; whole cow's milk, 33 c.c., water, to 100 c.c., calories = 0.89 per c.c.; *B*, butter-flour food II (Czerny-Kleinschmidt), butter, 4.2 gm., wheat flour, 4.2 gm., cane sugar 3.0 gm., whole cow's milk, 40 c.c., water to 100 c.c., calories = 0.87 per c.c.; *C*, butter-flour mixture (Moro), butter, 5.0 gm., flour, 7.0 gm., cane sugar, 5.0 gm., whole cow's milk, 100 c.c., calories = 1.52 per c.c.; *D*, whole milk butter-flour mixture (Moro), butter, 5.0 gm., wheat flour, 3.0 gm., cane sugar, 7.0 gm., whole cow's milk, 100 c.c., calories = 1.44 per c.c.; *E*, fat rich milk mixture (Kleinschmidt), butter, 3.5 gm., wheat flour, 3.5 gm., cane sugar 5.0 gm., Sk. buttermilk, 100 c.c., (fat, 0.5 per cent.), calories = 1.0 per c.c.

formulas the mixtures differ almost entirely only in concentration.   It is doubtful, however, if these mixtures were devised in any way as imitations of human milk, for they were adopted officially by pediatricians from the experience of Alpine peasants.[10]

---

9. The Kleinschmidt (Monatsch. f. Kinderh. **19**:369, 1920-1921) modification is an exception to this statement; it is really sour whole cows' milk, with 8 per cent. carbohydrate added in the form of sugar and flour.

10. Personal communication of Professor Feer of Zurich to Dr. E. A. Park.

COW'S MILK

Group 2.—In this group the percentage representation in the total calories of protein, carbohydrate and fat is approximately 20, 30 and 50 per cent., respectively. Cow's milk, evaporated milk, Cream-On, full strength Klim and goat's milk belong in this group. There appears to be no widely used infant feeding mixture which is actually an imitation, conscious or otherwise, of cow's milk; the tendency has always been away from unmodified cow's milk although it has been fed successfully to many infants. From the experience of Budin and his followers, there can be no doubt that sterilized whole cow's milk can

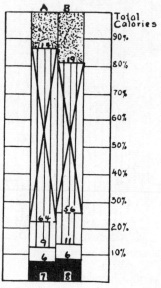

Chart 10.—Two malt-soup mixtures expressed in terms of the percentage of total calories in milk protein, vegetable protein, carbohydrate and fat: *A,* wheat flour, 5.0 gm., malt-soup extract, 10.0 gm., whole cow's milk, 33.0 gm., water 100 c.c., calories = 0.71 per c.c.; *B,* wheat flour, 5.0 gm., malt-soup extract, 10.0 gm., whole cow's milk, 50.0 gm., water 100 c.c., calories = 0.83 per c.c.

be successfully fed to some infants. That it is not extensively used is testimony, however, to the fact that it is not the most easily tolerated artificial food for infants.

WHEY

Group 3.—Here the percentage representation in the total calories of protein, carbohydrate and fat is approximately 13, 74 and 13 per cent., respectively—about three fourths of the calories being in carbohydrate and the remainder about equally allotted to protein and fat. The removal of the casein and enmeshed fat in the preparation of whey has the same effect on the caloric constitution of the mixture as that of adding 15 per cent. carbohydrate to half-skimmed milk. Many familiar friends are found in this group, the most prominent of which are the malt-soup mixtures (Chart 10). Nestle's Food, Horlick's Malted Milk and Eskay's food (when used without added milk) if not within the group are near relatives. Protein milk with 15 or 20 per cent. added sugar (Chart 12) also qualify for membership here, although the name makes these mixtures appear to be entirely unrelated.

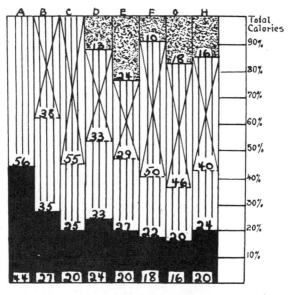

Chart 11.—Effect on the percentage of total calories in protein, carbohydrate and fat in various modifications of skimmed milk. *A*, skimmed milk (protein, 3.5 per cent., carbohydrate 4.5 per cent.), calories = 0.32 per c.c.; *B*, skimmed milk, cane sugar, 5 per cent., calories = 0.52 per c.c.; *C*, skimmed milk, cane sugar, 10 per cent., calories = 0.72 per c.c.; *D*, skimmed milk, cane sugar, 5 per cent., butter 1 per cent. (fat, 0.85 per cent.), calories = 0.6 per c.c.; *E*, skimmed milk, cane sugar, 5 per cent., butter, 2 per cent. (fat, 1.7 per cent.), calories = 0.68 per c.c.; *F*, skimmed milk, cane sugar, 10 per cent., butter, 1 per cent. (fat, 0.85 per cent.), calories = 0.8 per c.c.; *G*, skimmed milk, cane sugar, 10 per cent., butter, 2 per cent. (fat 1.7 per cent.), calories = 0.88 per c.c.; *H*, Holländische Säugingsnahrung (protein, 2.7 per cent.; carbohydrate = 3.5 per cent., fat, 1 per cent.), cane sugar, 5 per cent., wheat flour, 5 per cent., calories = 0.55 per c.c.

SKIMMED COW'S MILK

Group 4.—The percentage representation in the total calories of protein, carbohydrate and fat in members of this group approach those of completely skimmed milk: 45, 55 and 0 per cent., respectively (Chart 11). Completely skimmed milk, either as sweet milk or as lactic acid milk, is the simplest food used in infant feeding in the sense that it contains only two energy yielding food components. Because of this very simplicity, which depends on a deficiency, skimmed milk may be regarded as an abnormal food. Its extreme position, as shown in Charts 7 and 8, far removed from human milk, and indeed from all natural milks, would corroborate this view. On the other hand, skimmed milk serves as a convenient simple base for building up more adequately balanced foods and many successful feedings may be most easily looked on as modifications of skimmed milk. The "Holländische Säuglingsnahrung" [11]—widely and successfully used—is a sour skimmed milk containing 1 per cent. fat with sugar and flour added. Dryco and half-strength Klim are skimmed milks containing some fat; so also is Mammala but with added carbohydrate also. The success attributed to these dried, partially skimmed milks may be due in part to the fact that the removal of fat from whole milk not only reduces the proportion

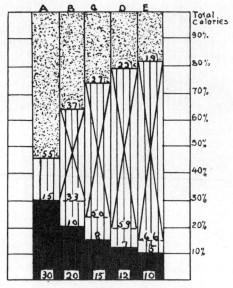

Chart 12.—Various protein milk mixtures expressed in terms of the percentage of total calories in protein, carbohydrate and fat. *A*, protein milk, calories = 0.37 per c.c.; *B*, protein milk, cane sugar, 5 per cent., calories = 0.61 per c.c.; *C*, protein milk, cane sugar, 10 per cent., calories = 0.81 per c.c.; *D*, protein milk, cane sugar, 15 per cent., calories = 1.01 per c.c.; *E*, protein milk, cane sugar, 20 per cent., calories = 1.21 per c.c.

of the total calories in that component, but, at the same time, has the effect of raising the proportions in protein and sugar. Chart 11 illustrates the simplicity and abnormality of skimmed milk and the effect on it of various modifications, most of which fall within the confines of the majority group of mixtures used in infant feeding. These mixtures are fairly high in protein and mixed carbohydrate and relatively low in fat.

---

11. Finkelstein, H.: Lehrbuch der Säuglingskrankheiten—Zweite Auflage, Berlin, J. Springer, 1921.

PROTEIN MILK

Group 5.—Like skimmed cow's milk, protein milk stands apart as a unique food; 30 per cent. of the total calories are allotted to protein, 15 to carbohydrate, and 55 to fat (Chart 12). The picture is exactly the reverse of the whey group of mixtures with their high sugar and low protein and fat. Even the addition of 5 or 10 per cent. sugar does not completely efface the peculiar makeup of this freak mixture. With the addition of 10 per cent. sugar, protein and fat are still well represented in percentages of the total calories. By name, whether in English or in German, attention is called to the high protein content of protein milk, but it ought to be equally well known that the fat content of this food is high. This fact is shown by its percentage composition, but is strikingly brought out when food components are graphed in terms of percentages of total calories. The percentage of total calories in fat (55) is the highest existing in any mixture used in infant feeding. As breast milk combines high fat with the lowest protein found in any milk mixture, so protein milk combines the highest fat with very high protein. Without the addition of carbohydrate, albumin milk is being less and less frequently used in infant feeding.

SWEETENED CONDENSED MILK

Group 6.—Here the percentage representation in the total calories of protein, carbohydrate and fat is approximately 10, 65 and 25 per cent., respectively; the caloric value of the added carbohydrate is 50 per cent. of the total calories (Chart 13). These mixtures are known in the Pirquet nomenclature as "dubo," because one-half the calories are in milk and one-half are in added carbohydrate. Some of the familiar members of this group may be enumerated in the order of their admitted orthodoxy in infant feeding as follows: one-third strength whole cow's milk with 5 per cent. added sugar, one-half strength whole cow's milk with 8 per cent. added sugar, two-thirds whole cow's milk with 10 per cent. added sugar, full strength cow's milk with 17 per cent. added sugar, and, lastly, sweetened condensed milk itself. These mixtures differ from each other only in concentration, a striking fact probably not generally appreciated and not easily demonstrable in the usual percentage manner of evaluating and comparing foods. These mixtures probably contain the minimum of fat and perhaps less than the minimum of protein which it is safe to give to any child for any considerable period of time.

MAJORITY GROUP

Group 7.—There is a final group which includes practically all other milk mixtures used in the artificial feeding of infants and, since it includes many of the mixtures commonly used in practice, it may be termed the majority group. The members of this group, although heterogeneous in their ancestry and constitution, cluster around the sweetened condensed milk family just described. The percentage of the total calories in protein varies between 10 and 20 per cent. and in fat between 15 and 30 per cent. Thus, the mixtures which are given to most artificially fed children contain somewhat more than 10 per cent. of the total calories in protein, and at least 15 per cent. of the total calories in fat. These values probably represent fairly satisfactory levels for these food components. In whole milk modifications, these requirements are met if 60 per cent. of the total calories are in milk, and 40 per cent. are in added carbohydrate. The European

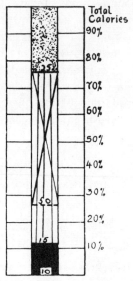

Chart 13.—Milk mixtures which seem widely different but which are identical when expressed in terms of the percentage of total calories in protein, carbohydrate and fat: whole cow's milk, 1 part, water, 2 parts, cane sugar, 5 per cent., calories = 0.42 per c.c.; whole cow's milk, 1 part, water, 1 part, cane sugar, 8 per cent., calories = 0.66 per c.c.; whole cow's milk, 2 parts, water, 1 part, cane sugar, 10 per cent., calories = 0.84 per c.c.; whole cow's milk, cane sugar, 17 per cent., calories = 1.3 per c.c.; sweetened condensed milk, calories = 3.3 per c.c.

rule of giving one tenth of the body weight in whole milk and one one-hundredth of the body weight in sugar as a daily ration is but the expression of a definite feeding allowance of a mixture which is actually whole cow's milk with 10 per cent. added sugar. This formula, when analyzed, shows that 13 per cent. of the total calories are in protein, 30 per cent. in fat, 18 per cent. in lactose and 39 per cent. in added carbohydrate. In other words, 60 per cent. of the total calories are in whole milk and 40 per cent. in added carbohydrate. In skimmed milk modifications, the protein and fat requirements are probably adequately met, if sugar and fat are added in amounts corresponding to 10 and 2 per cent., respectively, of the volume of the mixtures. Whatever the optimum protein intake of artificially fed infants may be, whether fairly fixed, or shifting with nutritional status, the fact remains that many infants have thriven on skimmed milk whether sweet or sour, reinforced with mixed carbohydrate and sufficient fat to cover fat soluble A requirements. Some milk fat is required because of its intimate association with vitamins and some is useful because of its high energy value. The relationship between fat and mineral metabolism is close. It is not established to what extent fat and carbohydrate are not isodynamically interchangeable in the infant's metabolism, but they are to a considerable degree.

Chart 8 demonstrates the intermediate position of the majority group of milk mixtures as determined on an ascending scale of protein percentages of the total calories. As already pointed out, it is obvious that the feedings in this group are similar to sweetened condensed milk; they differ chiefly in their somewhat higher protein content. The majority group is situated also next to the whey group from which it differs, calorically speaking, chiefly in having a greater percentage of the calories in fat. The majority group is thus intermediate between sweetened condensed milk on the one hand and the wheylike foods on the other. This would seem to be a surprising fact. *A priori,* one would not expect the majority of milk mixtures commonly used in infant feeding to be fashioned after freak mixtures such as skimmed milk or protein milk, but one would expect them to be much like human milk. That such is not the case is brought out in Chart 8. In contrast to human milk, which combines the lowest percentage of total calories in protein with the highest percentage in fat, the majority group mixtures show higher values for the percentages of total calories in protein and carbohydrate and a lower value for that of fat. The only natural milk to whose caloric percentage pattern the members of the majority group conform is that of the ass. It is of interest to point out that some French pediatricians hold ass's milk next in favor to human milk as an infant food.[12] The milk mixtures which conform to the caloric percentage distributions of the majority and sweetened condensed milk groups are widely used, because experience has shown that most infants thrive on one or another of them. If one mixture in the group does not seem satisfactory, then another mixture is tried and perhaps still another and probably, finally, sweetened condensed milk itself. Physicians little realize that these mixtures differ but little from one

12. Czerny, A., and Keller, A.: Des Kindes Ernährung, Ernähungsstörungen und Ernahrungstherapie, Leipzig and Wein, Franz Deuticke, 1923.

another except in the amount of dilution and degree of cooking. It is an astonishing fact that one-third strength cow's milk with 5 per cent. sugar—a mixture universally used in infant feeding and regarded as orthodox by pediatricians of all schools—differs from sweetened condensed milk as it comes from the can only in degree of dilution and extent of denaturization by cooking and storage. On no mixtures in the other groups discussed have large numbers of average infants been fed successfully for considerable lengths of time.

This method of food analysis may be carried out to the most minute detail. For example, not only may the percentage of the total calories in protein be determined and graphed but the protein calories

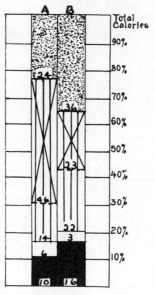

Chart 14.—Two Mellin's Food mixtures expressed in terms of the percentage of total calories in milk protein, vegetable protein, carbohydrate and fat: *A,* whole cow's milk, 1 part, water, 3 parts, Mellin's Food, 5 per cent., calories = 0.33 per c.c.; *B,* whole cow's milk, 3 parts, water, 1 part, Mellin's Food, 5 per cent., calories = 0.65 per c.c.

may be further analyzed. A graphic analysis of two Mellin's Food formulas are shown in Chart 14. The two mixtures graphed contain a rather high percentage of the total calories in protein, due to the fact that Mellin's Food contains vegetable protein. The vegetable protein is easily shown distinct from the milk protein. In the future, vegetable protein may be shown to give the carbohydrate mixtures containing it a distinct nutritive value. Malt-soup and butter-flour preparations are other noteworthy mixtures containing vegetable protein. In a similar manner, all forms of added protein, carbohydrate and fat may be estimated and charted and the importance of the individual constituents to infant nutrition may be determined.

One outstanding revelation of this method of approach to the problems of infant feeding has been that large numbers of supposedly different foods are similar, even identical, in all respects save their water content. The question of the relation of water to the digestibility of foods is thus brought to the forefront. Without doubt, there is an undetermined minimum of water required for digestion. There are, however, no exact data to indicate to what extent dilution is a benefit. There is no doubt that dilution is often an evil. Frequently infants fed on extremely dilute mixtures have become dystrophic either because the bulk of the food required to give the child sufficient energy for growth has been greater than it could take, or else the required amount has been taken and as promptly vomited from mechanical causes. The end-result is the same in either case. The influence of water on the digestibility of food needs further study, but primarily the infant's requirement of water must be considered rather than his food's requirement to increase its digestibility. Furthermore, no fixed standard for the comparison of various foods can be set up so long as the water content (that is, total volume) is used as the basis.

Our knowledge of vitamins at present does not permit an experssion of their quantitative values. Cow's milk, the basis of practically all infant foods, contains several vitamins, the potency and quantity of which are probably determined to a considerable degree by the dietary and seasonal changes to which cows are subjected. Mixtures very low in milk content or deficient in certain components of milk may be incomplete foods in this sense and probably require reinforcement by the independent administration of vitamins. In the hope of making the protein or fat of milk more digestible by dilution with water, pediatricians have lost sight of the serious consequences which may result from reducing thereby the vitamin content of the food, for it is the custom to enhance the nutritional value of the diluted milk only by the addition of and, therefore, further dilution with a nonvitamin fuel component. that is, sugar. The following quotation from Osborne and Mendel[13] is of interest in this connection:

From a practical standpoint a more precise understanding of the quantitative relations of the vitamins is highly desirable. The fact that such diverse cellular structures as yeast, wheat embryo, corn germs, and glandular tissues show a surprising richness in growth-promoting properties aside from their protein and mineral content, is of immediate significance at a time when milk is still so uniquely valued for its nutrient virtues. . . . A particular case of this kind is that of an infant feeding where it is customary to reinforce the supply of calories by diluting top milk and adding milk sugar. Under these circumstances the child is supplied with a food that contains a relatively smaller proportion of the water-soluble vitamin than does the original cow's milk. While milk

13. Osborne, T. B., and Mendel, L. B.: Milk as a Source of Water-Soluble Vitamin, J. Biol. Chem. 34:3, 1918, 543.

thus modified may contain sufficient vitamin as long as the food intake is normal, if for any reason the child's appetite fails the vitamin supply is reduced and endless dietary troubles may easily result. . . . This is a practical question which deserves prompt investigation, for the best way to reinforce the vitamin content of the diluted milk is not yet evident, chiefly owing to our still limited knowledge of the distribution of this vitamin in nature. Such investigations as have been made demonstrate that the proportion of water-soluble vitamin in the various vegetable and animal tissues differs greatly, and it is probable that sooner or later some way will be found to a solution of the problem of successful infant feeding.

In regard to the salt content of infant feeding mixtures, it may be stated that in general the mineral constituents of most of them parallels the milk content. When milk is diluted with water and the requisite calories of a milk mixture made up with salt-poor food components, the actual mineral intake is greatly reduced. The salt content of milk mixtures may be so expressed to bring out its relationship to the total energy value of the food or to that of any one of the food components. For example, in human milk there are 2.7 mg. of inorganic salts for every calory of milk, and 33 mg. for every calory of protein.[14] In comparing the mineral content of various foods as Shohl[15] has pointed out, the salts may "be calculated in common terms, namely, as normal solutions. The analogy to energy metabolism is obvious. Salts can be evaluated in cubic centimeters of normal solution just as grams of protein, carbohydrate and fat can be reckoned in calories. The calcium requirement can be expressed in cubic centimeters of normal solution or percentage of the total cubic centimeters of salt, just as the protein requirement can be stated in calories or in percentage of the total calories. Given the total requirement, the extent to which salts are interchangeable must be determined for the various radicals, just as isodynamic quantities of fat and carbohydrate can be calculated. Amounts of minerals can be compared directly as chemical equivalents."

Not only do infant feedings of identical or similar caloric percentage pattern differ in their water, vitamin and mineral content but also they may be very unlike in the chemical and biologic values of all the various food components. In grouping milk mixtures on the basis of similar caloric constitution for the food components, this vital aspect of the nutritional problem is neither ignored nor relegated to the background; on the contrary, it is brought into prominence. Indeed, milk mixtures shorn of their water relationships and reduced to caloric expression, present themselves for study, not alone from the point of view of energy values but also from that of the biochemical values of the

14. Computation on the basis that 100 c.c. of human milk contains 200 mg. of inorganic salts and has an energy value of 73 calories of which 6 are supplied by protein.

15. Shohl, A. T.: Mineral Metabolism in Relation to Acid-Base Equilibrium, Physiol. Rev. **3**:509 (Oct.) 1923.

various components. The wide range of opinion among clinicians as to the effect both in health and disease of this or that form of protein, carbohydrate or fat, is eloquent testimony to the fact that few data are actually established which correlate qualitative differences in food components with physiologic response. The energy unit is thus perhaps not the ultimate basis for a helpful classification and accurate study of infant feedings but just now its use would seem to be a step toward that simplicity which must prevail, if progress is to be rapid in the correlation of food with nutritional status and disturbance. Cathcart [14] says:

No one will, of course, seriously maintain that nutrition can ultimately be reduced merely to the satisfying of the energy demands; the calory factor may be regarded as strictly secondary to the supply of material. We do not live on calories, yet all our general estimates of food requirements are quite properly for the most part made in terms of calories. Calory value is simply a very convenient physical standard for the assessment of diets, but merely because such a standard has proved of great utilitarian value there is no real justification for placing this standard as the foundation stone of hypotheses framed to offer an explanation of cellular activity.

SUMMARY

The constitution of a great number of the milk mixtures commonly used in infant feeding has been expressed in terms of the percentage of each energy-producing nutrient in the total energy value of the food as fed. This method of food evaluation has been the means of extricating these heterogeneous mixtures from a maze of quantitative relationships which are metabolically meaningless, and has made them available for comparative study on a significant basis in terms of the standard unit of nutritional currency—the calory—and without regard to water content. In this simple way, a host of apparently dissimilar milk mixtures have lost an artificial individuality and have been classified in seven distinctive groups. Here individual differences may be studied where they actually exist, that is, in mineral content, chemical and biologic values of protein, carbohydrate and fat, degree of denaturization and water content.

CONCLUSIONS

The following points may be emphasized in concluding this study:

1. The dilution of milk mixtures with water affects the calories per unit of mass, but not the percentage relationships of protein, carbohydrate and fat in the total calories.

2. The addition to milk mixtures of an energy yielding nutrient affects not only the total calories per unit of mass, but also diminishes the proportional representation in the total calories of the protein, lactose and fat.

---

14. Cathcart, E. P.: The Influence of Fat and Carbohydrate on the Nitrogen Distribution in the Urine, Biochem J. **16**:747, 1922.

3. The magnitude of any food component in a mixture, as expressed by its percentage representation in the total calories, is relatively increased by the removal or reduction of any other food component.

4. An energy-yielding nutrient, if introduced in a ratio fixed with relation to the other energy-yielding components of mixtures made increasingly dilute with water, does not affect the representation in the total calories of the other components.

5. On the other hand, an energy-yielding nutrient, if introduced in a ratio fixed with relation to the total constant volume of mixtures made increasingly dilute with water, brings about a reduction in the values of the protein, lactose and fat percentages of the total calories.

6. When the multitude of milk mixtures commonly used in infant feeding are reduced to the caloric percentage formulation, it is perceived that many of them are essentially alike or identical excepting in concentration, degree of denaturization by cooking or souring and qualitative differences in protein, carbohydrate, fat and salts.

7. Practically all milk mixtures may be found in one of seven groups.

8. A great number of mixtures which experience has shown to be particularly successful in feeding infants fall into a majority group which approaches the caloric percentage pattern of the food mixtures in the sweetened condensed milk group: about 60 per cent. of the total calories are in whole milk and 40 per cent. in added carbohydrate.

9. One-third milk with 5 per cent. added sugar, and other somewhat less frequently used mixtures, have the identical caloric percentage configuration of sweetened condensed milk and of whole milk to which 17 per cent. sugar has been added.

10. Human milk, cow's milk, whey, protein milk and skimmed milk are the most prominent representatives of the remaining five groups.

11. The Czerny-Kleinschmidt and Moro butter-flour mixtures have the same proportions of the total calories in protein, carbohydrate and fat as has human milk.

12. It is a striking fact that the vast majority of successful milk mixtures used in infant feeding are unlike human milk, which stands apart from all other foods; indeed the popular mixtures are as unlike human milk as they are unlike unmodified cow's milk.

THE METABOLIC BASIS FOR THE INDIVIDUALIZED FEEDING OF INFANTS, PREMATURE AND FULL-TERM

Harry H. Gordon, M.D., and S. Z. Levine, M.D.

New York, N. Y.

IT IS the purpose of this paper to review certain data derived from metabolic studies which bear directly on the practice of infant feeding. This choice was dictated by the trend of modern practice toward what Powers in 1935 called the "psychological era" in infant feeding.[1] This swing has gained momentum from the over-all increase in psychiatric orientation of general medical practice and especially from the protestations of Aldrich[2] and others against dogmatic and anxious misapplication of metabolic data. The importance of satisfying the emotional needs of young infants has received growing recognition. Without minimizing these tenets of the "nutrition of the soul," the coordinate importance of the basic principles of the nutrition of the body needs re-emphasis. As a matter of actual fact, valid interpretation of metabolic data gives added support for the individualized feeding of infants, but for such proper appraisal one needs to know more rather than less about the principles of nutrition.

An optimum diet has been defined as one in which no change can promote greater health and well-being of the populace. What are some of the methods for studying the dietary needs of infants and how close are we to this goal?

Diets customarily eaten by infants have been correlated with their state of health. This type of dietary survey, consisting of records of body weight before and after large numbers of breast feedings, furnished early German investigators with original data on the approximate caloric and fluid requirements of breast-fed infants. These observations and more recently those of Davis[3] and Gesell and Ilg[4] have stressed the wide variability in the requirements of both breast and artificially fed infants and children.

Other methods of study attempt to relate the levels of intake of the substance under scrutiny with levels in blood or other body fluids (plasma and urinary concentration of ascorbic acid) or with physiologic function (vitamin A and light adaptation; iron and hemoglobin formation).

The method of balances furnishes the main source of the data presented in this paper. This method measures the total income and outgo of a given substance and thereby affords an estimate of body retention at different levels of intake. Balance studies give valuable in-

From the New York Hospital and the Department of Pediatrics, Cornell University Medical College.

The Borden Award, American Academy Pediatrics, St. Louis, Mo., Nov. 11, 1944.

formation on nutritional requirements but they are subject to inherent limitations of method and interpretation. These include errors in chemical methods, difficulties in collection of excreta, the necessity for few and often short observations because of technical obstacles, exposure of the infant to an unaccustomed and restricted environment, and possible misinterpretation of maximum for optimum retentions. As Gamble has stated,[5] it is a mistake to apply too rigidly the results of balance studies to the feeding of infants. Properly interpreted, however, they provide basic data for setting up dietary standards and normal variations.

WATER EXCHANGE

The first data deal with water requirements. The relation of water retention to gain in body weight of a group of premature infants fed human or cow's milk is presented in Table I. On both types of diet, containing from 102 to 141 calories and from 1.9 to 6.3 Gm. of protein per kilogram of body weight, water retentions varied only from 54 to 70 per cent and averaged 65 per cent of total weight gain. This average figure approximates the water content of the infantile body as obtained by direct chemical analysis. It is noteworthy that both human and cow's milk varying markedly in organic and inorganic content resulted in water retentions which constituted a relatively constant and desirable fraction of the body weight gain.

TABLE I

RELATION OF WATER RETENTION TO BODY WEIGHT CHANGE
(PER TWENTY-FOUR HOURS)

SUBJECT	DAYS OB- SERVED	CALORIES	PROTEIN (GM.)	WATER (GM.)	WATER RETEN- TION (GM.)	BODY WT. CHANGE (GM.)	WATER : WT. (%)
			Human Milk				
R. L.	3	141	2.1	182	13	20	65
N. O.	6	118	2.9	149	20	30	67
E. C.	3	126	1.9	158	15	22	68
E. M.	3	102	4.5	135	19	29	65
Average 4	15	122	2.9	156	17	25	66
			Cow's Milk				
N. O.	3	108	2.5	166	12	19	63
E. M.	3	120	4.8	136	23	33	70
L. O.	12	119	4.2	150	24	45	54
E. C.	4	124	6.0	130	41	65	63
H. L.	12	133	6.1	126	24	42	56
R. L.	2	134	6.3	160	43	61	70
Average 6	36	123	5.0	145	28	44	63

In Fig. 1 it is shown that variations in dietary fluid above maintenance levels with the solid constituents held constant result also in relatively constant water retentions. In both premature and full-term infants, reduction in fluid intake from average levels of approximately 170 to 130 Gm. per kilogram did not lower either their water balances or their loss through feces and skin and lungs. The urinary output, on the other hand, fell markedly and it is this concentrating ability of the

466

kidneys which sustains proper osmotic relationships in the body in the face of wide fluctuations in fluid and electrolyte intake or in output by extrarenal routes as in sweating, vomiting, or diarrhea. That there is a limit to this defensive mechanism is indicated by the negative water balances and development of fever when the fluid intakes were further reduced to 74 and 85 Gm. per kilogram.

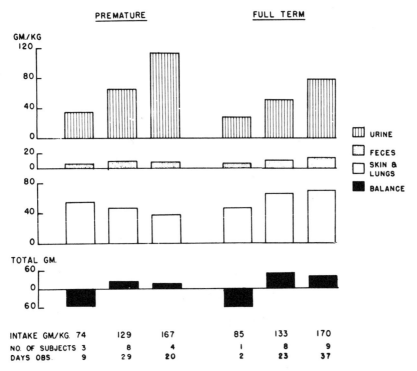

Fig. 1.—Effect of changing intake on water balance.

A partial explanation for this fever is the failure of the infant to compensate by adequate increase in evaporative loss for his increased heat production attributable to the crying of thirst and discomfort. This lack of sweating may in turn be due to hemoconcentration but unfortunately no direct measurements were made in these infants.

The primary role of the kidney in regulating the composition and volume of body fluids[6] prompted an assessment of renal function in young infants. In Table II is presented data on the urea clearance of young premature and full-term infants. The average clearance of 15 c.c. per square meter per minute with a range of from 5 to 24 c.c. for premature infants is significantly less than the 20 c.c. found for full-term infants, both sets of figures being less than the average of 38 c.c. reported by Schoenthal for older infants[7] and the average standard and maximal clearances of 30 and 40 c.c. reported for adults. Moreover, a 25 to 100 per cent augmentation of urinary output had no effect on the clearances of four infants, thereby demonstrating that their low

TABLE II

UREA CLEARANCE (CUBIC CENTIMETERS PER SQUARE METER PER MINUTE)

	OBSERVATIONS (NO.)	AVERAGE	RANGE	FREQUENCY DISTRIBUTION	
				UNDER 20 (NO.)	OVER 20 (NO.)
Premature (Under 2 months)	30	15*	5-24	25	5
Full Term (Under 2½ months)	10	20*	14-31	6	4
Full Term† (2 to 12 months)	9	38	23-55	0	9
Adult		30-40 C_s C_m			

*No change with urine flow increased 25 to 100%.
†Schoenthal.

values represented maximal clearances. Such impairment of renal function must handicap the young infant in his selective excretion of water and solids under stress. More precise definition of this impairment awaits completion of studies on renal tubular activity in young infants. Preliminary observations of the effect of pitressin on urinary specific gravity and chlorides are too equivocal to permit interpretation at the present time.

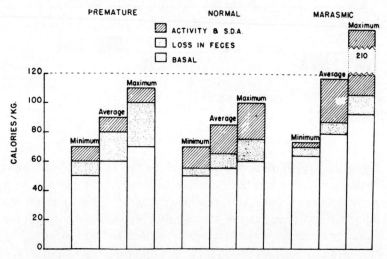

Fig. 2.—Approximate energy expenditure of normal, premature, and marasmic infants.

ENERGY EXCHANGE

In Fig. 2 is presented data on the energy exchange of premature, normal, and marasmic full-term infants. The figures for normal infants were determined in 24-hour calorimeter observations; those for premature and marasmic infants were calculated from shorter calorimeter studies combined with 24-hour minute-to-minute records of activity. The difference in calories between the dotted line representing normal caloric intake (120 per kilogram) and the height of columns representing the total caloric output is the energy quota available for growth. It is evident that some infants will gain, others will maintain, and still others will lose weight on this fixed intake.

The explanation for the differences in energy expenditure in the three groups of infants clarifies the need for individualization of feeding within each group. The low basal metabolism and low activity quota of some premature infants, characteristic for the first two weeks of life, are adequately covered by intakes well below 120 calories per kilogram. Premature infants who do not gain on such intakes of customary cow's milk mixtures usually fail to do so because of excessive loss of calories as fecal fat. Dietary calories should not be increased; dietary fat, rather, should be reduced (Fig. 3 and Table III).

TABLE III

EFFECT OF VARYING AMOUNT OF DIETARY FAT ON EXCRETION OF FAT

DAYS	DIETARY FAT (GM./KG.)	FECAL FAT		WEIGHT GAIN (GM./KG.)
		(GM./KG.)	DIETARY CALORIES (%)	
		Infant P. A.*		
10	1.8	1.0	9	14
8	1.9	0.8	7	15
7	4.7	1.9	16	7
9	2.1	0.7	5	16
		Infant H. A.†		
11	2.2	1.2	10	13
8	2.1	1.1	9	15
7	4.1	3.3	27	5
9	2.1	0.7	5	14

*108 to 114 calories per kilogram in diet.
†111 to 118 calories per kilogram in diet.

The variations in caloric expenditure of full-term infants are of a different nature. A wiry, active infant may have both higher basal and activity quotas per kilogram of body weight. If he is given insufficient food, hunger will further raise his energy quota for activity and his intake may become even more calorically deficient for growth. Satiation of appetite actually decreases the caloric output of such an infant. Conversely, a fat, placid baby whose basal and activity quotas are initially low may become more obese and sluggish if given the same intake as required for satisfactory gain in the thin, active infant. Appetite is a safe gauge for both thin and fat infants if one keeps in mind that satiety is conditioned not only by caloric adequacy but also by such mechanical factors as conditions of sucking and by nervous tensions transmitted from the environment.

The marasmic infant presents still other problems. His basal metabolism per unit of weight is notably higher because of his paucity of relatively inert body fat. Moreover, querulousness and sleeplessness often raise the activity quota. As a result, a diet of 120 calories per kilogram of actual weight is frequently inadequate. Higher caloric intakes, prevention of infections with accompanying increases in fecal loss and in basal metabolism (if fever is present) and good nursing care to decrease restlessness are required to produce satisfactory weight gains in these infants.

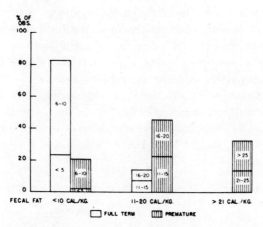

Fig. 3.—Excretion of fat by young full-term and premature infants.

FAT EXCRETION

In Fig. 3 is summarized the data of forty-eight observations on the frequency and magnitude of defective fat absorption in premature infants compared with data of twelve observations in young full-term infants. In all observations, the diets of whole milk mixtures contained from 35 to 50 per cent of the total calories as fat. The fecal caloric loss was less than 10 calories per kilogram in only 21 per cent of the observations on premature infants as against 83 per cent for the observations on full-term infants. Moreover, the former infants lost more than 20 calories per kilogram as fecal fat in one-third of the observations. Qualitative alterations in dietary fat—human milk, cow's milk, and cow's milk mixtures in which olive oil replaced the butter fat—had no effect on the heightened fecal loss of fat. Quantitative reduction of dietary fat, on the other hand, consistently led to diminished excretion of fecal fat as illustrated in Table III. In two male members of a set of triplets, augmentation of the fat intake by substituting iso-caloric whole mixtures for half-skimmed ones resulted in striking increases in fecal fat and corresponding decrements in weight gain from 13 and 15 Gm. to 5 and 7 Gm. per kilogram per day. Return to the half-skimmed milk mixtures promptly decreased the fecal fat and raised the weight gains to the control levels.

NITROGEN ABSORPTION AND RETENTION

In contrast to this defective absorption of fat, the capacity of premature infants to absorb and retain nitrogen is highly efficient. The data in Table IV indicate that premature infants absorb the nitrogen from cow's milk at least as well as that from human milk and that raising the protein intake from 2.8 to 4.7 and in one observation to 9.1

TABLE IV

ABSORPTION OF NITROGEN BY PREMATURE INFANTS*

MILK (TYPE)	OBSERVATIONS (NO.)	DAYS (NO.)	AVERAGE PROTEIN INTAKE (GM./KG./24 HR.)	COEFFICIENT OF DIGESTIBILITY† (%)
Human	11	69	2.3	79 (65-87)
Cow's	5	25	2.8	88 (84-92)
Cow's	21	118	4.7	91 (87-95)
Cow's	1	4	9.1	93

*Age, 3 to 60 days, weight 1.4 to 2.8 kilograms.

$$†\frac{\text{Dietary}-\text{Fecal Nitrogen}}{\text{Dietary Nitrogen}} \times 100$$

Gm. per kilogram did not lower the coefficient of digestibility, approximately 90 per cent being absorbed at each level of intake. This figure is well within the normal range of nitrogen absorption of adults.

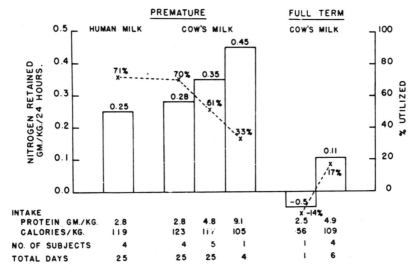

Fig. 4.—Nitrogen retention by premature and full-term infants—effect of changing intake.

In Fig. 4 is portrayed the data on nitrogen retention. Isocaloric diets of human and cow's milk of equivalent and low protein content (2.8 Gm. per kilogram) resulted in absolute retentions and percentages of utilization of similar magnitude in the premature infants. At this level of intake, presumably well above the minimum, no advantage in terms of nitrogen balance accrued for the protein of human milk. Furthermore, higher protein intakes in the form of cow's milk caused correspondingly higher retentions of nitrogen.

Despite lack of evidence from these data that such high retentions are necessarily beneficial, it is of interest that the levels of nitrogen balance of the premature infants fed approximately 5.0 Gm. of protein per kilogram were threefold those for older full-term infants on similar intakes. The evidence suggests that the heightened retentions in young infants are related to their increased rate of growth. Further evidence

337

of the value of high protein diets for young infants may be inferred by analogy from the data later presented on calcium retention.

CARBOHYDRATE METABOLISM

In Table V is recorded respiratory quotients obtained in infants fed customary whole milk mixtures. If the respiratory quotient is accepted as an index of the composition of the metabolic mixture, the high average and maximum quotients obtained in both premature and full-term infants indicate the ease with which carbohydrate is utilized by these subjects.

TABLE V

AVERAGE RESPIRATORY QUOTIENTS

| INFANTS | | OBSERVATIONS | RESPIRATORY QUOTIENTS | |
(AGE)	(NO.)	(NO.)	AVERAGE	RANGE
Premature:				
Less than 9 days	10	18	0.88	0.77-0.95
More than 9 days	16	38	0.91	0.87-0.95
Full term:				
1-12 mo.	15	19	0.88	0.77-0.94

CALCIUM METABOLISM

Data on calcium retention by three premature infants fed human milk and three fed cow's milk are given in Fig. 5. This figure is adapted from a diagram in Stearns' review[8] to illustrate the relation of observed retentions to certain theoretical requirements.

The heavy line A was obtained by Stearns from published data on analyses of fetuses. It shows the rise in body calcium with rising body

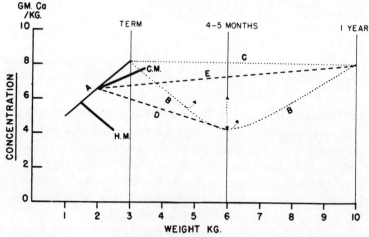

Fig. 5.—Effect of human and cow's milk on calcium stores of premature infants.

A, Fetal growth
B, Effect of human milk }from the literature*
C, Effect of cow's milk
D, Minimum standard for premature infant
E, Higher standard for premature infant

*A, constructed from a diagram in Stearns' review.[8]   B and C, constructed from composite data reported in the literature (references now unobtainable).

338

weights from 1 to 3 kilograms.   After birth, body retention of calcium is dependent on diet.   Curve C portrays the calcium storage by full-term infants fed cow's milk who have successfully maintained birth concentrations of 8 Gm. per kilogram.   The line in Stearns' diagram representing the average performance of full-term, breast-fed infants falls to a minimum of approximately 6 Gm. per kilogram at 4 months of age. In Fig. 5, the corresponding line B has been drawn to the lower level of 4 Gm. per kilogram to include the lowest level of retention reported for a young, rapidly growing, nonrachitic, full-term infant.   This baby was breast fed and received no added vitamin D.   A body content of 4 Gm. of calcium per kilogram at 4 months of age is obviously exceedingly low since doubling of the birth weight at this age with concomitant halving of body concentration of calcium implies no calcium deposition from birth.   It seems fair to assume, then, that a body calcium content of 4 Gm. per kilogram in a full-term infant is at or near the critical level below which optimal mineralization of bone is unlikely.

Against this background three hypothetic rates of calcium storage may be plotted to serve as a basis for establishing the dietary requirements of the premature infant.   The first, along line A, is perhaps the most natural rate since it corresponds to the one which would have been followed had he remained in utero to term.   If he follows the second lower rate, represented by line E, the diet would have to supply sufficient calcium so that from birth to 1 year of age he would systematically correct his initial deficit.   If he follows the lowest rate, D, the diet would be called on to supply only enough calcium to prevent depletion of the stores below the level of 4 Gm. per kilogram.

It is evident that human milk failed to meet any of the requirements, D, E, or A (Fig. 5); with the cow's milk mixture, on the other hand, the retentions of all three infants surpassed the lowest requirement, D, and for two exceeded the middle requirement, E.   Similar calculations can be made both for phosphorus and nitrogen.   The data indicate that human milk is too low in these three constituents to cover the increased needs of premature infants conditioned by their low stores at birth and their increased rate of growth.

VITAMIN REQUIREMENTS

Studies conducted in our clinic of the increased needs of premature infants for fat-soluble vitamin A[9] combined with their previously mentioned defect in fat absorption and their heightened calcium requirements confirm the clinical impression that these infants require relatively greater amounts of vitamin D.

More direct evidence will now be presented of the specific role of vitamin C in the metabolism of aromatic amino acids by premature infants.   When these infants are fed cow's milk mixtures of high protein content (5 Gm. or more per kilogram) the intermediary products, 1-p-hydroxyphenyllactic and p-hydroxyphenylpyruvic acids, appear in their urine in significant amounts.   The excretion of these or-

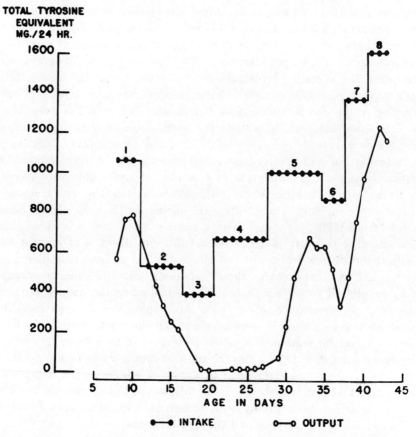

Fig. 6.—Effect of intake of aromatic amino acids on the urinary excretion of intermediary products.

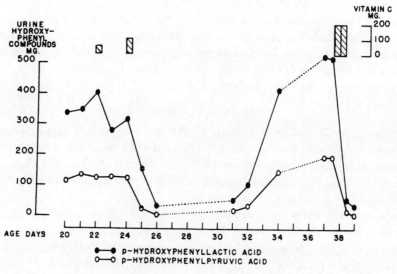

Fig. 7.—Effect of vitamin C.

ganic acids was found to vary directly with the dietary intake of phenylalanine and tyrosine (Fig. 6). These abnormal products were not routinely present in the urine of full-term infants but they could be produced by a single large dose of either amino acid, presumably by disrupting the enzymatic mechanisms responsible for the complete oxidation of these aromatic amino acids.

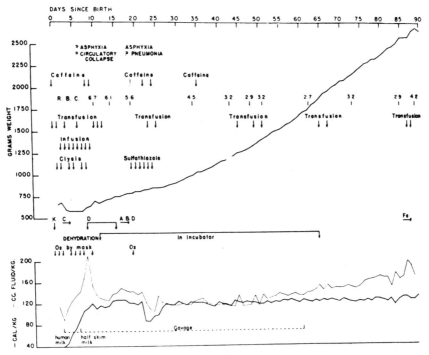

Fig. 8.—Clinical course, feeding, and therapy of a 662-Gm. infant during first three months of life.

Despite the well-known action of thiamine on pyruvic acid excretion in animals, this vitamin as well as all the other known fractions of the vitamin B complex was wholly ineffective in abolishing the defect in premature infants.

The administration of from 100 to 500 mg. of ascorbic acid, on the other hand, was followed by a dramatic disappearance of abnormal products (Fig. 7). They frequently subsided in the absence of any significant rise of the extracellular levels of ascorbic acid, plasma measurements ranging from 0 to 0.3 mg. per cent after therapy. It is evident that an extreme degree of depletion of body stores existed in these infants and that this depletion was demonstrable as early as the sixth day of postnatal life. It is recommended that ascorbic acid be added to the diet of premature infants shortly after birth.

COMMENT

The selected data which have been presented permit two reflections of a general nature. The first is embodied in a statement with which Dr.

James Ewing, late professor of pathology at the Cornell Medical College, was wont to introduce many of his lectures: "Variations is our theme." Appreciation of these variations and proper interpretation of their pathogenesis provide the physiologic background for proper individualization in the feeding of infants, sick and well, premature and full-term.

The second generalization relates to the feeding of premature infants. For many years, human milk which is relatively high in water and fat and low in calcium, phosphorus and protein, has been the feeding of choice for these subjects. The reported data suggest the desirability for critical reevaluation of this clinical impression which may actually be a mistaken one because of the many complicating factors which confuse the picture: degree of prematurity, amount and quality of nursing and medical care, environmental temperature and humidity, and incidence of infections. Well-controlled and prolonged clinical studies should provide the answer. In cooperation with the Children's Bureau, such a study has been in progress for the last five years in the New York Hospital. All premature infants are being fed in rotation according to birth, weight, sex, race, and plurality of birth, isocaloric diets of human milk, a simple evaporated milk mixture and a half-skimmed milk mixture, similar to the one originally recommended by Powers.[10] The results are awaiting tabulation but, as shown in Fig. 8, even an infant whose birth weight was only 662 Gm. (1 pound, 7 ounces) can thrive on a properly prepared artificial feeding.

The work reported in this paper represents the combined effort of many persons: physicians on the attending and house staffs, technicians, and nurses connected in the past and at present with the pediatric department of the Cornell University Medical College. We are especially indebted to Dr. O. M. Schloss, whose foresight made possible the establishment of the metabolic unit; to Miss E. Marples, Miss H. McNamara, and Dr. H. E. Benjamin, who contributed ideas as well as technical aid throughout the work; to Miss M. Kelly, whose faithful nursing was invaluable; and to Dr. E. C. Dunham of the Children's Bureau, whose knowledge of and interest in premature infants made much of the later work possible.

REFERENCES

1. Powers, G. F.: J. A. M. A. 105: 753, 1935.
2. (a) Aldrich, C. A.: J. A. M. A. 89: 928, 1927. (b) Aldrich, C. A.: J. PEDIAT. 1: 413, 1932. (c) Aldrich, C. A.: J. PEDIAT. 15: 578, 1939.
3. (a) Davis, Clara M.: Am. J. Dis. Child. 36: 651, 1928.
   (b) Davis, Clara M.: Am. J. Dis. Child. 40: 905, 1930.
4. Gesell, A., and Ilg, F. L.: Feeding Behavior of Infants, page 93, Philadelphia, Pa., 1937, J. B. Lippincott Company.
5. Gamble, J. L.: The General Terms of the Food Requirement, In Brennemann's, Practice of Pediatics, Vol. I, Chap. 23. Hagerstown, Md., 1944, W. F. Prior Co., Inc.
6. (a) Gamble, J. L.: Bull. Johns Hopkins Hosp. 61: 151, 1937.
   (b) Gamble, J. L.: Bull. Johns Hopkins Hosp. 61: 174, 1937.
7. Schoenthal, L., Lurie, D., and Kelly, M.: Am. J. Dis. Child. 45: 41, 1933.
8. Stearns, G.: Physiol. Rev. 19: 415, 1939.
9. Henley, T. F., Dann, M. D., and Golden, W.: Am. J. Dis. Child. 68: 257, 1944.
10. Powers, G. F.: Am. J. Dis. Child 30: 453, 1925.

Part VIII

SAFE, CLEAN MILK

Editor's Comments
on Papers 31 and 32

31   **ROTCH**
The Artificial Feeding of Infants

32   **TAYLOR and ROBERTS**
Whole Lactic Acid Evaporated Milk Does Not Require a Refrigerator

The battle to legislate for clean unadulterated milk illustrates the perennial struggle for social reform waged between the exploiter of the public weal and the crusader. Had this movement not been eventually successful, none of the advances in chemistry, metabolic measurement techniques, and balance studies would have been to any avail.

One would be hard put to find an issue of *Lancet* in the latter part of the nineteenth century that did not detail a febrile gastrointestinal illness, the origin of which could be traced to a contaminated milk source—the farmer or his cow. Furthermore, the revolting conditions under which commercial milk cows were kept, the practice of feeding them brewers' mash produced as a by-product of the distilleries, the lack of supervision and any health inspection of those milking the cows, the dirty containers in which milk was transported, and the lack of refrigeration lead one to wonder how any "dry-fed" infant managed to survive.

If the filth and disease contamination were not hazard enough, the nutritive value of the milk was also eroded through conscious adulteration, first by the addition of water to stretch the volume and then by supplementation with a variety of additives—ranging from chalk to plaster of paris and tragacanth—to improve the color, the consistency, and the flavor, and to obscure the odor. No less than 37 means of adulterating whole milk are described as "the result of microscopial and chemical analyses of the solids and fluids consumed by all of the classes of the public" in the analytical sanitary commission report in the January 7, 1865, issue of *Lancet*.

By 1856 Gale Borden had initiated the procedure of condensing milk, the earliest advance in sanitary milk processing and the gateway to an easily available, safe base for prepared artificial feeding formulas. Although the terms "condensed" and "evaporated" are sometimes used interchangeably, condensed milk usually refers to milk that has been evaporated from one third to one half of its bulk, to which is added nearly an equal amount, 40 percent, of cane sugar. Evaporated milk is milk condensed to the same degree but unsweetened and sterilized.

Henry Coit agitated successfully for the production of "certified" milk from rigidly inspected herds, with sanitary supervision of personnel and bacteriologic standards of safety. His standards remain the basis of the present sanitary code for purity. Although pasteurization was commercially available in Denmark in 1890, and was practiced in New York City in 1898, it was not required by law in New York State until 1912. The epidemiologic detective work, such as that detailed in the 53-page documentation by Theobald Smith and J. Howard Brown, involved in the identification of the streptococcus in "presumably milk-borne epidemics of tonsillitis occurring in Massachusetts in 1913 and 1914," was finally irrefutable.

It was Rotch who introduced the means of home terminal sterilization of milk formulas at the same time as Soxhlet in Germany. Rotch's article (Paper 31) outlines how the terminal sterilization apparatus can be made and also describes the bottles and nipples to be used, along with a description of their care. The method is almost precisely that in use today. His insistence on the need for physical cleanliness in conjunction with sterilization has since been substantiated.

31

Reprinted from *Arch. Ped.*, **4**, 458–467 (1887)

THE ARTIFICIAL FEEDING OF INFANTS.*

BY T. M. ROTCH, M.D.,

Visiting Physician to the Boston City Hospital; Instructor in Diseases of Children
in the Harvard Medical School.

WHILE recognizing the importance of feeding infants during the early months of life by means of human milk, we must allow that in civilized communities the necessity of supplying the infant with food not directly from the human breast must often arise, and will in all probability be a demand which will increase rather than decrease as our civilization advances; and when in addition to this we consider the great proportionate mortality of the artificially-fed over the

---

* Read before the Obstetrical Society of Boston, May 28, 1887.

breast-fed, and the difficulties which are so frequently met with in adapting the food to the individual case, it manifestly becomes a duty to carefully investigate the different methods of artificial feeding, and adopt some more uniform plan for starting human beings in life than is met with among physicians as a class and the laity as a whole, for diversity and not uniformity is the rule.

With the exception of the very small proportionate per cent. of inherited diseases which occur at birth, this diversity of method in feeding is the most prolific source of disease in early infancy. The group of symptoms which for want of a better name is represented by dyspepsia, difficult digestion, occurs most frequently in the three periods when the infant's digestion is likely to be tampered with,—namely, in the early weeks of life, when experiments are being made to determine what food will be best to start with ; next, when in addition to the irritation arising from the beginning of dentition new articles of diet are added to the original food ; and, thirdly, at the time of weaning, when there is often a sudden and entire change in the character of the food.

The proper management of the first of these periods is of the greatest comparative importance, because it is the time when the function of digestion is being established and is in a state of unstable equilibrium, and therefore, following the rule of functional establishment, the stomach is in its most active period of growth, and hence the most careful regulation of the bulk of the food given is needed to correspond to this activity in order that we should not weaken the digestive function by overtaxing its capacity and yet provide the proper materials for nutrition, thus avoiding by prophylaxis the dyspepsia of the later periods of infancy and childhood, the seeds of which are continually being sown in this early transitional period.

We therefore have the question not only of infantile digestion but infantile development to deal with, and we should at once recognize the fact that the problem of artificial feeding is not a simple factor,—namely, which food shall we give to the infant, —but is a combination of factors, of which the kind of food is only one, and all these factors, from which we deduce the gen-

eral problem for the average infant and the especial problem
for the individual, must approach as closely as possible to the
analogous factors which nature freely presents to us for investigation,—that is, we must follow nature as closely as possible.
Our scientific knowledge and ingenuity have not yet enabled
us to follow nature exactly, and we therefore have not yet obtained an ideal method of artificial feeding; but we must, nevertheless, go as far as the present state of our knowledge will
allow, thus gaining a little ground every year; and we must
be especially careful not to be led astray by the fictitiously
brilliant results which are reported from time to time in favor
of certain foods, instances continually occurring where one
food will fail and another when substituted for it succeed;
and yet these successes are merely temporary, and the mortality always remains far above that of human breast-milk.

It is certainly wiser and more economical not to spare expense and trouble in arranging the infant's diet, for, as has
been explained above, the period of active growth of an organ
is the time when its function is readily weakened, and when
once weakened the digestive function is a prolific source of
annoyance and expense in childhood and adolescence. Cheap
foods and cheap methods of feeding, unless they are the best
that can be procured, should no more be tolerated, and in fact
not nearly so much so, in the early feeding of infants than in
adult life: we often, however, see a food recommended for a
young infant because it is cheap and easily prepared, and yet
where its well-known lack of nutritive ingredients would with
adults at once stamp it as unfit for use.

What are the general factors of the problem which constitutes nature's method of feeding? We have first a receptacle,
the human breast, which mechanically provides a fresh supply
of food at proper intervals, absolutely prevents fermentation
of the food before it enters the infant's mouth, forms the
mouth by the process of sucking, incites to action the necessary digestive fluids, avoids a vacuum by collapsing as it is
gradually emptied, thus allowing the food to flow continuously,
and finally is practically self-regulating as to the amount of
daily food according to the infant's age. Second, the food
itself adapted to the infant's digestive function and for its

development, by its temperature, 98° to 100° F., its alkaline reaction, and its chemical constituents. Given these factors, how nearly can we approach them artificially? Human ingenuity has not yet been able to devise anything which approaches the perfection of nature's receptacle, and the best that we can do to offset this complex mechanism is to adopt that which is exactly the reverse,—namely, a receptacle of absolute simplicity,—and thus combat the tendency to fermentation by, through perfect cleanliness, preventing the receptacle from becoming a source of fermentation. To meet this demand I have had made what are practically enlarged test-tubes, which not having any angles are readily cleaned.

The receptacle, however, has to receive a food which usually is non-sterilized, and hence, where the factor of fermentation appears to be prominent in disturbing the infant's digestion, the food should be sterilized before it is given to the infant.

The process of sterilization is most simply accomplished by placing the food in one of the above spoken of feeding-tubes, adjusting the rubber nipple as on any nursing-bottle, then drawing tightly over the nipple and well down on to the tube a strong rubber cot, which, not being perforated, completely excludes the air. The tube is then exposed to steam confined in any vessel for twenty minutes, which is sufficient to render it sterile, in the sense of destroying the developed bacteria and thus making it correspond to human milk; at the same time, so far as my investigations on this subject have gone, the steam, while it sterilizes, does not apparently alter the chemical attributes of the food, as is essentially the case where the sterilization is accomplished by boiling; then again, in the steaming process the receptacle is sterilized as well as the food, so that when the rubber cot is removed we have the food enter the infant's mouth as free from bacteria as has been shown to be the case with human milk by Esherich,[*] who experimented with the milk of twenty-five healthy women, and found, by keeping it in sterilized tubes, that it remained sterile for some weeks, while, on the contrary, in women whose temperature was raised from fissures and excoriations of the

* Baumgarten's Jahresbericht. Erster Jahrgang, 1885, p. 34.

nipple and by general puerperal infection, bacteria were found in abundance. It is thus seen that this factor of sterilization is likely to be found of considerable importance in the future, and should certainly be called to our aid in those cases where the other factors of our problem are as nearly correct as we can make them, and, if for no other reason, because nature plainly tells us that a perfect food should be sterile, and, in fact, our practical clinical experience for years has taught us to withdraw the infant from the breast in exactly that class of diseases where we now know bacteria to occur in the milk. Reference has been made above to the developed bacteria; if it is desired to prepare the food so that it shall remain sterile for some time, it is necessary to sterilize for several days in succession, for the first sterilization, according to Dr. Harold Ernst, Demonstrator of Bacteriology in the Harvard Medical School, only destroys these developed bacteria, while the spores are left to develop later. Dr. Ernst also kindly placed one of my tubes in which there was a mixture of cream, milk, lime-water, and milk sugar in his sterilizer for twenty minutes and then in his incubator for twenty-four hours, and at the end of this time no change could be detected in the mixture, either in color, odor, or taste, all of which appeared to exactly correspond to a freshly prepared mixture of the same kind.

I have devised a simple apparatus for household use, which can be made at any tinsmith's at small expense, and answers for the purpose of sterilization very well.

It is a round tin pail, eight inches in diameter and fourteen inches deep, raised on three legs, sufficiently high to allow an alcohol lamp to stand under it; four inches from the bottom of the pail on the inside is a perforated tin diaphragm on which the feeding-tubes stand while being sterilized.

The pail has a cover and handle. Water is placed in the bottom of the pail, and when heated by the lamp the tubes are soon enveloped in steam.

The process of sucking is accomplished by the rubber nipple as by the breast, and a small hole near the end of the feeding-tube prevents a vacuum being formed and regulates the rapidity of the flow, while it allows it to be continuous; this is done by rolling up the edge of the rubber nipple from the hole with the finger, or letting it cover the hole according to the demand shown by the infant when feeding.

The artificial receptacle is not self-regulating, and hence we must first determine anatomically the amount of food in bulk which nature provides for the average infant at different ages, and from these average figures deduce the proper amount for the especial infant, having also the feeding-tubes graduated for the more important periods of growth, for the purpose of continually impressing, upon the mother and nurse, what the physician only has the opportunity of telling them at the beginning of the nursing period,—namely, that the error is in giving too much food rather than too little, an error also which naturally results when, as is commonly the case, the usual eight-ounce nursing-bottle is provided as the receptacle at the very beginning of infantile life.

Diagram I. represents the stomach of an infant five days old, in life-size.

DIAGRAM I.   DIAGRAM II.

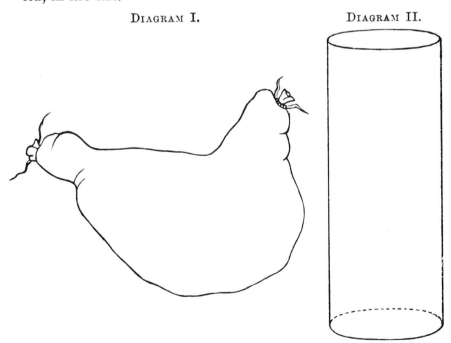

The specimen was prepared by Dr. C. W. Townsend, and was found to hold twenty-five cubic centimetres.

Diagram II. represents the size of the tube, which is

sufficiently large for each feeding during the first week; and when we consider the space which would be needed to represent the full-sized nursing-bottle, these two diagrams express better than can be explained by words the disproportion between the size of the infant's stomach and the amount which the mother supposes it should hold to keep her child from being starved.

Frolowsky's* investigations show that the activity of growth in the stomach's capacity can be represented by the ratio of one for the first week, to two and one-half for the fourth week, and three and one-fifth for the eighth week, while it is only three and one-third for the twelfth week, three and four-sevenths for the sixteenth week, and three and three-fifths for the twentieth week.

We thus see that there is a very rapid increase in capacity in the first two months of life, while in the third, fourth, and fifth months the increase is slight. Guided by these data, which we find correspond closely with the results of clinical investigations bearing on this point, we should rapidly increase the quantity of the food in the first six or eight weeks, and then give the same quantity up to the fifth or sixth month, unless the infant's appetite evidently demands more, when of course a gradual increase should be made. A considerable increase in the quantity needed, also, usually takes place between the sixth and tenth month.

Ssnitkin, after a series of careful investigations in the Children's Hospital at St. Petersburg to determine the amount which should be given in the first thirty days of life, finds that the greater the weight the greater is the gastric capacity. His general results also show that one one-hundredth of the initial weight should be taken as the starting figure, and to this should be added one gramme to each day of life. This, for example, gives the following amounts for each feeding, which closely correspond to the average figures which I have computed and introduced in Table I. on the basis of three thousand grammes as the initial weight. Thus, one one-hundredth of three thousand would be thirty grammes for

---

* Inauguraldiss., St. Petersburg, 1876.

the early days, and at thirty days the amount given would be $30 + 30 = 60$ grammes, about two ounces.

Table I.

The average initial weight of infants is 3000–4000 grammes = about 6–8 pounds.
The average normal gain per day in the first 5 months is 20–30 grammes = about 1 ounce.

General Rules for Feeding.

Age.	Intervals of Feeding.	Number of Feedings in 24 Hours.	Average Amount at each Feeding.	Average Amount in 24 Hours.
1st week	2 hours.	10	1 ounce.	10 ounces.
1–6 weeks .	2½ hours.	8	1½ to 2 ounces.	12 to 16 ounces.
6–12 weeks, and possibly to 5th or 6th month . .	3 hours.	6	3 to 4 ounces.	18 to 24 ounces.
At 6 mos. .	3 hours.	6	6 ounces.	36 ounces.
At 10 mos. .	3 hours.	5	8 ounces.	40 ounces.

The weight, as well as the age, is necessary to determine the amount for each feeding in the individual infant, the rule being $\frac{1}{100}$ of the initial weight + 1 gramme for each day during the first month.

Illustrations of above rule to serve as guides for especially difficult cases.

Each Feeding.

Initial Weight.	Early Days.	At 15 Days.	At 30 Days.
3000 grammes.	30 grammes (about ℥1).	$30 + 15 = 45$ grammes (about ℥1½).	$30 + 30 = 60$ grammes (about ℥2).
4500 grammes.	45 grammes (about ℥1½).	$45 + 15 = 60$ grammes (about ℥2).	$45 + 30 = 75$ grammes (about ℥2½).
6000 grammes.	60 grammes (about ℥2).	$60 + 15 = 75$ grammes (about ℥2½).	$60 + 30 = 90$ grammes (about ℥3).

The younger the infant the greater the metabolic activity, and hence the greater need for frequent feeding, for nutriment is required not only for the excess of waste but also for the rapid proportionate growth; this makes the intervals of feeding a factor of considerable importance in the management of the infant's diet.

The figures in Table I. are merely approximate average computations taken from the results of a number of Russian, German, and American observers and from my own experience during the past ten years, and are only intended to be a guide for the physician in his management of cases of difficult digestion, for of course some infants will have a greater appetite and a greater power for digestion than others of the same age and weight.

I have experimented with the glass-blower in having tubes of different sizes made, and finally out of a large number of samples the following have been chosen as the most practical

DIAGRAM III.   DIAGRAM IV.

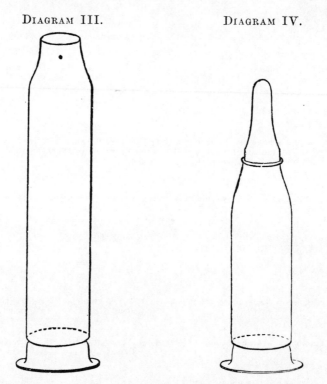

and the easiest to handle. For convenience I have had these tubes fitted to a box, which also contains directions for their use. The tubes as seen in Diagrams III. and IV. are merely enlarged test-tubes blown into a glass standard, and having a small hole at the mouth for the entrance of air.

A measuring-glass graduated to hold two ounces, and shaped like the larger tubes, is also in the box, and is used as a feeding-tube during the first six weeks, and later as a measure for the larger tubes. The smaller tube, Diagram IV., holds four ounces, has a calibre of one and five-eighths inches, and a height of six inches; it is to be used from the sixth week to the fifth or sixth month, and is intended to correspond to the above-described rapid growth of the stomach in the first two months, and its insignificant further increase in size up to the fifth or sixth month; it is represented in the diagram with the nipple adjusted for use. The large tube, Diagram III., has a calibre of one and six-eighths inches, a height of eight and three-fourths inches, and corresponds to the common half-pint nursing-bottle; it is represented in the diagram without the nipple, and shows the air-hole.

The box, besides the rubber nipple, contains a rubber cot for sterilization, test-paper for ascertaining the reaction of the food, and a bottle of soda for keeping the tubes pure during the intervals of nursing.

A medium-sized tube, which does not come with the box, but can be had separately, has a calibre of one and six-eighths inches, a height of seven and three-fourths inches, and holds six ounces. It of course is not a necessity, but is intended to be used between the sixth and tenth month, merely to enunciate the importance of careful supervision of quantity throughout the first year, as where a food qualitatively correct is being used, the error, as a rule, is in giving too great an amount quantitatively than too little, and a food which otherwise would be digested perfectly well often fails if it is given in too large an amount or at improper intervals; we may, however, here notice that while in breast-feeding frequent feeding is contraindicated from its altering the character of the food, in fact, condensing it, this trouble does not of course arise in artificial feeding, the food remaining the same, and we thus have a little more latitude given us in our management than we can have in regulating the breast-feeding.

[*Editor's Note:* The remainder of the article has been omitted, as it is not relevant to our subject.]

32

WHOLE LACTIC ACID EVAPORATED MILK DOES NOT REQUIRE A REFRIGERATOR

MAJOR HARVEY G. TAYLOR, MEDICAL CORPS, ARMY OF THE UNITED STATES, AND FIRST LIEUTENANT ROBERT W. ROBERTS, JR., MEDICAL CORPS, ARMY OF THE UNITED STATES

NOW that refrigerators are "frozen," which is not intended as a pun, foods which can be kept at room temperature are necessary, especially for infants who are more susceptible to intestinal infections than are adults. As may be seen in Table I, whole lactic acid evaporated milk* can be left in open dishes at room temperature for three days before becoming infected with molds and for five days before bacteria appear. As the total feeding of evaporated milk made from the usual 13-ounce can* is always consumed by the infant within forty-eight hours, it is obvious that a refrigerator is unnecessary. As Rothey[1] has shown, the lactic acid acts as an antiseptic.

In addition to this advantage of its "keeping" qualities at room temperature, whole lactic acid evaporated milk, which was introduced by Marriott[2] and has been used for all of the infants in Duke Hospital for the past ten years, has the following merits:

Digestibility.—Infants thrive on whole lactic acid evaporated milk, at least as well as they do on breast milk.[3] The incidence of diarrhea, vomiting, and bacillary dysentery is lower in infants fed whole lactic acid evaporated milk than in those receiving any other food.

Safety of Source.—The evaporation process of the whole lactic acid evaporated milk removes the risk of brucellosis (undulant or Malta fever), diphtheria, dysentery, foot and mouth disease, scarlet fever, septic or streptococcus sore throat, tuberculosis, typhoid and paratyphoid A and B fevers, and other diseases which can be spread through dairies.

Safety in Home Handling and in the Infant's Intestine.—The demonstration by Rothey,[1] that dysentery, typhoid, and paratyphoid bacilli, when added in large amounts to whole lactic acid evaporated milk, are destroyed rapidly is an indication of bactericidal power which no other infant feeding process possesses. The antibacterial or lysozyme strength of breast milk is weak in comparison. Sweet milk and powdered milk mixtures, even when boiled in the nursing bottle, can be infected by the

---

From the Department of Pediatrics, Duke University School of Medicine, and Duke Hospital, Durham, N. C.

*The contents of a 13-ounce (390 c.c.) can of unsweetened evaporated milk are poured into a quart jar, previously "scalded" with boiling water, and the empty can nearly filled with boiling water, in which then are dissolved one teaspoonful of lactic acid (U.S.P.) and three level tablespoonfuls of sugar. As soon as this solution is cold, it is poured slowly into the quart jar containing the unsweetened evaporated milk while shaking the jar constantly. Although not necessary, it is advisable, in order for the lactic acid to accomplish its full bactericidal effect, that the mixture be kept six hours before being fed in required amounts to the infant. It should not be boiled or pasteurized as it will curdle. Infants of any age can be fed 100 c.c. (100 calories) of this mixture per kilogram of body weight (1½ ounces [15 calories] per pound) in twenty-four hours, divided into four to six feedings. If a child requires more than this amount (one can each of milk and water, a total of 780 c.c., 26 ounces), he also needs solid food.[5]

TABLE 1

DAILY CULTURES OF WHOLE LACTIC ACID EVAPORATED MILK EXPOSED IN OPEN DISHES
AT ROOM TEMPERATURE

CULTURE MEDIUM	DAYS OF EXPOSURE AND RESULTS OF DAILY CULTURES							
	1	2	3	4	5	6	7	8
Broth	0	0	0	0	+2	+2	+2	+2
Dextrose agar	0	0	0	0	0	0	+2	+2
Blood agar	0	0	0	0	0	0	+2	+2
Sabouraud's medium for fungi	0	0	+1	+1	+1	+1	+1	+1

[1]*Penicillium glaucum* and Aspergillus.
[2]*Bacillus subtilis.*

mother's hands while attaching the nipple; whole lactic acid evaporated milk, because of its bactericidal activity, cannot readily be infected. This bactericidal action also is useful in reducing the growth of bacteria in the upper intestines which accompanies diarrhea.[4]

Cheapness.—Whole lactic acid evaporated milk is cheaper than practically all other feedings, except breast milk, if it is assumed that breast milk does not cost anything, a premise with which no mother would agree. The cost of whole lactic acid evaporated milk is one-half that of any other infant feeding.

Universal Obtainability.—Whole lactic acid evaporated milk is available everywhere, while in some areas good dairy milk cannot be purchased.

Evaporated milk feedings also have the advantage of simplicity* and of being beneficial in eczema and allergy, as the heating process reduces its antigenic action. The only objections to whole lactic acid evaporated milk are the destruction of vitamins and altered taste. However, all children 8 days to 3 years of age, despite irradiation and regardless of their type of feeding, should receive percomorph or cod-liver oil and ascorbic acid or their equivalents. Some infants dislike whole lactic acid evaporated milk, especially those who previously have been fed with very sweet mixtures, but always, if the physician and mother cooperate, this difficulty can be overcome. In fact, later many of these same children, after they have become accustomed to whole lactic acid evaporated milk, refuse to drink sweet milk—a consummation much to be desired. The addition of flavoring extracts, such as chocolate syrup, improves the taste of evaporated milk, especially for older children and adults. The lead content of canned milk is of no hygienic significance.[5]

REFERENCES

1. Rothey, K. B.:   J. PEDIAT. 7: 60, 1935.
2. Marriott, W. M.:   J. A. M. A. 73: 1173, 1919; M. Clin. North America 4: 717, 1920.
   Marriott, W. M., Davidson, L. T., and Harshman, L. P.:   Arch. Pediat. 39: 361, 1922.
   Marriott, W. M., and Davidson, L. T.:   Am. J. Dis. Child. 26: 542, 1923; J. A. M. A. 81: 2007, 1923.
   Marriott, W. M.:   J. A. M. A. 89: 862, 1927.

Marriott, W. M., and Schoenthal, L.:   Arch. Pediat. **46**: 135, 1929.
Gerstley, J. R.:   Am. J. Dis. Child. **45**: 538, 1933.
Saldun, M. L.:   Arch. de méd. d. enf. **34**: 341, 1931.
v. Massanek, G.:   Jahrb. f. Kinderh. **60**: 756, 1904.
Wurtz, A.:   Med. Klin. **1**: 1391, 1904.
Rensburg, H.:   Jahrb. f. Kinderh. **59**: 74, 1904.
Rummel, O.:   Therap. d. Gegenw. **7**: 259, 1905.
Tada, G.:   Monatschr. f. Kinderh. **4**: 118, 1905.
Dercherf, Elie: Arch. de méd. d. enf. **8**: 1, 1905.
Dunn, C. H.:   Arch. Pediat. **24**: 241, 1907.
Klotz, M.:   Jahrb. f. Kinderh. **70**: 1, 1909.
Menschikoff, M.:   Monatschr. f. Kinderh. **9**: 491, 1910.
Stolte, K.:   Jahrb. f. Kinderh. **74**: 367, 1911; Monatschr. f. Kinderh. **11**: 49, 1912.
Langstein, L., and Meyer, L. F.:   Säuglingsernährung und Säuglingsstoffwechsel, Munich, 1914, J. F. Bergmann.
Ohta, H.:   Jahrb. f. Kinderh. **85**: 358, 1917.
Leichtentritt, B.:   Jahrb. f. Kinderh. **94**: 119, 1921.
Dohnal, E.:   Monatschr. f. Kinderh. **27**: 58, 1923.
Hainiss, E.:   Monatschr. f. Kinderh. **26**: 568, 1923.
Schiff, E.:   Therap. d. Gegenw. **70**: 90, 1929.
Vogt, H.:   Monatschr. f. Kinderh. **31**: 30, 1925.
Todd, T. W., and Kuenzel, W.:   J. Lab. & Clin. Med. **15**: 43, 1929.
Engel, S.:   Deutsche med. Wchnschr. **56**: 433, 1930.
3. Frank, L. C., Clark, F. A., Haskell, W. H., Miller, M. M., Moss, F. J., and Thomas, R. C.:   Pub. Health Rep. **47**: 1951, 1932.
Kositza, L.:   J. PEDIAT. **1**: 426, 1932.
Ross, J. B.:   M. J. & Rec. **136**: 276, 1932.
4. Davison, W. C.:   Am. J. Dis. Child. **29**: 743, 1925.
5. Davison, W. C.:   The Compleat Pediatrician, ed. 4, Durham, N. C., 1943, Duke University Press, pp. 328; Acta paediat. **16**: 387, 1933; Am. J. Dis. Child. **49**: 72, 1935.

Part IX

HUNGER, APPETITE, AND
FREEDOM OF CHOICE

Editor's Comments
on Papers 33 Through 38

When and at what intervals to feed an infant had long been the subject of much discussion. Physiologically, at least, Taylor established that the time required for the development of hunger in any one infant is fairly constant (Paper 33). This served as ample justification for those who prescribed rigidly timed feeding schedules. It took the practical wisdom of Aldrich to articulate what must have been obvious to many other open-minded practitioners, because in his persuasive discussion on the prevention of anorexia in children (Paper 34), he calls attention to the fact that only the chronological arrangement and the report of his own results were original. Nonetheless, his emphasis on the psychic importance of the seemingly nondirective methods proposed were to affect "the practice of infant feeding mightily."

The final selections serve primarily to illustrate the enormous adaptability of the human infant. Davis's article (Paper 35) established that the hungry infant will comfortably accept, grow, and develop well on at least four different formulas presented in series over a period of time. (Further reports on work with toddlers show a similar pattern, with self-selection of a balanced diet from an array of solids.)

The q4h feeding schedule with milk formula alone has been challenged by Sackett in his studies of the three feedings a day concept for the newborn (Paper 36). The baby-bottle-warmer companies would be permanently out of business if the general public were to adopt (as I, as a working mother, adopted) the refrigerator-to-mouth technique.

History's lesson is clear to those who would hear it. Despite the swings of the pendulum, of fashions in feeding, given an adequate caloric intake of potable milk in almost any form, with modest vitamin supplements of A, D, and C, and allowed to adjust its own intake, the normal infant will thrive.

33

Reprinted from *Am. J. Dis. Child.*, **14**(4), 233–257 (1917)

HUNGER IN THE INFANT *

ROOD TAYLOR, M.D., Sc.D.

Mayo Clinic

ROCHESTER, MINN.

Cannon and Washburn,[1] and Carlson and his colaborers have given us a proved method for studying hunger objectively; its time of occurrence, its intensity, its effects, and the means by which it may be produced or inhibited. They have shown that contractions of the so-called empty stomach cause the hunger sensation. These contractions depend in part on vagus tonus. They can be increased by chemical changes in the blood, but are primarily due to a gastric mechanism as purely automatic as is that of the heart.

Impulses set up by these contractions and carried to the higher centers are, in the normal consciousness, recognized as hunger. These impulses produce secondary effects such as restlessness and irritability. They increase the reflex excitability of the central nervous system, the heart beats faster, and there are changes in the vasomotor mechanism. Well fed, sedentary adults seldom experience hunger. The prime factor in their desire for food depends not on the basis of distress due to the contractions of a hollow viscus, but on "the memory processes of past experience with palatable foods." This psychic factor is appetite, and its absolute distinction from the physical factor, hunger, must be kept in mind.

Working on dogs, Patterson, in 1914, showed the gastric hunger contractions to be much more frequent and vigorous in young than in older animals. In 1915, Carlson and Ginsburg described the great intensity of hunger contractions in the human new-born. Previous to that year no productive analytic studies of the hunger sense in the human infant had been made. Appetite and hunger were not distinguished, and the sucking mechanism alone had been analyzed.

In 1888, Auerbach distinguished the infantile type of sucking from the voluntary inspiratory type employed by the adult, and in 1894 Basch, disproving the older theory of Preyer that sucking is instinctive, showed it to be entirely reflex.

---

* Submitted for publication Aug. 18, 1917.

* From the Department of Pediatrics, University of Minnesota.

1. All references to the literature will be found at the end of the article.

Czerny, in 1893, observed that an infant awakened a short time after taking his fill from the maternal breast, would again suck vigorously if placed on it, and concluded that sucking per se could not be considered as a sign of hunger. A few years later (1900) Keller wrote that, since the normal infant sleeps three hours after nursing, although its stomach is empty in two hours, the emptying of the stomach cannot be considered a positive criterion of need for food. Pies, in 1910, considered the reddening and eczema of the lower lip which occurs in undernourished infants as a sign of hunger, and referred it directly to the infant's fruitless sucking. In 1913 Schlossmann concluded from extensive observations on semistarved infants that the sensation of hunger exists only in the imagination.

Meyer and Rosenstern studied the results of starvation in the different types of alimentary disorder, recording particularly the pulse, temperature, respiration and weight changes. Rosenstern later (1911-1912) wrote extensively on the general subjects of hunger and inanition in infancy. These studies are all defective in that they do not distinguish the various factors concerned. Neumann, Pfaundler, Cramer, Süszwein, Barth, and Kasahara have discussed the subject of disturbances in the food urge largely from the point of view of imperfections in the sucking mechanism.

The present studies are concerned particularly with the gastric factors in the urge for food. The major of these, the hunger contractions, was studied by means of apparatus similar to that used by Carlson. A rubber balloon of about 20 c.c. capacity attached to one end of a small soft rubber catheter is inserted into the stomach and inflated, the catheter is attached to a bromoform manometer with a cork float and a writing pennant which records the gastric movements on smoked paper.

The material investigated included 5 premature infants weighing from 1,200 to 2,500 gm., 40 full term new-borns under 3 weeks of age, and 11 older babies, 5 between 1 and 2 months, 2 between 3 and 4 months, 3 between 4 and 6 months, and 1 boy of 2 years with a surgically induced gastric fistula made necessary by the effects of corrosive in the esophagus. The gastric movements of some of the infants were recorded only once; on others as many as twenty observations were made.

Carlson and Ginsburg refer to the readiness with which most infants accept and retain the tube and balloon. It is naturally impossible to secure a graphic record of the stomach movements of a raging infant. Carlson and Ginsburg did their work on full term new-borns. These infants, as a rule, sleep quietly when not disturbed. The present work was carried on in a dimly lighted, quiet room. I had less difficulty when the infant was left undisturbed in his crib than when I attempted innovations, such as threading a pacifier on the tube or having the infant held in the nurse's arms.

The older babies resent the presence of the tube, and with them it was often necessary to make repeated attempts to secure tracings. Some infants finally became accustomed to the presence of the tube and slept quietly, particularly if the experiments were conducted in the evening. Most of the tracings on the 2-year-old boy with the gastric fistula were made when he was awake. The greatest problem was to keep him sufficiently interested to prevent crying and restlessness and at the same time to prevent riotous hilarity. In his case the balloon was introduced directly through the fistula.

It is said that passage of the stomach tube in infants is apt to cause aspiration pneumonia. No ill results followed the procedure carried out in these studies.

Does the presence of the balloon in the stomach act mechanically to produce gastric contractions? Carlson states definitely that it does not, and gives the following reasons for his belief:

1. The presence of the distended balloon in the stomach between the contraction periods does not induce these contractions.

2. In Mr. V. [his gastric fistula case] the gastric contractions can be observed directly through the large fistula without any balloon in the stomach.

3. The contraction periods come on just as frequently without any balloon in the stomach and produce the same effect (hunger).

4. In pigeons the periodic strong contractions of the empty crop can be seen directly through the skin, and a balloon in the crop does not alter their frequency or intensity.

The results of this work fully confirm Carlson and Ginsburg's report that the stomach of the new-born infant exhibits greater hunger contraction than does that of the adult. The intervals between the contraction periods are often less than five minutes and usually not longer than from ten to twenty minutes. The first contraction period after a nursing is apt to consist of from five to twenty separate contractions and to last from two to eight minutes. The succeeding contraction periods frequently endure from thirty minutes to an hour or even longer. The duration of each contraction is about twenty seconds. In many of the infants the contraction time of the more powerful contractions, especially in those periods ending in partial tetanus, was about eighteen seconds. Except in the first contraction period after a nursing, endings in partial tetanus were frequently observed. Partial tetanus is sometimes present before the close of the period. With the apparatus used, the force of the single contractions usually sufficed to raise the column of bromoform 2 to 3 cm. During partial tetanus the bromoform may be raised 5 cm.

Patterson found practically continuous hunger contractions in premature pups. It is particularly easy to obtain graphic records of the

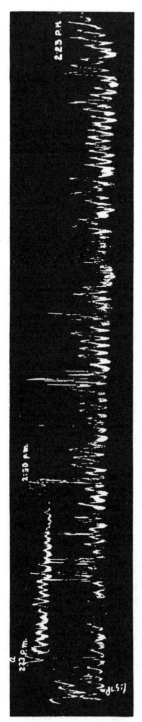

Fig. 1.—Hunger contractions in normal, new-born infant. Beginning of partial tetanus at extreme right in lower tracing.

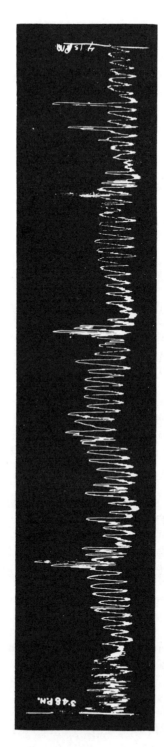

Fig. 2.—Prematurely born infant. Typical activity of the premature baby's stomach. Boy F., aged 15 days; weight, 1,536 gm.; getting 45 c.c. breast milk six times a day. Previous feeding at 2:30 p. m.

hunger contractions of the somnolent, prematurely born infant. The stomach of such an infant is in a state of nearly continuous contraction. The individual contractions require about the same length of time for their completion and are as powerful as those of the full term infant. In a tracing begun forty minutes after a feeding of 15 gm. of breast milk to a premature baby (Baby 5) weighing 1,510 gm., the record appears very like that obtained by Rogers from the crop of a pigeon in the second day of starvation. The periods of contraction last two or three minutes, with intervening periods of quiescence of about the same length. The individual contractions last twelve to fifteen seconds and raise the bromoform column 3 to 4 cm. Partial tetanus is frequent. Nine days later, when the infant was receiving more food, in spite of the fact that he had not gained in weight and that the tracing was begun five hours after his last feeding, the record obtained was similar to those from other infants.

Are the hunger contractions more frequent or more powerful in cyanosed infants? May they furnish a stimulus for crying with consequent better aeration of the lungs? In two such cases no significant increase or decrease in the hunger contractions could be observed. No records were taken from any cyanosed premature infants, although such infants are frequently slightly blue for the first few days.

Carlson, working on the adult, was unable to produce hunger contractions by any sort of stimulus acting directly in the mouth or in the stomach, except that he occasionally could, by suddenly distending the stomach, produce a few transitory contractions. He found, uniformly, that the only effect of such local stimulation was inhibitory. In general, the taste of salt, sour, bitter, or sweet; or the chewing of agreeable, disagreeable, or indifferent substances, all produce temporary inhibition of the gastric contractions. Chewing palatable foods by the adult when hungry causes an inhibition, made more lasting by the flow of appetite juice in the stomach.

Carlson found that acid and alkaline solutions, food and liquids in the stomach, all inhibit the hunger contractions. Inhibition from the stomach is less transitory than that from the mouth. Boldyreff showed that the periodic contractions of the empty stomach were inhibited by the presence of acid in the intestine. Brunemeier and Carlson completed and enlarged this work. They demonstrated inhibition from the presence of gastric juice or acid chyme in the small intestine. This inhibition from the stomach and intestine is reflex, partly through Auerbach's plexus, but mainly through the long reflex arc with the efferent path to the stomach muscles through the splanchnics.

Inhibition from the mouth is not present in the frog (Patterson). Carlson, who suspects that such inhibition involves conscious cerebral processes, has suggested experiments in infants to settle the point.

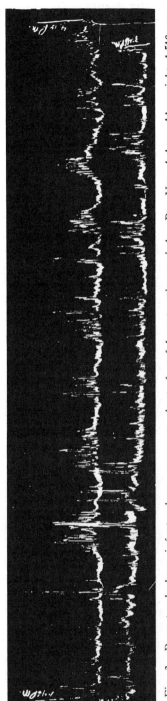

Fig. 3.—Prematurely born infant; shows numerous short, forceful contraction periods. Boy Von, 4 days old; weight, 1,510 gm.; birth weight, 1,715 gm.; at 2:30 p. m. received 15 c.c. breast milk.

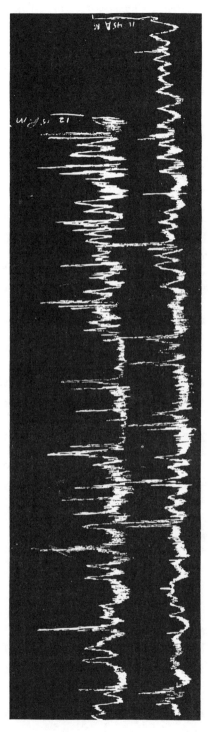

Fig. 4.—Baby Mi., 15 days old; tracing shows presence of hunger contractions in an infant who nursed poorly.

367

Repeated trials with breast milk, sugar water, common salt, quinin, and lemon juice in the mouths of premature and new-born infants in my study failed to produce inhibition of hunger contractions.

In general I obtained the same results in an infant of 8 weeks. A transitory inhibition occurred occasionally when sugar water was placed in his mouth. In none of the infants did chewing or sucking on the thumb or tube produce inhibition. Nor did such movements or the presence of sugar, breast milk or other substances in the mouth induce hunger contractions.

The boy of 2 years showed inhibition when sugar or protein milk (his diet at the time) was placed in his mouth. Quinin, dilute hydrochloric acid, small amounts of sugar water, table salt in crystals or solution, did not inhibit. Benzosulphinidum solution inhibited twice. It was not used subsequently. The sight of sugar did not inhibit. He began to cry when he saw his bottle if the latter were not given him immediately. Conseqeuntly the effect of his seeing the bottle on the hunger contractions could not be registered. During the periods of quiescence the sight of the nurse who fed him did not induce hunger contractions, although he began to whine and tease when she entered the room.

Apparently inhibition from the mouth was produced by those substances only which the child regarded as food. Quinin very evidently made a profound sensory impression, but did not inhibit the contractions. Dilute hydrochloric acid did not inhibit, while unsweetened protein milk (which is slightly sour) did.

Carlson's hypothesis as to the need of conscious cerebration for the production of inhibitory reflexes from the mouth would appear to offer the correct explanation. It seems to be agreed that the new-born infant leads a subcortical reflex existence (Soltmann-Cramer). Kussmaul and Thiemich note that the new-born infant accepts sugar and rejects salt, food that is sour and bitter — action which is almost certainly purely reflex on the part of the infant.

My work shows that when 20 c.c. of water or milk are introduced into the stomach during a contraction period inhibition follows invariably. This was found true in infants of all ages. With small amounts of water the inhibition often lasted only three or four minutes, when the contraction period would be resumed.

On the other hand, it was not unusual to recover from 15 to 40 cm. of clotted milk through the stomach tube even an hour after vigorous hunger contractions had begun. This is a considerable portion of the infant's meal, and in these cases would represent from one-sixth to one-fourth of his total intake at the previous feeding. Soltmann showed that the inhibiting nervous mechanism of the heart is much less effectual in the new-born infant than in later life. It seems possible

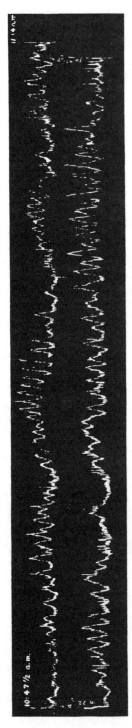

Fig. 5.—Baby Ri., 6 days old, with congenital myxedema; tracing shows presence of hunger contractions in a babe who nursed poorly.

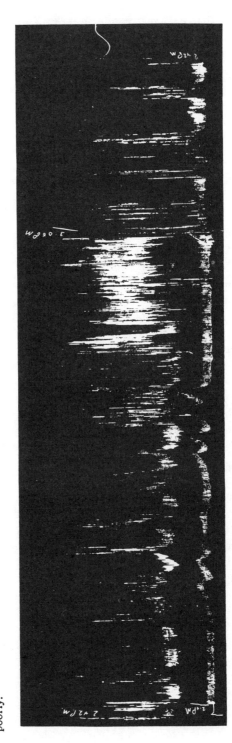

Fig. 6.—Baby J., 4 months old. Tracing shows development of hunger contractions during the interval following a feeding.

369

that the nervous apparatus for the inhibition of the gastric hunger movements may likewise be immature. Or the tissue hunger may be so great as to overcome any but the strong inhibition of a heavily laden stomach and duodenum.

The vagi form the sensory pathway from the stomach to the brain. The first reflex centers are the sensory nuclei of the vagi in the medulla. A second center, possibly that for conscious hunger, is located in the optic thalami. Rogers has shown that the picking reflex in the pigeon (analogous to the sucking reflex in the babe) is abolished on removal of the thalami.

The reflex irritability (as indicated by the knee jerk) is increased synchronously with each hunger contraction (Carlson). No observations have been made on the infant's knee jerks during the hunger state; but Zybell has shown that the electrical irritability increases during the first eighteen hours of starvation.

Let us summarize the events from the close of one meal till the end of the next. The infant sleeps. The upper stomach musculature maintains a tonic grasp on the contained food. The pyloric antrum is traversed by peristaltic waves (Cannon). The stomach gradually empties. The point of origin of the peristaltic waves rises higher and higher. The tonus rhythm of the fundus begins. The stomach empties itself more completely, the tonus rhythm becomes more intense, and the first hunger contractions appear (Rogers and Hardt).

The first contraction period is apt to be short. After a wait of perhaps twenty minutes a longer and more intense hunger period arrives; then another and another. The infant's sleep becomes lighter. He is more easily awakened by external stimuli or by gastric discomfort. He is put to the breast, nurses vigorously, becomes fatigued (Schmidt, Cramer, Pfaundler), or experiences satiety from distention (Neisser and Bräuning) and again goes to sleep.

What constitutes the hunger state? Does it result from the sum· mation of impulses with an increasing psychic and reflex irritability? The evidence is to the contrary. The increase in the reflex excitability is synchronous with the contraction phase of the stomach, and is absent in the intervals between the contractions. In the infant who has been some hours without food the hunger contractions are nearly continuous, and it would be expected that the reflex excitability would be nearly continuously high.

In the absence of hunger contractions the infant often sucks vigorously on the tube attached to the balloon. The receptive mechanism for the institution of the sucking reflex is so delicate that it is impossible to provide, artificially, a minimal stimulus. During the hunger state, when presumably a rapid succession of hunger contractions maintains a low reflex threshold, there may often be observed a succession of

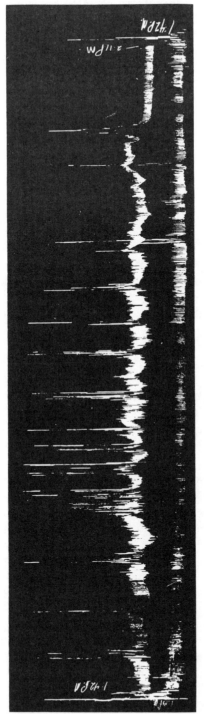

Fig. 7.—Same as Figure 6.

371

automatic sucking movements involving the lips, tongue and lower jaw, each movement providing the necessary stimulus for its successor.

The lay mind is prone to think that the crying infant is hungry. Comby and Czerny and Keller believe that hunger is a minor cause of crying. Rosenstern notes that in hunger young babies are usually quiet, but that the older infants cry more. Schlossmann remarks that the normal infant endures hunger well.

Observations on this point extending over sixteen months of study of the hunger sensation lead me to believe that in normally thriving breast fed infants, except when more than three or four hours have elapsed since the last feeding, neither the hunger contractions themselves nor the increased irritability due to them are ordinarily immediate factors in the production of crying. Young infants sleep throughout strong contraction periods. Older infants often do the same, and are frequently quiet even from twelve to sixteen hours after a feeding. Mental factors produce crying at a very early age. And the fact that crying ceases when food or water is administered may only mean that the infant's attention is diverted to the performance of a pleasurable act.

It may be noted in this connection that the 2-year-old boy was happier when allowed to take food into his mouth, and that his outlook on life was much more cheerful on days when he could take nourishment by mouth than on other days when the esophageal constriction increased, and it became necessary to introduce the food through the gastric fistula. This feeding through the fistula was without pain, and the child submitted to it with some pleasure.

What is the time interval between feeding and the first appearance of gastric hunger contractions? Ginsburg, Tumpowsky and Carlson studied this point in thirty normal breast fed infants under 4 weeks of age. They gave no data as to gain in weight and did not determine the amount of food taken, but stated that the babes nursed till satisfied. They found the average time between nursing and the appearance of hunger contractions to be two hours and forty minutes, with a minimum of two hours and twenty minutes and a maximum of three hours and thirty minutes. My observations on twelve new-born infants under like conditions yielded these results; a minimum of one hour and thirty minutes, a maximum of three hours and thirty minutes, and an average of about two and one-half hours.

Many infants in the first two weeks do not receive a sufficient supply of breast milk. This is particularly apt to be true of the time the babe and the mother remain in the hospital. Consequently, observations made under the conditions so far outlined may be misleading. Table 1 (A, B and C) gives the results of all satisfactory tracings obtained from normally thriving babies on whom sufficient data as to food intake and weight gain were obtained.

372

TABLE 1.—INTERVAL FOR DEVELOPMENT OF HUNGER

A. PREMATURE INFANTS

Name	Age, Days	Food	Feeding Interval	Quantity at Feeding	Interval Before Tracing	Time for Development of First Hunger Period	Remarks
Sw.	7	Breast milk	4 hours 5 times a day	35 c.c.	None	40 min.	Premature Wt. 2,140 gm.
Sw.	11	Breast milk	4 hours 5 times a day	50 c.c.	20 min.	1 hr., 20 min.	Wt. 2,240 gm.
Sw.	20	Breast milk	4 hours 5 times a day	90 c.c.	52 min.	2 hours	Wt. 2,470 gm.
Sw.	25	Breast milk	4 hours 5 times a day	75 gm.	38 min.	1 hr., 50 min.	Wt. 2,565 gm.
St.	13	Breast milk	4 hours 5 times a day	30 c.c.	None	1 hour	Premature Wt. 2,270 gm.
St.	14	Breast milk	4 hours 5 times a day	50 c.c.	None	40 min.	Wt. 2,280 gm.
St.	25	Breast milk	4 hours 5 times a day	90 c.c.	1 hr., 13 min.	1 hr., 15 min.	Wt. 2,450 gm.
St.	28	Breast milk	4 hours 5 times a day	90 c.c.	38 min.	1 hour	Wt.
St.	36	Breast milk	4 hours 5 times a day	100 c.c.	52 min.	1 hr., 50 min.	Wt. 2,720 gm.
Fre.	9	Breast milk	4 hours 6 times a day	45 c.c.	1 hr., 38 min.	1 hr., 38 min.	Premature Wt. 1,380 gm.
Fre.	15	Breast milk	4 hours 6 times a day	45 c.c.	1 hr., 18 min.	1 hr., 18 min.	Wt. 1,530 gm.
Fre	16	Breast milk	4 hours 6 times a day	45 c.c.	23 min.	1 hr., 15 min.	Wt. 1,535 gm.
Fre	21	Breast milk	4 hours 6 times a day	65 c.c.	2 hours	2 hr., 20 min.	Wt. 1,710 gm.

B. FULL TERM NEW-BORN INFANTS

Name	Age, Days	Food	Feeding Interval	Quantity at Feeding	Interval Before Tracing	Time for Development of First Hunger Period	Remarks
H.	8	Breast milk	4 hours 5 times a day	?	1 hr., 22 min.	3 hr., 50 min.	Wt. 3,500 gm.; gain in 4 days, 90 gm.
Dav.	8	Breast milk	3 hours 8 times a day	75 gm.	1 hr., 55 min.	2 hr., 25 min.	Wt. 4,100 gm.; gain in 5 days 260 gm.; 10 c.c. of milk clot removed from stomach 1 hr. after beginning of hunger contractions
Dav.	9	Breast milk	4 hours (for preceding 24 hours) 5 times a day	?	2 hr., 30 min.	2 hr., 30 min.	Wt. 4,200 gm.; gain in 6 days, 300 gm.; ½ c.c. thick mucus removed from stomach ½ hr. after beginning of hunger contractions
Wes.	8	Breast milk	4 hours 5 times a day	100 gm.	1 hr., 30 min.	3 hr., 10 min.	14 hours fast previous to last feeding
A.	9	Breast milk + cow's milk 8% lactose aa	3 hours 8 times a day	70 gm.	1 hr., 45 min.	2 hr., 10 min.	Wt. 3,610 gm.; gain in 6 days 230 gm.; 20 c.c. of thick soft milk clot removed from stomach 50 min. after beginning of hunger contractions
A.	10	Breast milk + cow's milk 8% lactose aa	....	70 gm.	1 hr., 52 min.	2 hours	15 c.c. of fluid and curds removed from stomach 30 min. after beginning of hunger contractions
Wal.	10	Breast milk	4 hours 5 times a day	95 gm.	1 hr., 30 min.	4 hours	Wt. 3,240 gm.; gain in 6 days, 260 gm.
D.	12	Breast milk	4 hours 5 times a day	115 gm.	2 hr., 30 min.	2 hr., 30 min.	Wt. 3,720 gm.; gain in 7 days, 400 gm.

C. NORMAL INFANTS OVER TWO WEEKS OF AGE

Name	Age, Days	Food	Feeding Interval	Quantity at Feeding	Interval Before Tracing	Time for Development of First Hunger Period	Remarks
Gor.	18	Breast milk	4 hours 5 times a day	85 gm.	2 hr., 23 min.	4 hours	Wt. 3,500 gm.; gain in 13 days, 70 gm.
Gor.	19	Breast milk	4 hours 5 times a day	110 gm.	1 hr., 58 min.	3 hr., 25 min.	
Way.	3.5 Mos.	Buttermilk + flour + saccharose	4 hours 5 times a day	150 c.c.	2 hr., 27 min.	3 hr., 12 min.	Wt. 4,960 gm.; gain in 7 days, 440 gm.
Way.	3.5	Buttermilk + flour + saccharose	4 hours 5 times a day	150 c.c.	57 min.	3 hr., 20 min.	40 c.c. of thick white materal removed from stomach 20 min. after beginning of contraction period
Way.	3.5	Buttermilk + flour + saccharose	4 hours 5 times a day	150 c.c.	2 hr., 3 min.	4 hr., 35 min.	
Herm.	4	Breast milk	2 or 3 hours irregular	?	2 hr., 45 min.	3 hr., 30 min.	Well nourished; gaining in weight; normal baby; cared for at home; not in hospital
J.	4	Breast milk	5 times a day	?	2 hr., 15 min.	3 hr., 30 min.	Well nourished; gaining in weight; normal baby; cared for at home; not in hospital
Ad.	4	Malt soup	4 hours 5 times a day	125 c.c.	2 hr., 37 min.	3 hr., 30 min.	Wt. 3,500 gm.; gain in 2 weeks, 200 gm.; prematurely born; 1,600 gm. at birth

The time required for the development of hunger in the premature infant is noticeably short. In the case of the full term new-borns the figures obtained agree fairly well with those given by Ginsburg, Tumpowsky and Carlson, but are definitely greater than those obtained by me (mentioned in a preceding paragraph) from infants whose food intake was not accurately known.

The time required for the development of hunger in any one infant is fairly constant over a short period of time, provided the amount and kind of food is not changed. This conclusion rests not only on the results shown in Table 1, but on a dozen other observations on infants whose feeding conditions remained constant during the time in which studies were made.

With the older infants difficulty in maintaining quiet, after the insertion of tube and balloon, limits the number of observations which give positive evidence as to the first appearance of hunger contractions. Many less successful observations on healthy, normally developing infants yield this negative evidence that in such infants more than a month old I did not observe the development of hunger before the end of three hours.

It should be noted further that the contraction period, the first appearance of which is recorded in Table 1, is the first one to develop after feeding. This period is usually short and is not made up of forceful contractions. With Infants J. and A. more intense and more nearly continuous contractions did not begin for four and four and a half hours, respectively.

Habits as to feeding interval affect the time required for the development of hunger chiefly as they influence the emptying time of the stomach. It has been shown that the speed of gastric emptying is proportional to the length of time during which the individual has been without food (Tobler, Haudek and Stigler), and that large feedings are emptied with relatively greater rapidity than small ones (Tobler and Bogen). Habits undoubtedly exert a more powerful influence on the mental factors associated with appetite than on hunger itself.

Tables 2, 3 and 4 illustrate the shorter time required for the development of hunger in infants with chronic nourishment disturbance, and indicate that the presence of hunger contractions is not in itself evidence that the stomach is ready for food.

In the columns headed "Remarks" in Tables 1, 2, 3 and 4, there are notes as to material recovered with the stomach tube after the onset of gastric hunger contractions. In normal babies, however, there probably does exist a relation between the emptying time of the stomach and the interval for the development of hunger.

Observations on the emptying time in infants, so far reported, have been made either with the relatively stiff catheter, the stomach tube,

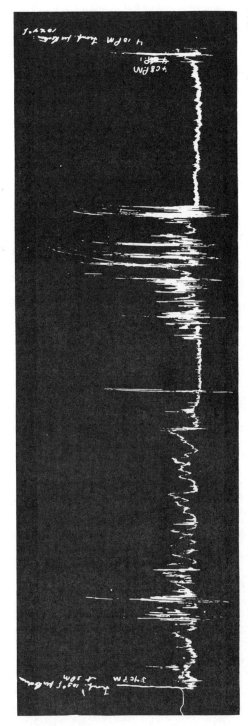

Fig. 8.—N. N., a 2-year-old boy with typhoid fever. Hunger contractions present when rectal temperature ranges between 104.4 and 105 F.

or the Roentgen ray. The flexible tube introduced by Rehfuss should replace the catheter for this purpose; it was used in my work. The literature contains no reports of the time required for gastric digestion in the premature infant. The emptying time in normal breast-fed infants under 1 week is usually less than one hour (Leo). The Roentgen-ray observations of Ladd and of Tobler and Bogen would indicate that in normal breast-fed infants the stomach is frequently not empty until after two to three hours. The figures obtained with the use of the stomach tube by Epstein, Czerny, Keller and Cassel indicate a delayed emptying time in gastro-intestinal disease.

TABLE 2.—HUNGER IN ATROPHY RESULTING FROM CONTINUED STARVATION

N. N., aged 2 years; gastric fistula; weight fluctuating between 6,800 gm. and 7,200 gm.; typhoid fever Dec. 1 until Dec. 14, 1916.

Date 1916	Food	Time of Last Feeding	Beginning of Tracing	
10/19	Diluted cow's milk + general diet	6 a. m.	10:15 a. m.	Practically continuous hunger periods until 10:50 a. m.
10/20	Diluted cow's milk + general diet	10 a. m.	2:12 p. m.	Practically continuous hunger periods until 3:15 p. m.
11/ 1	....	10 a. m.	2:16 p. m.	One hunger period at 2:45 p. m. to 2:50 p. m. Hunger contractions practically continuous after 3 p. m. until 4:50 p. m.
11/10	160 c.c. cow's milk at preceding feeding	2 p. m.	2:45 p. m.	Observations continued until 5:10 p. m. No hunger periods, but child cried or was restless over half of the time
10/11	160 c.c. cow's milk at preceding feeding	2 p. m.	9:00 p. m.	Practically continuous contractions until 11 p. m.
11/11	200 c.c. protein milk + 7% dextrimaltose	5 p. m.	10:12 p. m.	Practically continuous contractions until 11 p. m.
11/12	200 c.c. protein milk + 7% dextrimaltose	5 p. m.	8:41 p. m.	First hunger period at 9:30; practically continuous from 9:45 on until 10:44 p. m.
11/29	200 c.c. protein milk + 7% dextrimaltose	1 p. m.	4:02 p. m.	First hunger period began at 4:35 p. m.; practically continuous from 5 p. m. on until 5:42 p. m.
12/27	200 c.c. protein milk + 7% dextrimaltose + cereals	9 a. m.	12:34 p. m.	Hunger periods practically continuous until 1:30 p. m.
12/28	200 c.c. protein milk + 7% dextrimaltose + cereals	9 a. m.	12:22 p. m.	Hunger periods began about 12:50; hunger periods became continuous after 1:20 p. m.
12/30	200 c.c. protein milk + 7% dextrimaltose + cereals	5 a. m.	10:13 a. m.	Practically continuous hunger periods until 11:20 a. m.

Major, using the Roentgen ray, finds the emptying time delayed in dyspepsia, but accelerated in decomposition. With the same method Pisek and LeWald found the emptying time to be shorter in infants with chronic disturbances of nutrition.

These last findings, taken in conjunction with the already quoted reports of Tobler, and of Haudek and Stigler, that the emptying time is shortened by hunger, are suggestive of the results here obtained experimentally; that is, the greater gastric hunger contraction in infants with chronic nourishment disturbance.

Not only is the interval for development of hunger shorter in such infants, but the contractions become much more intense. Nov. 10,

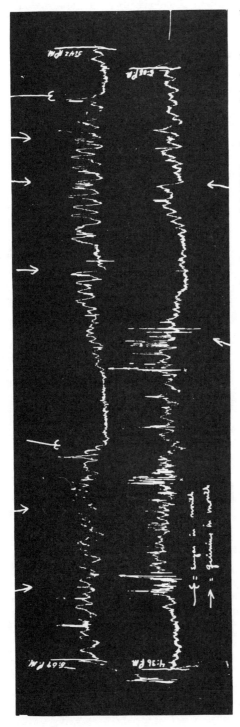

Fig. 9.—N. N., 2 years old. Tracing shows inhibition from sugar in the mouth; absence of inhibition from quinin in the mouth.

377

1916, the 2-year-old boy (Table 2), whose weight in spite of a calorically sufficient intake had remained stationary, and whose temperature had been irregular, developed fever and diarrhea. After eight hours of starvation, with temperature normal, the graphic record of his gastric activities resembled those of the starving pigeon and of the premature infant already mentioned. The contractions were continuous and required only twelve seconds for their completion. Next day the child was put on protein milk and thereafter improved.

It is generally agreed that mixtures with high fat content leave the stomach most slowly, while those with low fat and high carbohydrate

TABLE 3.—Hunger in Exudative Diathesis

Aus., 7 weeks old, Dec. 19, 1916.   Feeding interval 4 hours, 5 times a day.

Date	Weight, Gm.	Food: Breast Milk + Buttermilk + Flour Saccharose, C.c.	Time of Last Feeding	Beginning of Tracing	
12/19/16	4,450	100	1 p. m.	3:28 p. m.	Hunger contractions began at 3:30 p. m. Hunger contractions continuous from 3:55 to 4:37 p. m.
12/22/16	4,460	100	9 a. m.	11:49 a. m.	Hunger contractions present at 11:49 a. m. Hunger contractions continuous until 12:50 p. m.
12/22/16	4,460	150	1:15 p. m.	3:34 p. m.	Hunger contractions began at 5:45 p. m.
1/6/17	4,640	125	8 a. m.	10:55 a. m.	Hunger contractions began at 10:55 a. m. Hunger contractions continuous until 12:21 p. m.
1/8/17	4,640	125	8:40 a. m.	11:51 a. m.	Hunger contractions began at 12 m. Hunger contractions strong and continuous after 12:18. Babe was restless
1/11/17	4,650	125	8:45 a. m.	11:11 a. m.	Hunger contractions present by 11:45 a. m. Hunger contractions continuous until 1:35 p. m.
1/13/17	4,740	150	8:20 a. m.	11:03 a. m.	Hunger contractions began at 11:45 a. m. Hunger contractions continuous from 12 to 1 p. m.
1/15/17	4,770	150	8:45 a. m.	11:01 a. m.	Hunger contractions present at 11:20 a. m. Hunger contractions continuous from 11:30 a. m. until 12:50 p. m.
1/15/17	4,770	150	12:50 p. m.	3:21 p. m.	Babe cried a large part of time; no evidence of hunger periods until 5 p. m.

leave most rapidly. In Infants A. and W. the time interval for the development of hunger contractions was much longer when they received low fat and high carbohydrate, and shorter when they received high fat and low carbohydrate. This would be paradoxical if the gastric hunger contractions depended exclusively on the emptying time.

It is, then, only in normal babies, receiving well tolerated food in sufficient quantity, that the development of hunger waits on the emptying of the stomach.

The interval necessary for the development of hunger depends in part on the form of nourishment and is shortest with that food which least satisfies the infant's tissue need (Table 4). The question as to whether the rapid development of hunger in qualitatively poorly

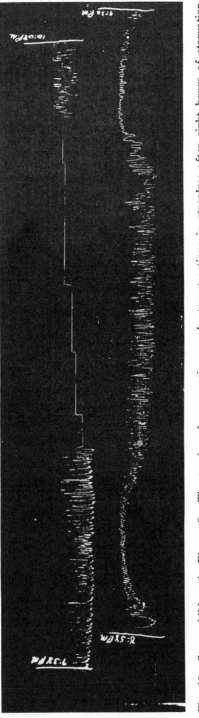

Fig. 10.—Same child as in Figure 9. The tracing shows continuous short contractions in atrophy; after eight hours of starvation.

379

nourished infants depends on the administration of food deficient in carbohydrate in particular, or on the giving of food poorly tolerated in general, is not answered. Records of the gastric contractions in infants suffering from the chronic nourishment disturbance due to long continued carbohydrate overfeeding (the "Mehlnährschaden" of Czerny) would help to settle this point.

TABLE 4.—INTERVAL FOR DEVELOPMENT OF HUNGER IN INFANTS WITH CHRONIC DISTURBANCE OF NUTRITION AND SHOWING INFLUENCE OF CHANGE IN FORM OF NOURISHMENT

Name and Date	Age, Mo.	Diagnosis	Weight, Gm.	Food	Interval Before Tracing	Time for Development of First Hunger Period	Remarks
Til.	3	Atrophy............	Stationary 4,080	120 gm. protein milk + 7% dextrimaltose 5 times a day	....	....	Hunger periods with partial tetanus less than 3 hours after feeding
Ad. 2/26/17	4	Chronic alimentary disorder due to overfeeding with milk	3,300	150 c.c. ½ milk + 10% saccharose 5 times a day	....	....	Hunger contractions present in 2 hours and 20 minutes
Ad. 3/8/17	4	Chronic alimentary disorder due to overfeeding with milk	3,500	125 c.c. malt soup 5 times a day	....	....	Babe improved clinically; hunger contractions first appear in 3½ hrs.
Way.	3	Chronic nourishment disturbance with eczema	....	Mixture containing 8% fat. Feeding intervals short and irregular. After entrance to hospital fed 5 times a day	....	....	Entered hospital April 14, 1917
4/14/17	..	....	4,200	150 c.c. ½ cow's milk + 10% saccharose	2 hr., 7 min.	2 hr., 7 min.	Stomach emptied 3 hours after feeding; ½ c.c. of mucus and thick curd obtained
4/23/17	..	....	4,510	150 c.c. ½ cow's milk + 10% saccharose	2 hr., 10 min.	2 hr., 10 min.	Eczema increased; 40 c.c. of clotted milk and clear thin fluid recovered from stomach 3 hours and 25 minutes after feeding
5/1/17	..	....	4,960	150 c.c. buttermilk + flour + saccharose	2 hr., 3 min.	4 hr., 35 min.	Eczema has disappeared
5/2/17	..	....	4,960	150 c.c. buttermilk + flour + saccharose	2 hr., 27 min.	3 hr., 12 min.	
5/3/17	..	....	4,960	150 c.c. buttermilk + flour + saccharose	57 min.	3 hr., 20 min.	40 c.c. of thick white material removed from stomach 20 minutes after beginning of first contraction period

Attention has already been called to the heightened electrical reactions found by Zybell in hungry infants. I also wish to mention the findings of Finklestein, Thiemich and Japha that the electrical irritability is frequently heightened in artificially fed infants, and of Czerny and Moser that there is an increase in the electrical irritability of infants suffering with "Mehlnährschaden." It is possible that the heightened electrical irritability in all depends on the increased hunger contractions due again in part to the constant chemical stimulation reaching the stomach from the semistarved tissues.

Most premature infants and many young infants nurse poorly. The consequent effect on lactation and on the babe's nourishment is serious. An extensive literature on this subject has been developed in German, but there is surprisingly little in French and in English.

In 1888 Auerbach described the infantile manner of sucking, which depends on the chewing muscles, and Escherich showed its teleologic importance. The reflex paths and center in the medulla were demonstrated in 1894 (Basch). Cramer, Suszwein, Finklestein, Rott, Rosenstern, Barth and Kasahara have further studied the question and report results which in general support the theory that the inability to nurse well is to be attributed primarily to an imperfect nervous mechanism and not to muscular weakness.

For further elucidation of the question, tracings of the movements of the empty stomach were taken in two infants who were extreme examples.

The first baby (Baby M.), weighing 2,700 gm. at birth and presenting no anatomic peculiarities, took very little from the mother's breast during the first three weeks, although sufficient milk was expressed therefrom to feed the baby and to complement the feedings of other babies.

The second infant (Baby T.), aged 3 months, had weaned himself from the breast, had developed dyspepsia and atrophy on artificial feeding, and could be made to take his food from the bottle only with great difficulty. He seemed able to fix his attention on anything other than the act of feeding.

In these infants as well as in the five prematures, and in one typical case of congenital myxedema, hunger contractions of at least normal force and duration were present. At the time they were studied, none of the infants was able to nurse successfully. In all, the sucking reflex was qualitatively present.

This study does not solve the problem as to the causation of feeble nursing, but does limit the field of possibilities by excluding derangements of the primitive hunger apparatus.

Carlson reports Rupp's finding that hunger contractions persist during the fever excited by the administration of typhoid vaccine. The boy with the gastric fistula contracted typhoid fever from a carrier. Tracings taken while his rectal temperature ranged between 104.4 F. and 105 F., show the presence of hunger contractions.

Carlson and Ginsburg found hypertonicity and hypermotility in the stomachs of two infants with pylorospasm and stenosis. From a six weeks' old infant (Baby S.) with pyloric stenosis, I obtained records which agree with Carlson and Ginsburg's description of periods of tetanus lasting several minutes interspersed with vigorous contractions of normal duration.

Carlson suggests that pylorospasm and stenosis may be an expression of gastric hypermotility. His cases were seen late, as was the one here reported. In the absence of tracings taken at the beginning of the disease, it is likely that the hypermotility results from the inanition following the obstruction at the pylorus. And without definite knowledge that the stomach was washed empty, the long periods of tetanus observed may represent the so-called visible gastric peristalsis.

SUMMARY

The study of fifty-six infants from birth to 2 years of age gives the following results:

1. Confirmation of previous work, that hunger contractions are greater in the new-born infant, with description of these contractions.

2. Determination of the still greater hunger contraction in the stomachs of prematurely born infants, with description of these contractions.

3. There is no relation between cyanosis and hunger contractions.

4. Inhibition of the hunger contractions from the mouth does not occur in young infants.

5. Inhibition of the hunger contractions from the mouth in older infants is present only as the result of stimuli, which the babe has learned to recognize as food. It does not occur with substances producing equally strong sensory impressions, but which are not considered by the infant as food.

6. Inhibition from the mouth is psychic in character.

7. Reflex inhibition from the presence of food in the stomach is present in infants of all ages.

8. This reflex inhibition from the stomach may be only partially developed in young infants.

9. Successive automatic sucking movements — each sucking act serving as the stimulus for its successor — are present during the hunger state, when the reflex threshold is kept almost constantly low by a rapid succession of hunger contractions.

10. In normally developing breast fed babes, hunger is not ordinarily an immediate cause of crying.

11. The average time required for the development of hunger in healthy infants gaining in weight and receiving a known sufficient amount of food is, in prematures, under one month, one hour and forty minutes, with a maximum of two hours and twenty minutes and a minimum of forty minutes; in full term infants under two weeks, two hours and fifty minutes, with a maximum of four hours and a minimum of two hours; in infants from two weeks to four months,

three hours and forty minutes, with a maximum of four hours and thirty-five minutes and a minimum of three hours and twelve minutes (Table 1).

12. The time required for the development of hunger in any one infant is fairly constant over a short period of time provided the amount and kind of food is not changed (Tables 1, 2, 3 and 4).

13. The time required for the development of hunger in infants with chronic nourishment disturbance is shorter than in normal infants (Tables 2, 3 and 4).

14. The time required for the development of hunger is shorter when the infant receives food which is poorly tolerated (Table 4).

15. Hunger contractions occur in these infants long before the stomach has emptied. Consequently their presence is not in itself an indication that the stomach is ready for food.

16. The feeble nursing exhibited by most prematures and by many older infants is not due to derangement of the primitive hunger apparatus. Hunger contractions are present and of normal intensity in such infants.

17. Hunger contractions were present in one infant with congenital myxedema.

18. Hunger contractions were present in a 2-year-old boy with typhoid fever when the rectal temperature ranged between 104.4 F. and 105 F.

19. Confirmation of previous findings of increased hunger contractions in infants with pyloric stenosis.

I wish to express my sincere thanks to Dr. A. J. Carlson of the University of Chicago for suggestions which aided materially in carrying out these studies; to Dr. E. P. Lyon and Dr. A. D. Hirschfelder for the loan of apparatus from the departments of physiology and pharmacology; to Dr. F. H. Scott and Dr. F. B.. Kingsbury for advice and assistance in the construction of apparatus; to Dr. F. W. Schultz for the use of material from the Infant Welfare Clinic; to Dr. N. O. Pearce, teaching fellow in pediatrics, and to head nurses Barber and Wenck, who cheerfully assisted in preparing the little patients for examination.

To my chief, Dr. J. P. Sedgwick, who first suggested this problem, and who allowed the free use of his material in the service at the university hospitals, I wish to express my grateful appreciation for constant stimulating interest and helpful suggestions.

REFERENCES

1. Auerbach, L.: Zur Mechanik des Saugens und der Inspiration. Arch. f. Anat. u. Physiol., 1888, p. 59. Quoted by Uffenheimer: Ergebn. d. inn. Med. u. Kinderh., **1**, 307-309.

2. Barth, H.: Untersuchungen zur Physiologie des Saugens beim normalen und pathologischen Brustkindern. Ztschrc. f. Kinderh., 1914, **10**, 129.

3. Basch, K.: Die Centrale Innervation der Saugbewegungen. Jahrb. f. Kinderh., 1894, **38**, 68.

4. Boldireff, V. N.: Periodic Work of the Digestive Apparatus in an Empty Stomach, Arch. Soc. de biol., 1905, **11**, 1. Quoted by Carlson, Footnote 9.

5. Brunemeier, E. H., and Carlson, A. J.: Contributions to the Physiology of the Stomach; XIX. Reflexes from the Intestinal Mucosa to the Stomach, Am. Jour. Physiol., 1914-1915, **36,** 191.

6. Cannon, W. B.: A Consideration of the Nature of Hunger, Harvey Lecture, Phila., 1911-1912, **7,** 130.

7. Cannon, W. B., and Washburn, A. L.: An Explanation of Hunger, Am. Jour. Physiol., 1911-1912, **29,** 441.

8. Cannon: The Mechanical Factors of Digestion, New York, Longmans, 1916.

9. Carlson, A. J.: Contributions to the Physiology of the Stomach; I. The Character of the Movements of the Empty Stomach in Man, Am. Jour. Physiol., 1912-1913, **31,** 151.

10. Carlson, A. J.: Contributions to the Physiology of the Stomach; II. The Relation Between the Contractions of the Empty Stomach and the Sensation of Hunger, Am. Jour. Physiol., 1912-1913, **31,** 175.

11. Carlson, A. J.: Contributions to the Physiology of the Stomach; III. The Contractions of the Empty Stomach Inhibited Reflexly from the Mouth, Am. Jour. Physiol., 1912-1913, **31,** 212.

12. Carlson, A. J.: Contributions to the Physiology of the Stomach; IV. The Influence of the Contractions of the Empty Stomach in Man on the Vasomotor Center, on the Rate of the Heart Beat, and on the Reflex Excitability of the Spinal Cord, Am. Jour. Physiol., 1912-1913, **31,** 318.

13. Carlson, A. J., Orr, J. S., and McGrath, L. W.: Contributions to the Physiology of the Stomach; IX. The Hunger Contractions of the Stomach Pouch Isolated According to the Method of Pawlow, Am. Jour. Physiol., 1914, **33,** 119.

14. Carlson, A. J., and Ginsburg, H.: Contributions to the Physiology of the Stomach; XXIV. The Tonus and Hunger Contractions of the Stomach of the New-Born, Am. Jour. Physiol., 1915, **38,** 29.

15. Carlson, A. J., and Ginsburg, H.: Contributions to the Physiology of the Stomach; XXX. The Tonus and Contractions of the Empty Stomach of Infants With Congenital Pyloric Stenosis, Pylorospasm and Chronic Vomiting (Merycism), Am. Jour. Physiol., 1915, **39,** 310.

16. Carlson, A. J.: The Control of Hunger in Health and Disease, University of Chicago Press, 1916, p. 228.

17. Carlson, A. J.: The Control of Hunger in Health and Disease. See Footnote 16.

18. Cassel, J.: Zur Kenntnis der Magenverdauung bei Atrophia infantum, Arch. f. Kinderh., 1891, **12,** 175.

19. Comby, J.: Traite des malades de l'enfance, Paris, Masson, 1902, p. 5.

20. Cramer, H.: Ueber die Nährungsaufnahme der Neugeborenen. Deutsch. med. Wchnschr., 1900, **26,** 32.

21. Cramer: Quoted by von Reuss, A.: Die Krankheiten des Neugeborenen, Berlin, 1914, Enzyklop. d. klin. Med., p. 66.

22. Czerny, A.: Die Ernährung des Säuglings auf Grundlage der physiologischen Functionen seines Magens, Prag. med. Wchnschr., 1893, **18,** 495, 510.

23. Czerny, A., and Moser, P.: Klinische Beobachtungen an magendarmkranken Kindern im Säuglingsalter, Jahrb. f. Kinderh., 1894, **38,** 430.

24. Czerny and Keller: Des Kindes Ernährung, 1906, Part 1, p. 582.

25. Epstein, A.: Ueber Magenausspülungen bei Säuglingen, Arch. f. Kinderh., 1883, **4,** 325.

26. Escherich: Ueber die Saugbewegung beim Neugeborenen, Sitzungsb. d. Gesellsch. f. Morphol. u. Physiol. in München, 1888, **4,** 72.

27. Finklestein, H.: Lehrbuch der Säuglingskrankheiten, Berlin, Kornfeld, 1905.

28. Ginsburg, H., Tumpowsky, I., and Carlson, A. J.: The Onset of Hunger in Infants After Feeding; A Contribution to the Physiology of the Stomach, Jour. Am. Med. Assn., 1915, **64,** 1822.

29. Haudek, M., and Stigler, R.: Radiologische Untersuchungen über den Zusammenhang zwischen Austreibungzeit des normalen Magens und Hunger gefühl, Arch. f. d. ges. Physiol., 1910, **133,** 145.

30. Kasahara, M.: The Curved Lines of Suction, Am. Jour. Dis. Child., 1916, **12,** 73.

31. Keller, A.: Ueber Nährungspausen bei der Säuglingsernährung, Centralbl. f. Inn. Med., 1900, **21,** 393.

32. Kussmaul: Untersuchungen über die Seeleben des Neugeborenen, Quoted by von Reuss, 1859, p. 65. Die Krankheiten des Neugeborenen, Berlin, 1914.

33. Ladd, M.: Gastric Motility in Infants as Shown by the Roentgen Ray, Am. Jour. Child. Dis., 1913, **5,** 345. Ibid., The Influence of Variations of Diet on Gastric Motility in Infants, Arch. Pediat., 1913, **30,** 740.

34. Leo, H.: Ueber die Function des normalen und kranken Magens und die therapeutischen Erfolge der Magenausapülung im Säuglingsalter, Berlin. klin. Wchnschr., 1888, **25,** 981.

35. Luckhardt, A. B., and Carlson, A. J.: Contributions to the Physiology of the Stomach; XVII. On the Chemical Control of the Gastric Hunger Mechanism, Am. Jour. Physiol., 1914-1915, **36,** 37.

36. Major, R.: Roentgenologische Beobachtungen am Säuglingsmagen, Ztschr. f. Kinderh., 1913, **8,** 340.

37. Meyer, L. F., and Rosenstern, J.: Die Wirkung des Hungers im den verschiedenen Stadien der Ernährungsstörung, Jahr. f. Kinderh., 1909, **69,** 167.

38. Neisser, E., and Bräuning, H.: Ueber normale und über verzeitige Sättigung, München. med. Wchnschr., 1911, **58,** 1955.

39. Neumann, H.: Ueber erschwerte Nährungsaufnahme bei kleinen Kindern, Therap. Monatsh., 1893, **7,** 220. Abstr. in Arch. f. Kinderh., 1897, **22,** 152.

40. Patterson, T. L.: Contributions to the Physiology of the Stomach; XIII. The Variations in the Hunger Contractions of the Empty Stomach With Age, Am. Jour. Physiol., **33,** 423.

41. Patterson, T. L.: Contributions to the Physiology of the Stomach; XXXVI. The Physiology of the Gastric Hunger Contractions in the Amphibia and the Reptilia, Am. Jour. Physiol., 1917, **42,** 56.

42. Pfaundler: Ueber Saugen und Verdauen, Wien. klin. Wchnschr., 1899, **12,** 1012.

43. Pies: Zur Physiologie des Neugeborenen; Ueber die Dauer, die Grösse und den Verlauf der physiologischen Abnahme, Monatschr. f. Kinderh., 1910, **9,** 514.

44. Pisek, G. R., and Le Wald, L. T.: The Further Study of the Anatomy and Physiology of the Infant Stomach Based on Serial Roentgenograms, Am. Jour. Dis. Child., 1913, **6,** 232.

45. Preyer: Die Seele des Kindes. Quoted by Baach, K.: Jahrb. f. Kinderh., 1894, **38,** 68.

46. Quest, R.: Ueber den Einfluss der Ernährung auf die Erregbarkeit des Nervensystems im Säuglingsalter, Wien. klin. Wchnschr., 1906, **19,** 830. Quotes: Finklestein: Fortschr. d. med., 1902, **20**; Thiemich: Revue d' hyg. et de méd. d. inf., 1903, **2**; Japha, A.: Ueber den Stimmritzankrampf der Kinder. Berl. klin. Wchnschr., 1903, **40,** 1126.

47. Rehfuss, M. E.: A New Method of Gastric Testing, With a Description of a Method for the Fractional Testing of the Gastric Juice, Am. Jour. Med. Sc., 1914, **147,** 848.

48. Rehfuss, M. E., Bergheim, O., and Hawk, P. B.: Gastro-Intestinal Studies; The Question of the Residuum Found in the Empty Stomach, Jour. Am. Med. Assn., 1914, **63,** 11.

49. Rogers, F. T., and Hardt, L. L. J.: The Relation Between the Digestion Contractions of the Filled, and the Hunger Contractions of the "Empty" Stomach, Am. Jour. Physiol., 1915, **38,** 274.

50. Rogers: The Hunger Mechanism in Birds (Preliminary Report), Proc. Soc. Exper. Biol. and Med., 1916, **13,** 119.

51. Rosenstern, I.: Ueber Inanition im Säuglingsalter, Ergebn. d. inn. Med. u. Kinderh., 1911, **7,** 332.

52. Rosenstern, I.: Hunger im Säuglingsalter und Ernährungstechnik, Deutsch. med. Wchnschr., 1912, **38,** 1834.

53. Rott: Zur Ernährungstechnik frügeborener Säuglings, Ztschr. f. Kinderh., 1912, **5,** 134.

54. Schlossmann: Ueber das Verhalten des Säuglings im Hunger. Verhandl. d. Versamml. d. Gesellsch. f. Kinderh. . . . deutsch. Naturf. u. Aerzte, 1913, Wiesb., 1914, **30,** 143.

55. Schmidt, A.: Brustsaugen und Flaschen saugen. München. med. Wchnschr., 1904, **51,** 2141.

56. Soltmann: Experimentelle Studien über die Funktionen des Grosshirns der Neugeborenen. Jahrb. f. Kinderh., 1876, **9,** 106.

57. Soltmann: Uber das Hemmungsnervensystem des Neugeborenen. Jahrb. f. Kinderh., 1877, **11,** 101.

58. Süsswein, J.: Zur Physiologie des Trinkens beim Säugling. Arch. f. Kinderh., 1904, **40,** 68.

59. Thiemich, M.: Ueber die Diagnose der Imbecillität im frühen Kindesalter. Deutsch. med. Wchnschr., 1900, **26,** 34.

60. Tobler: Ueber die Verdauung der Milch im Magen. Ergebn. d. inn. Med. u. Kinderh., 1908, **1,** 495.

61. Tobler and Bogen, H.: Ueber die Dauer der Magenwerdauung der Milch und ihre Beeinflussung durch verschiedene Faktoren. Monatschr. f. Kinderh., 1908-1909, **7,** 12.

62. Zybell: Beiträge zur Behandlung der Spasmophilie. München. med. Wchnschr., 1911, **58,** 2357.

34

Reprinted from *JAMA*, **89**(12), 928–931 (1927)

PREVENTION OF ANOREXIA
IN CHILDREN*

C. A. Aldrich, M.D.
Winnetka, Illinois

Before outlining the method of preventing poor appetites, to be presented here, I should like to mention the thoughts that suggested its use. In the first place, lack of appetite was so common a condition and its results so disastrous to the physical and mental welfare of many children that I became interested in its treatment and prevention. In treating other abnormalities, it has been customary to begin with a study of normal function, but in the matter of hunger and appetite our textbooks, until recently, have afforded little information. One gathers from this lack of attention to the subject that eating has been assumed to be instinctive. Perhaps some of our difficulties in the management of anorexia have been due to this vague conception of the eating mechanism.

Since hunger and appetite are the main stimuli to eating, it is worth while to investigate their nature. According to Webster's dictionary, hunger is a painful sensation due to lack of food, while appetite is a desire for gratification. Carlson[1] widens our knowledge as to their nature. Hunger, a purely physiologic function, is due to vigorous contractions of the empty stomach. Appetite, however, is a much more complex mental

* Read before the Section on Diseases of Children at the Seventy-Eighth Annual Session of the American Medical Association, Washington, D. C., May 20, 1927.

1. Carlson, A. J.: The Control of Hunger in Health and Disease, Chicago, University of Chicago Press, 1916.

387

process, dependent on pleasant memories of feelings, tastes, odors and sights. Hunger merely brings into consciousness the fact that we need food, whereas appetite transforms this sensation into a desire to eat. Hunger is appeased by the first few mouthfuls ingested, but appetite continues to urge us to eat throughout many courses. Not only does appetite control the amount of food eaten, but also it aids in digestion through its stimulation of salivary and gastric secretions.

This cursory consideration of the attributes of hunger and appetite led me to think that we eat because of the following hypothetic reflex or mechanism: When the stomach is empty, contractions occurring in its wall give rise to uncomfortable sensations interpreted as hunger. Since food has previously afforded relief from this sensation, consciousness of its need is thereby aroused. Then we begin to think of different kinds of food; of where, when and how we are to get our next meal. This is appetite, under the stimulus of which salivary and digestive juices begin to flow. When we sit down to eat, appetite urges us on to take our fill, long after the pangs of hunger have ceased, until satiety, by some unknown mechanism, stops our desire for food. Completed digestion and emptying of the stomach stimulates hunger waves and the process is repeated.

Such a conception of the mechanism of eating brings into relief many important points which are useful in any consideration of anorexia. Space does not permit me to do more than mention these questions.[2] Hunger and appetite are different, and may be treated separately by different methods. Physiologic stimuli will, in all probability, most affect hunger. Psychologic influences will probably be more important in developing good appetite, which insures adequate intake of food. Good appetite is, therefore, an important end in itself. What are the physiologic and psychologic factors most important in maintaining these two stimuli normally active? Obviously, to prevent anorexia, one must do the things which aid in maintaining their activity and avoid those which inhibit them.

The prophylactic technic here described is an attempt to fulfil these requirements. It does not contain any new elements. Many of these methods have been frequently mentioned by various writers. Brennemann[3] recently emphasized many of the points. Only in the chronological arrangement and in the report of results is this paper original. Six years ago I began to apply the embryo of this plan to all the infants with whom I came in contact. It has been gradually expanded into the technic here described. It will be noted that most of the methods were important from the psychic standpoint.

TECHNIC

1. *Propaganda.*—Mothers and nurses were instructed as to the nature of anorexia while their babies were young, at 2 or 3 months of age. They were emphatically told never to urge their children to eat except under express orders, and were asked to report refusal just as they would report vomiting or loose stools. This resulted in my being able to combat anorexia before it had become chronic. Prophylaxis thus had a chance.

2. *Treatment of the First Attack.*—This always consisted in a reduction of food. It should be taught that anorexia is usually the first symptom of infection and that it precedes all other signs of the common cold. Therefore, when a baby first refused its bottle the

2. Aldrich, C. A.: Cultivating the Child's Appetite, New York, Macmillan Company, 1927.
3. Brennemann, Joseph: Some Neglected Practical Points in the Technic of Infant Feeding, Arch. Pediat. 40: 359 (June 19) 1923.

mother was told to reduce the feedings and to look out for an illness. I now consider this the most important part of prophylaxis. Many instances occur in which chronic anorexia dates from the onset of an ordinary cold. Instead of reducing the diet, mothers frequently become determined in their efforts to force feedings, and from this unpleasant struggle over the bottle at a time when the child is physically not fit to eat, aversion for food on a psychologic basis develops. He first associates unpleasantness with food. Appetite is menaced. If left alone with the appetite as a guide, the baby in a few days would become hungry and make up for lost time; but, forced to eat, psychologic aversion dulls the returning appetite and the basis for a prolonged illness is established.

3. *Prevention of Weaning Difficulties.*—Since it was soon found that many cases had their beginning at this period, prevention of weaning difficulties became important. To this end, all babies were given an occasional bottle from birth, often enough so that they remembered the bottle as a friend. This practically eliminated difficulty in getting babies to take bottle food.

4. *Prevention of Trouble Due to Changes in the Character of Food.*—Since it was often difficult to get babies to make such marked changes as from cereal to vegetable, these variations were made gradually and mothers were instructed not to force new food on them. Cod liver oil and orange juice were given from the first few weeks of life to avoid later struggles.

5. *The Avoidance of Overfeeding.*—All babies were put on the minimal diet which would cause a satisfactory gain in weight. If such a gain was being made, no increase in formula was allowed simply because the baby seemed hungry. This part of the routine involved considerable education of parents, because what seemed satisfactory to me did not always appear so to them. The neighborhood baby race is a great obstacle to conservative pediatrics.

6. *Not Prescribing Definite Amounts of Food after One Year.*—After the first year, diet lists were given but parents were told to allow the child's appetite to be the sole judge as to the amount of food to be taken. No caloric diets were prescribed. By this method it was hoped to prevent psychologic aversion due to forced feeding in older children.

7. *Management of the Meal.*—Mothers were told to leave their children alone at mealtime as much as possible and not to talk about eating. They were told to try to develop a detached attitude toward the child at mealtime and never to force food.

8. *Allowing the Child's Appetite Play in Choice of Food.*—In the main the child was humored in this regard. This is not to be interpreted that he ate anything he pleased, but that when there was a choice between two equivalent foods, the one he liked best was most often given. It was not considered advisable to "make the child eat everything so that later on he would like everything." In my experience this is more likely to mean that the child will not enjoy eating anything because the repetition of struggles that result from insisting on especially disliked food tends to produce psychologic distaste for all food.

9. *Avoidance of Emotional Stress at Meals.*—Parents were instructed that nothing could be worse for appetites than pitched battles over meals. Unpleasant subjects were not to be brought up at such times.

10. *Reading of Psychologic Works.*—When the child was about 1 year of age, all parents were asked to begin

reading books on child psychology, and a list of some of these was recommended. In this way I hoped to be able to educate parents to see troubles early when prevention could be used.

11. *Nourishment Between Meals.*—This was not advised for any child.

QUESTIONNAIRE

The report of the results of this technic is based on the statistics gleaned from a questionnaire sent to the mothers of 215 consecutive children over 18 months of age. In selecting these cases I simply went through the files and took the first 215 histories of children whom I had seen from birth until the present time. No exceptions were made on account of chronic or acute disease of any sort. It was hoped that this might show whether or not it paid in appetites to take the trouble to go through the previously outlined routine. The following questions were asked:

1. Does your child usually eat:
   - (a) Hungrily?
   - (b) Willingly?
   - (c) Reluctantly?
   - (d) With aversion for food?
2. What is the approximate weight with clothes on?
3. What is the age in years and months?

RESULTS

Of the 215 letters sent out, 199 were returned. In assembling the results it has seemed best to present them in the form of three tables, one a summary of the entire group, one a detail of those who are underweight, and another a detail of those who ate reluctantly. In the subsequent discussion it will be taken for granted that the children who ate hungrily or willingly do not present an appetite problem. It was gratifying that none were said to have aversion for food and that none habitually vomited meals.

Statistics as to the prevalence of anorexia are few in spite of its widespread occurrence. Studies made by Maclay[4] and Mosely[5] in the Department of Home Economics of the University of Chicago, however, offer some basis for comparison. The children examined in these researches were of preschool age and were from approximately the same type of homes as are those reported here. Among 100 children, Miss Mosely found only nineteen who were good eaters.

TABLE 1.—*Results in the Entire Group*

Age Period	Number of Cases	Hungrily	Willingly	Reluctantly	Aversion	Number Underweight	Average Pounds Overweight
18 mo.-2 yrs..	43	19	21	3	0	1	3.8
2-3 years....	56	18	29	9	0	2	3.8
3-4 years....	43	16	22	5	0	3	3.7
4-5 years....	33	6	18	9	0	8	3.0
5-6 years....	24	12	8	4	0	7	3.7
Totals....	199	71	98	30	0	21	
Per cent (approx.)		35.5	49	15	0	10	3.61 lbs.

Consideration of these statistics must take into account the possibility that some parents, discouraged by failure, may have sought other advice, in which event this report would comprise most of the successes and leave out some of the failures. Furthermore, there is no way of telling how these children were actually treated. Judgment of results must be based on a consideration of what was told the parents, rather than on what may be assumed

4. Maclay, Eleanor: A Study of the Prevalence of Lack of Appetite in One Hundred Preschool Children, Chicago, August, 1924.
5. Mosely, Marion R.: Reaction to Food of Children of Preschool Age, Chicago, June, 1925.

to have been done for the child. If it can be shown that children whose parents are not so instructed have poorer appetites than those reported here, then some prophylactic merit may be claimed in the technic.

Table 1 summarizes all the replies according to the different age periods. There were more reluctant eaters above 2 years of age. The entire group averaged 3.6 pounds (1.7 Kg.) overweight for age. It would have

TABLE 2.—*Underweight Children*

Case Number	Pounds Underweight	Appetite*	Comment
19	1	R	Congenital heart disease
51	1	H	Premature baby
63	3	R	
129	3	R	Recurrent vomiting
125	2	W	
130	3	H	Premature baby
146	2	W	
148	2	H	
152	3	R	Celiac disease
158	3	W	
163	2	W	Chronic pyelitis
167	5	R	Chronic pyelitis
168	2	W	Chronic pyelitis
173	1	W	
180	6	W	Chronic tonsillitis with hypertrophy
187	3	R	Chronic tonsillitis with hypertrophy
191	1	R	
192	1	R	
195	6	R	Chronic tonsillitis with hypertrophy
197	4	H	
198	4	W	

* In this column, H, R and W signify that the respective child ate hungrily, reluctantly or willingly.

been more satisfactory to include in the questionnaire a query as to the height, but I felt that with so large a number the height would probably be about average. If I had anticipated that these children would average so much overweight, the height question would certainly have been added. This table demonstrates that it is safe for the pediatrician to advise strongly against forced feeding, provided he applies such measures as have been outlined.

Table 2 summarizes the statistics obtained for the underweight children. Of these twenty-one children, thirteen were less than 10 per cent underweight, and in eleven of them there was an adequate physical cause for the nutritional condition. Closer study showed that of the children free from physical disease, only three were more than 1 pound (0.5 Kg.) underweight for their height (cases 125, 146, 158), and that these children all ate willingly. The table indicates that in the entire group of 199 children there were none seriously underweight because of poor appetite alone.

In table 3 are summarized the data recorded for the reluctant eaters, the failures in this attempt to produce good appetites. Of the thirty children, nine had physical causes which may reasonably explain the anorexia. Of the remaining twenty-one, only three were underweight for age (cases 63, 191, 192). Two of these were only a pound underweight, and the other was overweight for height and quite plump. It is evident that among these poor eaters the difficulty has not reached proportions severe enough to produce malnutrition in any case.

Investigation as to the cause of failures was illuminating. In the first place I found to my surprise that several mothers had never heard of the problem and had gone on forcing down food because they thought "of course it was the proper thing to do." In spite of good intentions, my work was imperfectly done. On the other hand, there were parents who did not follow instructions. Some undoubtedly tried to leave their children alone at meals but just couldn't do it. Many parents are so constituted that they have to see to it that what their children do is done because they sugge-

vise it. They need a lot of education. In many instances I did not "sell" my ideas strongly enough. Popularization of the subject would have helped in these instances. The bogey of malnutrition has been so strongly upheld and the advantages of proper feeding so admirably demonstrated that many parents lack perspective and reason when it comes to a consideration of *how* their children eat. In this community, as in many others, the enlightened were dominated by the idea that children

TABLE 3.—*The Reluctant Eaters*

Case Number	Age	Pounds Underweight	Pounds Overweight	Comment
19	1	1	.	Congenital heart disease
24	1	.	1	
42	1	.	1	
49	2	.	6	
52	2	.	3	
56	2	.	2	
57	2	.	2	
63	2	3	.	
70	2	.	3	
86	2	.	2	
90	2	.	5	
91	2	.	5	
106	3	.	4	
115	3	0	0	
120	3	3	.	Recurrent vomiting
138	3	0	0	
139	3	0	0	Chronic pyelitis
142	4	.	9	
144	4	.	2	
151	4	.	2	
152	4	3	.	Celiac disease
154	4	0	0	
156	4	.	5	
164	4	0	0	Congenital spastic paralysis
167	4	5	.	Pyelitis
170	4	.	3	Chronic tonsillitis with hypertrophy
187	5	.	3	Chronic tonsillitis with hypertrophy
191	5	1	.	
192	6	1	.	
195	6	6	.	Chronic tonsillitis with hypertrophy

must eat definite, set formulas prescribed by the physician, nurse, government health bulletin or what not.

Therefore, instilling the ideas here presented was particularly difficult. It was hard to make parents understand that my advice was prompted by a desire that proper food should be eaten, and was not given because I did not care what they ate. The aid of propaganda is evidently necessary for complete success.

In meeting the widespread anorexia revolt now being staged by children, we must squarely face this issue: Are we to insist that children eat certain prescribed amounts of food in an effort to make them all attain prescribed statural goals, or are we to make an intelligent effort to develop appetites so that each child will voluntarily eat sufficient food to insure his own best development?

SUMMARY

1. Good appetite is an important end in itself for which to strive.

2. A hypothetic natural hunger-appetite mechanism or reflex controlling eating is outlined.

3. It is possible, by following a prophylactic technic, to prevent interference with this normal reflex.

4. The results of such prophylactic treatment, as shown by statistics obtained in 199 consecutive cases, demonstrate that (*a*) in this series it was not harmful to the nutrition of the children to advise strongly against forced feeding, as the group averaged 3.6 pounds above weight for age, and (*b*) there were no children in this group who were malnourished except those suffering from physical disease.

5. It is necessary in order to combat successfully the condition of chronic anorexia that propaganda as to the proper technic of presenting food be broadcast.

545 Lincoln Avenue.

35

Reprinted from *Am. J. Dis. Child.*, **50**, 385–394 (1935)

CHOICE OF FORMULAS MADE BY THREE INFANTS THROUGHOUT THE NURSING PERIOD

CLARA M. DAVIS, M.D.

WINNETKA, ILL.

During the course of an experimental study of self-selection of diet by newly weaned infants [1] carried on for several years in a nursery organized for this purpose the question of whether a new-born child could successfully exercise a choice of formula and regulate the quantities taken at feedings naturally suggested itself. This report outlines the experiment (also carried on in this nursery) designed to investigate that question and presents the results obtained during 1930 and 1931 with three breast-fed infants taken from lying-in hospitals at the ages of 10, 8 and 7 days, respectively, and subjected continuously to the experiment for periods of from seven and one-half to eight months.

Since there were obvious difficulties involved in presenting to such young infants a large number of formulas for choice at each feeding, it was decided to use for the experiment only four formulas which would be more or less representative of the types of feeding commonly in use and to offer all four at each feeding throughout the nursing period. The four formulas were as follows:

1. A proprietary "reconstructed" milk (Similac) in which for cow's milk fat there has been substituted a mixture of homogenized fats the physiochemical properties of which more nearly approach those of the fat of woman's milk and in which some readjustment of the salts in the direction of the salt content of woman's milk has been made and sufficient lactose added to make the total approximately that of woman's milk. Reliquefied according to the manufacturer's direction, its percentage composition and caloric value are stated to be: fat, 3.4 per cent; carbohydrate, 6.8 per cent; protein, 1.5 per cent; salts, 0.4 per cent, and calories per ounce, 19.

2. Fermented lactic acid milk, made daily from whole pasteurized milk to which 5 per cent of Blue Label Karo corn syrup was added. Its percentage composition and caloric value are approximately: fat, 3.5

---

1. Davis, C. M.: Self Selection of Diet by Newly Weaned Infants, Am. J. Dis. Child. **36**:651 (Oct.) 1928.

per cent; carbohydrates, 8 per cent; protein, 3.5 per cent; salts, 0.75 per cent, and calories per ounce, 23.

3. A simple milk dilution formula made as follows:

Whole milk, boiled ten minutes	20.0 ounces
Water	10.0 ounces
Lactose	1.5 ounces

The percentage composition and caloric value are: fat, 2.33 per cent; carbohydrate, 8 per cent; protein, 2.33 per cent; salts, 0.5 per cent, and calories per ounce, 19.1.

4. An orange juice, egg yolk, sugar, milk and water formula (J. Hess) made as follows:

Whole milk, boiled ten minutes	20 ounces
Egg yolks	1
Orange juice	2 ounces
Water	8 ounces
Cane sugar	1⅓ ounces

The approximate percentage composition and caloric value are: fat, 3 per cent; carbohydrate, 8 per cent; protein, 2.45 per cent; salts, 1.785 per cent, and calories per ounce, 21.4.

No change in the "strength" of any formula was made at any time regardless of the age of the infants.

Four bottles of the same make and size, marked, 1, 2, 3 and 4 to indicate the formulas, were offered at each feeding according to a schedule so arranged that a formula offered first at one feeding would have second, third and fourth place at successive feedings, and so on, thus equalizing the influence of greater hunger at the beginning of feedings. The nipples were of the same brand, size and shape throughout the experiment, and each was tested before feeding to see that it delivered well. During a period of eighteen days midway in the experimental period of the first infant the nipples were numbered, 1, 2, 3 and 4 and alternated on the bottles according to a fixed schedule in order to make sure that a favorite nipple was not a factor in choice. No evidence was found that one nipple was preferred above others.

During feedings the bottles were kept warm by a small water bath, and the infant was held on the nurse's lap and allowed to nurse as long as he wished from the first bottle. When he stopped sucking or if he did not suck, the second bottle was offered, and so on, all four bottles being offered at each feeding. A bottle emptied during the feeding was promptly refilled to insure that the infant had all that he wished of that formula, but no effort was made to get the infant to take more than he wished, the quantities of the feedings being left wholly to him. Intervals of feeding were at first every three hours during the day and whenever the infant waked at night. These intervals were lengthened from time to time as the infant showed a tendency to sleep over the feeding time or for several days in succession showed little interest in one feeding during the day, the desire being to conform the schedule as closely as possible to the satisfaction and comfort of the infant. Thus the number of feedings in twenty-four hours declined

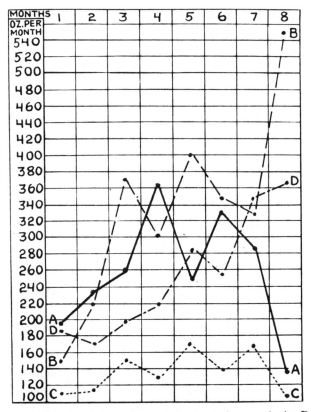

Fig. 1.—Quantities of each formula taken in successive months by Rosemary L. In this and the following charts *A* indicates Similac; *B*, lactic milk and Karo corn syrup; *C*, milk dilution; *D*, egg yolk, orange juice and milk (Hess).

from a maximum of nine (with one infant for one day only) in the first week to four and occasionally three in the last (eighth) month.

To make available ample quantities of antiscorbutic vitamin without compelling the infant to take the orange juice, egg yolk and milk formula (number 4), undiluted orange juice was offered twice daily between feedings to be taken in any amount wished. The reliquefied proprietary milk (number 1), according to the manufacturers' statement, contains 7 drops (0.4 cc.) of cod liver oil per liter. In addition to this,

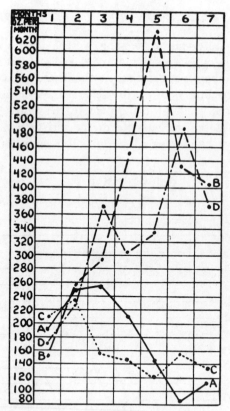

Fig. 2.—Quantities of each formula taken in successive months by Shirley S.

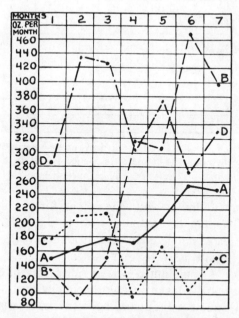

Fig. 3.—Quantities of each formula taken in successive months by Robert H.

cod liver oil was given to the first infant for two periods of twenty-one and sixteen days, respectively, during the first three months, being discontinued at the end of each of the periods because of her evident dislike of it. Cod liver oil was not administered to the other two infants, nor did any of the three receive viosterol, ultraviolet irradiation or sun-baths. Dietary supplements, such as the cereals and vegetables commonly added to the diet at 5 or 6 months of age, were omitted.

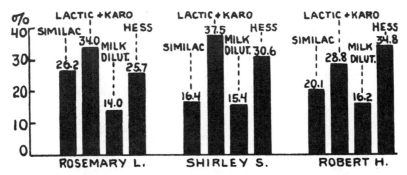

Fig. 4.—Percentage of each formula in the total quantity taken by each infant during the entire nursing period.

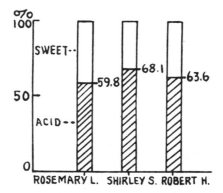

Fig. 5.—Percentages of acid and sweet milks in the total amount taken by each infant during the entire nursing period.

The respective quantities of the four formulas taken by the infants, the range in size and frequency of feedings, the calories consumed per month and the monthly weights of the infants are shown in the accompanying figures and tables, which are self-explanatory.

That differences in taste were appreciated early in the first week was unmistakably evidenced by the behavior of the infants. Lactic acid milk often caused unhappy grimaces and sometimes a distinct shudder on its first entrance into the mouth. Often after a few eager sucks from the first bottle the nipple would be pushed out by the tongue and what

TABLE 1.—*Number of Daily Feedings Taken by Rosemary L. in Successive Months and Their Minimum, Maximum and Average Size.*

Month	Number of Days	Number of Feedings per Day	Minimum Ounces at Any Feeding	Maximum Ounces at Any Feeding	Average Quantity per Feeding, Ounces	Total Number of Feedings in Month
1 (Jan.)	31	9 to 7	0.50	5.75	2.76	232
2	28	8 to 6	0.50	8.75	3.83	197
3	31	6 to 5	1.00	11.50	6.14	160
4	30	6 to 4	2.50	10.50	6.70	150
5	31	5 to 4	1.00	15.00	8.06	136
6	30	4	3.50	14.50	8.99	120
7	31	4	1.75	15.50	9.09	120
8	31	4	2.25	18.50	9.50	120

TABLE 2.—*Number of Daily Feedings Taken by Shirley S. in Successive Months and Their Minimum, Maximum and Average Size*

Month	Number of Days	Number of Feedings per Day	Minimum Ounces at Any Feeding	Maximum Ounces at Any Feeding	Average Quantity per Feeding, Ounces	Total Number of Feedings in Month
1 (Aug.)	31	8 to 6	0.75	6.75	3.20	226
2	30	8 to 5	0.75	9.00	4.83	201
3	31	7 to 5	1.00	11.00	6.16	174
4	30	6 to 5	1.50	11.00	7.31	151
5	31	5	1.50	15.00	7.94	155
6	31	5 to 4	3.00	15.00	8.72	133
7	28	4 to 3	2.50	15.75	10.52	98
8	17	3	6.00	18.00	12.55	51

TABLE 3.—*Number of Daily Feedings Taken by Robert H. in Successive Months and Their Minimum, Maximum and Average Size*

Month	Number of Days	Number of Feedings per Day	Minimum Ounces at Any Feeding	Maximum Ounces at Any Feeding	Average Quantity per Feeding, Ounces	Total Number of Feedings in Month
1 (April)	31	8 to 5	1.00	6.00	3.19	233
2	30	7 to 6	2.75	8.50	4.81	187
3	31	6 to 5	0.00	9.50	5.51	174
4	30	5 to 4	1.00	10.00	5.95	149
5	31	5	0.00	13.50	6.75	155
6	31	5	2.50	12.00	7.12	155
7	30	5 to 4	4.50	12.50	8.33	136
8	13	4	6.00	13.00	9.41	52

TABLE 4.—*Average Size of Feedings (in Ounces) Taken in Successive Months by the Three Infants*

Month	Rosemary L.	Shirley S.	Robert H.	Average
1	2.76	3.20	3.19	3.05
2	3.83	4.83	4.81	4.46
3	6.14	6.16	5.51	5.94
4	6.70	7.31	5.95	6.59
5	8.06	7.94	6.75	7.65
6	8.99	8.72	7.12	8.24
7	9.09	10.52	8.33	9.31
8	9.50	12.55	9.41	10.15

TABLE 5.—*Minimum, Maximum and Average Daily Quantity (in Ounces) Taken by Rosemary L. in Successive Months*

Month	Number of Days	Minimum Daily Quantity	Maximum Daily Quantity	Average Daily Quantity
1	31	12.50	27.75	20.600
2	28	18.00	39.75	26.800
3	31	25.75	39.00	31.485
4	30	28.50	44.25	33.525
5	31	23.50	41.75	35.600
6	30	25.75	43.75	35.940
7	31	15.50	44.75	36.380
8	31	23.25	50.50	37.700

TABLE 6.—*Minimum, Maximum and Daily Quantity (in Ounces) Taken by Shirley S. in Successive Months*

Month	Number of Days	Minimum Daily Quantity	Maximum Daily Quantity	Average Daily Quantity
1	31	14.25	30.50	23.30
2	30	26.00	39.75	32.39
3	31	27.25	41.25	34.57
4	30	30.00	40.75	36.80
5	31	33.00	46.75	39.69
6	31	29.25	46.75	37.45
7	28	31.75	43.25	36.83
8	17	31.25	45.25	37.65

TABLE 7.—*Minimum, Maximum and Average Daily Quantity (in Ounces) Taken by Robert H. in Successive Months*

Month	Number of Days	Minimum Daily Quantity	Maximum Daily Quantity	Average Daily Quantity
1	31	16.75	32.75	22.96
2	30	25.75	34.00	29.97
3	31	24.25	34.50	30.90
4	30	24.50	37.50	29.60
5	31	27.00	40.50	33.80
6	31	29.00	42.75	35.62
7	30	29.75	44.00	37.77
8	13	33.50	39.75	37.65

TABLE 8.—*Average Daily Quantities (in Ounces) Taken in Successive Months by the Three Infants*

Month	Rosemary L.	Shirley S.	Robert H.	Average
1	20.60	23.30	23.00	22.30
2	26.80	32.40	30.00	29.70
3	31.50	34.60	30.90	32.30
4	33.50	36.80	29.60	33.30
5	35.60	39.70	33.80	36.40
6	35.90	37.45	35.60	36.30
7	36.40	36.80	37.80	36.90
8	37.70	37.65	37.65	37.66

was in the mouth allowed to run out, after which the infant took the next bottle eagerly. As the infants grew older a bottle might be refused without tasting, probably from a perception of the distinctive and familiar odor of its contents. But in general the keener hunger at the beginning of a feeding resulted in the taking of at least a small amount of the first formula offered.

TABLE 9.—*Average Calories per Kilogram of Weight per Day*

Month	Rosemary L. January	Shirley S. August	Robert H. March
1	114.20	151.21	153.20
2	122.30	151.76	145.90
3	118.00	133.20	127.50
4	115.65	122.00	108.30
5	105.90	113.90	113.70
6	96.50	97.70	108.60
7	93.70	90.00	109.20
8	93.00	87.50	104.60

TABLE 10.—*Amount of Orange Juice (in Ounces) Taken by Each Infant During the Entire Period*

Name	Amount Taken as Such	Amount in Hess Formula	Total Ounces	Average Ounces per Day
Rosemary L.	283.75	134.78	468.53	1.70
Shirley S.	428.00	162.10	590.10	2.58
Robert H.	104.50	168.50	273.00	1.25

TABLE 11.—*Number of Egg Yolks (in Hess Formula) Taken by Each Infant*

Name	Number of Yolks
Rosemary L.	67.60
Shirley S.	81.66
Robert H.	84.26

TABLE 12.—*Cod Liver Oil (in Drachms) Taken by Each Infant During Entire Period*

Name	Administered as Such	Amount Incorporated in Similac	Total Drachms
Rosemary L.	69	7.20	76.20
Shirley S.	0	4.51	4.51
Robert H.	0	4.25	4.25

The infants were wholly free from digestive troubles, such as diarrhea, vomiting, constipation and colic, and they slept soundly, seldom cried and exhibited the vigorous yet serene and contented behavior that is characteristic of the adequately fed and well cared for breast-fed infant. R. L., at the age of 6 weeks, contracted from her night attendant a streptococcic infection (of the upper respiratory tract) which resulted in bilateral suppurative otitis media, with drainage for four weeks. This was not accompanied by any digestive disturbance or interruption of steady gain in weight. S. S. had one mild cold and R. H. no illness of any kind.

Their nutritional condition appeared to be excellent in every way. Their turgor, muscular development and tone were all that could be desired; their hair was abundant, soft, glossy and fine and grew rapidly. Monthly roentgenograms of their bones for evidence of rickets gave negative results with one exception: The report on S. S. at the age of 5 months was "possibly early slight rickets." The next month, however, the report was "normal; no evidence of rickets," as were subsequent reports.

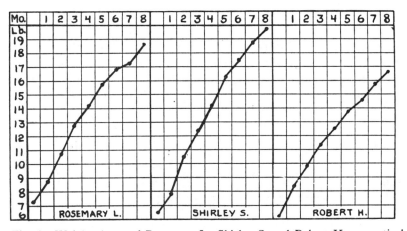

Fig. 6.—Weight charts of Rosemary L., Shirley S. and Robert H., respectively.

COMMENT AND CONCLUSIONS

In view of the fact that healthy vigorous infants have been reared on each of the four formulas and that all are in general well liked by infants, it is not surprising that the preferences shown were moderate in degree, a result to which the necessity of offering bottles successively instead of simultaneously also doubtless contributed.

That all three infants took relatively much less lactic acid milk during the first two months of life than later corroborates the findings of those pediatricians who have reported that this milk is not as readily taken by new-born infants as by older infants. It would be interesting to know why less was taken of the milk dilution formula than of any other. An outstanding difference in its composition from that of all the others is that its fat content is the only one which falls below the 3 per cent that seems to be the base line for this element in the milk of all species.

The most striking feature of their performance, however, is the wide variation in the quantities taken at a feeding. The maximum quantity taken at single feedings in every month seems large, especially in the first three months, for which the figures are: first month, from 5.75 to 6.75 ounces; second month, from 8.5 to 9 ounces; third month, from 9.5 to 11.5 ounces. But with the minimum feedings relatively small—on some occasions little more than a taste—the averages are not out of line with current practice. This pattern of eating behavior, i. e., occasional "stuffing" and meals of widely varying quantities is, of course, the natural one not only of mammalian young in general but also of the breast-fed baby. Furthermore, it is not merely an infantile pattern but one that continues to a greater or less degree throughout life. Artificially fed infants appear to be the only large group on whom identical quantities for successive meals are meticulously imposed, and one cannot but wonder whether the comfort of these infants who exercised choice not only of formulas but of quantities and their complete freedom from digestive discomforts and symptoms of any sort were not due rather. to the following of this natural eating pattern than to the combinations made by their choices of formulas.

SUMMARY

An experiment in which three infants were allowed their choice of four formulas from the first week throughout the nursing period is reported, with figures and tables showing the performance of each infant and comments on the results.

695 Prospect Avenue.

36

RESULTS OF THREE YEARS EXPERIENCE WITH A NEW CONCEPT OF BABY FEEDING*

Walter W. Sackett, Jr., M.D.
Miami, Florida

During the past three years I have been employing in my practice a baby feeding schedule which revolves about a 6-hour feeding interval from birth with the introduction

*Read in Section on General Practice, Southern Medical Association, Forty-Sixth Annual Meeting, Miami, Florida, November 10-13, 1952.

*From the Medical Research Department of the University of Miami, Miami, Florida.

of solid foods as early as the second day of life. The story of the origin of such a revolutionary schedule along with the *raison d'etre,* its details, advantages and results will be the subject of my paper today.

The reading in one of the medical journals in 1942 a paper which emanated from New Orleans, so exaggerated my dissatisfaction with the manner in which I had been taught to feed babies that I shortly began to deviate from the milk-for-five-months diet to one marked by the early introduction of solid foods. Consequently, I found myself putting infants of three to four months on a three-meal-a-day diet. Inquiry among pediatricians of recognized ability in my locality as to what was bad about such an idea (having already been convinced : s to what was good about it) brought forth the very unscientific reply, "We do not think their little stomachs are big enough to hold sufficient food at this age to carry them through." Strangely these same pediatricians have long since adopted these then seemingly radical ideas.

A continued pursuance of a practice, general in every sense of the word, gradually brought me to the realization that many of the present day physical and functional disorders seen, are directly due to the tension and fears of present day living. A conviction that many modern mothers fall into this category, mainly because of their undue concern as to the welfare of their babies, plus the fact that they are always tired and fatigued as a result of constant care for the demands of their babies, with the resultant loss of sleep and rest, started me to thinking how such a situation might be remedied. Naturally in general practice there are many babies with minor illnesses that are of little import, or with behavior and feeding problems. I was impressed by the profound disturbance of mothers over these minor problems, and through a gradually evolutionary process of thought on these matters I became convinced that we physicians lay too much stress on the baby's welfare and pay too little attention to the effect of these matters on the mother. I wondered whether one could not discover a feeding method, or should I say a baby care routine, which would take the stress off the mother, would simplify her obligations towards the baby and still produce a healthy, contented infant. A study of infant feeding

procedures through the ages and in different geographical locations was impressive in one common denominator: the continued healthy survival of infants despite what feeding practices were employed. The natural process was then to hit upon one that, without jeopardizing the baby's health in any way, would be less demanding on the mother's time, patience and good nature. The process of these ruminations led me into many contiguous fields which had to do with customs and procedures involved in baby care all of which resulted in the firm conviction that it is rather difficult to find anything that will hurt a normal newborn. These mental gyrations were all part of a subconscious process involving years of baby care on my part and with it the stress I laid on babies became less and less and at the same time their feeding routines became more and more simple. It is my feeling that when the mother manifests signs of over attention, indecision and insecurity the baby in time becomes affected by these manifestations. In other words, to me an unstable mother will insure an unstable baby.

An expression of my ideas on baby feeding to a receptive obstetrical patient, the mother of four other children, resulted in her asking following delivery, that her infant be put on three meals a day. To my delight and that of the nurses the idea worked to a degree far exceeding expectations. The second infant to be put on a three-meal-a-day schedule was a 5 pound 12 ounce infant which I had the good fortune to follow daily because of a continued hospitalization period, resulting not from any physical ailment but because the baby was up for adoption. Again I was pleased by the very normal neonatal course this baby followed while on this new schedule.

As I continued to put more and more babies on this routine (at first all were the babies of volunteer mothers) I found I had many critics in the guise of grandparents, well meaning friends and neighbors, particularly those of the apartment house variety. In order to placate some of the neighbors, relatives and apartment house dwellers who could understand and condone the crying of a baby fed frequently but not that of an infrequently fed baby, a midnight feeding was added to the three-meal-a-day schedule, thus making it a 6-hour interval schedule.

At this time, all babies under my care are on this 6-hour schedule. I would estimate that 300 babies have been and are being raised on this new regimen. I first introduce my new obstetrical patients to my baby feeding ideas at one of their early prenatal visits. I encourage them to observe these babies as the opportunity presents itself in my waiting room and to feel free to question the mothers of the babies on the 6-hour schedule.

At the time I discharge my obstetrical patients from the hospital I spend quite a little time, either singly or in groups, going over in great detail the favorable points of this schedule. I first impress upon them the idea that this is truly a philosophy of baby feeding rather than any new idea or system. I often admit that I have only borrowed from the mother with 8, 10, or 12 children her ideas of baby feeding, altered as they are by her restricted time, and polished them up a little for the modern mother with her much smaller family. I try to impress these mothers with the idea of training the baby to fit into their lives rather than embarking on a life in which they are constantly and frequently altering the course of their own lives to fit into the baby's life. I admit readily these babies will cry, but steadily maintain that at no time any more than other babies, with the added assurance that shortly the amount of crying will lessen as the baby learns that the crying gains him naught. Indeed, in my experience in private practice along with that of 6 years of caring for institutional babies I am sincere in my belief that the normal baby will fit into any given routine; it is the mother who has trouble fitting into a routine.

In instructing the mothers I then enter into the details of the schedule impressing upon them that this is a strict 6-hour feeding interval schedule whether it be at the suggested 6, 12, 6, 12 or one of their own choosing such as 8, 2, 8, 2. It might be well here to outline the essential details of the feeding routine which I use but which could be adapted to the individual variations of any physician (Table 1).

Schedules are discussed in general. All foods are started with one teaspoon amounts. I admonish these mothers to continue to awaken their babies for the midnight feeding until they themselves are ready to drop that feeding regardless of the protestations of the

baby. While many mothers do it before, I suggest a time of 17 days for dropping this midnight feeding and give them signs, namely the difficulty of awakening and the diminishing amount taken at that feeding as criteria of the baby's readiness for such an omission. Moreover, I warn them, if they go into this phase of dropping the midnight bottle with the mental reservation of giving a bottle if the baby cries, not to drop this feeding but to continue it at its regular time. However, once this feeding is dropped it is never to be resumed.

Once these babies are on a three-meal-a-day routine, I then suggest to the patient that these babies are no longer on a strict schedule but are eating three meals a day; however, at times chosen for the mother's convenience and not at the baby's insistence. It is my urging that by 3 to 4 months these babies will be taking breakfast anywhere from 7 to 9 in the morning, lunch at anywhere from 12 to 2, and dinner anywhere from 5 to 7 in the evening, indeed a flexible and most desirable routine to most mothers. I stress to these mothers that I want them to be independent mothers with only a minimal amount of guidance from me. It is my practice to see these normal babies formally only twice in the first year, once at the time I give the mother her 6 weeks postpartum check and again at the 5 to 6 months period for checking and the start of their immunization injections. On each of these occasions

---

SIX-HOUR FEEDING SCHEDULE

Given Mothers at Time of Leaving Hospital

Feedings at 6:00 a.m., 12:00 noon, 6:00 p.m. and 12:00 midnight. Water between feedings.

At 2-3 days of age: Cereal at 6:00 a.m. and 6:00 p.m. (Oatmeal and barley suggested as starters.)

At 10 days of age: Strained vegetables at 12:00 noon. (Peas, beans, carrots suggested as starters.)

At 14 days of age: Concentrated cod liver oil, 2 drops a day to start. Increase one drop a month up to 5 drops daily.

At 17 days of age: Strained fruits at 6:00 p.m. (Applesauce, peaches, pears suggested as starters. May decrease cereal.)

Midnight feeding may be dropped at any time.

At weekly intervals add:
   3 weeks—Orange juice and sterile water, equal parts of each, up to 2 ounces of each at 6:00 a.m.
   4 weeks—Strained meats
   5 weeks—Custards
   6 weeks—Soups
   7 weeks—Mashed banana
   8 weeks—Egg

Formula as indicated.

TABLE 1

weight and hemoglobins are taken. In addition to these visits the mothers are encouraged to bring their babies in so that my nurses may weigh them and get hemoglobins on them frequently. These mothers are also encouraged to call one of the nurses in my office who is completely familiar with this routine, if any questions arise on which they are in doubt.

Individual charts, in addition to the usual office records are kept on these babies showing weight increments and blood levels. From these charts I have attempted to draw conclusions as to weights and blood trends. The weight would seem to follow a pattern with a lesser initial weight loss, a slower primary rise and finally a delayed but definite rise to average levels. The babies on this schedule have represented a wide variation in initial weight. The smallest baby was 4 pounds 12 ounces at birth but quite normal. The largest was well over 10 pounds. Blood levels seem to follow those on control regimes. For our subtropical Miami clime no blood standards have been set up so our work on this score is handicapped. Regardless of the use or non-use of vitamins and mineral preparations these findings seem to undergo wide fluctuations. I recently saw a 5-months-old baby with a hemoglobin of 76 per cent which represented a rise of 26 points from 52 per cent at 2 months, on no hematinic therapy whatever.

RESULTS

Whereas all this may sound wonderful on paper the inevitable question arising is one concerning results. Unfortunately it is impossible to reduce to statistics the constant flow of favorable comments and enthusiasm which is forthcoming from these mothers both directly and indirectly. However, blood levels and weight charting seem to be the main concern of those who set the standards for evaluating babies. A routine check on these aspects would tend to prove that these 6-hour babies follow closely the physical standards set up by control babies, namely those on a more conventional type of feeding regime. In a preliminary survey on well over 100 babies, overwhelmingly favorable reports were given on observations as to time of sitting, standing and walking, appearance of first tooth, on questions as to ease of management, incidence of bowel upsets and allergies and the ease of new food introduction. One of the most startling results to come out of this preliminary survey was the finding that 99 per cent were able to follow the early introduction of foods closely or moderately well. It is probably this phase of the regime which has the greatest popular appeal and approbation but it remains my observation that the acceptance of this phase spells for success of the 6-hour phase. It is my feeling that the two phases of this program are reciprocals one of the other in determining the success of the whole program.

At a long time glance it is my feeling that these babies as they continue to grow will present less in the way of feeding problems particularly if the parents will continue to follow the principles of this regimen. It has been and always will be my insistence that hunger is the best, but most commonly neglected, tonic in the presence of feeding problems in infants and children.

The majority of mothers with babies on this schedule are wont to maintain that the infants are healthier, faster developing babies, but naturally I am reluctant to accept this plaudit. I am content to maintain that they are just as healthy.

The criticism of this concept centers about four main points, namely: (1) question of nursing, (2) frequency of allergies, (3) question of the baby's ability to swallow and assimilate these foods, and (4) allegation of the omission of the opportunity to manifest parental love. These are all well taken but can easily be answered and in my opinion all refuted.

On the question of nursing I find my percentage of mothers nursing successfully quite low, but still no lower than it was when I was using a 4-hour schedule. The mothers who nurse have no more difficulty going 6 hours than my nursing mothers during the war who often nursed only morning and evening on the resumption of their wartime jobs, this often as early as 3 to 4 weeks following delivery.

If one is to accept the new basic concepts of allergies, particularly as viewed by Rinkle one cannot help deciding that with the early introduction and rotation of foods there should be fewer allergies. Indeed what could have more allergenic potentialities than a diet restricted for months to one single food substance such as milk, other than the mother's own milk.

As to the question of swallowing solid foods, I find absolutely no inability on the part of mothers who feed solids from a spoon when started practically at birth. This is in direct contrast to the troubles my mothers used to have when waiting until 6 or 8 weeks to start solids. On the question of the assimilation of these foods I found a willing and most progressive ally in the guise of one of the baby food houses who produced scientific article after scientific article, all favorable, when asked the question concerning what work would have to be done to prove ability to assimilate foods on the part of these babies.

It is not my intention to omit any opportunity for the manifestation of the parental instincts. Rather it is my desire to advise more wisely the time for such manifestations. I urge my patients to fondle, cuddle, love and rock their babies, but only when they are happy and not when they are crying. It is my own feeling, the child psychiatrist notwithstanding, that by granting a child what it wants when it cries, be it only food, that we are fostering a definite pattern of demand which will be continued throughout childhood.

The applicability of such a routine has far exceeded my narrow field of visions. I have had a number of requests for details of this idea from countries where milk is not readily available, namely West Africa, the Dominican Republic, and Paraguay. These countries, primitive as we may picture them to be, still encounter the problem of insufficient lactation on the part of the mother. At the present time the governments of the Dominican Republic and Paraguay are having the original article translated into Spanish for distribution throughout the maternal and well baby centers in the hope that with the early introduction of foods the infants getting insufficient breast milk can be started on solids rather than depend upon the importation of expensive canned or powdered milks for supplementary feedings. You may be sure I shall follow this work with great interest.

In summary I might say that use of a baby feeding regimen that is comprised of a 6-hour feeding interval which is rapidly converted to a three-meal-a-day regimen, along with the introduction of food other than milk as early as the second day of life continues to be a source of gratification to its users and also a source of medical interest as these babies continue to follow closely and sometimes even surpass the physical standards set up by babies on a more conservative routine. A more detailed survey, now in progress, which will cover some 300 babies would seem to emphasize the results of our preliminary survey done over one year ago. In addition these results would seem to be equally satisfactory in babies not under my direct supervision as the schedule reaches out to friends and relatives in my own locality, in other states and in foreign countries.

DISCUSSION (Abstract)

Dr. Benjamin M. Cole, Orlando, Fla.—With Dr. Sackett's 300 personal case records, and because many of us with a smaller series are just as enthusiastic, I am convinced that he has a concept that is sound and logical and that is gaining supporters everywhere.

As I listened to him today and as I have reviewed his past work, it seems to me that there are several pertinent points to be brought out. First is the fundamental philosophy of this new concept. It has been our custom in the past to remind the family that a frail new baby was coming and that they were to conform to a whole new schedule of living when it arrived. The father was to feed it at night so mother would be fresh and rested for the constant daily routine. In the daytime other members of the household had to be quiet so baby could sleep or they must postpone their meals so baby could eat exactly on time.

To me the idea of having a baby conform to the family routine, rather than having the whole family conform to the baby is a wholesome, stable thing to do. It contributes to the stability of the family, the mother and the baby.

Second, the very early supplementary feeding of solid food has many merits. We see many new mothers who have insufficient milk early. The milk just does not come down as it is supposed to do in sufficient quantity to keep baby full. The mother puts him to breast often to stimulate the flow and stop the hungry child from crying. Often times during these early days there is no increase and mother winds up instead with sore, cracked nipples and baby is given a supplementary bottle. He learns immediately that he gets more milk and gets it more easily this way and the result is another mother who cannot nurse her baby. By offering solid food early we can dispense with this early bottle, keep baby satisfied and spare mother's breasts until she produces milk and adjusts to nursing. By the same token we see bottle babies who will not take enough milk at a nursing to last to the next feeding. They are just not interested in sucking. Some solid food in their stomachs will carry them much longer. Third, there may be those who ask how you can teach a newborn to eat. To this I reply that they learn faster than at any other age and offer the following evidence. Recall if you will how easy it is to instill the first medication in a newborn's eyes. But in the seconds it takes to get to the other eye he has already learned that the medication is unpleasant and has it squinched up as tight as wax.

He learns just as quickly to eat solid food. I tell my patients to mix the cereal very thin at first and to use an after dinner coffee spoon instead of their own baby spoon or one that relatives provide to the newly arrived one. When the spoon touches baby's lips he will suck the contents out and before you know it he will be eating.

Fourth, I should like to mention the matter of sensitivity. In my series I have encountered some cases of sensitivity. I am inclined to agree with Dr. Sackett that we shall have less of it when we offer a more varied menu. I am not qualified to discuss the subject even if I thought it posed any great problem. I should like to describe some interesting cases for you to tell you of my very personal series of one who is one year old no :. However, suffice it to say that I feel Dr. Sackett has worked out a system of infant care that is safe, simple and satisfactory. I hope more of you will give it a trial and report your results so that next time he can report 3,000 cases instead of this rather imposing 300 personal cases.

Dr. John E. Crews, Orlando, Fla.—About two years ago I began feeding my babies cereal, banana, fruits, and vegetables at six weeks of age. This program was so successful that one year ago I instituted a three-meal-a-day program, beginning when the infants were three weeks old. At first there was an extreme amount of criticism from some of the parents, from most of the grandparents, and in general from most other physicians. Most of the criticism from the parents and the grandparents has been largely overcome. However, there are still many physicians who object to this program. The following is a schedule which I give to the mother when the baby is three weeks old:

6:00 a.m. (1) Cereal: cerevim® or pabeena.® Begin with one tablespoon, increase as tolerated. (2) Banana. Be sure it is ripe. Up to one-half banana. Whip with fork until light. (3) As much formula as baby desires.

9:00 a.m. Orange juice. Strain and dilute with equal amounts of water, gradually increase to full strength. Give baby up to two ounces. Multi-vitamin drops.

12:00 noon. (1) One or two vegetables: choice of spinach, carrots, peas, string beans. Warm and season very lightly with butter or oleomargarine and salt. Baby may have as much as one-half jar of each. (2) As much formula as baby desires.

3:00 p.m. Orange juice, same as 9:00 a.m.

6:00 p.m. (1) One or two fruits: choice of pears, peaches, apricots, prunes, applesauce. Give as much as baby desires. (2) Cereal as for breakfast. (3) As much formula as baby desires.

Offer your baby water three or four times daily between meals. After the evening meal, do not give the baby formula or water until breakfast the next morning. Keep the baby's diapers dry during the night and he will sleep better. If you will follow the program persistently for one week your baby will be sleeping through the entire night. Remember the success of this program depends upon the parents, not upon the baby.

Mothers who wish to nurse their babies can very easily do so. Their breasts can very easily be trained to this three-meal-a-day program. At first during the night it was difficult for some mothers as their breasts did become a little engorged and uncomfortable. However, if the mother would relieve the engorgement by pumping the breast until the tension

was relieved, the breast would soon be trained satisfactorily to the three nursings a day and none during the night. In general the babies on three meals a day have fewer feeding problems, have less colic, and appear to be happier babies.

It is my contention that babies, even though they are fed on a three or four-hour schedule of nothing but milk for several months are still hungry babies, even though their weight gain may be satisfactory. In my series of about 100 babies on the three-meal-a-day program, all have gained weight satisfactorily, are happier babies, and they seem to be less susceptible to upper respiratory infections. A baby in this series, at three and one-half weeks of age had an operation for pyloric stenosis. Ten days later he was placed on the above three-meal-a-day program and has progressed satisfactorily in weight and growth. Another baby in this series was started on the three-meal-a-day program at seven days. This baby nursed the breast at midnight for one week. Since then the baby has been on the strict three-meal-a-day program.

I wish to commend Dr. Sackett for his program of early feeding. Its results are very satisfactory.

Dr. Sackett (closing).—With my dietary schedule, I encounter no more allergies than I have seen before in babies on other feeding routines.

Dr. Cole said something about the consistency of food. It has been my observation on one of my own babies and in my practice that these babies handle thicker foods better than foods of a watery consistency. Routinely I advise my mothers to make the foods, particularly the cereals, of a consistency to their liking and then rapidly to thicken it. Most of them will report back, as in my own personal experience, that newborns can take cereal from the spoon in a consistency similar to putty.

Concerning the giving of orange juice in midmorning and midafternoon, I could give Dr. Crews a sly dig. If you once start them on orange juice in the middle of the morning the next thing you know when they are a year or two or three old, there will be adding a cookie, or a slice of bread to the orange juice. This practice could result in a schedule with a three-hour interval.

37

REACTION OF 150 INFANTS TO COLD FORMULAS

JOHN P. GIBSON, M.D.

ABILENE, TEXAS

THE young mother asked, "Will cold milk hurt my baby? I gave him an ice-cold formula the other night. I was so tired I didn't realize what I was doing, but he liked the milk cold and now prefers all his bottles straight out of the refrigerator. Will it hurt him?"

The baby, 6 weeks old, seemed perfectly healthy and happy, so what was the answer to her question? After this same inquiry came from several other mothers following similar incidents, I began to ask questions. I soon found that quite a few mothers had stumbled into this same practice of giving cold formulas, and that a surprising number of infants were being given ice cream, all with obvious enjoyment, and none with any apparent harmful results.

Questions presented themselves for further study:

1. Is the practice of warming formulas based upon necessity or tradition?

2. What is the acceptance rate on the part of young infants to cold formulas?

3. Do cold formulas have any harmful effect on the babies?

Information on these points would be important to mothers who prepare about 1,400 bottles of formula during the first 8 months of the baby's life. Do they need to warm all those bottles? This question becomes still more urgent in the middle of the night and on trips. It is of importance to us as physicians to know whether cold formulas are harmful to infants.

METHODS

Since no studies could be found in medical literature dealing with the problem of giving cold formulas to infants, I began with my own patients in private practice. As the mothers would bring their babies to the office for their regular monthly examinations I would ask, "Mother, wouldn't it be nice if you didn't have to warm all those bottles?" She would respond, "Oh, that would be wonderful! Tell me more." I would then suggest that if she would warm each bottle a little less each time, before long the baby might prefer his bottle either cool or straight out of the refrigerator. No time schedule was suggested and bottle temperatures were not taken. The enthusiasm with which the mothers acted on this suggestion was remarkable.

At the monthly visits, the infants were weighed, measured, and given a complete examination, and the mother reported on her experiences. The mothers described a cool formula as one that had been removed from the refrigerator and allowed to stand in the kitchen "until the chill was off" or "until it approached room temperature." A cold bottle was one taken directly from the refrigerator and given to the baby. Usual temperatures of formulas from refrigerators are about 40° F. or 5° C. All of the babies were changed gradually from warm to cool to cold bottles.

There are 150 infants in my private practice who have been offered cold formulas. Of these, 69 are males, 81 females. All are white except for 1 Negro and 1 Mexican. Their ages range from 15 hours to 7 months.

convinced that the cold formulas had "cured the colic" for their babies. In the other 9 there was apparently no change. In 3 other babies, not in this group, the mothers felt that the cold formulas had caused the babies to have "gas pains," so no further effort was made to give them cold bottles. This group is too small to be of significance.

In assessing the developmental progress of the 134 infants who accepted cool and cold formulas, a complete ex-

ACCEPTANCE RATE

TABLE I. ACCEPTANCE OF COOL AND COLD FORMULAS BY 150 INFANTS

AGE GROUP	NUMBER	REFUSED COOL OR COLD MILK	ACCEPTED COOL MILK	ACCEPTED COLD MILK	AVERAGE INTERVAL FOR CHANGE (DAYS)
1 day to 3 weeks	43	3	17	23	7
1 to 3 months	68	6	20	42	6
3½ to 7 months	39	7	4	28	7
Totals	150	16	41	93	average 6-7

TABLE II. SUMMARY OF WEIGHT CURVES OF 120 INFANTS CHANGED TO COOL OR COLD FORMULAS, AND FOLLOWED FOR AN AVERAGE OF 6.7 MONTHS AFTER THE CHANGE

AGE GROUP	CONSISTENT WEIGHT CURVES				WEIGHT CURVE DEVIATIONS	
	NUM-BER	ABOVE AVERAGE	AVERAGE	BELOW AVERAGE	UPWARD	DOWN-WARD
1 day to 3 weeks	38	18	15	1	4	0
1 to 3 months	56	34	16	3	3	0
3½ to 7 months	26	16	8	2	0	0
Totals	120	68	39	6	7	0

It was noted that the acceptance rate for cold formulas varied from about 50 per cent (23 of 43) for the very young infants to about 75 per cent (28 of 39) in the older group. For the whole group of 150, the acceptance rate for cool or cold formulas was 89 per cent, within an average period of one week.

EFFECT OF UNHEATED FORMULAS ON INFANTS

There were 11 infants in the group who could be classified as "gassy" or "colicky." Two of the mothers were

amination was made each month. Weight records were plotted on a chart with the average curve starting at 7½ pounds, curving up to 14 pounds at 5 months, and 20 pounds at 12 months. More attention was given to a consistent weight curve parallel to the average than to actual poundage. Weight curves were classified as: (a) consistently above average, both before and after the change to unheated formulas; or (b) consistently average, before and after the change; or (c) consistently below average, before and after the change.

All of these curves were considered satisfactory, if consistent, and if the infant's general condition was good. Search was made for deviations in the weight curve either upward or downward that coincided with or followed a change to unheated formulas.

All of the weight curves were consistent before and after the change to unheated formulas, except for 7 infants who had a marked deviation upward in their weight curves coinciding with the change. No infant had a downward deviation.

EFFECT ON BODY TEMPERATURE

One mother who had just been delivered of her second baby requested, "Please train my baby to take his formula cold while he is in the nursery; my first child did so well on cold formulas." This presented an opportunity to record body temperatures after taking a cold formula. The infant (6 pounds, 11 ounces) had received one warm bottle when he was 12 hours old, taking it well. At the age of 15 hours, rectal temperature was taken and an ice-cold formula offered, which he also took well (about 2 ounces). Rectal temperatures were then taken immediately after feeding, and at intervals of 5, 10, and 30 minutes later. This was repeated for the next 8 cold formulas, average $1\frac{1}{2}$ to 2 ounces each. In the 25 postformula temperatures there was no reduction of temperature in 12; a reduction of 0.2 degree in 6, a reduction of 0.4 degree in 1, and a reduction of 0.6 degree in 2, a reduction of 0.8 degree in 2, and an elevation of 0.2 degree in 1.

This infant started to gain weight on the second day. At the age of 13 days, the weight was 7 pounds, and at 1 month it was 8 pounds, 10 ounces, with general condition excellent.

CONCLUSIONS

1. In a group of 150 infants, cool or cold formulas were accepted by 89 per cent.

2. In 120 of the infants accepting cool or cold formulas and followed for an average of 6.7 months, development proceeded normally.

3. No harmful effects could be found in the infants accepting the cool and cold formulas.

38

Reprinted from Am. J. Dis. Child., **108**, 601–604 (Dec. 1964)

Milk or Formula Volume Ingested by Infants Fed ad Libitum

SAMUEL J. FOMON, MD; GEORGE M. OWEN, MD; AND LORA N. THOMAS, RN, IOWA CITY, IOWA

Because of a paucity of published data on amounts of food ingested by normal infants fed ad libitum, the following summary is presented.

Subjects and Feedings

The data pertain to observations made during the course of metabolic balance studies with normal fullterm infants. At the time of each balance study the infant was judged to be in excellent health; even mild rhinorrhea was considered a contraindication to proceeding with the balance study. The occurrence of fever, loose stools, or vomiting during the three days of a balance study resulted in immediate termination of the study, which was then rescheduled for the next week. In studies performed between 1954 and May, 1959, all infants lived continuously in the metabolism ward. After May, 1959, infants lived at home and were admitted to the metabolism ward only as necessary for performance of 72-hour balance studies. The majority of the infants were studied at intervals of two weeks from 2 or 3 weeks of age until 5 months of age.

Nurses experienced in metabolic studies fed the infants and recorded volumes of intake. The data are therefore more accurate than could be obtained by questioning of mothers.

Table 1 presents a classification of the feedings. Human milk or cow milk formula served as the sole source of calories and fluid, providing approximately 67 calories/100 ml with 7% to 14% of the calories from protein, 42% to 46% of the calories from carbohydrate, and 40% to 51% of the calories from fat. Supplementary vitamins and iron were usually given.

Received for publication Aug 14, 1964.

Samuel J. Fomon, MD, Department of Pediatrics, University Hospitals, State University of Iowa, Iowa City, Iowa.

Department of Pediatrics, State University of Iowa.

This investigation was supported in part by Public Health Service research grant HD-00383, research career program award 5-K3-HD-2465 and graduate training grant 5-T1-AM-5246, and in part by grants from Ross Laboratories, Columbus, Ohio, Evaporated Milk Association, Chicago, and the Borden Special Products Company, New York.

Although data on volumes of intake are presented as milliliters per day (or milliliters per kilogram per day), it must be emphasized that the observations were actually made during intervals of three days and that in most instances results of two (sometimes three) such three-day studies were averaged. If intervals of observation had been only 24 hours in duration, more variability would have been anticipated.

Results

Volume of Intake in Relation to Age, Sex, and Body Weight.—The relation of volume of intake to body weight and age is presented in the Figure. During the age intervals 8 to 30, 31 to 60, 61 to 90, 91 to 120, and 121 to 150 days, the regressions[7] of volume of intake on weight were as follows: $y = 223 + 0.137x$, $y = 418 + 0.095x$, $y = 586 + 0.056x$, $y = 598 + 0.055x$, and $y = 899 + 0.010x$, where y is volume of intake (milliliters/day) and x is body weight (grams). From the Figure it would appear that the influence of body weight on volume of intake is greatest when body weight varies between 3 and 5 kg. Mean volumes of intake increase relatively less as body weight increases from 5 kg to 7 kg.

The relation of volume of intake to weight and sex is shown in Table 2. It may be seen that volumes of intake by boys weighing between 4 and 6 kg are somewhat greater than those by girls of equal weight. There was no remarkable influence of type of feeding on volume of intake.

The relation of volume of intake, expressed as milliliters per kilogram per day, to age is presented in Table 3. When expressed in this manner, volumes of intake by boys and girls were similar. Median values for boys were 196, 189, 175, 158, and 148 ml/kg/day, respectively, during the age intervals 8-30, 31-60, 61-90, 91-120, and 121-150 days. Corresponding median volumes of

TABLE 1.—*Classification of Feedings*

Feeding Group	No. of Subjects	No. of 3-Day Observations	Subject-Months of Observation	Description of Feeding *
I	13	75	46	Pooled human milk (1); approximately 7% of calories from portein, 51% from fat, and 42% from lactose
II	13	87	46	Formulas 1257 (2) and 1257A (3); approximately 7% of calories from protein of cow milk, 42% from lactose, and 51% from vegetable oils
III	20	119	77	Formulas 22-3 (4), S-26 (4), 657, 359, Similac PM 60/40, and SMA S-26; approximately 10% of calories from protein of cow milk, 44% from lactose, and 46% from vegetable oils (and for formula S-26 and SMA S-26, oleo oils); protein partially demineralized and ratio of lactalbumin to casein adjusted to resemble that of human milk
IV	21	114	75	Liquid Similac (5); approximately 11% of calories from protein of cow milk, 42% from lactose, and 47% from vegetable oils
V	8	52	29	Powdered Similac with iron (6); approximately 11% of calories from protein of cow milk, 42% from lactose, and 47% from vegetable oils
VI	7	46	25	Formula 3086A; approximately 14% of calories from protein of cow milk, 46% from carbohydrate (lactose, dextrins, and maltose), and 40% from vegetable oils

* References (numbers in parentheses) to published reports are given. Other data are unpublished.

intake by girls were 199, 190, 169, 158, and 150 ml/kg/day.

Caloric Intakes.—Since all feedings employed in the study provided approximately 67 calories/100 ml, caloric intakes could be calculated. The data are summarized and compared with those from reports by other investigators [8,9] in Table 4.

Volume of Intake During Metabolic Balance Studies and in Intervals Between Balance Studies.—Because metabolic balance studies were performed only at times when the infants were considered to be in excellent health, it seemed possible that amounts of food ingested during the course of these studies might be somewhat greater than amounts ingested during the intervals between balance studies. This possibility was explored with respect to 28 infants who lived continuously in the metabolic ward dur-

TABLE 2.—*Intake of Milk or Formula in Relation to Weight and Sex*

Wt, Kg (Lb)	Sex	No. of Subjects	Mean Wt, Gm (Lb)	Vol of Intake, Ml/Day, Percentiles		
				25th	50th	75th
3.000-3.999	M	25	3,708 (8 3/16)	660	720	800
(6 5/8-8 13/16)	F	29	3,621 (7 15/16)	690	730	800
4.000-4.999	M	33	4,520 (9 15/16)	800	860	930
8 13/16-11)	F	34	4,429 (9 3/4)	750	830	880
5.000-5.999	M	49	5,477 (12 1/16)	880	920	1,020
(11-13 1/4)	F	38	5,468 (12 1/16)	830	870	900
6.000-6.999	M	37	6,391 (14 1/8)	900	960	1,030
(13 1/4-15 7/16)	F	22	6,345 (13 15/16)	890	950	990

TABLE 3.—*Intake of Milk or Formula in Relation to Age*

Age, Days	No. of Subjects	Vol of Intake, Ml/Kg/Day, Percentiles				
		10th	25th	50th	75th	90th
8-30	56	172	184	199	220	224
31-60	62	164	174	189	205	220
61-90	69	145	155	174	190	199
91-120	62	134	148	158	170	188
121-150	49	132	138	149	158	172

TABLE 4.—*Intake of Calories in Relation to Age*

| Age, Days | No. of Subjects | | | Intake of Calories, Calories/Kg/Day | | | | | | |
| | | | | 25th Percentile | | 50th Percentile | | | 75th Percentile | |
	Beal (8) *	Rueda-Williamson & Rose (9) *	This Report	Beal	This Report	Beal	Rueda-Williamson & Rose	This Report	Beal	This Report
8-30	22	—	56	105	123	118	—	133	144	147
31-60	26	—	62	122	117	130	—	127	146	137
61-90	26	67	69	108	104	119	124	117	127	127
91-120	29	67	62	102	99	110	117	106	119	114
121-150	28	67	49	98	93	104	114	100	115	106

* Parentheses indicate reference numbers.

ing 98 subject-months of observation. Median volumes of intake by these infants during balance studies were 192, 194, 171, 158, and 150 ml/kg/day, respectively, in the age intervals 8-30, 31-60, 61-90, 91-120, and 121-150 days. Median volumes of intake in the intervals between metabolic balance studies were similar to those recorded during the balance studies: 200, 197, 168, 158, and 148 ml/kg/day, respectively, for the five specified age intervals. However, these infants remained in the same environment and were fed by the same group of experienced nurses whether or not they were serving as subjects of metabolic balance studies. The recorded intakes of milk or formula by the infants who lived at home during the intervals between balance studies may have been less representative of average monthly intakes by these infants.

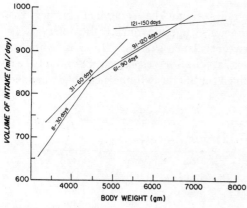

Regression of volume of intake on body weight during the age intervals 8 to 30, 31 to 60, 61 to 90, 91 to 120, and 121 to 150 days.

Comment

Infants serving as subjects of studies summarized in this report did not receive foods other than milk or formula and therefore almost certainly ingested more milk or formula than would have been the case had they received precooked cereal or strained foods commercially prepared for infants.

The attitude of the individual who feeds the infant is undoubtedly reflected to some extent by the volume of formula consumed. Infants in this study were fed the largest volume of milk or formula they would accept consistently rather than the least amount that would seem to relieve hunger. In this regard the observations of Brown et al [10] * are of interest. Fifty-six infants between 29 and 56 days of age were offered approximately 165 ml/kg/day of formula, and this volume was not increased unless excessive crying between feedings suggested that the infants were dissatisfied.[11] Under these circumstances, the median intake was 168 ml/kg/day; the 10th percentile value (158 ml/kg/day) was only 10 ml/kg/day less than the 50th, and the 90th percentile value (186 ml/kg/day) was only 18 ml/kg/day greater than the 50th. By contrast, in the present study generally greater volumes of intake and more variability in volumes of intake were encountered. The 10th, 50th, and 90th percentile values for the corresponding age interval (31-60 days) were

* Dr. Brown supplied complete tabular data so that the average volumes of intake by each infant could be calculated.

164, 189 and 220 ml/kg/day, respectively (Table 3).

Intakes of calories by infants serving as subjects in this study were generally similar to those reported by Beal[8] on the basis of dietary histories taken in Denver between 1946 and 1953 and those reported by Rueda-Williamson and Rose[9] on the basis of dietary histories taken in Boston between 1959 and 1960. In the study by Beal, cereal was generally introduced into the diet between 2 and 3 months of age, fruit and vegetables between 3 and 4½ months of age.[12] The slightly greater intakes of calories reported by Beal[8] than by Rueda-Williamson and Rose[9] may reflect the trend between 1946 and 1960 toward increasingly early administration of cereal and strained foods. Similarly, the somewhat lesser intakes of calories in the present study may be a reflection of the fact that milk or formula served as the sole source of calories.

Summary

Data are summarized from observations during 298 subject-months of observation of normal fullterm infants receiving milk or formula ad libitum as sole source of calories. Volumes of intake of milk or formula increased rather rapidly as weight increased from 3 to 5 kg but showed relatively little increase with increase in weight from 5 to 7 kg. Median volumes of intake by boys weighing between 4 and 6 kg were slightly greater than those by girls of similar weight.

Median volumes of intake were 199, 189, 174, 158, and 149 ml/kg/day, respectively, during the age intervals 8-30, 31-60, 61-90, 91-120, and 121-150 days. Caloric intakes were slightly less than those reported in two comparable studies in which cereal and strained foods were permitted.

REFERENCES

1. Fomon, S. J., and May, C. D.: Metabolic Studies of Normal Fullterm Infants Fed Pasteurized Human Milk, Pediatrics 22:101-115, 1958.
2. Fomon, S. J.: Comparative Study of Adequacy of Protein From Human Milk and Cow's Milk in Promoting Nitrogen Retention by Normal Fullterm Infants, Pediatrics 26:51-61, 1960.
3. Fomon, S. J., and Owen, G. M.: Retention of Nitrogen by Normal Fullterm Infants Receiving Autoclaved Formula, Pediatrics 29:1005-1011, 1962.
4. Fomon, S. J.; et al: Calcium and Phosphorus Balance Studies With Normal Fullterm Infants Fed Pooled Human Milk or Various Formulas, Amer J Clin Nutr 12:346-357, 1963.
5. Fomon, S. J., and May, C. D.: Metabolic Studies of Normal Fullterm Infants Fed Prepared Formula Providing Intermediate Amounts of Protein, Pediatrics 22:1134-1147, 1958.
6. Owen, G. M., and Fomon, S. J.: Use of Iron-Fortified Milk Formula During the First Three Months of Life, abstracted, J Pediat 63:490-491, 1963.
7. Wilks, S. S.: Elementary Statistical Analysis, Princeton, NJ: Princeton University Press, 1956, p 240.
8. Beal, V. A.: Nutritional Intake of Children: I. Calories, Carbohydrate, Fat and Protein, J Nutr 50:223-234, 1953.
9. Rueda-Williamson, R., and Rose, H. E.: Growth and Nutrition of Infants: Influence of Diet and Other Factors on Growth, Pediatrics 30:639-653, 1962.
10. Brown, G. W., et al: Evaluation of Prepared Milks for Infant Nutrition: Use of Latin Square Technique, J Pediat 56:391-398, 1960.
11. Brown, G. W.: Personal communication to the authors.
12. Beal, V. A.: On Acceptance of Solid Foods, and Other Food Patterns, of Infants and Children, Pediatrics 20:448-456, 1957.

SELECTED BIBLIOGRAPHY

Biedert, P. H. (1905). *Die Kinderernährung im Säuglingsalter.* Ferdinand Enke, Stuttgart.

Bosworth, A. L., Bowditch, H. I., and Giblin, L. A. (1918). Is the amount of calcium usually given in dilutions of cow's milk injurious to infants? A reply to Holt, Courtney, and Fales. *Am. J. Dis. Child.,* **16,** 265.

Bowditch, H. I., and Bosworth, A. W. (1913). Casein in infant feeding. Experiments in exact percentages. *Am. J. Dis. Child.,* **6,** 394.

Brennemann, J. (1923). Artificial feeding of infants. Chapter 23 in I. A. Abt, *Pediatrics,* Vol. II. W. B. Saunders Company, Philadelphia.

——— (1949). *Practice of pediatrics.* W. F. Prior Company, Inc., Hagerstown, Md.

Burr, G. O., and Burr, M. M. (1930). On nature and role of fatty acids essential in nutrition. *J. Biol. Chem.,* **86,** 587.

Clark, W. M. (1915). Reaction of cow's milk modified for infant feeding. *J. Med. Res.,* **31,** 431.

Clements, F. W. (1949). *Infant nutrition: its physiological basis.* Bristol: John Wright and Sons Ltd.; London: Simpkin Marshall Ltd.

Cowie, D. M. (1912). A graphic chart method of studying and teaching the principles of infant feeding with special reference to the importance of the energy line. *Am. J. Dis. Child.,* **14,** 360.

Czerny, A. D., and Keller, A. (1909). *Des Kindes Ernährung, Ernährungstörungen, und Ernährungstherapie.* Franz Deuticke, Leipzig.

Davis, C. M. (1928). Self selection of diet by newly weened infants: experimental study. *Am. J. Dis. Child.,* **36,** 651.

Davis, J. A., Harvey, D. R., and Yu, J. S. (1969). Neonatal fits associated with hypomagnesaemia. *Arch. Dis. Child.,* **40,** 286–290.

Finkelstein, H., and Meyer, L. F. (1910). Ueber Eiweissmilch. *Jahrb. Kinderh.,* **21,** 655.

Finkelstein, H. (1912). *Lehrbuch der Säuglingskrankheiten.* Verlag von Julius Springer, Berlin.

Gamble, J. L. (1937). Extracellular fluid: extracellular fluid and its vicissitudes. *Bull. Johns Hopkins Hosp.,* **61,** 151.

415

—— (1937). Extracellular fluid: renal defense of extracellular fluid; control of acid–base excretion and the factors of water expenditure. *Bull. Johns Hopkins Hosp.*, **61**, 174.

Gordon, H. H., and Ganzon, A. F. (1959). On the protein requirements of infants. *J. Pediatr.*, **54**, 503.

Hansen, A. E. (1933). Study of iodine number of serum fatty acids in infantile eczema. *Proc. Soc. Exp. Biol. Med.*, **30**, 1198.

Holt, L. E., Courtney, A. M., and Fales, H. L. (1918). Is the amount of calcium usually given in dilutions of cow's milk injurious to infants? A reply to the article on "Calcium in its relation to the absorption of fatty acids," by Bosworth, Bowditch, and Giblin, in the *American Journal of Diseases of Children*, June, 1918. *Am. J. Dis. Child.*, **26**, 52.

——, Courtney, A. M., and Fales, H. L. (1919). Fat metabolism of infants and young children. II. Fat in the stools of infants fed on modifications of cow's milk. *Am. J. Dis. Child.*, **17**, 423.

Howland, J. (1911). The fundamental requirements of an infant's nutrition. *Am. J. Dis. Child.*, **2**, 49.

—— (1913). The scientific basis for the artificial feeding of infants. *Am. J. Dis. Child.*, **5**, 390.

Jelliffe, D. B., and Jelliffe, E. F., eds. (1971). The uniqueness of human milk. Symposium. *Am. J. Clin. Nutr.*, **24**, 968–1024.

Levine, S. Z., McEachern, T. H., Wheatley, M. A., Marples, E., and Kelly, M. D. (1935). Respiratory metabolism in infancy and in childhood. Daily energy requirements of normal infants. *Am. J. Dis. Child.*, **50**, 596.

McCollum, E. V., and Davis, M. (1915). The nature of the dietary deficiencies of rice. *J. Biol. Chem.*, **23**, 181.

——, Simmonds, N., Becher, J. E., and Shipley, P. G. (1922). Studies on experimental rickets. XXI. An experimental demonstration of the existence of a vitamin which promotes calcium deposits. *J. Biol. Chem.*, **53**, 293.

McCulloch, H. (1944). Use of evaporated milk without added sugar for the feeding of infants. *Am. J. Dis. child.*, **67**, 52.

Meyer, H. F. (1955). An appraisal of present day artificial infant feeding. *Symposium on Diagnosis by Presenting Symptoms. Pediatric Clinics of North America.* W. B. Saunders Company, Philadelphia.

Osborne, T. B., and Mendel, L. B. (1915). The comparative nutritive value of certain proteins in growth, and the problem of the protein minimum. *J. Biol. Chem.*, **20**, 351–378.

Pemell, R. (1653). *De morbis puerorum or, a treatise on the diseases of children: with their causes, signs, prognosticks, and cures, for the benefit of such as do not understand the latine tongue.* London.

Powers, G. F. (1935). Infant feeding: historical background and modern practice. *JAMA*, **105**, 753.

Rominger, E., and Meyer, H. (1927). Mineral metabolism studies on infants: I. Salt retention of healty breast-fed and bottle-fed infants. *Arch. Kinderh.*, **80**, 195.

Routh, C. H. F. (1879). *Infant feeding and its influence on life, or the causes and prevention of infant mortality.* William Wood and Company, New York.

Rubner, M., and Heubner, O. (1898). Die natürliche ernährung eines sauglings. *Z. Biol.*, **1**, 36.

Shaftel, N. (1958). A history of the purification of milk in New York. How now brown cow. *N.Y. State J. Med.*, **58**, 911.

Smith, T., and Brown, J. H. (1915). A study of streptococci isolated from certain presumably milk-borne epidemics of tonsillitis occurring in Massachusetts in 1913 and 1914. *J. Med. Res.*, **31**, 455.

Soxhlet, F. (1886). Ueber Kindermilch und Säuglings-ernährung. *Munch. Med. Wochenschr.*, **15**, 253.

Stearns, G., and Stringer, D. (1937). Iron retention in infancy. *J. Nutr.*, **13**, 127.

Still, G. F. (1931). *The history of pediatrics.* Oxford University Press, London.

Waddell, J., Elvehjem, C. A., Steenbock, H., and Hart, E. B. (1928). Iron in nutrition. VI. Iron salts and iron containing ash extracts in the correction of anemia. *J. Biol. Chem.*, **77**, 777.

AUTHOR CITATION INDEX

Naismith, D. J., 163
Nauyn, B., 73
Neisser, E., 123, 385
Nelson, M. V. K., 36, 277
Neumann, H., 385
Neumann, J., 123
Neville, A., 258
Newburgh, L. H., 226
Newcomer, H. S., 214
Nicloux, M., 120
Niemann, A., 74, 122, 129
Noll, A., 123
Nygaard, K. K., 294, 295

Ohta, H., 358
Oppel, A., 123
Orgler, A., 123
Orr, J. S., 384
Orr, W. J., 202, 208
Osborne, T. B., 36, 129, 252, 256, 257, 261, 262, 275, 327, 416
Overton, 123, 191
Owen, C. A., 294
Owen, G. M., 413

Panos, T. C., 163
Park, E. A., 203
Patek, A. J., Jr., 210
Patterson, T. L., 385
Peacock, W., 212
Peiser, J., 129
Pemell, R., 416
Pennell, S., 74
Pentler, C. F., 295
Perley, A. M., 38
Peterman, M. G., 283
Peters, J. P., 36, 239
Peterson, W. H., 210
Pflaundler, M., 385
Pflüger, 123
Philips, F., 123
Phillips, G. E., 49
Pick, 121
Pies, W., 385
Pisek, G. R., 385
Pitz, W., 261, 275
Plant, O. H., 123
Platenza, B. P. B., 73
Plauth, 120
Plum, P., 294
Poncher, H. G., 277
Porter, T. E., 283
Powers, G. F., 342, 416
Poyner-Wall, P., 60
Pratt, E. L., 163
Preyer, 385

Price, J. W., 49

Quest, R., 183, 385
Quick, A., 295

Raczynski, 123
Ramlingaswami, V., 162
Randoin, L., 87
Rapheal, F., 73
Rapoport, M., 282, 283
Ratner, B., 41
Raudnitz, R. W., 123
Ravdin, I. S., 41
Rehfuss, M. E., 385
Reicher, K., 119
Reid, D. E., 211
Rensburg, H., 358
Reuss, A. v., 73, 115
Reyber, 123
Rice, E. E., 38
Richter, C. P., 49
Ridout, J. H., 41
Rietschel, H., 123
Rivkin, H., 229, 277
Roberts, H. K., 212
Roberts, L. J., 40, 283
Robertson, T. B., 170
Robinson, H. W., 49
Robscheit-Robbins, F. S., 38
Roby, C. C., 211
Rodda, F. C., 294
Rogers, F. T., 385, 386
Rohmann, 170
Rominger, E., 36, 74, 416
Roper, M., 36
Rose, H. E., 413
Rose, M. S., 40
Rose, W. C., 38, 40
Rosenberg, 123
Rosenfelt, 123
Rosenstern, I., 386
Rosenstern, J., 385
Ross, J. B., 358
Rotch, T. M., 318
Rothberg, 123
Rothey, K. B., 357
Rott, F., 386
Rousselet, 123
Routh, C. H. F., 416
Rubner, M., 121, 123, 299, 416
Rueda-Williamson, R., 413
Ruh, H. O., 318
Rummel, O., 358
Rumpf, F., 74

Saldun, M. L., 358

SUBJECT INDEX

About the Editor

DORIS H. MERRITT is Professor of Pediatrics at Indiana University School of Medicine and Director of the Indianapolis Sickle Cell Center. She is the Dean for Research and Sponsored Programs of Indiana–Purdue University at Indianapolis.

A Phi Beta Kappa graduate of Hunter College of the City University of New York, she received her M.D. in 1952 from George Washington University, where she returned as a teaching and research fellow in Pediatrics after an internship at Duke University Hospital. In 1954 she returned to Duke University as Assistant Resident in Pediatrics and later as a USPHS Heart and Lung Institute fellow. Immediately before coming to Indiana University, she was Executive Secretary of the Cardiovascular and General Medicine Study Sections of the National Institutes of Health.

Formerly chairman of the Biomedical Library Review Committee of the National Library of Medicine, Dr. Merritt serves as a consultant to the USPHS, the National Institutes of Health, and the Health Manpower Programs. A consultant for the American Association of Medical Colleges and the American Council of Education, she is contributing to the President's Biomedical Research Panel report on the impact of federal funds on educational institutions. She is a member of the subcommittee for maternal and child health research evaluation, National Academy of Science–National Research Council.